CW01638717

Practice

Clinical management in General Practice

Edited by

Jack Cormack MD, FRCGP
General Practitioner, Edinburgh

Marshall Marinker MD, FRCGP
Director, MSD Foundation

David Morrell OBE, MB, BS, FRCP, FRCGP, FFCM
Wolfson Professor of General Practice, United Medical and Dental Schools of Guy's and St Thomas's Hospitals

Kluwer Medical **London**

British Library Cataloguing in Publication Data

Practice: a handbook of primary care.
1. Medicine 2. Family medicine
I. Marinker, Marshall II. Morrell, David
III. Cormack, J.J.C.
610 R130

ISBN 0 903393 59 X

First published in Great Britain in 1976 in loose-leaf format by

Kluwer-Harrap Handbooks, 1 Harlequin Avenue, Great West Road, Brentford, Middlesex TW8 9EW
1st bound edition 1982
2nd bound edition 1987

Printed in Great Britain by Marshment & White, Bradford-on-Avon, Wiltshire

Preface

When we were asked to edit a loose-leaf book for general practitioners designed to solve the common problems presenting in general practice, we envisaged a continuing relationship with our subscribers. We knew that the facts we presented would be constantly revised as more knowledge was acquired about the interpretation of symptoms presenting in primary care. We invited a dialogue with our subscribers and in this we have not been disappointed. As a result we have been able to update regularly the original text, and will continue to do so.

In the context of this dialogue we have, however, learned that *Practice* is used, not only as a regularly updated work of reference, but also as a textbook by trainees and undergraduates. Those of us concerned with examining for the MRCGP are aware that it is of particular value to candidates preparing for this examination, and those of us concerned with undergraduate education recognize that it can present for medical students a new and realistic approach to the common symptoms of illness.

We still believe that the loose-leaf, regularly updated version of *Practice* provides a particularly valuable contribution to continuing education in general practice, and that it is ideally suited to accommodate the increasing amount of research from general practitioners. We are, however, aware that there is a demand for a more modestly priced textbook which can be used by undergraduates, trainees and young principals in general practice.

We hope that those who use *Practice* will continue to support our work by looking very critically at the contents and advising us of new information which should be incorporated in the updating material. We particularly value the contributions we have received from trainers who have used individual chapters from *Practice* for small group discussions among trainees and have pointed out our shortcomings and the need for new information.

In producing a bound copy of *Practice* we are not wavering from our original objective that the loose-leaf version should provide the most up-to-date information required by general practitioners in managing the common symptoms presented to them. We are, however, trying to accommodate the needs of new entrants to our discipline.

We are very grateful for the assistance and support of many colleagues in the development of this work and we would like to express our particular thanks to our publishers for their continuing friendly and helpful cooperation, which has resulted in this second edition of bound *Practice*. This edition incorporates all the updated material issued in the past five years for loose-leaf *Practice* and also data from the Third National Morbidity Survey.

JACK CORMACK
MARSHALL MARINKER
DAVID MORRELL

Outline of contents

Contributing authors

John Bain MD, PhD, FRCGP, DCH, D(Obst.)RCOG

Is Professor of Primary Medical Care at Southampton University and a Principal in General Practice at Aldermoor Health Centre, Southampton. He was formerly in practice in Livingston New Town and Senior Lecturer in General Practice at the University of Aberdeen. His research interests include the study of the natural history and treatment of ear, nose and throat disorders in children and the role of practice nurses in primary care. Co-editor of *Colour Atlas of Mouth, Throat and Ear Disorders in Children* and *Child Care in General Practice*, and has written numerous articles on child care in the setting of general practice.

John Bennison MB, BChir, FRCGP

Practises in partnership with his wife in rural Essex, where they both take part in many community activities. He has always been interested in education for general practice, and most of his writing has been to this end. He has been Associate Regional Adviser for Essex, Chairman of the Education Committee and Vice Chairman of the Council of the Royal College of General Practitioners.

Graham Buckley MB, ChB, BSc, FRCPE, FRCGP, D(Obst.)RCOG

Is a general practitioner in the Livingston New Town Health Service with a special interest in Geriatrics. Hospital practitioner in Geriatric Assessment Unit. Associate Adviser in General Practice in the South-East Scotland Region. Editor, *Journal of the Royal College of General Practitioners.*

Aubrey Colling MD, FRCGP

Is a general practitioner in Stockton-on-Tees and a former Regional Adviser in General Practice. He was a member of the Teesside Coronary Survey Team and also of the Joint Working Party of the Royal College of Physicians and the British Cardiac Society on rehabilitation after cardiac illness. Has written articles on coronary care, the 'sick family' and the community responsibility of the general practitioner.

J.J.C. Cormack MD, FRCGP

Is a general practitioner in Corstorphine, Edinburgh. Formerly part-time lecturer in the Department of General Practice, Edinburgh University. After qualifying worked in mission hospitals in Labrador and Malawi. He was for 12 years an examiner for the MRCGP, and for two years an examiner for the DCCH. Author of *The General Practitioner's Use of Medical Records* and papers on medical records; editor, *Teaching General Practice.*

David F. Coulter MD, FRCGP

Is a general practitioner in Bridgend, Mid Glamorgan. An originator and organizer of the Bridgend General Practitioner Vocational Training Scheme. Graduated in 1946 at the University of Glasgow and after several hospital posts and service in the RAF Medical Branch settled in South Wales. Is co-editor and contributor to *The Practice of Family Medicine* and examiner for the Royal College of General Practitioners. Has a continuing interest, amongst many others, in the diagnosis and management of ear disease in general medical practice.

Michael Courtenay MA, MB, BChir, FRCGP

Is a general practitioner in Battersea and Senior Research Fellow in St Thomas's Hospital Department of General Practice. Entered general practice soon after qualifying (having served as an army engineer in the war). Worked for the Family Planning Association for 10 years. Author of *Sexual Discord in Marriage* and numerous articles on the emotional aspects of illness in the general practice setting.

Denis Craddock MD, FRCGP, D(Obst.)RCOG

Is a general practitioner in Croydon. Member of the Royal College of Physicians' Working Party on Obesity and member of the DHSS working party on very low calorie diets. After house jobs and National Service in the Royal Navy, he went into general practice. After eight years in general practice, he was appointed to a single-handed practice in Croydon in 1958 and is now senior partner of a group of four doctors. He is the author of *Obesity and Its Management*, *The BMA Slimmers Guide*, *A short Text Book of General Practice*, and several journal articles.

A.G. Donald OBE, MA, MB, ChB, FRCGP, FRCPE

Is Regional Adviser in General Practice for South-East Scotland concerned with the continuing education of established general practitioners as well as vocational training of new entrants. Had undergraduate teaching experience for some years in association with Edinburgh University Department of General Practice. Past Chairman of Council, Royal College of General Practitioners and past Chairman, Joint Committee on Postgraduate Training for General Practice.

Derek Doyle, OBE, MB, ChB, FRCPE, FRCGP

Is Medical Director of St Columba's Hospice in Edinburgh, a Member of the Clinical Teaching Staff of the University of Edinburgh, Editor-in-Chief of *Palliative Medicine* and currently Chairman of the Association of Palliative Care and Hospice Doctors of Britain and Ireland. He has worked as a medical missionary in South Africa, and as a general practitioner with hospital appointments. He is the author of *Domiciliary Terminal Care* and *Coping with a Dying Relative* and editor of *Palliative Care: The Management of Far-Advanced Disease*.

Allan Forsyth MB, ChB, MRCGP

Is a general practitioner in Perth, tutor in general practice at the University of Dundee and Medical Officer to Strathallan School. His special interest in varicose veins began as a Surgeon in the Royal Air Force in Ely, Uxbridge and the Indian Ocean and continued after he completed a five year Short Service Commission and returned home to general practice in Scotland.

John Fry OBE, MD, FRCS, FRCGP

Is a general practitioner in Beckenham, Kent. He is also an Elected Member and Senior Treasurer of the General Medical Council, a Trustee of the Nuffield Provincial Hospitals Trust and past Chairman of the Board of Censors and Education of the Royal College of General Practitioners. He has worked in the same practice for 40 years and is author of *The Catarrhal Child*, *Profiles of Disease*, *Common Diseases* and many papers on clinical and operational research from his own practice, and co-editor of *NHS Data Book* and *Disease Data Book*.

George Gomez FRCGP

Qualified at The London Hospital in 1945. Squadron Medical Officer in the RAFVR. Hospital Practitioner (allergy) ENT Department and Honorary Senior Lecturer in the Department of General Practice at St George's Hospital. Staff doctor for Borough of Wandsworth, Acting Regional Chairman of a GP Sub-committee. Has published numerous articles including 'Training a Trainee', '100 cases of Asthma in General Practice', and several on ear disease.

Ian Gregg DM, FRCP, FRCGP

Is a senior research fellow in the University of Southampton and was formerly Director of the Department of Clinical Epidemiology in General Practice of the Cardiothoracic Institute (Brompton Hospital). He has carried out research in three general practices, mostly concerned with the pathogenesis of asthma and chronic bronchitis, with particular reference to the roles of infection by viruses and bacteria and of host factors in these and other respiratory diseases. He is the author of numerous articles on these subjects and other topics of an epidemiological nature.

Julian Tudor Hart MB, DCH, FRCGP

Is a general practitioner in the Welsh mining village of Glyncorrwg. He has a research attachment to the Medical Research Council, and has published numerous papers on preventive and anticipatory work in primary care, and the changes in medical education and the delivery system required for this. He was Milroy Lecturer to the Royal College of Physicians in 1974, Delamar Lecturer to Johns Hopkins University and Butterworth Gold Medallist of the Royal College of General Practitioners in 1975, Visiting Professor at the University of Birmingham in 1976, and at the University of North Carolina in 1981 and 1986. He is medical adviser to the National Union of Mineworkers and a member of the Council on Epidemiology and Prevention, the International Federation of Cardiology.

John C. Hasler OBE, MD, FRCGP, DA, DCH

Is a general practitioner at Sonning Common Health Centre in South Oxfordshire and Regional Post Graduate Adviser and Clinical Lecturer in General Practice at the University of Oxford. From 1978 to 1983 was Honorary Secretary and from 1985 to 1987 Chairman of Council of the Royal College of General Practitioners. He has published and lectured widely on general practice.

David Holton MB, ChB, DCH, DRCOG, FRCGP

Is a member of a group practice in Corstorphine, Edinburgh. Developed a particular interest in paediatrics during hospital attachments and is now a paediatric trainer and Honorary GP Tutor to the School of Community Paediatrics attached to the Royal Hospital for Sick Children in Edinburgh as well as a research assistant in the Department of Paediatrics at the Western General Hospital, Edinburgh. Currently a member of the Panel of Examiners for the RCGP.

J.G.R. Howie MD, PhD, MRCP(Ed.), FRCGP

Is Professor of General Practice at the University of Edinburgh. After qualifying, spent four years in laboratory medicine followed by four years as a principal in a Glasgow general practice. He spent ten years in the University Department of General Practice in Aberdeen before moving to his present post in 1980. Author of articles on appendicitis and its management, and the use of antibiotics in respiratory illness in general practice. Author of *Research in General Practice* published in 1979.

F.M. Hull MB, FRCGP

Was formerly in general practice in Warwickshire from 1960 to 1984. He is professor of General Practice at the Free University of Amsterdam and Senior Lecturer in the Department of General Practice in Birmingham University Medical School. In 1973 he was Visiting Professor in Family Medicine at the University of North Carolina. He is currently chairman of the General Practitioners Writers Association. Published work on a wide range of topics includes a book on infective disease in primary care and papers on morbidity coding, diagnostic method and comparative care in different countries.

David Illingworth CVO, MD, FRCP(Ed.)

Was a general practitioner in a National Health Service Group in Edinburgh. Three years in the Royal Navy Medical Service were followed by four years in hospital medicine. Since then many years have been spent in part-time teaching in the General Practice Unit of Edinburgh University. Latterly he has joined the Rehabilitation Department of Edinburgh University. Formerly a Travelling Fellow of the Nuffield Foundation, his medical contributions have mainly been related to the diagnosis, detection and prevention of cancer and coronary arterial disease. Joined Royal Medical Household in 1970 (LVO 1980, CVO 1987). Prematurely retired from National Health Service, through ill-health, in 1980.

Donald Irvine CBE, MD, FRCGP

Is a general practitioner in Ashington, Northumberland. Is Regional Adviser at the University of Newcastle upon Tyne and past Chairman of the Council of the Royal College of General Practitioners.

Cyril Josephs MD, FRCGP, DCH

Senior Medical Officer to Nightingale House, a large home in South London for elderly Jewish people. Retired from general practice in South London in 1985. Lately member of the British Geriatric Society. After qualifying in 1943 worked for several years in hospital where he developed a particular interest in geriatrics and paediatrics. Author of various chapters and articles on such subjects as paediatrics and rheumatoid arthritis. Lately medical editor and regular contributor to *Geriatric Medicine*. An occasional lecturer on problems encountered in the care of the elderly in general practice. Examiner in the Diploma in Geriatric Medicine of the Royal College of Physicians of London.

Ann-Louise Kinmonth MD, MRCP, MRCGP

Is a senior lecturer in the Department of Primary Medical Care at Southampton University and a general practitioner at the Aldermoor Health Centre. Her research interest in diabetes began with studies of the management of children with diabetes and has developed through studies on the delivery of care to young adults with diabetes to a project concerned with the process and outcome of developing general practice care for non-insulin-dependent diabetic patients. She is an editor of *Care of the Child with Diabetes* and author of original papers and review articles on the management of diabetes in different age groups.

James D.E. Knox MD, FRCP(Ed.), FRCGP

Professor of General Practice at the University of Dundee. After qualifying, spent three years in the Royal Air Force Medical Service, followed by five years in teaching hospitals in Edinburgh. Thereafter became a principal in a group practice in Edinburgh from 1960 to 1970. During the past decade has been establishing a Department of General Practice in the Dundee Medical School. Currently is a principal in the Medical School Teaching Practice. Is author of *Presentations in Primary Care* and various articles on general practice subjects.

Brian R. McAvoy MB, ChB, BSc, MRCP, MRCGP

Is senior lecturer in the Department of Community Health at Leicester University and a Principal in general practice in Leicester. He qualified at Glasgow in 1972 and after completing vocational training, spent a year as a Teaching Fellow in the Department of Family Medicine at McMaster University, Hamilton, Ontario. He has a special interest in role-play and simulated patients and their application in the teaching of clinical and communication skills and Asian health care.

Pauline A. McAvoy MB, ChB

Is a general practitioner in Leicester and a lecturer in the Department of Community Health at Leicester University. She qualified at Glasgow in 1973 and after three years' training for general practice spent a year as a Clinical Fellow in the Department of Family Medicine at McMaster University, Hamilton, Ontario. Her current interests include informal caring and family violence.

John McEwan MB, BChir, FRCGP

Is a general practitioner in Southwark and part-time Consultant in Family Planning at King's College Hospital. Since 1962 he has been concerned with the development of Family Planning services in South East London and for nine years has been teaching this subject at King's. Joint author with Peter Diggory of *Planning or Prevention? — the new face of family planning.*

Marshall Marinker MB, BS, Hon.MD, FRCGP

Was in general practice in Essex for some 15 years until 1974, when he was appointed to the Foundation Chair in the Department of Community Health, University of Leicester. In 1982 he was appointed Director of the MSD Foundation. He is a member of the Council of the Royal College of General Practitioners and became Chairman of its Education Division in 1982. His published work is concerned with medical education, clinical problem solving and the doctor-patient relationship. Editor, *Teaching General Practice*.

Judith Millac MRCGP, DCH, D(Obst.)RCOG

Is a general practitioner in Leicestershire, Scheme Supervisor Leicester Vocational Training Scheme, and member of the Panel of Examiners for the Royal College of General Practitioners. After qualifying, spent four years in hospital practice, concentrating on general medicine and paediatrics. Author of articles on paediatrics, general practice and training.

David Morrell OBE, FRCP, FRCGP, FFCM

Wolfson Professor of General Practice at United Medical and Dental Schools of Guy's and St Thomas's hospitals. He spent three years as a physician in the RAF Medical Branch and subsequently five years as principal in general practice in Hoddesdon, Hertfordshire. In 1963 he was appointed Lecturer in General Practice in the University of Edinburgh and in 1967 Senior Lecturer in General Practice at St Thomas's Hospital Medical School. His first book, *The Art of General Practice*, was published in 1965 and has since published extensively on patterns of illness in general practice and factors influencing the demand for primary medical care. He is an editor of *Teaching General Practice* and associate editor of *Laboratory: A manual for the medical practitioner.*

H. R. Patterson MD, MB, BChir, FRCGP, D(Obst.)RCOG

Is a general practitioner in Glenfield, Leicestershire. He is a part-time Lecturer in the Department of Community Health in the University of Leicester and Postgraduate Adviser in General Practice for Leicestershire and Lincolnshire and Regional Adviser in General Practice for Trent. He has published several articles mainly on hypertension e.g. 'Sources of Error', Management of Hypertension in General Practice' and 'The Epidemiology of Hypertension'.

Raymond Pietroni MB, BS, BSc, DCH, MRCGP

Is a general practitioner at the Elephant and Castle, London, with a particular interest in children, and is medical adviser to the Church of England Children's Adoption Society.

Margaret Pollak MD, BS, D(Obst.)RCOG

Formerly Senior Lecturer in Educational and Social Paediatrics at King's College Hospital, Department of Child Health. She is author of *Today's Three-year-olds in London* and numerous papers on child health, developmental screening, paediatrics, the menopause and sickle cell disease.

M.E. Preston-Whyte MB, BChir, MRCGP, DA

Is a general practitioner in Leicestershire and is a Lecturer in General Practice at Leicester University. After qualifying, went as an externe to the Hôpital Necker in Paris and then to the MRC Pneumoconiosis Research Unit in South Wales. Subsequently specialized in anaesthetics and spent two years at Grooteschuur Hospital, Cape Town, before returning to the United Kingdom and entering general practice.

Martin O. Roland BM, BCh, DRCOG, MRCP, MRCGP

Following his vocational training, spent four years as Lecturer in the Department of General Practice at St Thomas's Hospital Medical School where he carried out a study of the natural history of back pain. He is now a principal in general practice in Cambridge.

Mairi G.B. Scott MB, ChB, MRCGP

Is a general practitioner in Glasgow and is widely involved in medical education and research in general practice. She is an elected member of the Council of the Royal College of General Practitioners.

Deborah Sharp MA, BM, BCh, MRCGP

Is a general practitioner in Lambeth. Qualified in Oxford in 1976 after previously completing a biochemistry degree. After finishing vocational training, she spent two years in Holland working for a pharmaceutical company. In 1983 she was appointed Lecturer in General Practice at St Thomas's Hospital Medical School. Her main clinical interest is in obstetrics, gynaecology and women's mental health and this led to the award of a Mental Health Foundation Fellowship (held in conjunction with the General Practice Research Unit at the Institute of Psychiatry) to study childbirth-related affective disorders in the primary care setting.

J.S.K. Stevenson MB, ChB, FRCGP, D(Obst.)RCOG

Has been a Senior Lecturer in the Department of General Practice at Edinburgh University since 1968. Was for eleven years before this a general practitioner in Stevenston, Ayrshire. Is author of numerous articles, mostly related to practice organization.

Ian Tait MA, MD, FRCGP

Is a general practitioner in Aldeburgh, Suffolk. He has been active in the field of vocational training for general practice for many years. He is particularly interested in medical records in general practice and their use in education. He was the Jephcott Visiting Professor to University College Hospital Medical School in 1977, and Visiting Professor to the Royal Australian College of General Practitioners 1980–1981.

Michael Macdonald Tellis MB, ChB, FRCGP, D(Obst.)RCOG

Is a general practitioner in Measham, Leicestershire. He is a clinical teacher at the University of Leicester and is interested in malignancy and was closely attached to the Radiotherapy Department, Queen Elizabeth Hospital, Birmingham, for eight years.

John H. Walker MD, FRCGP, FFCM, DPH

Qualified in Newcastle in 1954. After several house jobs, spent a year as a trainee assistant in general practice, and returned to the University to do epidemiological and clinical research in haematology. Was appointed Lecturer in General Practice in the University of Newcastle, with responsibility for developing an undergraduate course in Family and Community Medicine. Since 1968 he has been head of the Department of Family and Community Medicine, responsible for teaching community medicine, general practice and the behavioural sciences in relation to medicine, and in addition has maintained an interest in paediatrics. He was involved in the establishment of vocational training for general practice, was for several years a member of the Joint Committee on Postgraduate Training for General Practice, became Honorary Examination Secretary of the Royal College of General Practitioners in 1972 and was Chairman of the Membership Division from 1981–83. He continues an interest in assessment of training.

Chris Watkins PhD, MRCGP

Is a general practitioner in Lambeth. Is Reader in General Practice at St Thomas's Hospital Medical School. He has conducted experimental research into factors influencing demand for medical care, the measurement of quality of general practitioner care, and into respiratory illness during the first year of life. Author of 'Measuring the quality of General Practice' and papers on Respiratory Illness in Children.

Pauline E. Watson MB, ChB, MRCGP, MRCPsych.

Qualified at Glasgow in 1965 and subsequently worked in the Western Infirmary, Glasgow, before going into general practice. Having worked in general practice in Leicestershire for ten years, she is now a consultant psychiatrist in Newcastle upon Tyne.

C.A.H. Watts OBE, MD, FRCGP, FRCPsych., D(Obst.)RCOG

Was a general practitioner in rural Leicestershire for 30 years. He qualified at Durham in 1934, and, after house jobs, both he and his wife went to Africa to run a mission hospital. During the war he served with the SAMC and ended up as a graded psychiatrist. He came back to Britain determined to apply this special training in general practice. For twelve years he worked on the Standing Mental Health Advisory Committee of the Ministry of Health. He made a special study of depressive disorders in the community, and has written widely on psychiatry in general practice. In 1974, just before he retired, he was elected a Fellow of the Royal College of Psychiatrists.

Luke Zander DCH, DRCOG, FRCGP

After five years in hospital medicine, joined the Department of General Practice in Edinburgh in 1966 and five years later was appointed Senior Lecturer in the General Practice Teaching Unit at St Thomas's Hospital. Since then he has been actively involved in both undergraduate and postgraduate teaching. His main research interest has been concerned with the development of an information system for general practice, including the introduction of microcomputers. Another interest has been the interface between the General Practitioner and specialist services with particular reference to maternity care. He has taken an active part in the Royal College of General Practitioners and is a past president of the General Practice Section of the R.S.M. His many publications include articles on confidentiality in general practice, the role of the general practitioner in obstetrics and medical records. In 1979 he spent one year as a visiting associate professor in the Department of Family Medicine, University of Western Ontario.

The use of *Practice*

The Editors

Originally *Practice* was produced in loose-leaf form, not so much because we expected that the facts of general practice would be rapidly revised, but because we were anxious to modify our text in the light of the way in which our subscribers to the loose-leaf edition used our book as a tool for everyday practice. We therefore invited a dialogue with our subscribers and in this we were not disappointed. In the context of that dialogue we were pleasantly surprised to find that *Practice* was being used in a variety of ways which we had not envisaged. In our thirteenth instalment we included many of these new uses of *Practice*, and we reproduce them here in this preliminary chapter.

You will note that this bound edition of *Practice* is supplied with an index. This had not been our intention when we first produced the loose-leaf version. We thought then that the symptom chapter headings would themselves constitute a sufficient key for using the book. But our readers pointed out that they could not use the book in this rather simple way.

Sometimes the situation is quite straightforward. If a patient presents with persistent diarrhoea, and the symptoms have failed to respond to simple medication, the doctor may well wish to consult Chapter 3.46, to refresh his memory. Sometimes the presentation will be less simple and a hunt for a diagnosis becomes even more open-ended than the layout of *Practice* suggests. A patient presents with recurrent mid-abdominal pain, intermittent diarrhoea and the passage of fresh blood. If he is a 20-year-old man, perhaps a tense university student who has a past history of asthma or eczema, the practitioner may consider the possibilities of ulcerative colitis, or Crohn's disease. The index allows the doctor to check on both these disease processes in relation to a number of important presenting symptoms. This permits a cross-checking between the symptoms with which the patient presents and the diagnostic possibilities which the reader already has in mind.

Patients often present not with one or two symptoms, but with a cluster that may be instantly recognized. A 30-year-old travelling salesman with a drawn expression and nicotine-stained fingers, presents with upper abdominal pain made worse by hunger, heartburn and recent vomiting. The pain is relieved by antacid tablets which he has been buying across the chemist's counter. It is unlikely, with this kind of presentation, that the general practitioner will need recourse to *Practice*.

Goethe says that man sees what he already knows. A patient may complain of difficulty in seeing, and on close questioning describe rainbow-coloured rings around objects when he tries to focus. If the symptoms are associated with frontal headache, the doctor may leap to a diagnosis of migraine, and dismiss the more likely diagnosis of glaucoma. If he recognizes the patient's description as a 'halo' then recourse to the index will lead him to this diagnostic possibility. On the other hand, if he begins with headache, the index will direct him to Chapter 3.18, a reading of which may help him to recall the diagnostic characteristics of glaucoma and separate them from migraine and other forms of visual disturbance, red eye and so on.

Inevitably each chapter will contain material which may not accord with the experience of the reader. There may be controversial ideas, or material which the writer has merely treated in a fairly perfunctory way. Even in a chapter written by some imagined paragon, whose experience of general practice is large, whose clinical knowledge is broad and whose powers of communication are excellent, each reader will find deficiencies. If the reading has been stimulated by the need to sort out a clinical problem, it will be more critical, more sharply observed, and the deficiencies more glaringly obvious. If the contributor can develop the habit of annotating his own copy of *Practice*, each chapter will become something more relevant than simply the communication of the author's ideas. The meeting of the printed word and the reader's written comments constitutes more than mere communication. In this way the chapters can become a dialogue between writer and reader. Every writer writes from what he knows, from what he does not know and from his own peculiar value system. The reader's different distribution of knowledge, ignorance and values, is confronted in a particularly revealing way, when writer and reader meet in an attempt to use the book to solve a particular problem.

We need to know much more about how our colleagues are in fact using *Practice* in the consulting room. Many readers seem to make a note of a particular problem, or series of problems and then read through a chapter at the end of the surgery or the end of the day. This seems to be at least as common as, if not more common than, consulting the book at the time of the consultation. Because of the continuing nature of care (see Chapter 4.1), it is often useful to consult *Practice* in the interval between two consultations concerned with the same episode of illness. A woman of fifty presents with upper abdominal colicky pain, some nausea and minimal weight loss over the past six months. She is depressed, and begins to weep when she tells the doctor that she also has a vaginal discharge. This presentation supports the need for a number of consultations to sort out the various clinical problems and the relationship of one to the other. It is in this sort of instance that recourse to a number of chapters in *Practice* may be useful to the doctor between one consultation and the next.

Medical education

Text books are a basic tool of all education, but little is said about their use. For example, any one of the larger comprehensive textbooks of internal medicine contains most of the material which the undergraduate and postgraduate student needs to know. Yet despite the excellent quality of these texts, and the large number of them available, most medical schools, at a considerable cost in teachers' time and resources, continue to provide a programme of topic teaching. Why are the textbooks not considered to be a sufficient resource for this sort of learning? Medical textbooks set out the currently believed facts about diseases. In order to do this in a coherent way, they present facts the validity of which range from the result of clinical research to the inheritance of enshrined belief. Not all texts distinguish between these different sorts of facts, nor can it be claimed that the writers of *Practice* have themselves always drawn such important distinctions.

It is currently fashionable to demand the evidence for any and every statement of opinion in medicine. Without such questioning, medicine would quickly slip back from its present scientific status to what it was not so very long ago – an informed practice of old superstitions and mythologies.

Medicine, however, is neither a science nor a philosophy alone – it is also a code of behaviour. It encompasses practical skills and it still has to employ arbitrary rules in the solving of pressing and practical problems. The statement that both the upper and the lower facial muscles are affected in Bell's palsy is a fact whose validity relies on the evidence of clinical observation, but also on what we know about the structure and function of the nervous system. The statement that steroids should always be given as soon as the symptoms appear, or a statement about the dose and route of the drugs, has a rather different sort of validity. They include an element of opinion, a judgment about the balance of risks.

Clinical problem solving

Such matters as advice, in coronary thrombosis, about bed rest, the decision to admit to a coronary care unit, or the indications or inadvisability of giving xylocaine if the pulse rate becomes irregular while arrangements are being made for the patient's admission, are an amalgam of data from empirical research and judgments about the interpretation of such data. In some areas of medicine the boundary between what we know from empirical research and what we believe from our own observations or prejudices is even harder to define. Decisions about the management of chronic backache, the diagnostic criteria and plans for the management of depression, the decision about whether to reduce the blood pressure of a 30-year-old man with a persistent diastolic of 95 mm Hg, all these will rely as heavily on opinion and belief as on facts.

The hope of the editors of *Practice* is that it will help individual practitioners to develop their own individual style of clinical problem solving. The facts contained in this book, whether derived from current research, or current belief, change (though not as quickly as some believe) and envisaged revisions of the chapters will reflect these changes. More important than the changes in facts, however, will be a refinement in the way in which we use them. In this sense the pages of *Practice* begin as a statement by their authors, but can be transformed into a mode of communication between general practitioners who are trying, perhaps for the first time, to develop a common logic of clinical problem solving.

The wish that all facts in medicine should be empirical and validated, that those facts which reflect only belief or habit or ethic should either be replaced or disavowed, is a very naive one. A medicine which could not use facts based on belief would be very restricted, might avoid some of the unwanted effects of the contemporary bio-technology, but would fail to answer much human distress.

What binds together the different sorts of facts which doctors use, what lends scientific status to the practice of modern medicine, is the logic of clinical thinking. It is the quality of the judgments that we make, the rules that we set for ourselves about how we come to a judgment that distinguish good from bad medical practice. In each of the chapters of this book, the authors have attempted to display their own internal logic. Because the approach of each writer has of necessity been idiosyncratic, has displayed a personal choice of facts, perhaps a preference for one drug over another or for a particular set of diagnostic criteria, each reader will find much with which to disagree. In many ways it is the points of disagreement rather than those passages which can be read with an appreciative nod of recognition, which provide the greatest opportunity to learn.

Practice as a tool for continuing education

Much has been written in recent years about clinical audit. In a thoughtful review of North American reports Brook[1] has suggested that explicit audit, that is the drawing up of detailed protocols of diagnosis and treatment for defined conditions like coronary thrombosis, gall bladder pain, or thyroid disease, create as many problems as they solve. Because these lists are drawn up by experts, anxious to leave no stone unturned, or rather no Achilles' heel exposed, these protocols for sound clinical behaviour are lengthy, overwhelmingly comprehensive, and expensive. Far from ensuring quality (some of the research showed that there was little concordance between different experts reviewing the same clinical records) this form of explicit audit simply ensured a growth of technical manipulations and an approach to clinical problem solving which was exhaustive, rather than purposeful. Crombie[2] and others have taken the view that implicit audit has much more to offer.

Many general practitioners are now trying to establish such implicit audit of their own work. For example the doctors in a group practice or the members of a particular professional society or postgraduate centre, or vocational training scheme, meet together in order to share what they know about a particular clinical problem and how they approach the problems of diagnosis and management. This is a very different model from much that now goes on in the name of continuing education: that is the instruction of the generalist in practice by a series of experts in a particular specialist subject. The limitations of such a method are obvious. The problems selected by the expert are not always the problems with which the general practitioner has to deal. Even when the selection of problems is appropriate, the fact that the specialist meets these problems in a different setting, and has a different set of resources available to him, again limits the value of his contribution.

Group discussion

The value of the peer group review is that all the members of the group share a similar clinical setting, and are beset with similar problems. What transforms the meetings of such groups from a vapid exchange of personal prejudices into a constructive pooling of knowledge and skills (particularly intellectual skills) are the rules of discipline which the group agrees to obey.

Because this method is still so new, the less dogma that is propounded about it the better. But these groups would do well to learn something about the characteristics of small group behaviour.[3,4] Next there should be certain implicit rules which govern the contributions which group members make. The status of facts presented should always be challenged. Facts which are based on belief, or preferences, or idiosyncratic choice, are admissible only if their status is declared. Time and again in trying to come to a conclusion about how a particular condition should be managed, or on what basis a particular diagnosis is agreed, doctors will have recourse to such beliefs and choices. The choice of penicillin V in the management of an exacerbation of chronic bronchitis is unacceptable as a preference or belief; there is empirical evidence that *Haemophilus influenzae* is an important pathogen and that this organism is not sensitive to penicillin V. On the other hand, the choice between oxytetracycline and co-trimoxazole is an open one. So is the policy of supplying the chronic bronchitic with appropriate antibiotics to be taken when the sputum turns yellow. When the evidence is uncertain, and the status of that uncertainty is explored and discussed, so-called 'clinical freedom' can display its proper credentials. What marks the quality of such discussions and enhances the quality of decision-taking is the willingness of the group to adhere to rules which stem from the logic of science and clinical medicine. These rules are best constructed and agreed by the members of the group themselves.

Methods of problem solving

In the same way the solution of clinical problems may be submitted to the following catechism:

1. Is the resolution of the problem obtained in the shortest possible time?
2. Have the number of problem solving steps been reduced to a minimum consonant with safety?
3. Has the simplest technology been employed?
4. Has the cheapest effective medication been used?
5. Does the management cause the minimum harm or risk of harm?
6. Has there been optimum use of health-care personnel?
7. Have self-care and family care been fully mobilized?
8. What realistic criterion of success is acceptable?

The chapters of *Practice* can be used to serve these purposes in two ways. First the symptom chapters provide examples of this approach to clinical standards. In this way, the reading of a chapter by members of the group can provide a useful starting place. Members may then agree to produce a series of records from each of their practices, to look at what happened when patients presented with, say, backache, or sore throat, or abdominal pain. The clinical record becomes in this way, an essential tool for the construction of clinical standards (Chapter 1.4).

The views of group members, like the views of the *Practice* authors, should be submitted to the sort of catechism outlined, the status of facts should be established, and the logic of clinical argument should be used to bridge the gap between what is known, and what must be conjectured for the good of the patient.

The development of clinical standards in this way is a major challenge for general practice.[5] We believe that this is so important that we have added a new chapter following the chapter on medical records, entitled 'Performance review'. Without adequate records review is difficult and the new material therefore fits comfortably in that section. In addition future authors who are updating chapters will add as appendices examples of the way a group of doctors may develop a practice policy for the management of the common symptoms encountered in general practice. The appendix to Chapter 3.51, for example, describes how a group can develop a policy for the management of the symptoms of dysuria and frequency of micturition, against which they can measure their performance.

The role of *Practice* in vocational training

Similar exercises may be carried out during vocational training. A group of trainees may be set a particular task or, better still, asked to identify a standard-setting task which they themselves regard as being important.

Vocational trainees will need to use a number of resources: for example, their clinical teachers both in general practice and in the hospital, and sometimes specialists in fields like pathology or community medicine. *Practice* can provide them both with written resources and with alternative models of clinical standards with which they can compare their own work. Vocational training schemes could devote part of their half-day release course to a programme of learning based on the chapters in this book.

Undergraduate education

Lastly, *Practice* can provide a valuable teaching tool for the general practitioner who accepts medical students into his practice. Part 1 provides the student with a useful introduction to the concepts of health, the distribution of clinical problems which manifest themselves in general practice, and the approach to the management of these problems, which is unique to general practice.

For the medical student, this field of work, and the clinical logic which stems from it, will constitute a dramatic contrast with what he has learned in the setting of the teaching hospital. Students may be invited to look at symptoms such as cough, chest pain, weight loss and so on, and construct their own approach to the problem. The medical student is likely to generate a problem solving flow-chart based on assumptions which are more or less appropriate to the setting of the hospital ward, but are quite unrealistic in the setting of general practice. Much self-directed learning can occur if the group of students is then invited to compare their approaches with those taken in the chapters of this book. The status of the facts used by both can be explored. When a patient presents with cough as a major symptom, the distribution of possibilities and probabilities in the general-practice setting can be compared with the likely distribution in the setting of the teaching hospital. In this way the medicine practised in both settings can be shown to be scientific, logical and relatively safe, although the actions taken by the doctor in general practice will be very different from the actions appropriately taken by the doctor in hospital.

Practice in the future

The reasons for choosing to publish *Practice* in the alternative bound form we give in the preface to this second edition. In particular we hope that this version will make the material more readily available, not only for general practitioners in training, but for other clinicians and senior students who may increasingly feel the need to study medicine from the important setting of general practice.

At the time of writing senior medical students are already being offered clinical secondments in general practice immediately preceding qualification. There are also some experimental preregistration posts in general practice which seem to be successful and may give rise to a much broader inclusion of general practice in that period of training. Lastly, a number of Royal Colleges are showing an increasing interest in the participation of general practice in general professional training for future specialists.

Practice is intended to be a tool in the consulting room and a resource for the small group. If the shape of that tool is to change, if its structure is to become more relevant to the tasks to which it is put, we need to share our experience of using it.

These bound editions, derived from the updates which we continue to produce for the loose-leaf version, are influenced by the way our readers use the book. The editors are anxious to continue the same sort of dialogue with those who read our bound edition as we have already established with the subscribers to our updating service and in this way we hope that a broad spectrum of the profession will contribute to future editions.

References

[1] Brook, R.H. (1973): Critical issues in the assessment of care and their relationship to HMOS. *Journal of Medical Education*, *48* Suppl. III, 114–32

[2] Crombie, D.L. (1972): Cum Scientia Caritas. *Journal of the Royal College of General Practitioners*, *22*, 7

[3] Beard, R. (1970): *Teaching and Learning in Higher Education*. London: Penguin

[4] Bion, W.R. (1968): *Experience in Groups*. London: Tavistock

[5] Stevens, J.L. (1977): Quality of care in general practice: can it be assessed? *Journal of the Royal College of General Practitioners*, *27*, 455–66

1
The Diagnostic Process

1.1 Health and unhealth

Marshall Marinker

Traditionally, doctors are concerned with patients who present problems about their health. What doctors have studied, and what they know about, are diseases, their diagnosis, natural history and treatment. In those branches of medicine where the behavioural or psycho-social component of illness is seen to be important, for example, in paediatric and geriatric medicine, psychiatry and general practice, it is still the deviations from the norm that concern the doctor. Just as he thinks in terms of physical pathology so also he is concerned with the psychopathology and the social problems of his patients' lives.

In general practice the pressures of work, the shortage of time and the struggle to keep up to date with advancing technology are such that the doctor has little incentive to turn from the consideration of illnesses and their management to the consideration of his own therapeutic goal. Medical textbooks and learned journals are full of descriptions of diseases and accounts of their management. The study of the individual without disease has been, and continues to be, peripheral to the training and the continuing education of clinicians. And yet, unless the doctor is aware of what we all mean by the term 'healthy', unless he is prepared to study and make explicit the ways in which health and unhealth are defined, he cannot really say what is the object of diagnosis and treatment. There is an assumption that health is the universal clinical goal, but in reality clinical goals are much more short term and pragmatic. The doctor's goal for a patient with acute appendicitis is to make an early diagnosis and to remove the appendix with sufficient skill to cause minimal upset to the patient's system. Clinical problems like acute appendicitis and clinical skills like those needed to perform an appendicectomy do not call into question the philosophical basis of medical care, nor does the successful management of the patient demand from the surgeon an awareness about definitions of health. Acute appendicitis, however, is a poor model for understanding the nature of ill health and the nature of medical care. For the most part, patients do not bring to their doctors acute, well-defined illnesses for which finite and successful treatments are readily available.

A contrasting model is the child who is brought repeatedly to the doctor because his mother is concerned about his night cough. Is this child healthy or unhealthy? If a disease process cannot be identified, and usually it cannot, who defines the health status of the child or of the mother? Is a man with an amputated leg healthy; or the woman who has just been delivered of a mongol child? Is the well-controlled epileptic a healthy man or not? A young happily married woman who chooses to become pregnant may be defined as blooming with good health. Is she similarly healthy when she delivers of her fifth child, even though the physiology of the pregnancy is normal and the child is wanted? And who decides? The mother of a six-year-old child who is physically severely deformed and imbecile calls a doctor because the child has developed a fever and a rash. The mother says; 'I thought it was probably measles. She just wasn't well yesterday and the day before'. Questions about the meanings which this mother gives to the word 'well' raise fundamental issues about the approach of doctors to patients, ways in which patients define themselves as being ill, and the ways in which society tries to deal with the ethical dilemmas of medical intervention.

Definitions

Past attempts by doctors to define health by edict have been less than successful. Most often quoted is the Utopian definition of the World Health Organization: 'Complete physical, mental and social well being, and not merely the absence of disease and infirmity'. Few of us would feel confident in describing ourselves as healthy by such stringent criteria. When Sigmund Freud said that the healthy man is a very dark horse indeed, he was not simply making an ironical joke about the social realities of the concept 'health', he was also hinting at the weakness of the frontier between health and unhealth, and at the predatory habits of the medical profession in making forays across the border to establish new territorial claims. More recently, sociologists like Zola have commented on this 'medicalization' of society. Illich goes further and talks of the doctors' expropriation of the patient's health. The absence of disease, or the absence of symptoms, including psychological symptoms, is a biological concept. The often quoted epigram (of which no clinician is prepared to admit authorship) that the healthy man is one who has been insufficiently investigated illuminates the limitations of a purely biological approach.

Health is not only biological but also a social concept. Society as a whole characterizes certain human experiences and certain human behaviours as healthy and unhealthy. As society changes, as its structure and function are modified, so these definitions of health and unhealth shift. In the early middle ages when the madman did not threaten the political integrity of a society which could tolerate a wide range of human behaviours, madness was not considered unhealthy. In a 20th century monolithic political system, the political dissenter may be labelled mentally ill. Ivan Illich confronts us more starkly with the social nature of health when he says that health is not a commodity which doctors dispense to their patients, it is simply an expression of the culture in which we live.

From the point of view of therapeutic goals, health is best thought of as the optimum adaptation of the individual to his environments, physical, psychological and social. In this sense the child with a night cough, her mother, the man with the amputated leg, and the woman with her mongol baby, all experience health, in terms which are real to them as an internal experience, and real to the society in which they live. Although this definition takes us further than that of the World Health Organization, it still begs many difficult and awkward questions. What do we mean by optimum adaptation?

The environments to which the individual must adapt may themselves be manipulated. The old woman with severe osteoarthrosis and chronic bronchitis who lives alone on the third floor of a crumbling tenement building might be faced with a very different task of biological adaptation, if society as a whole, and her family in particular, were more caring. It was the so-called diseases of civilization that became manifest during the social changes of the industrial revolution in this and other European countries, which led to the development of public health. In the 19th century the new growth of biological science in medicine was accompanied by a growing awareness of the social dimension of health. The view which Rudolf Virchow, and so many other pioneers of public health, held in the mid-19th century is summarized in his rhetorical statement that 'medicine is a social science and politics nothing but medicine on a grand scale'. The clinical management by the general practitioner of the old woman with osteoarthrosis and chronic bronchitis demands not only technological skills but also political action. The consequence of the general practitioner's willingness to make his diagnoses simultaneously in physical, psychological and social terms is that he will reflect in his management, not only a concern for the individual's adaptation to the environment, but also a manipulation of that environment in such a way as to be helpful to his patient.

Modes of unhealth

There are three sorts of departure from health which the individual experiences, and society recognizes. As doctors, we respond, and differently, to all three, but an imprecision in differentiating one from another can lead us into all sorts of therapeutic traps.

The first mode of unhealth is disease. This is a pathological process, most often physical as in throat infection or cancer of the bronchus, sometimes undetermined as in schizophrenia. The quality which identifies disease is a deviation from structural and functional biological norms. It is true that the concept of biological norms only takes us a little way. In a now famous controversy about hypertension, Platt held the view that high blood pressure was a distinct disease entity. He believed that we could say either that the patient had hypertension or that he did not, in much the same way as we can say that a patient either has or does not have influenza or an inguinal hernia. Pickering argued that blood pressure was a biological measurement that is continuously distributed in the population; that blood pressure was a measurement like weight or height. The general practitioner is aware that in his practice population there are not two distinct groups, one thin and one fat, but rather that the weights and heights of his patients are continuously distributed: those at either end of the scale he recognizes as being 'underweight' or 'obese'. Pickering demonstrated that the same is true for measurements of blood pressure: in statistical terms the distribution is not bi-modal but uni-modal. The Bedford survey of diabetes mellitus revealed a similarly continuous distribution of blood-sugar measurements. The cut-off point, the moment when the label switches from healthy to unhealthy can no longer be sharply marked. It is negotiated in relation to a host of factors. These include the believed prognostic significance of the measurement at a particular moment in the life span of the individual; the ability of the individual to avoid the predicted consequences; the availability of a specific remedy; the morbidity of the treatment in terms of unwanted side-effects of drugs; the social cost; the future dependence of the individual on health care and so on.

There is an objectivity about disease which doctors are able to see, touch, measure, smell. For this reason diseases and their management are the central facts of a medical education. Even though every disease is a unique event in the life of a unique individual, diseases are studied as ideal textbook models. The presence of a disease reveals itself to the doctor, in so far as the unique event in the patient resembles the ideal model the doctor recognizes from the literature. It is in this sense that the patient has been described as the accident of the disease.

The second mode of unhealth is illness. Illness is a feeling, an experience of unhealth which is entirely personal and interior to the patient. It most often accompanies disease, but may be entirely absent in the early stages: for example, tuberculosis, or cancer, or hypertension. Sometimes illness is experienced where no physical disease can be found. Doctors (and sometimes patients too) find this state of affairs hard to tolerate. Often the problem is 'resolved' by instituting a plethora of investigations, and when these have not yielded the description of a recognized disease, labelling the patient with a psychiatric disease like 'hysteria' or 'neurosis'.

The third mode of unhealth is sickness. If illness is an interior and personal experience for the patient, sickness is the external and public display of unhealth. Sickness is a social role, a status, or a negotiated position in the world. It is a bargain struck between the person henceforward called sick, and the society which is prepared to recognize and sustain him. The security of this role depends on a number of factors. The most important is to be in possession of a disease. Sickness based on the presence of illness alone is a very uncertain status.

Disease alone, however, guarantees nothing. The status accorded the sick person is influenced by the disease from which the individual suffers. The chronic sick are much less secure than the acute; the old than the young; the psychiatric than the surgical. The role of the doctor may be to cure diseases or to relieve illness: in contrast, society recognizes and legitimates sickness. At every consultation the doctor establishes, maintains, terminates or denies the sick role to his patient.

The system of medicine presented in this book is based on the detection of disease processes from the symptoms presented. Many of the disease processes to be described will differ from the fully worked out ideal models of the standard medical textbook. Sometimes these disease processes will be fragments of the ideal models. The collection of symptoms and physical signs will not constitute a recognized disease, but rather a cue for action. Less will be said about illness and sickness. As with almost all medical textbooks, the goal of returning the patient to a state of health will be implicit, but the nature of that state of health will not be further examined. Nonetheless questions about the definition of health raised in this chapter, and the three basic modes of unhealth here described, constitute the framework within which medical care takes place. The general practitioner should relate everything which follows to the different expressions of unhealth with which his patients may present, and to the culture values within which the individual patient identifies his state of health.

1.2
Clinical problem solving in general practice

Marshall Marinker

In previous attempts to define the clinical work of the general practitioner[1] a number of salient characteristics have been identified. These include the wide range of problems brought to the general practitioner by his patients, the early presentation of symptoms which may or may not develop into a picture of a well-recognized disease, and the relative importance which the general practitioner gives to the psychological and social (including family) components of illness. Inevitably such characteristics have been compared and contrasted with clinical work done by specialists in the hospital setting. Sometimes these differences have been exaggerated because of the need to train doctors for general practice, whose education has been entirely within the hospital. For example, the good clinician in any setting will attempt to approach the patient as a whole person and to deal with the disease process which is part of his specialty in relation to the whole of the patient's life. What differentiates the work of the general practitioner more sharply from the clinical work of the specialist in the hospital is not so much his concern for the whole man, as the nature of the problems that are brought to him. The technical resources available, the unorganized nature of the problems that are brought by the patient, and the degree to which these problems are organized by the process of diagnosis into diseases, reflect other differences.

Take for example the case of a young woman of 20 who complains to the doctor that she passes her water frequently, and that this is accompanied by a burning sensation. It is Friday at 18.00 hours and the local pathology laboratory has closed down for the weekend, apart from hospital emergency work. How does the general practitioner approach this problem?

His immediate response will be that 'this young woman has cystitis'. Why does he think this? The symptoms which she describes are typical of a lower urinary-tract infection. But what has caused the infection? And what does the general practitioner mean by 'caused'? If he asks a question about micro-organisms, then only laboratory investigation can give him a confident answer. On the other hand, previous studies on the epidemiology of lower urinary-tract infection can also provide him with a guide. They can tell him how likely it is that this infection is caused by a virus or by a bacterium. Epidemiology can give the general practitioner no information whatsoever about this young woman at this particular time with these particular symptoms: it can only help him to make an intelligent guess, which is more likely to be right than if he tries to use the clinical history as a guide or tosses a coin. Epidemiology can tell him which micro-organism is most likely to be present. Logic, rather than the laboratory, can then help him to decide what to do.

In thinking about causes, however, the general practitioner may have in mind not so much the nature of the bladder infection as the reason why the lower urinary tract is put at risk. He may elicit the history of recent sexual intercourse, perhaps for the first time, perhaps accompanied by feelings of guilt, or shame, or fear of pregnancy. In general practice the chances are that the doctor will have known the patient over a number of years. Fragments of this past knowledge, some of it recorded in her own notes or the notes of other members of her family, some of it simply implicit in the relationship that he has with her, will be included in the data which he processes in solving the immediate problem.

By contrast, in specialist medicine the information that is processed by the doctor ranges over a narrow spectrum of the patient's life and experience, but is profound. There is a concentration of data not only accumulated by a history and examination which focuses on the particular system or organ, but also supported by increasingly sophisticated medical technology. In general practice the information about the patient and the illness ranges over large areas of the patient's life, but is relatively shallow, and is pieced together from a series of consultations. The information gathered may cover many years of the patient's life and many episodes of illness. On the basis of this fragmented information, the general practitioner needs to formulate the problem at the time of the consultation in such a way as to be able to take action which will help his patient. The setting of general practice is such that the area of the patient's life with which the doctor deals may be a very broad one. The point in time in the natural history of the illness is relatively early, and the level of diagnostic certainty is relatively low. These differences between specialist medicine and general practice are differences that are appropriate to the different settings, and reflect the different problems to be solved. They are essential differences, not differences of quality of care.

Classically, the process of diagnosis is described as the taking of a full and careful history, beginning with the presenting complaint, and then embracing symptoms relevant to all the body systems. This is succeeded by a physical examination which follows the same pattern, from the particular to the general. The collection of further relevant information is by laboratory investigations (and in the hospital setting this often includes 'routine' blood counts and chest x-ray). The final stage is a diagnosis which best fits all the facts that have been gathered. This process, which bears a strong resemblance to inductive reasoning in science, is an excellent model for teaching about applied pathology and therapeutics, but it bears little resemblance to the work of clinicians, either in hospital or in general practice. Clinical work (as opposed to clinical teaching) is not inductive, but rather hypothetico-deductive. This simply means that the doctor on the basis of incomplete evidence makes an informed guess, and then attempts to see whether his guess fits the reality of the patient's problem. In the words of Sir Peter Medawar:[2] 'Imaginative conjecture and criticism, in that order, underlie the physician's diagnosis of his patient's ailments'.

What characterizes clinical thinking is informed guesswork. The doctor does not delay making a provisional diagnosis until all the pieces of the diagnostic jigsaw puzzle have been assembled by him. It begins with a word, a clue, a symptom, the age and sex of the patient, the time of year and the illnesses which are prevalent in his practice, the memory or a note about the patient's past, the way in which the patient walked into the room and sat down, the look of pain or sadness, or fear. The so-called 'hunch' of the experienced doctor, or clinical intuition, is simply the working out of such presentations in terms of a diagnostic statement. Far from being unscientific, this way of thinking and working is of the essence of science. Science is simply the process of examining the way in which the world is put together by guessing and testing. The careful and complete clinical model presented by such classical educational texts as *Hutchison's Clinical Methods* is scientific only in its insistence on careful observation, scrupulous techniques and unambiguous statement. As a method of making a diagnosis it is, in its essence, unscientific. In its essence science is not about methods of measurement, or the type of phenomena that are measured, but about the way in which we think, and the honesty with which we test our hypotheses.

Simple representation of the way in which doctors solve clinical problems is given in figure 1.

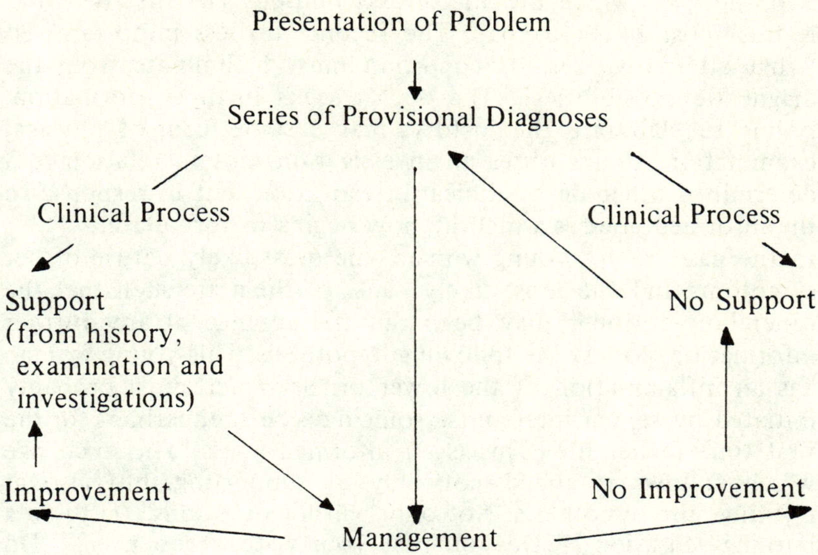

Figure 1. – Diagnostic method

If we take the example of the young woman presenting with urinary symptoms, her first statement might have been 'I'm having trouble passing my water'. At this stage in the consultation what other information is available to the doctor? Perhaps he notices only that she is an attractive rather anxious young woman. The medical record reveals no previous history of urinary symptoms, but there is a note of painful periods when she was in late adolescence. She is 20 years old, unmarried, wears no engagement ring and the doctor remembers that she is an only child still living with rather quiet elderly parents. So far as the doctor is aware she has never consulted for oral contraception. It is this sort of not-quite-random information, a partial picture of the patient and the environment, with which the doctor begins his diagnostic work. On this basis what sort of a diagnosis can he make? The answer, in terms of a classical clinical training, is that he can make no diagnosis because the information is too incomplete. After all, the complaint, 'I'm having trouble passing my water', might suggest a whole range of possible causes, from retrocaecal appendicitis to a phobic anxiety state.

The inductive method of thinking demands that the total information precedes firm diagnosis. But this is not the way in which doctors think and work. From the first presentation of the problem the doctor begins to formulate a series of tentative or provisional diagnoses. These hypotheses are formed in relation to two questions which the doctor asks himself. The first is: 'What is this most likely to be?' The second, no less important, is: 'What alternative serious condition must I eliminate from the diagnostic possibilities?' The doctor seeks further information, begins to elaborate the history, makes some form of physical examination, or institutes an investigation, not in relation to a determined schedule of clinical investigation, but in response to the informed guesses which he now begins to formulate.

In the case of this young woman, the most likely nature of her symptoms and the most likely cause of them are such that the general practitioner may begin, in the absence of any further information, to test the following hypothesis. This young woman has an inflammation of the lower urinary tract, most probably initiated by sexual intercourse some days before, perhaps for the first time in her life. This is an informed guess. The exchange which follows is aimed not only at supporting, but also at refuting, the hypothesis. Not only will his questions ('Is there a burning sensation?'; 'Do you pass your water frequently?'; 'Do you pass your water frequently during the night?') focus on the possibility of cystitis, but he may, if his patient allows him, open up the subject of the patient's sexual experience, perhaps her anxiety about this, perhaps her need for contraceptive advice. Given that this area of the patient's life may be a highly sensitive one for her, it may be that, on this first occasion, little will be asked and little will be told.

At the same time, other factors from the family history may be entering into the problem solving pathway. The fact that there is a strong family history of diabetes mellitus may alter the priorities that the doctor gives to looking for causes, or to the presentation of advice (should this become necessary) on contraception. The fact that the patient was brought up in a strict religious household, with strongly held convictions on the part of her parents and herself concerning sexual behaviour will also modify the sort of information that the doctor might seek (or avoid making explicit) and the sort of counselling that he will give. Diagnosis, in this case, may well be expressed in terms of an epidemiological survey as 'acute cystitis'. But the real formulation of the problem will be less secure in terms of the exact pathology or the identity of the micro-organism responsible, and more specific to the patient's life situation at this particular time, of which the urinary symptoms are but one component.

It is a classical precept of clinical teaching that the history is all important. Once the hypothetico-deductive nature of clinical problem solving is grasped, it becomes clear that the history is not simply the gathering of data in a systematized form. It is a rapid process of finding support for, or probing for refutation of, the possible diagnoses created in the imagination of the doctor. In the case of the young woman under discussion, the sort of questions which will be asked will depend on the possibilities which the doctor is considering. If the doctor was to take a 'full clinical history' he would, of course, also ask about the possibility of chest pains, disturbances of balance or sensation, symptoms of indigestion and so on. But answers to such questions will not help the doctor to solve the patient's problem. At best or at worst, the answers to these questions will only generate fresh problems whose resolution may be a priority for the doctor, but not necessarily for the patient.

The physical examination is simply an attempt to collect more data in a different way from the history. It is neither systematized nor random, but problem oriented. The physical examination is rarely diagnostic: it is rather a way of supporting or refuting the diagnosis which has already been reached by the doctor from the history that he has taken. Sometimes, for example in the case of this young woman, the physical examination may not be a necessary step in problem solving. Of course, the doctor might elect to examine the abdomen, to test for renal tenderness, or even attempt a vaginal or rectal examination in order to rule out local causes. There are no prescriptions for correct conduct at this sort of consultation. But it is at least arguable that none of these examinations is relevant and that some of them can be positively harmful to the patient, and to the doctor-patient relationship at this stage. In other situations, for example the history of a lump in the breast or abdominal pain, the physical examination is much more important. But even here the history is paramount. If the examination of the breast reveals none of the signs of a carcinoma, but a simple cystic swelling, in the last analysis the diagnosis will still depend on histological examination. An inconclusive series of findings on abdominal and rectal examination of a patient who gives a classical history of acute appendicitis will probably be insufficient to persuade the surgeon that he should not operate there and then.

It is true that not all physical examinations are strictly problem oriented. It is highly unlikely that the patient who presents to the general practitioner with a history of a pain in the chest will receive not only an examination of the cardiovascular system, but also a rectal examination. On the other hand, a middle-aged man presenting for the first time in many years with a history of rectal bleeding may well have his blood pressure taken. The taking of the blood pressure, however, does not refer to the problem of rectal bleeding. It refers to the problem of middle age and the possible utility of picking up hypertension at an early and treatable stage. General practice affords an excellent setting for this sort of early diagnosis and problem detection. Hodgkin[3] has suggested that, in the case of the elderly, vigilant care of patients who present to the doctor obviates the need for population screening programmes. The underlying notion here is that there are two sorts of problems with which the doctor is presented. First there is the problem that the patient presents (and included here are those psychological problems which the patient has unconsciously translated into physical terms). Secondly, there are problems which the doctor identifies either because of the appearance of the patient or from what the patient has to say, or simply from the patient's age and sex, occupation or other risk factor. An obese middle-aged man may consult for a certificate because he is recovering from influenza. His obesity is in itself a problem which the doctor identifies: the possibility of high blood pressure and diabetes mellitus will also have to be explored.

At its best this clinical method is characterized by its economy. There is an economy of time, information elicited, and disturbance to the patient. One of the worst characteristics of the modern clinical method, particularly in the hospital setting, is the plethora of technological investigations which seem to bear no relationship at all to the problem which the patient presented. Clinical medicine is not a game of hunt the thimble: the doctor who reacts to the problem of a patient with a characteristic abdominal pain by ordering an electrocardiogram, barium meal, cholecystogram, barium enema and intravenous pyelogram, has already disengaged his mind from the scientific method. His report on the patient may be impressively technological, but the finding of a small hiatus hernia, a poorly functioning gall-bladder or a diverticulosis will probably create more problems than it will solve.

It is a useful maxim that no investigation should be instituted unless the result is likely to alter materially the doctor's management. The question of whether or not to x-ray a chest when the patient coughs, or estimate the haemoglobin when the patient complains of tiredness and so on will be dealt with in succeeding chapters of this book. One example of the relationship between laboratory investigations and clinical problem solving may suffice here. What investigations should the general practitioner carry out in the case of the young woman who presents with urinary symptoms at 6 o'clock on Friday evening? He may decide to test the urine then and there for the presence of albumin. Its presence may support the diagnosis of a urinary-tract infection, but its absence will take him no further. Microscopy of the urine there and then will be of much greater value. The usefulness of making a bacteriological examination of a midstream specimen of urine at this stage is more questionable. If the infection is bacterial, and sensitive to antibiotics, then there is a nine to one chance that the organism is *E.coli.* It is almost certain that this organism will be amenable to treatment by trimethoprim, and that such treatment should now be instituted. If after forty-eight or seventy-two hours the symptoms are unchanged, then the chances are that the organism was not *E. coli*: now an examination of a midstream specimen of urine can be instituted, and a broad-spectrum antibiotic like ampicillin or cotrimoxazole substituted while confirmation is awaited from the laboratory. Laboratory confirmation that the urine is free of bacteria is more important some four weeks after the symptoms have resolved than at the time of presentation.

Conclusion

Clinical problem solving does not require a totality of data. Indeed too much information may impede rather than help the process. A knowledge of probabilities (stemming from epidemiological studies) is the first essential: a knowledge of the early presentation of life-endangering conditions is the second. It is the quality of thinking and not the quantity of facts that is likely to lead to the resolution of clinical problems.

References

[1]Working Party of the Royal College of General Practitioners (1972): *The Future General Practitioner. Learning and Teaching*. London: Royal College of General Practitioners

[2]Medawar, P.B. (1969): *The Art of the Soluble.* Harmondsworth: Penguin Books

[3]Hodgkin, K (1966): Good General Practice without Routine Screening Examinations: In Symposium on Preventive Medicine in General Practice. *Journal of the College of General Practitioners,* Supplement No. 1, pp. 100–112

1.3 Symptom perception and reporting

David Morrell

This book is concerned with the interpretation of symptoms of illness presented to the general practitioner. Previous chapters have dealt with the process of becoming ill and the diagnostic pathways in general practice. This chapter deals with information that has been collected about the perception and reporting of symptoms in the community. The experienced general practitioner has always used his knowledge of the probabilities of disease in respect of different presenting symptoms to direct his further diagnostic action and decision making. In order to define this knowledge in such a way that it may be communicated to others it is necessary to quantify much that has hitherto been accepted as 'experience'.

Sources of information

A variety of sources of information has been explored to provide the data used in this book. In order to interpret this information, it is necessary to appreciate the value and limitations of these data.

Some of the data are derived from studies of random samples of the population. In these cases it is important to know the characteristics of the population from which the sample was taken in terms of age, sex, social class and cultural characteristics. The population of, for instance, a south coast seaside resort would be very different from that of a 'new town' or a mining community. It is also important to know the proportion of the population sampled who co-operated with the study. In some cases this is as low as 50 to 60 per cent and it is often impossible to tell the extent to which this response rate biased the results.

Many studies on which this work is based took place of necessity in individual general practices. The population sampled in these cases, even if randomly selected, is biased by the type of people attracted to that particular practice and the area in which it is situated. This is not to denigrate the value of these studies. The scientific method has been applied to general practice, with a few outstanding exceptions, for only three or four decades. The amount of knowledge available is necessarily limited and this book has had to depend for information on many small studies of selected populations. These are beginning to throw important light on the diagnostic process in general practice but the reader must beware of trying to take more out of the results than the original research workers claimed.

The areas of study which will be examined in this chapter are illustrated in Figure 1.

Incidence of Symptoms in the Community

↓

Decision to Seek Medical Care

↓

Symptoms Presented to the General Practitioner

↓

Distribution of Diseases diagnosed in General Practice

Figure 1. – Areas of study

Symptoms in the community

Three methods have been used to study this problem.

Prevalence studies. – These studies, in which random samples of the population are asked whether or not they are presently experiencing specific symptoms, are particularly used to study the relationship between symptoms and objective physical abnormalities. A good example of such a study is that carried out by Wood and Elwood,[1] who attempted to relate the traditional symptoms of anaemia to haemoglobin level. They found no relationship unless the haemoglobin level is below 10 G per 100 ml of blood. Similar studies have been carried out to clarify the symptoms of hypertension and chronic bronchitis.

Studies of symptom recall. – These studies attempt to measure the occurrence of symptoms over a set period of time. Patients are asked to respond to a questionnaire indicating whether or not they have experienced a particular symptom during the preceding two or four weeks. This is the method most commonly used to measure the frequency of symptoms in the community. It is subject to all the problems of sampling and in particular must be carried out throughout the year to avoid the seasonal fluctuations in symptoms. It has the added problem of depending on symptom recall. The method has most often been used to relate symptoms to the use of medical care services.

The study carried out by Dunnell and Cartwright[2] into medicine taking is an example of research of this type, and is a source of information which will be used in this book. The sampling method was complex but covered fourteen parliamentary constituencies throughout Britain. The response rate was 75 per cent. The period of symptom recall was two weeks. The percentage of respondents reporting a variety of symptoms is illustrated in table I in the appendix to this chapter.

The symptoms most commonly reported by adults were headache, coughs, aches or pains in muscles or joints, backache and 'nerves'. Age, over 21 years, had no consistent effect on the number of symptoms reported until the age of 65 years was reached. Over 65 years slightly more symptoms were reported. The type of symptoms reported did, however, vary with age. Headaches and nerves were much less common over 65, while aches and pains, breathlessness, constipation, indigestion and sleeplessness were more commonly reported. The variation in symptoms reported with age is illustrated in table II in the appendix.

Dunnell and Cartwright found no difference in the number of symptoms reported by boys and girls. Women over 20 years of age, however, reported more symptoms than men and the particular symptoms reported by the sexes also differed. The symptoms reported more often by women than men were constipation, faintness, headache, weight problems, nerves, backache and muscle and joint pains. This is illustrated in table III in the appendix.

Incidence of symptoms (Health diary method). – The use of health diaries to measure illness experience is relatively recent. Individuals are invited to keep a diary of their health over a period of time, usually one month, and to record each night any symptoms experienced during the day. The individuals co-operating may be asked to record other events occurring during the diary days, such as the action taken in response to symptoms or stressful events. The method is particularly useful for relating symptom recording to the subsequent action taken. It requires a high degree of co-operation from the study subjects and careful supervision, and is not really suitable for large samples. The frequency of symptom recording is higher using health diaries than using symptom recall. The results of a study using health diaries in a London general practice illustrate this method. The sample was drawn from women aged 20 to 44 years, registered with the practice. The response rate was a little over 60 per cent, who completed the dairies for a period of one month, but the social class distribution of responders in the sample did not differ significantly for that of women in this age-group in England and Wales. Findings from this study were used to examine associations within the group studied but care must be taken in making generalizations.

Symptoms are recorded in health diaries on about one day in three. About one symptom in thirty-eight leads to a consultation with a doctor. This finding is at variance with studies using symptom recall, which suggested that one symptom in four led to a consultation. Part of this difference is undoubtedly due to the method used for recording symptoms.

Decision to seek medical care

All the studies carried out on this subject have demonstrated that only a proportion of perceived symptoms lead to a demand for medical care. It has been demonstrated in one study that 23 per cent of patients reporting symptoms which they described as producing severe pain or disability, or which they regarded as serious, did not report these symptoms to the doctor. It has also been shown that the demand at primary care level does not precisely reflect the pattern of morbidity in the community. It has, for instance, been demonstrated that for symptoms of skin disease a high frequency of symptom reporting by women in general practice did not reflect a sex difference in the prevalence of skin disease in the community. Likewise, the highest reporting of hearing problems to the general practitioner occurred in the age-group 40 to 64 years, while the highest prevalence of hearing disorders occurs in patients over the age of 65 years. Similar discrepancies have been demonstrated in respect of social class. A number of studies have been carried out to identify some of the factors that influence demand for primary medical care. In summarizing some of these factors the work of Hannay,[3] who studied the prevalence of symptoms and action taken in response to these in a sample of 1,344 individuals in a general practice in Glasgow, and Morrell and Wale,[5] who used health diaries in a sample of women in London, have been used together with other research reported from general practice.

Certain biological factors, such as age and sex, inevitably affect demand in that they affect morbidity. High consultation rates are characteristic of the very old and the very young and of women in the age group 15–44 years.

Marital status has been shown in a number of studies to influence demand for medical care. Widows and widowers report symptoms and seek care more frequently than the married, while the divorced and separated report more symptoms, but this is not reflected in their demand for care.

There is a higher utilization of care in families of three or more children, but mothers of large families are less inclined to adopt the sick role than mothers of small families.

Educational levels have been shown to influence demand for medical care. There are lower demands among those who proceed beyond the age of 15–16 years in education, and they make more use of preventive services but less of emergency services.

Social class affects demand for medical care in a complex way, interacting with many other variables, and conflicting results have been reported. Morbidity and mortality rates are higher in the lower social classes, but this is not always reflected in higher uptake of primary medical care.

Not unexpectedly, the personality of an individual is important in determining when he or she makes a decision to assume the sick role. It has been shown there is a relationship between objective measures of anxiety and both the perception of symptoms and the reporting of symptoms to the general practitioner. High neuroticism scores measured by the Maudsley personality inventory are associated with high prevalence of symptoms but not independently with the propensity to consult the doctor. Introverted patients initiate a greater number of consultations than extroverted, and depressed patients both experience and report more symptoms to the general practitioner.

In different studies, a variety of factors, such as high mobility in the community, lack of active religious participation, dissatisfaction with housing and the community and moving into high-rise flats have been shown to increase the frequency of symptom perception and to increase the frequency of consultation.

These facts are derived from studies that have been devised to examine the factors which influence the individual perceiving symptoms to seek medical care, and they indicate the complexity of the subject. In the most general terms the perception of symptoms gives rise to anxiety. The anxiety generated is influenced by the individual's previous experience of illness, personality, cultural, religious, marital and family resources. Whether or not this anxiety leads to a demand for medical care is in turn influenced by cultural factors, family support, education, occupation, the accessibility of care and perhaps, above all, the individual's expectations of the general practitioner. Many of these factors inevitably interact. Different symptoms have a different potential to provoke consultation, and this is reflected in the proportion of symptoms perceived which lead to a demand for medical care.

This is illustrated in tables IV and V in the appendix, where the twelve most commonly perceived symptoms by a random sample of women aged 20 to 44 years are compared with the twelve symptoms most commonly presented to the general practitioner by the same sample of women.

In this study, the relationship between the symptoms presented to the general practitioner and the impact of these symptoms in driving the patient to assume the sick role has been further investigated. Assumption of the sick role might be reflected by the patient restricting her normal activities, by the patient being constrained to lie down in response to symptoms, or by self-medication. The symptoms in this group of patients that most commonly led the patient to restrict her normal activities were cough, changes in energy and disturbances of menstruation. Lying down occurred most often in response to changes in energy, backache and distubances of menstruation. Self-medication was more commonly carried out in response to cough, toothache, headache. These relationships are illustrated in table VI in the appendix. There is no clear relationship between any of these variables and the decision to seek medical care and it seems likely that this decision is influenced both by the anxiety engendered by the symptoms perceived, which is itself a product of many other factors, including the disability produced by the symptoms and the expectation that the doctor can provide relief, and that it is appropriate to seek his aid.

Symptoms presented to the general practitioner

The factors considered in the previous section determine the symptoms that are finally presented to the general practitioner at a consultation.

Surprisingly few studies have been carried out of the over-all pattern of symptom presentation in general practice, although in contrast large numbers of studies have reported the morbidity measured in general practice. There are no uniformly recognized methods of grouping or coding symptoms, as there are for handling morbidity data, and individual workers have developed their own coding for symptoms recorded in general practice.

Epidemiological studies of symptoms presented to the general practitioner must be looked at critically, as indicated earlier in this chapter, and the characteristics of the samples studied related to the over-all population. A further difficulty, however, arises in defining what is meant by a presenting symptom. A verbatim record of the patient's initial complaint does not necessarily reflect the deviation from normal health which he, or she, has perceived, and which has prompted the consultation, and indeed owing to the varied use of words by different cultural groups, this approach may lead to serious misinterpretation. In studying symptoms it is therefore necessary to develop a method which allows the doctor to exercise some judgment in recording the main deviation from normal health that led the patient to consult; this, in turn, leads inevitably to some inter- and intra-observer variation. Studies of symptoms may concern themselves with all the symptoms presented to the general practitioner, or may focus on the first, or most important presenting symptom only. They may be concerned with all symptoms recorded at all consultations, or they may limit themselves to those consultations where the patient is initiating a new contact with the doctor.

These problems may explain the relative paucity of data on this subject. Some information is available from a study carried out in a practice of 4,500 patients in London.[4] The age distribution of the practice was slightly biased towards the over-55 year age-groups, but the social-class distribution did not differ significantly from the social-class distribution of the population derived from census data.

The symptoms studied were the presenting symptom recorded at new patient-initiated consultations. These represented 25 per cent of all consultations (34 per cent of consultations of those under the age of 44 years and 15 per cent of consultations of those over the age of 45 years). The twelve most commonly recorded symptoms in this study are illustrated in table VII in the appendix.

With few exceptions, such as symptoms of trauma, the proportion of symptoms presented by women in the practice was greater than the proportion of women registered with the practice, which reflects the propensity for women to initiate new consultations with the doctor. This difference was particularly marked in symptoms reflecting changes in the emotional function, changes in appearance, changes in energy and disturbances of bladder function and balance.

Some symptoms were closely associated with age. Disturbances of bowel function, cough and rashes occurred most often under the age of 5 years and became less common with advancing years. Sore throat, headache and abdominal pain were most common in the age-group 5 to 34 years. Pain in the back, chest and joints became increasingly common with advancing years.

In respect of social class, after adjustment for age, pain in the back was more commonly presented in social class V, while symptoms of eye disease and gynaecological disorders were under-reported in this social class.

Analysing the incidence of symptoms in general practice has two purposes. First, it identifies the main areas of diagnostic activity of the primary physician and thus underlines the particular knowledge required by the doctor working in this field. Secondly, it identifies the mismatch between the prevalence of symptoms in the community, and the symptoms presented to the general practitioner. In this way it is possible to identify groups particularly vulnerable to disease, in whom this is not reflected in their demands for primary medical care.

Morbidity studies in general practice

These studies reflect the diagnoses applied by general practitioners to the symptoms presented to them. Many studies have been carried out in this field, the best known being those of the General Register Office, in co-operation with the Royal College of General Practitioners.[6] Morbidity studies in general practice present all the problems of other epidemiological studies. Only the best organized practices are able to co-operate in them, and this necessarily introduces an element of bias. A more serious problem, however, arises from the fact that these studies demand of the doctor a diagnostic label for each consultation, and it is well known that up to 50 per cent of consultations in general practice do not admit of a precise diagnostic label. The doctor recording in a morbidity study is to some extent constrained to make a diagnosis. Table VIII in the appendix summarizes the distribution into diagnostic groups of consultations recorded in the most recent National Morbidity Study.

Studies of morbidity more closely related to the objectives of this book are those in which presenting symptoms are related to the diagnosis recorded in response to them. Most textbooks of medicine are based on hospital experience. It is quite clear that the probability that particular symptoms will reflect a particular morbid process in hospital practice is totally different from the probability in general practice. It has been shown that only about one consultation in thirty in general practice leads to a contact with the hospital, and that while 70 to 80 per cent of a general practitioner's population have a contact with him during one year, only about 10 per cent have any contact with the hospital specialists. To quote just one example: cough in a child under the age of 5 years in general practice is almost always due to upper respiratory infection. The same symptom in the same age-group presenting in hospital practice more often reflects lower respiratory infection. Other common symptoms such as diarrhoea, vomiting, headache, anxiety and depression are subject to the same bias. Books on differential diagnosis based on hospital xperience are not therefore entirely appropriate for the doctor working in the community. In this book those who have carried out research in general practice will contribute their findings to clarify the interpretation of symptoms presented in general practice. Each author will use not only his own experience in the field but also the published results of other research workers in general practice. In this way, it is hoped that each symptom will be interpreted in a realistic way for the practising family doctor.

References

[1] Wood, M.M. and Elwood, P.C. (1966): Symptoms of Iron Deficiency Anaemia. *British Journal of Preventive and Social Medicine, 20,* 117

[2] Dunnell, K. and Cartwright, A. (1972): *Medicine Takers, Prescribers and Hoarders.* London: Routledge and Kegan Paul

[3] Hannay, D. (1979). *The Symptom Iceberg*. London: Routledge and Kegan Paul

[4] Morrell, D.C., Gage, H.G., Robinson, N.R. (1971): Symptoms in General Practice. *Journal of the Royal College of General Practitioners, 21*, 32

[5] Morrell, D. and Wale, C. (1976). Symptoms Perceived and Recorded by Patients. *Journal of the Royal College of General Practice*, *26*, 398–403

[6] Royal College of General Practitioners, Office of Population Censuses and Surveys, Department of Health and Social Security (1986): *Morbidity Statistics from General Practice 1981–82*. HMSO Series MB5, No. 1

Appendix

In this appendix a number of tables have been brought together which may be referred to, not only in reading this chapter, but in studying individual chapters on symptoms in this book. They illustrate the distribution of symptom incidence in the community, symptom reporting in general practice, action taken in response to symptoms and morbidity in general practice.

	Percentage reporting symptoms in a two-week period	
	Adults	Children
Sore throat	12	8
Breathlessness	15	1
Coughs, catarrh or phlegm	32	17
Cold, 'flu, or running nose	18	18
Constipation	10	6
Diarrhoea	3	3
Vomiting	3	6
Indigestion	18	1
Eye strain or other eye trouble	14	4
Ear trouble	7	3
Faintness or dizziness	8	1
Headaches	38	8
Pain or trouble on passing water	2	—
Loss of appetite	6	4
Any problem of being under- or over-weight	10	—
'Nerves', depression, or irritability	21	3
Pains in the chest	5	—
Backache or pains in the back	21	1
Aches or pains in the joints, muscles, legs, or arms	29	3
Palpitations or thumping heart	6	—
Piles	5	—
Sores or ulcers	4	2
Rashes, itches, or other skin troubles	13	12
Sleeplessness	16	4
Swollen ankles	8	1
Burns, bruises, cuts, or other accidents	9	16
Trouble with teeth or gums	7	12
Undue tiredness	16	2
Corns, bunions, or any trouble with feet	19	2
Women's complaints*	5	1
'A temperature'	2	3
Any other symptoms	6	3
Number of people (100%)	1,410	519
Average number of symptoms reported	3.9	1.4

*Only asked of women and girls over 10 years old

(Tables I, II and III are reproduced from Karen Dunnell and Ann Cartwright (1972): *Medicine Takers, Prescribers and Hoarders*. London: Routledge and Kegan Paul. Reproduced by courtesty of the Publishers.)

Table I. Symptoms reported by adults and children

	Age-group							
	21-24	25-34	35-44	45-54	55-64	65-74	75+	All adults
Percentage of adults reporting:	%	%	%	%	%	%	%	%
Sore throat	17	17	15	14	9	5	5	12
Breathlessness	5	8	12	17	20	22	19	15
Coughs, catarrh, or phlegm	27	27	34	30	34	35	35	32
Colds, 'flu, or running nose	25	23	19	17	15	15	15	18
Constipation	12	7	8	9	9	14	20	10
Diarrhoea	5	4	2	2	2	4	3	3
Vomiting	4	5	2	2	3	3	6	3
Indigestion	15	10	15	18	22	25	20	18
Eye strain	20	11	11	14	14	16	22	14
Ear trouble	4	3	6	6	5	17	13	7
Faintness or dizziness	6	7	7	6	7	12	14	8
Headaches	41	51	48	42	29	23	21	38
Pain or trouble on passing water	—	—	—	2	2	3	6	2
Loss of appetite	9	4	4	7	6	6	6	6
Any problem of being under- or over-weight	16	7	11	14	9	9	8	11
'Nerves', depression or irritability	27	27	24	22	16	13	19	21
Pains in the chest	5	4	4	6	6	9	3	5
Backache or pains in the back	21	17	22	21	21	23	17	21
Aches or pains in the joints, muscles, legs, or arms	21	20	23	29	34	39	45	29
Palpitations or thumping heart	1	5	4	7	6	11	3	6
Piles	5	4	2	6	5	6	6	5
Sores or ulcers	5	4	4	3	2	4	8	4
Rashes, itches, or other skin trouble	22	17	13	17	7	10	6	13
Sleeplessness	11	10	12	16	22	21	23	16
Swollen ankles	1	3	5	8	10	13	20	8
Burns, bruises, cuts, or other accidents	14	11	9	12	9	2	3	9
Trouble with teeth or gums	12	8	10	5	6	5	3	7
Undue tiredness	17	16	19	15	17	12	15	16
Corns, bunion, or any trouble with feet	17	13	10	15	23	35	33	19
Women's complaints like	23	18	12	14	2	1	—	10
period pain*	(47)	(123)	(141)	(138)	(139)	(106)	(54)	(748)
'A temperature'	2	3	2	4	1	—	—	2
Any other symptoms not already mentioned	6	6	4	5	5	8	10	6
Number of adults (= 100%)	81	230	289	269	258	194	86	1,410

*The figures in brackets are the numbers of women from which percentages were calculated.

Table II. Variation in symptoms reported with age

	Men	Women
Percentage reporting:	%	%
Sore throat	11	13
Breathlessness	13	17
Coughs, catarrh or phelgm	35	29
Cold, 'flu or running nose	18	19
Constipation	6	14
Diarrhoea	2	4
Vomiting	3	3
Indigestion	16	19
Eye strain	13	15
Ear trouble	8	7
Faintness or dizziness	6	10
Headaches	30	46
Pain or trouble on passing water	1	2
Loss of appetite	5	6
Any problem of being under- or over-weight	7	14
'Nerves', depression, or irritability	14	27
Pains in the chest	6	5
Backache or pains in the back	18	23
Aches or pains in the joints, muscles, legs, or arms	26	32
Palpitations or thumping heart	4	8
Piles	3	6
Sores or ulcers	3	5
Rashes, itches or other skin troubles	12	14
Sleeplessness	12	20
Swollen ankles	2	13
Burns, bruises, cuts, or other accidents	9	9
Trouble with teeth or gums	6	8
Undue tiredness	10	21
Corns, bunions, or any trouble with feet	15	23
Women's complaints like period pain	–	10
'A temperature'	3	2
Any other symptoms not already mentioned	6	5
Number of adults (=100%)	661	749

Table III. Variation with sex in reported symptoms

Symptom episodes recorded	Number
Headache	294
Changes in energy	146
Backache	85
Disturbance of gastric function	71
Disturbance of emotional response	69
Abdominal pain	63
Sore throat	46
Cold	40
Pain in lower limb	36
Disturbance of menstruation	32
Others	385
Total	1,267

Table IV. Symptom episodes from the diaries of 204 patients

Symptoms presented	Number
Sore throat	33
Cough	29
Abdominal pain	28
Skin rash	22
Disturbance of menstruation	21
Backache	21
Headache	20
Disturbance of bladder function	19
Bleeding or abnormal discharge from genital tract	16
Disturbance of bowel function	14
Chest pain	14
Disturbance of emotional response	14
Others	185
Total	436

Table V. Symptoms presented at 436 consultations in one year initiated by 204 patients keeping health diaries

Symptom days (1st recorded symptom)	Total days	Normal activities restricted	Lie down	Some form of medication
Headache	365	54 (15%)	58 (16%)	252 (69%)
Changes in energy, tiredness	207	54 (26%)	60 (29%)	84 (41%)
Backache	143	24 (17%)	33 (23%)	54 (38%)
Cold	128	31 (24%)	20 (16%)	80 (62%)
Disturbance of gastric function	100	7 (7%)	16 (16%)	42 (42%)
Disturbance of emotional response	100	21 (21%)	12 (12%)	61 (61%)
Sore throat	90	17 (19%)	14 (16%)	53 (59%)
Abdominal pain	88	19 (22%)	18 (20%)	46 (52%)
Cough	74	20 (27%)	14 (19%)	60 (81%)
Pain in mouth (toothache)	55	4 (7%)	1 (2%)	45 (82%)
Bleeding and abnormal discharge from nose	50	8 (16%)	3 (6%)	32 (64%)
Disturbance of menstruation	48	11 (23%)	11 (23%)	28 (58%)
TOTAL symptom days	2,027	366 (18%)	333 (16%)	1,157 (57%)
TOTAL non-symptom days	3,685	102 (3%)	44 (1%)	589 (16%)

Table VI. Action taken in response to the twelve most common symptoms reported in health diaries

Symptom	Males	Females	Total
Cough	240	287	527
Rashes	137	165	302
Sore throat	125	162	287
Abdominal pain	93	104	197
Disturbance of bowel function	93	94	187
Spots, sores, ulcers	79	103	182
Pain in back	82	90	172
Pain in chest	83	85	168
Pain in lower limbs	66	95	161
Pain in head	70	89	159
Pain in joints	66	75	141
Disturbance in gastric function	61	80	141
Others	1,068	1,633	2,701
Total	2,263	3,062	5,325

Table VII. The twelve most common symptoms reported in a general practice

Disease or condition	Males	Females	Total
Infective and parasitic diseases	162	199	181
Neoplasms	41	45	43
Endocrine, nutritional and metabolic disorders	51	97	75
Diseases of blood and blood-forming organs	8	24	17
Mental disorders	143	309	230
Diseases of nervous system and sense organs	244	273	260
Diseases of circulatory system	279	322	301
Diseases of respiratory system	583	550	544
Diseases of digestive system	128	141	135
Diseases of genito-urinary system	56	268	167
Complications of pregnancy, childbirth and puerperium	–	30	–
Diseases of skin	185	218	202
Diseases of musculo-skeletal system and connective tissue	245	331	290
Congenital anomalies	5	3	4
Certain causes of perinatal morbidity and mortality	0.6	0.3	0.5
Symptoms and ill-defined conditions	224	324	276
Accidents, poisoning and violence	194	171	182
Supplementary classification	205	713	471
All diseases and conditions	2,710	4,021	3,396

Data derived from 1981–82 Morbidity Statistics for General Practice.[6]

Table VIII. Consultation rate per 1000 population per year

1.4 The medical record

J.J.C. Cormack

The medical record is, or should be, the bridge which links the patient, within his environment of family, past medical history and social circumstances, and the doctor whom he consults. The consultation is the basic unit of all medical practice; it has been written of the patient at the time of his consultation with his doctor:

> '... At this moment behind him and around him, visibly or invisibly, stand his family and his habits, his genetic and personal past'.

It is this background of the patient's environment and his experiences which should be represented by the record.

The purpose of the record is to enable and promote the establishment and re-establishment of that relationship between patient and doctor which is central to the provision of all medical care. It can be used for administration and planning and for the prosecution of research, but all such uses should be subservient to the overriding aim of providing a basic tool for the day-to-day management of the patient and his problems.

Given this basic philosophy, the form of the record can conveniently be considered in two parts:

1. The summarized clinical information which any doctor (or nursing colleague) needs to know about the patient whenever he presents
2. The 'aide-memoire' record of succeeding consultations which has been neatly described as 'the note the doctor writes to himself for the next time he sees the patient'.

Necessarily these two aspects of the record overlap, but it is helpful to consider them, at least in the first instance, separately.

Summarized information

This can be further subdivided into three categories: 'essential', 'highly desirable' and 'desirable' data.

Essential clinical information.– Essential information can be defined as information which could be potentially life-saving when a patient is unconscious or otherwise unable himself to give an account of his history. In fact such items are surprisingly few. They comprise:

1. History of drug hypersensitivities
2. Current therapy – especially if this includes
   – anticoagulants
   – monoamine oxidase inhibitors
   – steroids
3. History of diabetes mellitus or other endocrine disorders such as Addison's disease or myxoedema
4. History of epilepsy
5. History of myocardial infarction or ischaemia
6. History of cerebrovascular accidents
7. Congenital neurological or cardiovascular disorders such as cerebral palsy or congenital heart disease.

Highly desirable information.– This comprises other information which would be included in a referral letter as a summary of important medical history:

1. Previous serious illnesses not included in the 'essential' category
2. Operations (other than very minor ones)
3. Blood group.

Desirable information.– This is information which may amplify the purely medical history and also provide clues to the patient's psychological and social background:

1. Occupation (in as detailed a form as practical)
2. Hobbies and recreations
3. Family structure and medical history.

It should be obvious that it is more important to know about the son killed in a road traffic accident or the sibling handicapped with severe neurological disease, than that the patient has had a sprained ankle or laryngitis.

All of these categories of information should be incorporated in a summary sheet or card which should be readily available and visible to the doctor on each occasion that the patient consults him (with the possible exception of 'current therapy' which may be listed on a separate drug sheet and/or be easily identifiable in the current continuation notes).

The aide-memoire record

The continual need to save time, energy and paper makes it

necessary, and in many ways desirable, that the clinical notes entered at each consultation should be relatively brief. As a minimum such notes should include:

1. Date of consultation
2. Problem or problems identified
3. Action taken.

Date.– The date of each consultation (and this should include instances where the patient is not actually seen, but action is taken, as, for instance, the issue of repeat prescriptions) is of obvious importance in establishing chronology and the sequence and duration of the 'extended consultation'.

Problems.– The problems identified at a particular consultation are not necessarily the problems overtly presented by the patient; they are rather the reasons elicited by the doctor in the course of that consultation for the presentation of these symptoms.
In perhaps the majority of cases such problems will be identical with 'diagnosis' in conventional terms, but in a substantial minority a more complex and less definitive formulation may more accurately reflect the true situation. The purist may demand more rigorous establishment of evidence to satisfy diagnostic criteria and both Weed,[1] and much earlier James Mackenzie himself, stressed the undesirability of applying diagnostic labels implying greater accuracy than the evidence warranted. In the pragmatic situation of the normal general practice consultation however, it is for the practitioner himself to decide how he can most usefully apply a diagnostic label which is, after all, simply a shorthand summary of his interpretation of the situation which provides the pointer for present therapy and future investigation and action. Thus an entry:

14.5.86 4/7 dysuria and frequency Micro: pus cells ++
R_X Trimethoprim 200 mg × 2 MSU 1/52 [UTI] 2/52

could quite sufficiently indicate to any practitioner subsequently seeing the patient that in this consultation the patient had presented with dysuria and frequency of four days' duration, pus cells had been detected on microscopy, it had been arranged that a midstream specimen of urine would be sent to the laboratory in one week's time and that two 200 mg tablets of trimethoprim had been supplied. The presumptive diagnosis (and it must be realized that all diagnoses are in a sense presumptive) was urinary-tract infection and a follow-up appointment had been made for two weeks ahead.

The subsequent entry might read:

28.5.86 VMI 0 symptoms *MSU: –ve* Adv on hygiene

[Urethral syndrome]

to indicate that the patient had very much improved with no symptoms now and that the midstream specimen of urine had failed to grow any organisms. Advice was given on hygiene and the 'diagnosis' now changed in the light of the further evidence from 'urinary-tract infection' to 'urethral syndrome'. This still lacks precision as debate continues on the definition and nature of the 'urethral syndrome', but the point is academic in so far as the label, 'urethral syndrome', is a sufficient indication of the practitioner's interpretation of the patient's symptoms in the light of the evidence he has.

A more complex situation might be represented by the entry:

14.5.86 4/7 dysuria and frequency Unprotected s.i. Wants pill 0 jaundice 0 F/H diabetes BP 110/70 MSU: Adv fluids R_x Microgynon 30 (1 pack) [OC] 2/52

Here the same symptoms were presented but the practitioner had detected that something more was behind the presentation. He had established that unprotected sexual intercourse had been taking place and that the girl wanted to go on the contraceptive pill and that this was the 'real' reason for the consultation. He had checked and recorded that there were no contraindications to prescribing the pill and had recorded a base-line blood-pressure reading. On this occasion a specimen of urine was not examined, but a midstream specimen of urine was arranged. He advised the patient to take fluids plentifully and prescribed one pack of pills, arranged follow-up for two weeks and recorded the label 'oral contraception'.

We might then see:

28.5.86 Came with anxious ma. – wants to know what's happening 0 symptoms *MSU: E.coli 10^6* Further MSU in 2/52 and review xpl 'germ in waterworks, need to investigate further' see pt alone n.t. Remind ma. re confidentiality [UTI] [Maternal anxiety]

The girl's symptoms have now settled, but her urine shows a significant bacteriuria. This is a problem, and the practitioner decides to temporize by arranging for another midstream specimen of urine in two weeks. An even greater problem arises with the appearance of the girl's mother obviously suspicious about what is happening. The doctor explains that there is a urinary infection and notes his request to see the girl alone next time while explaining to the mother the patient's right to confidentiality. The patient's problems are obviously not yet resolved, even less the doctor's. His formulation of the two problems however, as 'urinary-tract infection' and 'maternal anxiety' coupled with the 'oral contraception' label give sufficient warning to provide the basis for his further planning and action.

It will not have escaped notice that an important item of information in each of these cases would be the age of the patient. This, of course, can be derived from the date of birth which should form part of the basic registration data at the top of each continuation card or clinical note sheet, but it is often advantageous to work out and note the age of the patient (possibly entering it in a different coloured ink) in a space among the consultation date entries.

Action

The action taken at any given consultation may materially affect the conduct of the succeeding consultation in the same episode and may indicate the doctor's interpretation of the situation even more succinctly than the formal labelling of the problem, and therefore all such action should be recorded. Action may be any one of the following or combination of them:

1. Prescription for drugs (e.g. $FeSO_4$ bd (60))
2. Immediate therapy (e.g. Lignocaine and HCA injection)
3. Investigation (e.g. Ba. meal.)
4. Referral (e.g. Refer gynae.)
5. Advice (e.g. Adv stop smoking)
6. Explanation (e.g. Xpl need to follow up).

It is in this area of recording perhaps more than any other that there may conceivably be medico-legal implications. The National Health Service general practitioner's Terms of Service state that the practitioner

> 'is required to keep records of the illnesses of his patient and his treatment of them in such form as the Minister may from time to time determine after consultation with an organization which is in his opinion representative of the general body of medical practitioners'.

This is later amplified in the statement:

> 'The clinical record should contain all information that would normally be considered by general practitioners as necessary both to the doctor and to other practitioners who may subsequently be responsible for the care of the patient to enable proper and necessary treatment to be given . . . '.

The definition of 'all information that would normally be considered by general practitioners as necessary' has yet to be tested, but it is in those (happily rare) instances where disputes or difficulties arise that evidence of what the practitioner did (or did not) do or advise that is likely to be more important than his diagnoses or interpretation of the patients' problems.

Supporting data

Given the essential minimum of recording in day-to-day clinical notes of date, problems identified and action taken, how much or how little supporting data is it necessary or advisable to record? Possibly the simplest approach to this is to consider those items which the recording doctor feels it would be useful to note for the next doctor who is likely to see the patient. In the majority of instances the recording doctor himself will be maintaining continuity of care and will be the most likely to see the patient the next time. In such circumstances supporting data can be quite brief, and in general should include only positive symptoms or signs (such as nausea or morning stiffness or a cardiac murmur or suspicious abdominal mass) which can indicate fruitful lines of future enquiry or investigation. Negative symptoms or signs (e.g. good appetite, normal locomotion, pure heart sounds, no organomegaly) should probably be omitted, though it can be helpful to remind oneself that certain examinations have in fact been made: for instance ophthalmoscopy, palpation of breasts or rectal examination. It is, however, often useful for aide-memoire purposes to record items of a social nature such as an impending holiday or recently acquired hobby or the wedding of a close relative to provide a conversational 'opener' at the next consultation and strengthen the doctor-patient relationship by emphasizing one's interest in the patient as an individual and not a 'case'.

Fuller notes may be desirable when one is likely to be writing for a colleague: for instance when just about to go off on holiday. We all know our own routines – what questions we ask and what systems we examine in specified instances – but our colleagues do not always share this knowledge. It is, however, important to remember that an essay of twelve lines will be much less likely to be read and digested than a short statement of two or three.

What is of greater significance than the quantity of information recorded is its clarity. When recording basically for ourselves legibility may not be a problem: most of us can decipher most of what we write most of the time. Recording for the likely use of colleagues calls for a little greater effort in the interests both of courtesy and clinical care.

In theory, the typewritten record has much to commend it, but in practice it is not clear that a cost-benefit analysis would justify the expense in terms of the use of ancillary staff when dealing with the records of the majority of day-to-day patient contacts. It can even be argued that there are occasions when deliberate lack of clarity can be used to prompt the doctor's subsequent memory while at the same time preserving confidentiality. A much stronger case can be made for the typing of summaries.

The use of shorthand and abbreviations must be a decision for individual doctors or groups of doctors. Abbreviations can undoubtedly save time and nobody is going to write 'Blood Pressure' in full when 'BP' is understood by all. In a group practice the members of the group (one hopes) will see one another frequently and it will be easy to unravel an obscure abbreviation. The obscurity may not be so easily resolved when the records pass on to another practice, but this may not be of great moment provided really vital information is written in full – and ideally really vital information will all be contained in the summary.

Visual aids

The record is essentially a means of communication. Most of our communication in this setting is by the use of words, but the use of underlinings, diagrams and different colours can all greatly contribute to the clarity and usefulness of the record. Hodgkin[2] has emphasized the importance of 'boxing in' the diagnostic labels or problem definitions. Walford[3] has promoted the use of rubber stamps depicting body outlines to illustrate the localization of physical signs. Family structure and history can be illustrated in chart fashion[4] (see Figure I in Chapter 1.6). Different coloured inks can be used to highlight the recording of drug hypersensitivities, to underline laboratory results or to denote the patient's age. No one standard system is likely to be universally applicable to all practice circumstances, but any practitioner can devise or adapt his own methods to make the record more dynamic, more meaningful and more useful.

Accessibility of information

It can be beneficial to record certain items of information separately from the day-to-day continuation notes. Obviously, there is the summary, to which major importance has been attached throughout this chapter. If diagnoses or problem definitions are 'boxed in' they will be seen readily and will in due course, when appropriate, be transferred to the summary sheet or card. Drug therapy (especially long-term therapy) can be entered on a separate sheet or card, and this can form a model for a variety of flow sheets which can be devised: for instance for hypertensive patients, women on the oral contraceptive pill, asthmatics, post-gastrectomy patients, chronic bronchitics. The principle is already widely accepted in the use of special maternity record cards, and paediatric developmental assessment schedules and geriatric follow-up schemes are being devised. Immunization records are usually separate from the main body of the notes and provision can helpfully be made for the recording in sequence of common 'screening' parameters such as blood pressure, routine chest x-rays, cervical cytology, urinalysis and height and weight.

It is a matter for debate whether attached nurses or health visitors should record within the continuation notes of the medical records or on separate sheets. Logic would seem to be on the side of the former, but nursing administration may dictate the latter. The debate can only be resolved by discussion and it matters little if there is no national consensus provided agreement is reached at local or practice level.

Laboratory and x-ray and electrocardiographic reports present a further problem. Should they be filed in order among the hospital letters, or separated out into constituent categories: e.g. bacteriology, haematology, biochemistry, or mounted all together sequentially on a pathology report sheet? Once again there is no standard answer, but one recommendation can be made and that is that results should be entered in the body of the continuation notes (perhaps summarized and cross-referenced for fuller details) and really significant results should be reflected in an entry on the summary.

Hospital letters provide a great deal of the bulk of the record of any patient with a history of any complexity; the information contained in such letters is often of great value and relevance and almost invariably easily read, because typed. For maximum accessibility they should be filed flat, and this is one of the most cogent arguments for the introduction of A4 folders as opposed to medical record envelopes which were never designed as holders of substantial amounts of correspondence. If medical record envelopes are used considerable discipline is required by filing staff to see that letters are kept together (treasury tags are useful) and in chronological order. In either system therapy needs to be consistently applied to minimize the 'fat file' syndrome. As a profession we suffer from a squirrel instinct in regard to documents about our patients. So far as general practice is concerned this instinct may possibly be due to an unrealistic fear of the medico-legal consequences of destroying reports: unrealistic in view of the fact that almost all letters received will also be held in copy form at the source – and while microfilming may be practical (and necessary) in hospitals, it is unlikely to be so in general practice.

There is a phenomenon of information overload which may lead to a situation where the more data there is, the more daunting it is to analyse and the less likely it is to be used. Discharge notes can be discarded when they are superseded by the definitive discharge letters. Outpatient follow-up letters can succeed one another at three- or six-monthly intervals or even more often; in many cases the first letter and the most recent are all that need to be kept. Some surgeons send full operation notes in addition to a summarized discharge letter; after the period of possible immediate postoperative complications has passed, such operation notes are of doubtful value to the general practitioner. A normal chest x-ray report from five years ago does not need to be kept when there is another normal one this year. The information in a brief letter of a few lines with some important data may be transferred to the summary sheet or continuation record and the original note destroyed, to help to minimize the bulk of the file. The flow of input about our patients is not likely to diminish and the habit of 'pruning' records is one which the increasing bulk of our records will force us all to adopt.

Research uses

Medical records can provide valuable tools for the purposes of research – both clinical and operational, but rarely without the use of ancillary tools. In recent years a number of such tools have been designed. They include age-sex registers, the 'W' book, the 'E' book, the 'F' book, family registers on punch cards and computerized diagnostic indexes.[5] The Royal College of General Practitioners has involved 1,400 practitioners in a remarkable piece of collaborative research in the form of the Oral Contraceptive Study, but here, too, subsidiary documents are used. Any or all of these aids to recording and research can be employed by the interested practitioner, and from their use numerous important studies have evolved which have materially promoted the resurgence of general practice in this country in the past decades. Here we need do no more than note this potential for research; it has wide implications for epidemiology and patient care, but is not strictly relevant to our present concern which is clinical care: the care of the individual patient.

The contribution of computers to medical records

The introduction of microcomputers at reasonable prices has opened up new opportunities for general practitioners to store and retrieve information about their patients. At the same time, because many doctors who are currently in practice are unfamiliar with modern computer technology they create anxieties about such things as confidentiality, or at a more mundane level the ability of the general practitioner to adapt to these innovations.

Fully computerized medical records are feasible and have been developed in some experimental situations. In 10–20 years they may well become a normal way of keeping records. At the present time however, the microcomputer may be viewed simply as a more efficient way of keeping and developing a practice register.

Many practices currently maintain an age/sex register on index cards. When a new patient joins the practice a new card is produced and when a patient leaves, the card is removed. The card will usually record the patient's name, address, date of birth and in some cases occupation. Some general practitioners mark the cards of patients suffering with particular diseases, by using a coloured marker. In this way these patients may be reviewed at regular intervals or offered particular preventive procedures; chronic bronchitics for example, may be identified and offered influenza immunization each autumn.

The microcomputer can provide a similar system of registering each patient. When a patient registers, his name, address and date of birth can be typed into the computer. As extra information about the patient is collected, this can be added to that patient's record in the computer. There are many ways of collecting this information. On registering with the practice, patients may be asked to complete a questionnaire providing information about past medical history, allergies, etc. The fact that the patient is suffering from chronic and ongoing problems such as chronic bronchitis, diabetes, or schizophrenia, may thus be indentified. Another source of information is the incoming records of patients from the Family Practitioner Committee. These can be summarized and important information added to the computer. Finally, when services are provided, particularly in the preventive field, such as cervical cytology, immunization or a record of blood pressure, these can also be added to the register.

Ensuring that items of information which are important in the continuing care of patients are accumulated on the computer record demands good clerical support and disciplined methods of recording by the general practitioners and other members of the primary care team.

Once the information is recorded on the computer, it is then possible to take advantage of the technology to manipulate this information.

A typical patient file on a computer is illustrated diagramatically below.

Name	*Forename*	*D of B*	*Chronic problems*	
Smith	Mary	6.11.44	091/2	218/0

Last cervical smear	*Last B.P.*	*Immunization*		
		D	*Tet*	*Polio*
2.1.84	110/70	7.10.45	5.11.75	5.11.75

The computer may be asked to carry out a variety of tasks. It may for instance be asked to print out a list of the names of all female patients between the ages of 35–64 years who have not had a cervical smear carried out in the preceding 5 years. The doctor is then in a position to follow up these patients and offer the service.
The computer may be asked to list all those patients suffering from chronic bronchitis so that they may be offered vaccination against influenza.
The computer may be asked to list all the patients suffering from hypertension so that these patients' records can be reviewed in order to estimate the adequacy of the treatment which the practice is providing.
The use of the computer is not limited to improving the clinical care of patients. It can also improve the income of the practice by ensuring the doctor receives the maximum possible income from the items of service he provides. This helps to offset additional clerical help which must be employed to ensure that relevant information is stored on the computer record.
If computers are seen as no more than a rather sophisticated way of holding practice registers, they should hold no fears for the general practitioner. What they offer is the ability to manipulate information to provide, for example, good preventive care. Their effectiveness depends on adequate clerical support to provide them with the information and a disciplined way of recording this information by the members of the primary care team.

Medical record envelopes or A4 folders

The profession and the Health Departments have now accepted that in future A4 folders should be the normal method of record-keeping in general practice in the National Health Service. For economic reasons there is delay in effecting the change and medical record envelopes, first introduced in 1920, continue to be used in the majority of practices. There can be no reasonable doubt that systematic recording is much more easily accomplished and encouraged when using folders, but this is not to deny the possibility of achieving the same ends, albeit with more difficulty, within the system currently available. The general principles of summarizing and structuring the record remain the same and if they are conscientiously applied in the use of medical record envelopes the eventual task of converting to folders will be less intimidating.

Problem-oriented records

The work of Laurence Weed and his concept of Problem-Oriented Medical Records have created considerable interest on both sides of the Atlantic and there is no doubt that his system of recording has the virtues of clarity, logic and thoroughness. For all but the obsessional enthusiast, however, the prospect of attempting to operate the system in its entirety can be dispiriting. But it is from obsessional enthusiasts that we learn, and habits of systematic recording can be developed to suit individual circumstances. The summary of medical and family and social history suggested in this chapter, along with 'boxed-in' identifications of diagnoses or problems, parallel the 'data base' and 'problem list' of the Weed system. It is on questions of the amount of detail recorded, and examination of the use to which such detail is put, that the debate must be joined between those in general practice who are convinced that the problem-oriented system is ideal, and their opponents. Fuller detail in records than that suggested here may be desirable, or even essential when records are used for the purposes of education or audit. Records may indeed be usefully employed for both such purposes, but here we are concerned simply with practical patient care.

Conclusion

The principles enunciated in this chapter are quite simple: that the important data in a medical record should be available in summary fashion (important information being defined as that which is likely to be of use in the future management of the patient's problems); that selected items (such as long-term drug therapy, blood-pressure readings or data on chronic on-going conditions) should be sequentially recorded and easily identifiable and accessible; that routine day-to-day recording of consultations should be succinct and so structured that problems identified and action taken should always be clearly visible; that records should regularly be 'pruned'. The means by which such aims can be achieved are many and various, and it is neither necessary nor practical to attempt to design one detailed system which can be translated to all practice situations. Simplicity and accessibility should be the keynotes, and the basic purpose of the record as the tangible link between patient and doctor should always inform its structure and use. It is vital to avoid the situation where we may look more at the record than at the patient. We make the record to serve us and thus our patient. It must always be a link and never a distraction.

References

[1] Weed, L.L. (1969): *Medical Records, Medical Education and Patient Care*, Chicago: The Press of Case Western Reserve University

[2] Hodgkin, K. (1973): *Towards Earlier Diagnosis*. 3rd ed. Edinburgh: Churchill Livingstone

[3] Walford, P.A. (1962): The Art of Record Keeping in General Practice. *Journal of the Royal College of General Practitioners*, 6, 225

[4] Cormack, J.J.C. (1975): Family Portraits. *Journal of the Royal College of General Practitioners*, *25*, *520*

[5] *Eimerl, T.S. and Laidlaw, A.J. (1969): A Handbook for Research in General Practice*. 2nd ed. Edinburgh: Churchill Livingstone

1.5
Performance review

Marshall Marinker and David Morrell

Traditionally general practice has been concerned particularly with responding to the requests for care presented by the defined population of patients for whom the doctor has accepted responsibility. Over the past two decades there has been increasing recognition of the general practitioner's role in providing continuing care for chronic disease and in the prevention of diseases and disability.

The amount of time the doctor and the primary care team can devote to providing for the needs and demands of the community is necessarily finite. It is therefore essential to determine priorities in the use of this time. In so doing it is important to be able to state the objectives of care in terms of the outcome the doctor wishes to achieve. He must develop ways of evaluating his work in terms of costs (the use of necessarily limited resources) and benefits (the relief of illness and disability). Some of the ways of grappling with this very difficult equation are described in this chapter.

The development of any new discipline is bedevilled by the introduction of a new vocabulary designed to describe the innovations, and the discipline of performance review is no exception. This is always confusing and may be a major disincentive to those, who though actually aware of the need to prove that what they are doing is worthwhile, find it difficult to comprehend the new 'jargon'. In an attempt to overcome this problem we have tried to define some of the terms currently used by those involved in performance review.

Performance review: This is the generic term given to the whole process of determining specifically what it is that the practice or individual health care worker is attempting to achieve, how relative success and failure are measured, and what reforms of practice result from the exercise.

Medical audit: A synonym for performance review.

Standard: This is a statement about levels of performance (for example of diagnosis, or management, or some other aspect of health care like record keeping or continuity of care).

Base-line standards reflect the performance of the individual or the practice, before any organized attempt is made to move that performance in a desired direction. They may be described in terms of the mean and distribution of that current performance. In this sense, in a particular practice, the standard of care for diabetic patients may include the statement that 40 per cent of known insulin-dependent diabetics receive an annual estimation of glycosylated haemoglobin. This simply describes what is going on. In no way should it be seen as reflecting desirable performance.

For decades general practitioners in the National Health Service have been given data about the level of their own prescribing. These have been compared with the prescribing levels of their partners and of doctors in their area. If we just take the issue of cost, these data cannot suggest that low cost is in any sense 'better' than high cost or that there is some virtue in the local mean. These data are, in the real sense of the word, valueless.

So-called *normative standards* have nothing to do with arithmetic norms but rather refer to ideal situations. The standards that a practice adopts, however, may differ from such ideal statements, taking into account the practical limitations of resources, public expectations and so on.

Minimal standards are statements of performance, below which the quality is evidently unacceptable.

We will use the term *realistic standard* to describe a standard which has been agreed upon by the group, which takes into account the realistic limitations of time, personnel and other resources, but which is pitched considerably above minimal standards, in order to improve and augment the quality of care.

Criteria and targets: These terms are sometimes used to describe the components of an agreed *realistic standard*: for example a practice immunization rate for children of 90 per cent, or a mean diastolic reading of less than 100mm of Hg in the control of hypertension.

Indicator or markers: The standards, from among many in a particular practice, which are sampled in order to indicate the general level of performance. Here the notion is that excellence in one particular example is likely to suggest all-round excellence.

Priority: This simply reflects the rank order given to a particular standard, by the individual doctor or the group. It is a reflection of the importance accorded to the subject by those who determine the sequence in which new standards are to be sought and implemented.

Policy: This refers to the agreement which may be reached by a group about its priorities, the specific components of its standards, the method of monitoring and of introducing reform. More than anything else, the practice policy will reflect the values of the group.

Structure: This comprises those components of health care which form part of the resources. Examples would include the building, the equipment, the doctor/patient ratios, number and type of staff.

Process: This refers to the actions taken by health care workers. It would include measurements of numbers of consultations and home visits, record keeping, items of physical examination carried out, or drugs prescribed.

Outcome: This is the most important, often missing, element in measuring the success or failure of health care. Suicide and para-suicide rates might be used as an indicator of the success or failure of diagnosing and treating depression. School absence might be a useful outcome measure in assessing the diagnosis and management of childhood asthma. Because outcomes are so difficult and time consuming to measure, those conditions where the outcome has been reliably established (like the treatment of moderate to severe hypertension, or the achievement of high immunization rates) tend to be given a high priority.

Avedis Donabedian, one of the most influential scholars in the evaluation of quality in health care, first drew attention to the need to define and differentiate between structure, process and outcome.

Internal audit: A performance review voluntarily devised and carried out by those actually involved in providing the service to be audited.

External audit: An audit carried out by others.

Implicit audit: A reflective review (a prime example might be case discussions) in which judgments are based on shared beliefs, rather than on agreed, stated and validated criteria.

Explicit audit: Agreed, stated and validated criteria are used.

Developing management policies

Until the last decade or so, the comparative benefits of different patterns of management had seldom been tested in general practice. It is rarely satisfactory to translate the result of trials of treatment carried out in hospital to problems presenting in primary care and many of the management decisions concerned with prevention and early diagnosis are unique to the primary care setting.

A great deal has been written about the importance of auditing the care provided by general practitioners. This is clearly impossible until reliable research data have been collected which clarify the costs and benefits of the alternative forms of care available in general practice. This is now however rapidly becoming a practical proposition. The time has therefore come for general practitioners, individually or in groups, to draw upon the research findings from general practice and to develop practice policies which set out the criteria for optimum management of the common problems they encounter.

An approach to setting practice policies

In the hectic day-to-day work of general practice, it is very easy for a doctor to develop an habitual way of responding to the symptoms or diseases presented by his patients without looking critically at this response. Faced with a great deal of incurable illness he is also in danger of uncritically trying out the latest available drug which, it is claimed, will offer his patients some benefit over its predecessors. In planning his work, the doctor can easily develop a routine.

Despite all that has been written about the importance of planning and management in practice, the idea persists that good clinical care is only taking place during face-to-face consultations. It is now becoming increasingly evident that without time set aside for thinking through priorities and policies, the clinical encounters between doctor and patient in the practice remain haphazard, and the quality of that encounter in terms of health benefits to the patient, uncertain and unmeasured.

Doctors who wish to look critically at their care and establish management policies, must set aside a period of time at regular intervals. In group practice this should be relatively easy. For single-handed doctors it will mean developing a study group with their colleagues. At the meetings of the group, the doctors must establish the problems they wish to study. It is usually helpful to begin with common problems such as the management of otitis media or a policy for case finding of hypertensives.

Determining priorities

The very fact that there is such a wide variety of important new tasks to accomplish in general practice, can have a paradoxically stultifying effect. Whatever is proposed at a practice meeting, for example that the practice shall monitor the prescribing of hypnotics, or organize systematic paediatric surveillance, or run a well-woman clinic, there will always be countervailing arguments that other conditions or aspects of service should be given priority.

Agreements about priority simply determine the sequence in which innovations are introduced to the practice. There can be no absolute rules, nor absolute values given to any particular priority. The following approach was developed by Dr Marshall Marinker and Dr

David Pendleton for the 1984 MSD Foundation Leadership Courses:

> We suggest the following four questions, and list a number of issues raised by each of them.
>
> I Should the schedule be constructed for the individual doctor or for the practice?
> (1) Group practice or group of individual doctors?
> (2) Individual learning and/or small group learning?
> (3) What is the base population: the list of registered patients or the number of patients who actually consult?
>
> II How do we choose priorities and the sequence of their introduction?
> (1) Frequency of occurrence of the condition.
> (2) Potential danger of the condition or situation.
> (3) Controversial matters and topical issues (public relations).
> (4) Achievable tasks.
> (5) Exemplars from major areas of concern (e.g. chronic disease; acute infection; immunization; prescribing; monitoring of at risk group).
> (6) How crucial is the standard to the outcome of care?
>
> III How frequently should the performance be reviewed?
> (1) How likely is the standard to change (changes in medical knowledge; in society; in practice organization)?
> (2) How rapidly is the performance likely to deteriorate after each service?
> (3) What work load will be imposed on the practice by the review?
>
> IV How many items of performance should be reviewed?
> (1) The likelihood that standards will be contagious.
> (2) The desirable level of confidence for each standard.
> (3) The willingness to tolerate uncertainty.
> (4) Workload.

Standards may be set in relation to the results of empirical research, or they may be based on logic and the best guesses which we can make. They may be motivated by politics, philosophy, consumer demand or analysis of needs. They may require change in the consultation, in the organization of the practice or in the community.

Some such framework as the one which we suggest here will be necessary in order to make choices which are relevant to the needs of the practice population, and tolerable to those who work within the practice.

Why develop policies?

It may be argued that because medicine is as much an art as a science, and because it is concerned with a very personal response by one doctor to the unique condition of his patient, the very notion of priorities, policies and standards seems distasteful. There is an anxiety that the creation of policies may interfere with the doctor's freedom of choice, or with the special, personal, and unpredictable priorities which may suddenly arise in the course of a unique consultation, and in the setting of a unique doctor/patient relationship. Although these arguments have some merit they are grounded in an earlier era of medical practice, are more consonant with the ethic of paternalism than with the ethic of patient autonomy, and they ignore the growing critique of unbridled medical technology, and the rise of consumerism in health care.

The practice may decide to create a policy for many different reasons. For example:

(1) In order to ensure a common language: examples might include a definition of terms like asthma, peptic ulcer, eczema, osteoarthritis. These terms are used at a number of levels: speculative, presumptive, supported by established agreed criteria. Without a common language it becomes impossible either to create or monitor standards.
(2) In order to improve the treatment of conditions: examples would include determining the optimum medication, and agreeing on measures of outcome.
(3) In order to enhance so-called tertiary prevention: examples would include the monitoring of patients with known asthma or diabetes.
(4) In order to increase the margin of safety of what we do: examples of this might include the monitoring of dangerous drugs like cardiac glycocides, or hypnotics or anti-depressants.
(5) In order to develop new services: examples might include a well-woman clinic, a paediatric surveillance programme and so on.

Making and monitoring clinical standards

It is peculiarly difficult to construct a clinical standard in isolation. The use of a small group allows a variety of opinions to be voiced, and if the group is properly conducted, allows a rational discourse about evidence, opinion and predilection. Once a particular issue has been identified as a practice priority, one member of the group should be asked to review the relevant literature and to report his findings and recommendations. Reviewing the literature need not be too arduous. The librarian at the Royal College of General Practitioners has lists of references for many common problems. A good review article such as a leader in the *Journal of the Royal College of General Practitioners* or the *British Medical Journal* will usually append a series of references. Most of the important articles will have appeared in the commonly available journals at postgraduate centres or medical school libraries.

These articles must be read critically. It is important to establish that the study population is comparable with the practice population. In looking at trials of treatment it is important to clarify how the illness was defined, what criteria were used to establish a diagnosis and what tests were used to measure the outcome of the trial. It is also important to know whether there were built-in methods of ensuring compliance with treatment and ensuring accurate and complete data recording. In studying more broad-based management problems concerned with case finding or prevention, it is important to establish the resources available, how these were deployed and the way outcome was measured. There is little point in finding cases of a particular disease unless treatments or resources are available to influence the prognosis.

As a result of this enquiry, an individual member of the practice should be in a position to return to his group and recommend the 'best buy' in management. The practice may eventually be able to agree a policy and by studying a variety of problems establish a file setting out the practice policy for the management of the common or uncommon but important problems.

We suggest that a clinical standard should contain the following elements:

1. Specific criteria for diagnosis.
2. Reasons for choosing management.
3. Explicit statement of the aims of management.
4. Criteria for success and failure (the latter may be more important, and easier to define).
5. Tools for monitoring performance.

So far we have talked only about individual clinical problems. But general practice is concerned not only with an individual perspective but with the possibility of looking at a population. Here, interestingly enough, it becomes much more easy to identify agreed areas for concern.

There can be almost no argument about the need to ensure compliance with immunization schedules. Although there may be detailed countervailing arguments, we might all agree about the importance of finding and controlling moderate to severe hypertension. There is renewed evidence about the utility of cervical cytology (particularly in those women who currently are rarely screened) and so on. Most of the current rhetoric about clinical standards, performance review, audit or what you will, concentrates on this population aspect of general practice care.

A clinical standard in relation to populations may be (similarly) composed of the following elements:

1. Targets for performance (concerned with numbers of persons, time within which to accomplish the aims, biological targets, and so on).
2. Reasons for choosing these targets.
3. Criteria for success and failure.
4. Tools for monitoring performance.

Adherence to practice policy

The establishment of criteria for the management of common problems is just the first step in improving the quality of care provided. The next step is to ensure that the doctors concerned adhere to the agreed policy. In studying the management of specific diseases the easiest way to achieve this is to ask the doctors at regular intervals to complete (for perhaps one week) a simple encounter form during each surgery session. The form can be developed in practices using an appointment system from the list of patients booked for each surgery. The doctor is asked to record a diagnosis against each name on the list. One member of the group collects the lists and notes the names of patients who have presented with one of the diseases for which a practice policy has been agreed. He then withdraws the records of these patients and analyses the treatment prescribed. The results may then be presented at a subsequent meeting of the group. If there has been poor compliance with the agreed practice policy, this can be explored and if necessary the policy amended.

In studying compliance with practice policy concerned with the process of care rather than the treatment of specific diseases, a different approach is necessary. The practice may for instance have agreed that all asthmatic patients (the criteria will need to be explicit) should have an estimate made of peak flow at each consultation. In the case of children, such an estimate might be requested no less than twice a year. To check compliance with this policy the receptionist is asked to retain all the records of patients in the relevant age group over a period of a number of days (of the receptionist's own choosing). These records are then passed to one of the doctors who examines them for compliance. If a large number of records are incomplete, the doctor must try to determine why this is so and either try to improve the performance of the practice, amend the practice policy or seek some alternative way of attaining the agreed objectives.

This chapter has described in general terms an approach to establishing priorities, policies and standards. A detailed example is included as an appendix to chapter 3.51. The introduction of new material dealing with standards is one way in which the editors will take advantage of the loose-leaf format of *Practice.* Clearly this presents a unique opportunity for dialogue between editors, authors and readers. We therefore invite our readers, when shaping their practice policies to subject them to the kind of critical review which we have outlined in this chapter, test their ideas in the experimental setting of their own practices and let us know their conclusions. In this way we hope that *Practice* will not only become a resource for teaching and caring for patients but an instrument for the reform and development of general practice.

1.6
Anticipatory care

J. J. C. Cormack

This book is in the main concerned with the ways in which general practitioners use the patient's description of his symptoms as a starting point in the pathway which should lead to the construction of a hypothesis in which the patient's problems are identified and solutions proposed. The bulk of our work as general practitioners falls into this pattern: taking our first cues from the reported subjective sensations of our patients (their symptoms), and then adding to them our own assessment of what we perceive with the use of our senses, often extended by the use of instruments, and sometimes supplemented with the results of technical investigations. This process becomes so natural and routine to us that we rarely analyse its components; it is the standard framework within which we attempt occasional cure, frequent relief, and comfort as invariably as human frailty will permit.

However, our responsibility for patient care extends beyond this standard framework of response to presented symptoms to include also an informed approach to prevention of disease, when that is possible (e.g. by immunization), and anticipation, where that is rational (e.g. by the detection of raised blood pressure).

Screening or Case-finding?

The whole subject of screening in general practice has been reviewed very thoroughly.[1] Much information has been gathered from public health screening programmes in the 1960's, especially those in Salford, Bedford and Rotherham. The value of the 'one-off' check-up, however, is to say the least, debatable and is attacked by Ivan Illich as the 'medicalization of prevention'. He propounds the extreme argument that

> 'Even if people survive a positive laboratory diagnosis unharmed, they have incurred a very high risk of being submitted to therapy that is odious, painful, crippling and expensive.'

We do not need to subscribe fully to these sentiments to see an alternative and more rational way of providing what Tudor Hart describes as 'anticipatory care' within the framework of National Health Service general practice. Indeed, Hodgkin and Fry[2] claim that good British general practitioners already carry out an

effective screening function by their attention to continuity of care, combined with high rates of contact with their populations (65 to 75 per cent in one year, or 90 to 95 per cent over five years). This screening function is more properly described as 'case-finding'.
For the parameters of effective anticipatory care we must depend on the epidemiologists, and much still needs to be done to clarify the natural history of many if not indeed the majority of disease processes. It is only on good epidemiological data that we can base intelligent anticipation.
Planning for any form of presymptomatic screening requires to be based on the criteria clearly set out by Wilson[3]:

1. The condition sought should be an important problem.
2. There should be an accepted treatment for patients with recognized disease.
3. Facilities for diagnosis and treatment should be available.
4. There should be a recognized latent or early symptomatic stage.
5. There should be a suitable test or examination.
6. The test or examination should be acceptable to the population.
7. The natural history of the condition, including its development from latent to declared disease, should be adequately understood.
8. There should be an agreed policy on whom to treat as patients.
9. The cost of case-finding (including diagnosis and subsequent treatment of patients) should be economically balanced in relation to the possible expenditure on medical care as a whole.
10. Case-finding should be a continuing process and not a 'once for all' project.

The primary tools needed for anticipatory care include epidemiological information, an age/sex register and a recording system which will encourage the recording of data essential for such care (although often irrelevant to current symptoms) in easily identifiable form.
For the population as a whole the routine recording of certain data would be encouraged by the provision of a special recording sheet such as is suggested by the Joint Working Party on the Redesign of Medical Records. This could then be readily checked at each consultation to see that the selected parameters (appropriate to the patient's age, sex and/or special 'at risk' group) had been recorded (and were normal) within, say, the past five years. Lack of such data recorded within the arbitrarily decided time span should alert the doctor to arrange or carry out the appropriate examination at that consultation.
The criteria for routine estimation of the blood pressure, urine for

	Condition screened for	High risk
Blood pressure	Hypertension	See chapter 3.76
Glycosuria	Diabetes mellitus	"
Haemoglobin	Anaemia	"
Immunization status	Unprotected	Pre-school children, agricultural and other workers at special risk for tetanus
Rubella antibodies	Immunity to rubella	Women in child-bearing years; preferably pre-conception
Chest X-ray	Pulmonary tuberculosis Lung cancer	Elderly; immigrants; alcoholics; socially deprived Heavy smokers
Breast examination	Breast lumps, especially cancer	All women aged 25 to 60, especially nulliparous
Cervical cytology	Pre-invasive carcinoma	All women aged 25 to 60, especially multiparous, social class IV and V and those with early sexual experience
Weight for height	Obesity	Clinical impression of overweight
Smoking habits	Bronchitis Lung cancer Cardiovascular disease	All smokers

Table I. — Anticipatory care data

sugar and blood for haemoglobin are described in Chapter 3.80. Some other data which could usefully be elicited and recorded in this way are suggested in Table I.

Special groups

There are two groups of women who receive routine anticipatory care in the absence of known disease: pregnant patients and women on the oral contraceptive pill. The recording of such care has, at least for pregnant patients, been agreed either locally or nationally, and various forms are currently being devised for family planning. Developmental screening for pre-school children is being developed in general practice, where the broad aims are to monitor:

1. Neurological development
2. Visual defects
3. Squint
4. Hearing defects
5. Social adaptation
6. Maldescent of testicles
7. Congenital displacement of hips
8. Congenital heart disease.

At the other end of the age scale a number of practices have mounted geriatric screening programmes (especially in relation to any of their elderly population who have not had contact with the practice over the preceding year or eighteen months). Such programmes aim to assess:

1. Visual defect
2. Hearing defect
3. Locomotion (including care of the feet)
4. General health: e.g. early heart failure
anaemia
tuberculosis
5. Mental status: e.g. depression
dementia
6. Nutritional status
7. Social support.

A diagrammatic representation of a possible approach to anticipatory care on a purely age/sex basis is shown in Table II.

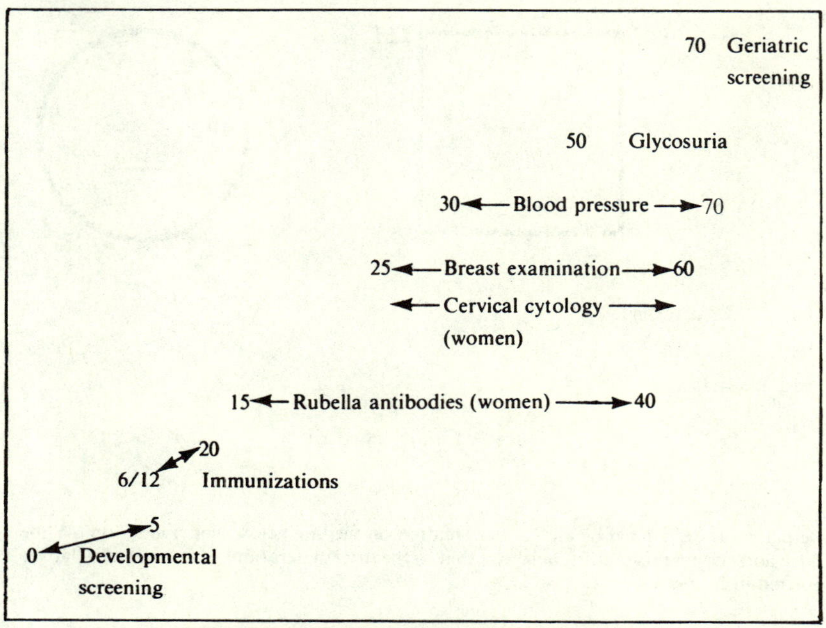

Table II. — Anticipatory care in age-groups

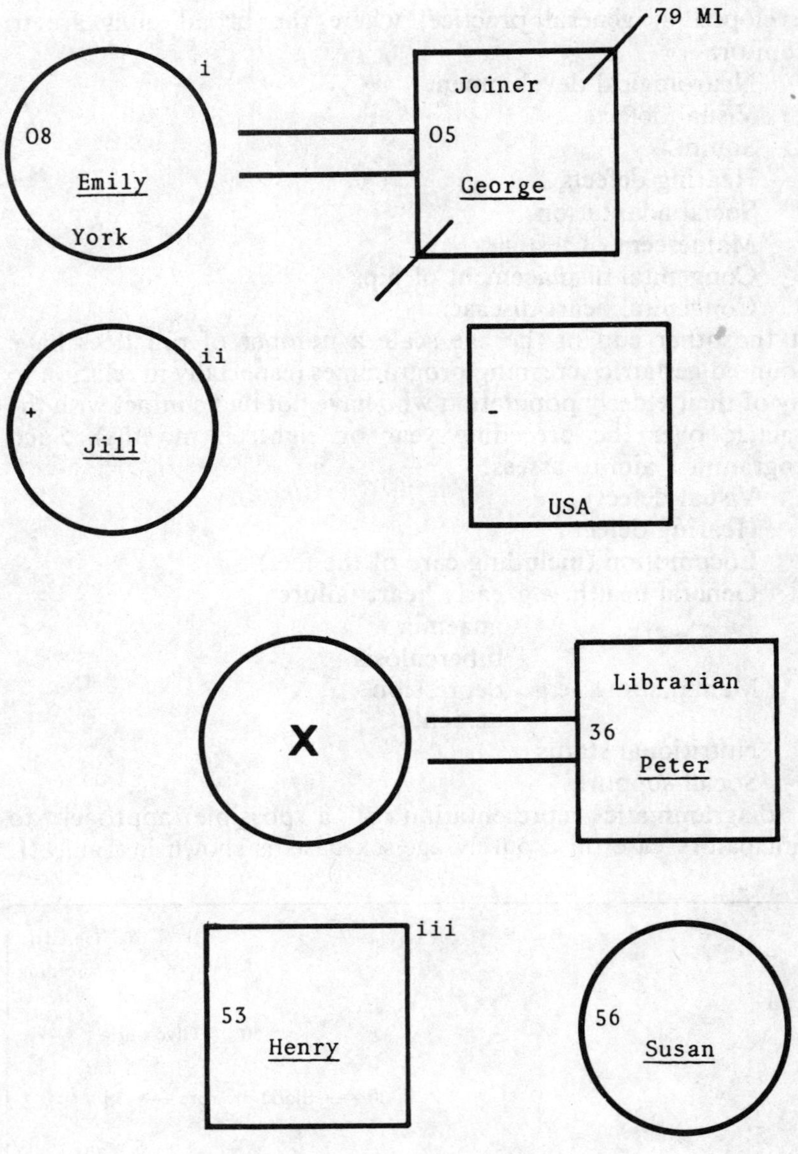

i) Glaucoma

ii) Diabetic

iii) Asthma

Figure 1. Family portrait[4]

Note
The patient is designated by an 'X', her children on the line below, her siblings on the line above and her parents on the line above that — the three generations of first degree relatives depicted in four lines.

There are a few special groups (in addition to those already mentioned) to whom extra attention should be paid in relation to anticipatory care. These include those with a family history of ischaemic heart disease, severe depressive illness, intestinal cancer and glaucoma. Indeed it can be argued that in all patients the adequate recording of the structure and the significant medical history of the patient's immediate family (i.e. first degree relatives)[4] should be an integral and basic part of anticipatory care, as it certainly is of effective family doctoring. An example of this sort of recording is shown in figure 1.

True preventive medicine involves intelligent anticipation based on scientifically established epidemiological data. It is at once the privilege and responsibility of the general practitioner in a National Health Service in which he serves a defined and identifiable population to mobilize the resources at his disposal to maintain, as well as to restore, his patient's health. The 'one-off' health check is not a satisfactory solution. By using our frequent contact with patients, allied with knowledge of normal development and disease processes, plus adequate records and an informed awareness of epidemiology, we aim at real continuity of care.

References

1 Hart, C.R. (1975): *Screening in General Practice*. Edinburgh: Churchill Livingstone

2 Hodgkin, K. and Fry, J. (1966): In *Surveillance and Early Diagnosis in General Practice* Ed. G.G. Teeling-Smith. London: Office of Health Economics

3 Wilson, J.M.G. (1966): Some principles of early diagnosis and detection. In *Surveillance and Early Diagnosis in General Practice* Ed. G.G. Teeling-Smith. London: Office of Health Economics

4 Cormack, J.J.C. (1975): Family Portraits — a method of recording family history. *Journal of the Royal College of General Practitioners*, *25*, 520

1.7 The doctor's bag

Graham Buckley

The general practitioner with his black bag has been an enduring image of the family doctor in this country. The external appearance of the bag may have changed little, with many doctors still using the Gladstone type bag. The contents however have changed dramatically over the years. This is particularly true of the drugs carried by the doctor, and continuing developments in the treatment of common medical emergencies demand regular review of the contents of the bag.

The drugs and equipment carried in the bag cannot be considered separately from the rest of the practice organization. This chapter will therefore not confine itself only to the clinical equipment that is capable of being carried in the doctor's bag. Equipment based in the practice premises and only occasionally taken into patients' homes will also be discussed. The essential requirement is ready access to appropriate diagnostic equipment and to effective therapy. A wide range of factors will influence whether equipment should be kept in the main surgery premises or carried by the doctor in his car, or in the bag.

The location of the practice determines, to a major extent, what equipment is to be carried by the doctor. Family doctors practising in the Scottish Highlands and Islands are equipped with suitable back-packs to enable them to carry heavy resuscitation equipment over rough terrain and in and out of small boats. In some rural areas, general practitioners routinely provide first-aid care at road traffic accidents. The organization and the equipment necessary for such work have been well described[1,2] and will be only briefly discussed in this chapter. Arrangements such as these would obviously be superfluous in an inner-city practice. The distance to the nearest hospital and the speed of response of the local ambulance service are of major importance when considering whether such things as portable oxygen and infusion fluids should be carried in the doctor's car.

Apart from the location of the practice, the size of the area served will also influence the content of the doctor's bag. Doctors with patients living a considerable distance from the surgery will be inclined to carry more equipment and drugs than their colleagues working in more compact practice areas. Each doctor must therefore plan the contents of his own bag and the clinical equipment to which he requires access, bearing in mind the conditions that he may encounter and be expected to deal with unaided.

Type of bag

Basically there are three different types of bag used by doctors; the Gladstone style, the square case with internal drawers, and the rigid fibreglass document case.

The Gladstone bag with its lack of internal divisions and compartments is an excellent holdall for bulky equipment such as sphygmomanometer, dressings, and resuscitation equipment. This makes it a useful container for emergency equipment and in such emergencies the whole of the contents can be rapidly emptied on to the bed or the floor. For more routine work its lack of compartments causes frustration with valuable time being wasted in trying to locate a particular item of equipment.

The second type of bag is the small square case fitted with various sizes of drawers, in addition to having an open section for the larger pieces of equipment. This case provides numerous compartments in a very practical way. It is easy to carry and fits well into the smallest of cars. Bottles, ampoules, dressings, and other items of equipment can all be carried safely and are readily accessible if the drawers are suitably labelled. It remains a popular case with doctors in dispensing practice because of the convenient way in which packets of drugs can be carried.

The third type of bag is the fibreglass case fitted with compartments for stationery, and lined in foam rubber which can be cut to provide compartments for any item of equipment or for small medicine containers. This flexible arrangement of the compartments means that similar cases, suitably adapted internally, can serve as the emergency, obstetric or routine bags. The contents are easily visible and rapidly located and the cases have the additional advantage of being light and very robust.

Even with the lighter cases and with the availability of smaller diagnostic instruments, the choice of contents of the doctor's bag is necessarily a compromise between the desire to cater for every possible emergency, and the need to keep the bags down to a convenient size.

The functions carried out by the doctor may be categorized under diagnostic, therapeutic, and administrative headings and it is convenient to consider the contents of his bag this way too. It is also useful to consider which items are necessary for emergencies and which are convenient for more routine home visits. In some practices it has been found helpful to separate these functions into separate bags. The duty doctor then keeps the 'emergency bag', and 'obstetric bag' in his car, in addition to his own personal bag which he uses for non-urgent home visits.

Diagnostic equipment

Basic equipment

- Stethoscope
- Auriscope/ophthalmoscope
- Tendon hammer
- Sphygmomanometer
- Torch
- Tuning fork
- Disposable gloves
- Disposable tongue depressors
- Urine-testing dip sticks (Ames Labstix and Dextrostix)
- Containers for blood and urine specimens
- A range of disposable syringes and needles
- 2 thermometers (1 low-reading)
- Disposable proctoscope and vaginal speculum
- Lubricant cream

The development of auriscopes, ophthalmoscopes, and stethoscopes small enough to fit into the pocket has made it more convenient for some family doctors to dispense altogether with the bag for initial assessment of the patient at home, keeping the bag in the car should further items of equipment be required. The pocket ophthalmoscopes now have a range of lenses almost as extensive as the standard ophthalmoscopes although they remain more expensive. The practice of carrying so much equipment in ordinary clothing may be criticised as being unhygienic, and the possibility of causing cross-infection by our diagnostic equipment is perhaps a neglected topic. Stethoscopes in particular have been identified as carriers of pathogenic bacteria. Disposable ear-pieces for the pocket auriscopes eliminate the risk of transferring ear infections.

In this list of basic diagnostic equipment, there are items which have provoked heated discussion when 'the doctor's bag' has been considered at clinical meetings. Many doctors regard vaginal specula and proctoscopes as impractical for use on home visits. Plastic disposable specula however are light and easy to use and may give an immediate diagnosis in cases of vaginal and rectal bleeding.

The frequency with which these simple diagnostic instruments are used gives an excellent insight into the way that we practise medicine. Some doctors take the temperature of the patient as part of their routine examination and find that this activity gives a useful period of silence in which to come to a decision about the immediate management of the patient. Other doctors argue that an isolated measurement of temperature is of little value (except in the diagnosis of hypothermia) and that taking the temperature encourages excessive emphasis on body temperature by the patient. All agree, however, that the thermometer should be carried in the bag. Such discussions do reveal that the practise of medicine remains an individual art and re-emphasizes the fact that each doctor has his own style of consulting.

Additional diagnostic equipment (available in practice premises)

- Electrocardiograph
- Tests for lung function (Wright's peak-flow meter or gauge. Vitallograph)
- Sigmoidoscope
- Head lamp (nasal and ear specula, mirrors for indirect laryngoscopy)
- Magnifying loupe
- Vision charts (Snellen test cards)
- Fluorescein (in solution or impregnated paper strips)
- Ishihara plates for colour vision
- Height rule
- Adult and baby scales
- X-ray viewing box
- Haemoglobinometer
- Ultrasound
- Foetal stethoscope
- Tape measure
- Clinitest kit and tablets
- Audiometer/audio-tester

Although this list is not exhaustive, few practices will have all these items of equipment available to them. Before a decision is made to purchase additional clinical equipment, several basic questions need to be posed. Will the equipment significantly influence the diagnosis and treatment of patients?; Are the doctors competent in the use of the equipment?; Is the equipment robust and reliable in use?; Does the frequency of use warrant the cost of purchase and maintenance?. As an electrocardiograph is often the item of equipment under consideration, the arguments for and against purchasing such a machine will be discussed in detail.

Will the equipment significantly influence the diagnosis and treatment of patients? Many doctors entering general practice will be accustomed to obtaining and reading electrocardiograms in their hospital work. In hospital, patients with suspected myocardial infarction have their electrocardiograms monitored for arrhythmias so that immediate appropriate therapy can be administered. Similarly in general practice the most common use of the electrocardiograph in an emergency is in the diagnosis of suspected myocardial infarction. It is well recognized, however,

that the electrocardiogram may be entirely normal in patients during the first few hours following myocardial infarction and the treatment and management of the patient are dependent on the history and physical findings rather than electrocardiographic changes. Atropine in patients with bradycardia and an intravenous lignocaine bolus in patients with a rapid irregular pulse can be given safely without benefit of an electrocardiogram. Treatment of the patient and transfer, if appropriate, to a coronary care unit need not be delayed by the taking of a cardiograph.
Previous surveys have indicated that the major use of the electrocardiograph in general practice is in the routine assessment of patients in the surgery rather than in an emergency in the patient's home.[3] Usually assessment is carried out in the practice premises for the convenience of the patient rather than for immediate therapeutic benefit.

Are the doctors competent in the use of the equipment? In both routine and emergency uses it is vital that the quality of tracings is good enough to allow consideration of the differential diagnoses, and that the doctors are competent in reading the tracings. Even in large group practices, however, the number of tracings will be insufficient to maintain the proficiency of general practitioners, and special arrangements must be made to obtain authoritative opinions on the tracings in doubtful cases. Informal links with the local hospitals and coronary care units have allowed many general practitioners to improve their competence in reading the tracings and to achieve a high technical quality of tracings. In such circumstances the availability of an electrocardiograph in a group practice or health centre does seem to be a logical development in encouraging general practitioners to investigate their patients as fully as possible.

Is the equipment robust and reliable in use? To arrive at a patient's home with an electrocardiograph that will not function creates more problems than to arrive without such equipment. It is therefore necessary to ensure a system of regular maintenance for the machine, and to have one that is small and robust, to withstand the handling involved in domiciliary use.

A decision to purchase and use additional diagnostic equipment, such as an electrocardiograph, may be made in the light of the foregoing discussion. The cost and frequency of use of the equipment are also important considerations.

Therapeutic equipment

Drugs

When constructing a list of suitable drugs for the doctor's bag, it is useful to think of the acute medical conditions for which urgent treatment is required: bronchial asthma, left ventricular failure, myocardial infarction (and other cardiac pain), hypoglycaemic and hyperglycaemic coma, biliary colic, renal colic, anaphylactic shock, acute poisoning, respiratory failure, shock from various causes, uterine haemorrhage, unexpected and precipitant labour, pneumothorax, epistaxis, hypothermia, grand mal and febrile convulsions, croup, and psychiatric emergencies such as overbreathing or acute paranoid illnesses. This list covers most of the acute conditions for which the general practitioner himself will be expected to give immediate therapy.

The choice between drugs with similar pharmacological properties is a personal one (Chapter 2.1). The following list should therefore serve merely as a check list for doctors in making their own choice of drugs. It is of great importance that the doctor should be familiar with his own range of drugs and of any possible adverse interactions between them.

Sedative, anti-convulsant, and anti-emetic preparations

Diazepam 10 mg ampoules and 5 mg tablets. The slow intravenous injection of diazepam (10 mg) is effective in status epilepticus, but care is required because of the risk of respiratory depression. The intramuscular and oral use of diazepam will be found useful in a wide range of anxiety states. The difficulties in administration of paraldehyde with the unpleasant smell and tendency to produce a prolonged hangover and the need to use a glass and not a plastic syringe have persuaded many doctors no longer to carry this anti-convulsant in their bags.

Phenobarbitone 200 mg ampoules. If intravenous treatment is difficult or inadvisable in status epileticus, intramuscular injection is a safe alternative to diazepam.

Chlorpromazine 50 mg ampoules (or other phenothiazine) and 25 mg tablets are useful to carry in the bag as an alternative to diazepam in the treatment of anxiety states. A parenteral phenothiazine will possibly be more often used in the control of persistent vomiting. The administration of large doses of phenothiazines in an acutely psychotic disturbed patient is difficult for the general practitioner to achieve unassisted. The help of the local psychiatric team in dealing with such patients is often required.

Prochlorperazine (Stemetil) suppositories, 5 mg and 25 mg, and 12.5 mg ampoules. Injection of prochlorperazine is useful initial therapy in severe vomiting (especially in Menière's disease), acute labyrinthitis and migraine.

Cyclizine 50 mg ampoules provide a useful anti-emetic when sedation is not desired. It should not be mixed in the syringe with opiates as the drugs may be precipitated out of solution.

Amylobarbitone sodium 200 mg tablets (or other barbiturate). The choice of a barbiturate hypnotic is justified on the grounds that barbiturates are more effective and more rapid in onset than the benzodiazepine hypnotics and are as safe, provided that their use is restricted to treatment in a crisis and that long-term treatment is not instigated. Both benzodiazepines and barbiturates may cause confusion in elderly patients.

Analgesics

Morphine sulphate injection 10 mg and Cyclimorph (10 mg or 15 mg of morphine – 50 mg cyclizine tartrate in 1 ml ampoules) are essential in any doctor's bag for the immediate treatment of the pain in myocardial infarction and for the relief of tachypnoea and anxiety in left ventricular failure.

Pethidine 100 mg ampoules and 50 mg tablets are both useful in relieving biliary and renal pain. In both these conditions the addition of anti-spasmodics, e.g. propantheline bromide 30 mg, may also help.

Pentazocine injections, 30 mg and 60 mg and 25 mg tablets are carried by some doctors as an alternative to pethidine, although the effectiveness of pentazocine is less predictable.

Paracetamol and dextropropoxyphene tablets. The combination of 325 mg paracetamol and 32.5 mg dextropropoxyphene (Coproxamol) is an effective analgesic for moderate pain: for example, following soft tissue injuries. The tendency for some patients to become habituated to dextropropoxyphene should be noted, but this is not a problem in the treatment of the acute injury.

The bag should also contain paracetamol 500 mg tablets and aspirin 300 mg tablets, preferably in a soluble form. Patients in ill-equipped households without these simple analgesics-anti-pyretics will not be impressed by the doctor who is similarly ill equipped.

Cardiovascular and Diuretic Drugs

Frusemide 20 mg ampoules and 20 mg and 40 mg tablets. It is particularly of value in the treatment of left ventricular failure, when it is administered intravenously.

Lignocaine 100 mg (5 mls solution), available in ampoules or in prepacked syringe (Xylocard). This amount of lignocaine can be given as an intravenous bolus for the suppression of multiple ventricular ectopic beats or ventricular tachycardia in a patient with a myocardial infarction. A single bolus of 100 mg can be given on clinical grounds alone and does not require electrocardiographic confirmation of the dysrhythmia. Toxic effects of lignocaine include agitation, sweating, fits, and asystole in patients with heart block. A 2 per cent solution is also appropriate for injection as a local anaesthetic.

Atropine sulphate 0.6 mg ampoules. This is one of the few drugs which continue to be prescribed in a quantity related to the grain (1/100 gr.) Following a myocardial infarction, bradycardia, especially if accompanied by hypotension, should be treated by atropine. It has a short duration of action and two ampoules require to be carried. It is also of use in the treatment of poisoning by organophosphorus pesticides (e.g. malathion).

Digoxin 0.5 mg ampoules and 0.25 mg tablets. For the treatment of heart failure and supraventricular tachycardias. Parenteral digoxin is sometimes required when vomiting accompanies cardiac failure. Care should be taken to ensure that the patient is not already receiving digoxin. Many of the dysrhythmias treated by digoxin can also be induced by digitalis toxicity.

Oxprenolol 2 mg injections and 20 mg tablets (or other β-blocker) occasionally require to be used in the treatment of supra-ventricular tachycardia, especially if the patient is already digitalized. Rarely a β-blocker is required in the emergency treatment of thyrotoxic crisis.

Glyceryl trinitrin 0.5 mg tablets for the immediate treatment and possible diagnosis of angina. The tablets should be frequently renewed as they lost their potency after about eight weeks in use.

Respiratory drugs

Aminophylline 250 mg in 10 ml can be given as an intravenous injection in the treatment of left ventricular failure and acute asthma.

Terbutaline sulphate 500 μg in 1 ml, also terbutaline inhaler. Subcutaneous or aerosol use of one of the newer sympathomimetics in the treatment of acute asthma is preferred to adrenaline because of their relative specificity for bronchial receptors (β_2). The dose of terbutaline for subcutaneous injection in children is 10 μg/kg body weight.

Drugs for use in hypersensitivity reactions

Adrenaline 0.5 ml ampoule, 1-in-1000 solution for subcutaneous injection. Adrenaline acts on both α and β receptors and is an effective bronchodilator. Because of its lack of specificity it has the serious side effects of hypertension, tachycardia, and cardiac dysrhythmias. It remains an excellent drug for the immediate treatment of anaphylactic shock because of the immediate onset of its effect. Dosage: children up to one year, 0.05 ml; one to five years, 0.1 to 0.4 ml; six to twelve years, 0.5 ml. If the patient is unconscious these doses may be exceeded and the injection given intramuscularly.

Hydrocortisone sodium succinate 100 mg and 500 mg ampoules for intravenous or intramuscular injection.

Chlorpheniramine maleate 10 mg ampoules and 4 mg tablets. Although useful, the effect of an intravenous or intramuscular injection is only apparent after about thirty minutes.

As these drugs are required in the treatment of anaphylactic shock and other hypersensitivity conditions, they should be available both in the doctor's bag and in the surgery premises.
Steroid tablets such as prednisone 5 mg are useful to have in the bag for the initiation of a short course of treatment in acute asthma.

Miscellaneous drugs for use in emergencies

Syntometrine intramuscular injection (0.5 mg ergometrine,

5 units synthetic oxytocin) for the control of post-partum haemorrhage or for use prophylactically in the immediate post-partum period.

Dextrose injection 50 per cent in 50 ml ampoules or bottles. The viscous fluid is difficult to draw up through a fine needle and it is much easier to draw up the fluid directly using the nozzle of the syringe. The bottles of dextrose are safer to carry in the bag than large ampoules.

Glucagon injection 1 mg. The ampoules of glucagon have a relatively short shelf-life and require to be renewed regularly.

Treatment of poisoning and drug overdose

Naloxone 400 μg in 1 ml for intravenous, intramuscular or subcutaneous injection is an antagonist in respiratory depression, especially if due to opiates. It has a short duration of action and may require to be repeated. Unlike nalorphine and levallorphan, it does not cause significant respiratory depression itself in therapeutic doses.

Vitamin K_1 (Konakion) 1 mg and 10 mg ampoules; 10 mg tablets. In patients bleeding due to overdosage with oral anticoagulants, doses of vitamin K_1 in excess of 20 mg are usually required.

Ipecacuanha emetic mixture B.P. is an effective and safe emetic for use in children. The dose is: 0–2 years, 10 ml; 2–5 years, 15 ml. An effect is usually observed within fifteen minutes.

Antibiotics

Although not essential it is often convenient to carry 'starter packs' of a range of antibiotics. *Penicillin V*, *amoxycillin*, *erythromycin* and *co-trimoxazole* can all easily be carried in tablet form and in 'starter packs' for children. An injectable form of penicillin is also useful: e.g. benzyl penicillin 1 mega-unit as powder and amoxycillin 250 mg in 1 ml.

Drugs acting on the gastro-intestinal tract

Anti-emetic injections and suppositories have already been considered. Diarrhoea, constipation, colic and indigestion are not usually medical emergencies. However, immediate treatment is sometimes appropriate and the doctor may wish to carry the following drugs.

Loperamide (Imodium) 2 mg tablets. The range of anti-diarrhoeals is very wide in terms of potency and cost. The choice of loperamide is justified by its requiring little space in the bag and because of its absence of side-effects.

Bisacodol suppositories 5 mg and 10 mg. In a patient with impacted faeces, it is of advantage to insert a suppository after carrying out a rectal examination and possibly manual removal of faeces.

Antacid tablets require little space and, in addition to providing immediate symptom relief, may help in the diagnosis of chest pain. Magnesium trisilicate tablets are cheap and, for the immediate relief of symptoms, as effective as the more expensive antacids.

Therapeutic equipment

It is in the range and sophistication of therapeutic equipment carried in the bag or the car that the greatest variation between doctors will occur. Doctors in urban practice may require only the following basic equipment.

Basic equipment

- Scissors
- Disposable scalpel
- Needle holder
- Sterile suture material
- Mucous extractor for neonates
- Brook-type airway
- Bottle of local anaesthetic
- Portable oxygen (e.g. Respirex Ox-Vital)
- Sterile dressings (e.g. gauze and Melolin non-adherent dressings)
- Adhesive tape
- Small adhesive dressings
- Ribbon gauze and angle forceps
- Range of needles and syringes
- Catheter pack
- Range of indwelling urinary catheters

For the urban general practitioner the main current debate is whether or not to carry an oxygen set in the car. There is now a wide range of small portable sets available. Oxygen is recommended as part of the initial treatment in myocardial infarction and in status asthmaticus. In severe asthma, oxygen therapy should precede the use of sympathomimetics and theophylline derivatives because of the risk of cardiac arrhythmias being provoked by these drugs when the myocardium is hypoxic. There will only be a small number of occasions when the individual general practitioner will wish to give oxygen and it may be that the speed of response of the local ambulance service is sufficiently good to avoid the necessity of purchasing such equipment. In many parts of the country, however, there may be considerable delay before the oxygen carried by the ambulance can be administered to the patient. If the general practitioner does have oxygen available, he should be aware of the possible dangers of oxygen therapy. High concentrations of oxygen are obtained by the majority of face masks available with portable oxygen sets and this is usually desirable, but, in respiratory failure in patients with chronic bronchitis, this may cause hypercapnia and so further depress respiration. Positive pressure ventilation is possible with many of the oxygen sets and is beneficial in attempting to resuscitate patients in shock due to myocardial infarction. Asthmatic patients occasionally develop a pneumothorax which may be aggravated by positive pressure ventilation.

Additional equipment required for resuscitation and first-aid treatment

Doctors who may be called upon to provide first-aid treatment at the scene of road traffic accidents, and doctors who practise in remote regions of the country, require to have specific training in resuscitation and to work in close co-operation with the emergency services.[1,2] The following check-list gives some idea of the extensive equipment that is required. Certain items in the list will be of general use: e.g. intravenous fluid giving set and plasma. At roadside emergencies white or light-coloured doctors' bags are preferred. Resuscitation equipment and dressings should be carried in separate containers.

Resuscitation

Portable oxygen with attachments and adaptors for face mask and endotracheal tubes
Endotracheal tubes (adult and child sizes)
Laryngoscope (adult and child sizes)
Face masks (adult and child sizes)
Bag and mask resuscitator (Ambu bag)
Brook airways
Mouth gag
Lubricant cream
Disposable tracheostomy tube
Artery forceps
Scalpel
Blunt scissors
Sharp scissors
Sutures
Range of syringes and needles and container for blood for cross-matching
Tourniquet
Alcohol swabs
Intravenous cannulae
Intravenous giving set
500 ml normal saline and 500 ml plasma or dextran

Dressings and splints and protective clothing and apparatus

- Inflatable splints
- Spinal board
- Cotton wool
- Sterile gauze
- Melolin dressings
- Large wound dressings
- Conforming bandages
- Crepe bandages
- Triangular bandages
- A large sharp knife for cutting clothing, etc.
- Adhesive tape
- Safety pins
- Fluorescent waistcoat
- Overalls, gloves, boots
- Waterproof suit
- Waterproof sheet
- Space rescue blanket
- Plastic container of water
- Plastic container of antiseptic
- Disposable gallipots

Further equipment carried on or in the car

- Four-way flasher
- Accident triangle
- Fire extinguisher
- Large torch

In addition to the above list, some doctors carry entonox apparatus to allow inhalational analgesia as an alternative to the use of opiates. Accurate records should be kept about the condition of injured patients and the timing of drug administration. Each case should therefore be equipped with a notepad and ball-point pen.

Equipment for home confinements

Although home confinements are decreasing in number, the obstetric bag is a necessity for doctors with practices remote from maternity hospitals. The Gladstone type bag is very suitable for midwifery because of the ease with which it can accommodate the larger pieces of equipment, such as obstetric forceps.

Obstetric bag

- Apron
- Sterile towels and sheets
- Cord clamp
- Mucous extractor
- Blunt and sharp scissors
- Artery forceps
- Identification tag
- Sutures
- Needle holder
- Syringes, needles
- Containers for blood tests
- Pudendal block needles
- Large torch or head lamp
- Disposable gallipots
- Plastic container of antiseptic
- Plastic container of sterile water
- Cotton wool
- Sterile gauze
- Ampoules of syntometrine
- Ampoules of Konakion (vitamin K_1)
- Ampoule of pethidine
- Ampoule of nalorphine
- Local anaesthetic
- Catheter pack
- Range of catheters

Entonox apparatus
(carried in car)
Child's laryngoscope
Endotracheal tube
Obstetric forceps

Plasma
Normal saline
Intravenous giving set
Intravenous catheters

Administrative equipment

Stationery

The prescription pad, the National Insurance certificates for sickness benefit, and a pen, are sometimes regarded by cynics as the only essential items of equipment in general practice. In addition to these items the bag should contain, in a tidy manner, the following:

Notepaper
Envelopes
Request forms for haematology, biochemistry, etc. with appropriate small plastic bags
N.H.S. claim forms for night visits, temporary residents, treatment of emergencies, treatment of patients whom you do not wish to join your list, treatment of dental emergencies
Protocol for recommended emergency admission to a mental hospital under the terms of the Mental Health Act. (This is obtainable from H.M. Stationery Office.)
List of useful telephone numbers, e.g. ambulance, local hospitals.
M.I.Ms. and/or British National Formulary
Medisc or other chart of adverse drug interactions

As the range of equipment and drugs available to general practitioners becomes more sophisticated, it is inevitable that the foregoing lists can merely serve as a guide and doctors will wish to adapt the content of their bags according to local requirements and their own individual experience.

References

[1]Snook, R. (1972): Accident Flying Squad. *British Medical Journal*, *3*, 569–74
[2]Aston, P. (1969): Equipment for use at roadside accidents. *British Medical Journal*, *4*, 214–17
[3]Peniket, J. and MacQuaide, D.H.G. (1973): A domiciliary ECG service for general practitioners. *Journal of the Royal College of General Practitioners*, *23*, 352–6
[4]Taylor, J.W. (1970): Equipment *in* Report of a Symposium on Group Practice. *Journal of the Royal College of General Practitioners*, *20*, Suppl. no. 2, 34–42
[5] Birch, C. Allan (1976): *Emergencies in Medicine Practice*, 10th edn. Edinburgh: Churchill Livingstone

2
Management

2.1 Principles of management

David Morrell and Marshall Marinker

The role of the general practitioner in the National Health Service in the United Kingdom is to identify and respond to the problems of the patients registered with him for medical care. Frequently new problems will be presented as new symptoms of illness, and his response will often be immediate, relatively specific and of short duration. He is, however, becoming increasingly concerned with problems resulting from chronic degenerative diseases which develop over many years, causing a variety of disabilities. Doctors are also becoming aware that treatment may be desirable before symptoms arise.

Diagnosis is considered throughout this book in physical, social and psychological terms. Management may conveniently be looked at in the same way. Having identified the patients' problems in these areas, the doctor must be prepared to respond appropriately. It would be simple to restrict this chapter on the Principles of Management to drug therapy. Such an approach, however, would ignore the wider possibilities for managing ill health in general practice.

The doctor as listener

Unless a doctor is a good listener, and can encourage his patients to express the anxiety provoked by their symptoms, he is unlikely to identify their problems, although he may diagnose their diseases. Listening is therefore a crucial part of the diagnostic process. It may also be therapeutic, particularly in the management of interpersonal relationship problems, chronic painful and disabling diseases, and terminal illness. By allowing patients to express their feelings of inadequacy, frustration or fear, the general practitioner who is a good listener will provide valuable therapy. Many patients who go to the doctor for advice really require an opportunity to verbalize their own thoughts and feelings, and if the doctor can listen he will often give them a chance to organize their thoughts and be better able to cope with their problems.

By listening, the doctor may become aware of areas of ignorance or confusion which are producing anxiety and fear and simple explanation or reassurance may remedy the situation. It is often assumed that patients attend their doctors for treatment with drugs and the doctor therefore feels constrained to write a prescription. It is wise to recall that many patients attend for reassurance that the symptoms they are experiencing do not indicate serious disease. This is likely to become more common as the population is educated to present with the early signs of illness. If patients are given time they will usually tell the doctor why they have come and this can save a lot of unnecessary prescribing and allow him to provide more appropriately for their needs.

The doctor as adviser

Whether or not the doctor prescribes for his patients, he is often required to provide advice. There are several important topics on which he must not only advise, but make it possible for his patients to accept his advice.

Rest. – This plays an important part in the management of many acute illnesses. Not only does the patient feel more comfortable at rest, but it is probable that rest also shortens the natural course of many illnesses. In the case of trauma particularly, rest allows healing to proceed and is an important component of treatment.

In the management of chronic illness, rest must be prescribed judiciously. During an acute flare up of an arthritic joint, or an acute exacerbation of chronic bronchitis, for instance, rest may be appropriate. Prolonged rest, particularly in the elderly, carries with it the risk of loss of mobility and deep venous thrombosis.

The patient who presents to the doctor complaining of tiredness and feeling in need of a good rest, is often the patient suffering from boredom or depression, whose real need is greater stimulation or involvement.

In many instances, rest necessitates withdrawal from employment, whether this is gainful employment in the factory, or the day-to-day responsibilities of the mother. In the elderly it may result in the patient becoming unable to provide for his or her day-to-day needs. For the patient to accede to the doctor's advice, it may be necessary for the doctor to provide an alternative form of income by using a certificate which entitles the patient to sickness benefit. In other circumstances he may have to call in 'home-help services', or in extreme cases arrange for the foster care of children. His responsibility therefore does not end with his advice: he must make is possible for his patients to accept his advice, and in doing so must often seek help from his health visitor, or the social services department.

Diet. – Specific dietary advice is needed by patients suffering from diabetes mellitus, peptic ulcer and some disorders of intestinal absorption. More often, the doctor is required to provide dietary advice in the management of acute infections, particularly of the gastro-intestinal tract. Many patients are unaware that it is possible to survive for long periods without solid food, as long as they have adequate fluids, and such patients insist on force-feeding, particularly pyrexial children who are experiencing acute infections. This often leads to vomiting, which may negate the benefits of drugs taken by mouth, and in time may lead to dehydration. Firm advice is necessary to offset this misguided approach to feeding.

The doctor has a serious responsibility in the prevention and treatment of obesity by giving advice on diet. There is little doubt that obesity often starts in infancy and childhood, and here the health visitor has special responsibilities. There are other times in life when excessive weight gain may occur. These are puberty, pregnancy and the puerperium, and middle age. The treatment of obesity is almost universally disappointing, and the general practitioner has therefore a special responsibility to prevent its occurring and to intervene at an early stage.

Exercise. – With increasing dependence on the motor car there is a tendency for people in developed countries to take insufficient exercise. This predisposes to such diseases as coronary thrombosis and it certainly encourages the development of obesity. The general practitioner can play an important part in encouraging his patients to take adequate exercise.

There are in addition many specific conditions where he will be asked for advice. How soon, for instance, after a coronary thrombosis, hernia repair or prolapsed intervertebral disc, should a patient exert himself physically? What sort of exercise should he take and how much? Surprisingly little is known about the effects of exercise on the outcome of disease or the results of surgical operations. There is, however, evidence that in the management of coronary thrombosis many doctors are over-cautious, and many patients become premature, and sometimes permanent, invalids.

Environment. – The doctor is often called upon to give advice on the effect of the patient's environment on the course of his disease. In some cases he may be asked whether a geographical change in environment would be beneficial to, for instance, a patient suffering from asthma. More often he is asked to adjudicate on the suitability of the patient's housing conditions. Not uncommonly, he may feel that such requests are inappropriate and that he is being forced to support, by medical argument, cases which should be judged on social merits. If he accedes to these requests he will weaken his position when he really wishes to advocate rehousing on medical grounds. There are many occasions where rehousing will make it possible for a housebound patient imprisoned by three or four flights of stairs to return to a less restricted way of life. He should therefore reserve his resources for this type of situation, and explain to other patients that the social services department is a more appropriate place to seek advice.

There are numerous situations where modifications in the patient's home will reduce the impact of disability. A close relationship with the social services department will facilitate the introduction of such modifications.

In introducing home nursing care, the doctor may also alter the patient's environment. A good district nurse has an enormous contribution to make, not simply in providing traditional nursing services, but in helping patients to adapt to their disabilities in the environment of their home.

Habits

Tobacco. – The habit of cigarette smoking usually develops insidiously in adolescents, and the pressures on the young to start smoking are very strong. The doctor has a role in combating this and where appropriate should make his patients aware of the risks they are taking. A major difficulty in advising about the dangers of smoking is the time interval that exists between starting the habit and the consequences. The prospect of chronic bronchitis or of cancer of the lung at the age of 50 years seems remote to the teenager attracted by the status which a cigarette confers on him among his peers. Until recently smoking was accepted as a social grace, and many friendships have started with the offer of a cigarette. There is some evidence that this influence is becoming less strong.

Once the habit of smoking is acquired, the doctor can offer little help to the addict who wishes to stop. Warnings of a remote danger provide little motivation. There are, however, certain events which occur in the lives of his patients when he can help. The onset of pregnancy should give the doctor an opportunity to advise about the risks of cigarette smoking to the unborn child. This may provide the motivation for the patient to give up smoking. If the parents can be introduced together to the admittedly more remote dangers of passive smoking by their prospective infant, it may provide an opportunity for both parents to abandon smoking. The occurrence of an acute chest infection during which the immediate effects of cigarette smoking become apparent may be used to motivate a young adult. The prospect of surgery, particularly hernia repair, has often been the time when individuals have given up smoking. The discovery of hypertension or coronary artery disease provides powerful motivation to stop smoking.

While making his patients aware of the dangers of tobacco, the doctor must at the same time avoid presenting unacceptable prohibitions. He must also recognize the right of the individual cognizant of the facts to make a free choice in the way he leads his life.

Alcohol. – Giving advice on the use of alcohol is much less easy than in the use of tobacco. Alcohol is a socially acceptable drug. In moderation it causes no harm, it contributes to easy social relationships at all levels of society and is used safely by many people as a tranquillizer in stressful situations. Unfortunately it can lead to addiction. When this occurs the individual indulges to excess, becomes dependent on alcohol and to obtain supplies will sacrifice himself and his family. The doctor must become sensitive to the early signs of alcoholic dependence. It may present to him under a variety of guises: a social problem, recurrent trauma, anorexia or impotence, to mention but a few. Early diagnosis is important because established alcoholism has a poor prognosis.

Sexual relationships

As with so many other diagnostic problems in medicine, the doctor sees what he is looking for. To a large extent the sexual maturity of the doctor himself and his attitude to these problems will determine the readiness of his patients to consult him. It will also influence his ability to identify the importance or otherwise of sexual difficulties in the etiology of his patients' symptoms. There can be few aspects of general practitioner care which better illustrate the need for a combined physical, psychological and social approach to diagnosis and treatment.

Problems about sexual behaviour arise from a variety of causes. Total ignorance of the 'facts of life' is now rare, but many patients are misinformed about the nature of sexual relationships which are viewed by some as an athletic performance rather than an act of love. This type of problem may be easily resolved by a sensitive general practitioner prepared to counsel his patients and encourage husband and wife to communicate with each other on a subject which heretofore they have found difficult to discuss.

Most commonly sexual unhappiness stems from psychological problems which prevent the patient establishing a loving relationship or the ability to experience sexual pleasure or give it to a partner.

There are many opportunities for the general practitioner to advise his women patients, created by his involvement in antenatal and postnatal care and in family planning, and it is apparent that women are usually more ready than men to seek advice in this field. Problems may, however, be equally experienced by male patients.

The doctor should be sensitive to their needs, as they may find it more difficult to present them. In the presence of such illnesses as depression, coronary thrombosis or major surgery, he should make a positive effort to enquire about problems in this area of human behaviour and provide appropriate support. (The reader is referred to Chapter 3.61, Difficulties with Sexual Intercourse).

The doctor as prescriber

It is a recurring theme in the criticism of modern medicine that doctors prescribe too many drugs and that patients make too many demands for them. In fact, a great deal of modern medicine is concerned with the treatment of the unwanted effects of this medication. In addition, the fact that doctors prescribe so readily for almost every complaint which their patients bring to them, reinforces the myth that modern medicine is omnipotent, and increases a demand for medical care, whereas self-care might be much more appropriate and is certainly more economical. When, for example, the general practitioner indiscriminately prescribes an antibiotic for the patient with acute diarrhoea he performs a disservice in a number of different ways. First he prescribes a medication which is not only unhelpful, but may actually prolong the illness. Second, he educates the patient to expect the services of a doctor and the prescribing of this sort of medication on future similar occasions. Finally, he involves the patient in a small, and the public purse in a larger, expense in the course of this disservice which he does to his patient, the profession and the public. In England the precursor of the general practitioner was the apothecary. Before the medical reforms of the 19th century, although the apothecary was allowed to make diagnoses and to give advice, the right to make a charge for these services was reserved for the physician. The apothecary was only allowed to make a charge for the drugs which he prescribed and provided. The expectation or the giving of a drug as an integral part of the act of consulting has therefore a long history in our culture, and antedates the explosive growth of contemporary pharmacology. In constructing a rational medical practice, a major task for the general practitioner is the development of a sensible policy of drug prescribing.

How can this be achieved when every year new and more sophisticated drugs are being invented and marketed? In a general sense, the doctor is aware of the dangers. He knows that drugs can do harm, but he also wants to do the best for his patient. If a new agent for the treatment of high blood pressure is said to be an improvement on previous ones, then he is tempted to make this available to those patients under his care. In support of their claims drug companies often quote an extensive literature detailing the results of drug trials, but it is simply unrealistic to expect the general practitioner to read these articles, let alone to make a judgement about the scientific rigour of the methods, or the interpretation of the results. More difficult still, the growing number of drugs available may cause trouble in any one, and any combination, of the following ways:

1. *Unwanted actions.* Because the target site of most drugs is cellular or molecular rather than organic, a drug prescribed with a specific action in mind (for example a beta-blocking drug prescribed for the alleviation of angina pectoris) will have an analogous pharmacological action at another site with the production of unwanted effects: for example a beta-blockade producing bronchospasm or urinary retention. As the pharmacological sophisitication of modern drugs increases, that is to say as the site of action becomes more specific in terms of cell biology, so a single specific drug may come to have an increasingly blunderbuss effect on cellular mechanisms in quite distant body systems and organs. Corticosteroids and many psychotropic drugs are examples of this. Sometimes the unwanted effects are simply those of local irritation: the effect of aspirin or ibuprofen on the gastric mucosa. Sometimes the action, which may be life-threatening, is more obscure: the actions of phenylbutazone and chloramphenicol on the blood-forming tissues.

2. *Unreliability of dose.* We are increasingly aware that so-called standard dosage schedules result in a wide variety of blood levels, and that the delivery of the drug to the target site depends on a wide variety of factors. A pharmacologically appropriate drug may therefore be totally inert in terms of its intended function (for example, phenoxymethylpenicillin prescribed for an alveolar abcess, because the antibiotic fails to penetrate the fibrous tissue surrounding the infection), although it may well produce an unwanted effect, such as diarrhoea. Similarly, digoxin given in the so-called routine dose of 0.25 mg twice daily may well cause slowing of the heart and arrhythmias when the serum potassium has been depleted, or when administered in such dosage to the elderly.

3. *Genetic idiosyncrasy.* Not a great deal is yet known about the genetics of pharmacology. We are aware that some families are resistant to treatment with anticoagulants and tricyclic anti-depressants and that families with porphyria are liable to severe damage if treated with barbiturates. It is more likely that when an anxious mother tells the doctor that her children never respond to penicillin, or the middle-aged housewife that she requires twice or three times the usual dose of a hypnotic in order to get an hour or two of sleep, the doctor is encountering a behavioural problem, or a

failure to reach an accurate diagnosis rather than a genetic idiosyncrasy. Nonetheless, the large range of responses to some drugs, for example in the treatment of Parkinsonism, suggests that there may be a strong constitutional variation in drug response.

4. *Acquired idiosyncrasy.* Hypersensitivity to drugs is a common problem in general practice. Perhaps the most common is penicillin allergy, when the patient, usually a child, is labelled as being allergic to oral penicillin because of the appearance of a rash shortly after its prescription. Often this judgement is made on scant evidence: the appearance of the rash, for example, may have been connected with the viral illness for which the penicillin was inappropriately prescribed. This over-hasty judgement not only rules out the use of perhaps the most appropriate and potent antibiotic, oral phenoxymethylpenicillin, but also the future use of the synthetic pencillins because of the potential danger of associated allergies. Most notoriously topical applications can cause severe local reactions. In particular, topical antibiotics, often presented in combination with a topical steroid, can cause a rash far more severe than the disease for which it was prescribed. Paradoxically, the antihistamine used topically in order to reduce the allergic reaction can be itself a powerful allergen.

5. *Interaction with disease processes.* The metabolism and clearance of drugs often depend on the integrity of the liver and the kidneys. Any disease affecting the organs concerned with drug metabolism may therefore interfere with the pharmacological action. Sometimes the interactions between a drug and a disease process can be highly specific and dramatic: the commonest example is the widespread and often severe rash caused by ampicillin in the patient with glandular fever. Sometimes a drug may potentiate a hitherto undeclared disease process: for example the precipitation of glaucoma by the administration of steroid eye-drops.

6. *Interaction with other drugs and chemical substances.* The problem of potential drug interaction is a large and growing one. There are now so many categories of drugs, and so many molecular variations within each category, that it becomes quite impossible for the general practitioner to be aware of all the possible synergistic and harmful drug interactions. In addition to this, drugs may interact with chemical substances contained in some foods. The interaction of M.A.O.I. antidepressants with the tyramine contained in such foods as meat extracts, certain cheeses, wines, broad beans and so on is the best known example.

There are a number of important additive and antagonistic effects. For example in the presence of oral iron preparations or calcium-containing foods like milk or medicines like antacids, tetracyclines are chelated and absorption reduced. There may be displacement of drugs by protein binding: aspirin is a very potent protein binder and may give rise to problems when the patient is receiving warfarin or phenytoin. Patients receiving warfarin are also at risk when phenobarbitone is prescribed. The anticoagulant effect of the warfarin may be potentiated, and this may continue for up to three weeks after stopping phenobarbitone. The dose of warfarin which had previously been stabilized may then be far too high and the anticoagulant therapy out of control.

These are only a few examples of what is becoming an increasingly complex problem.

Because it is simply not possible to recall all the potential drug interactions, it becomes highly important for the doctor to restrict his own pharmacopoeia. The fewer drugs that he employs the less likely it is that he will meet an unexpected and damaging interaction. The general practitioner must, however, be aware that the patient may be taking drugs, either in the form of self-medication or prescribed by some other agency (most often the hospital, or a previous general practitioner). It is therefore essential that the general practitioner should know the patient's current medication before prescribing a new drug. Unless there is a really excellent record system, the medical record alone cannot provide a safe guide. For this reason the prescribing of drugs after a telephone consultation between the patient and receptionist or nurse carries a particular hazard.

The prescribing of any new drug for a patient, and in particular a new drug which is likely to be taken for a chronic condition over a long period of time, should always be the signal for a complete review of the patient's drug therapy. Many district general hospitals are now staffed by information pharmacists, and they should be freely consulted about the problems of drug interactions. It is, of course, almost impossible for the modern general practitioner to prescribe for his patients without frequent reference to sources of information about drugs, such as the *British National Formulary, Treatment* (published as a companion volume to *Practice),* or M.I.M.S. It is a common experience that the patient accepts the making of such reference and welcomes it as an integral part of the consultation.

7. *Interaction with developmental processes.* The behaviour of drugs in the body depends also on the phase of the patient's development. The phase of human development may therefore alter the intended pharmacology, alter its unwanted effects and modify the way in which the drug is metabolized and excreted. The 'thalidomide disaster' highlighted the risk to the foetus from drugs prescribed during pregnancy. As a result both doctors and patients alike now tend to avoid the giving and taking of drugs at this time. More recently a sudden increase in the incidence of carcinoma of the

vagina in young girls has been attributed to the treatment of habitual abortion with high doses of oestrogen, some fifteen to twenty years ago. Certain common drugs are contraindicated during pregnancy: for example cotrimoxazole and the tetracyclines. Nitrofurantoin is contraindicated during the first month of life and also in old age when renal impairment may be present and result in severe peripheral neuropathy. Although there is only inconclusive evidence that steroids given in pregnancy may cause foetal abnormalities, the threat is sufficient to indicate that steroids should only be given to a pregnant woman when no other remedy is available for a life-threatening situation. Similarly, steroids given regularly before adult life may have a stunting effect on growth, in addition to the other well-known toxic effects of this group of drugs.

8. *The drug treatment of drug-induced disease.* Since drugs give rise to so many unwanted symptoms, and since treatment of symptoms by drugs is central to medical practice, the prescribing of drugs tends to be self multiplying. The doctor may prescribe an antacid mixture to treat the indigestion caused by ibuprofen. A tricyclic antidepressant drug may be prescribed for the depressed mood caused by methyldopa, and then digoxin added to the regime of the elderly patient whose tachycardia is not in fact related to the onset of hypertensive heart failure, but is simply a side-effect of the inappropriately prescribed tricyclic. It becomes clear that in any chronic condition, or for that matter in any clinical situation already under drug treatment, the cause of a new symptom should first be looked for in the patient's drug regime.

9. *Addiction and habituation.* These two terms are sometimes used loosely and patients are described as being addicted to drugs which are clearly not drugs of addiction.

Addiction implies a physical as well as psychological dependence on a drug, and the subsequent physiological upset when the drug is withdrawn. In general practice the most important drugs of addiction are the amphetamines; the major analgesics including morphine, pethidine and heroine: the barbiturates and the benzodiazepines. Until a few years ago the amphetamines were widely prescribed as tonics, antidepressants and for the suppression of appetite in the obese, or those who felt themselves to be obese. Widespread abuse of these drugs, particularly in the drug-taking subculture where they were obtained and used illegally, led to a public outcry and the present situation where amphetamines are hardly ever prescribed. It is now generally recognized that the amphetamines had no rational place in the control of obesity, which was the major ostensible reason for prescribing. It will probably never now be established whether or not the amphetamines in small doses were as effective or perhaps even more effective than the currently prescribed tricyclic drugs for the minor depressive disorders so common in general practice.

The danger which arises from the notoriously addictive nature of the opiates is a different one. Because the doctor is always aware that he may be introducing the patient to a drug of addiction, there is a danger that these drugs will not be prescribed or administered in sufficiently large doses when they are properly indicated. Such drugs are indicated in the presence of severe pain: for example, following injury, myocardial infarction or renal colic. The danger of addiction is not materially increased by ensuring that the patient is given a full dose of the appropriate drug: that is to say a dose sufficient to control the pain and shock.

The barbiturates have come under strong criticism because of their addictive nature. Some authorities recommend that the barbiturates should now only be prescribed in general practice as part of an anticonvulsant regime for the control of epilepsy. The availability of alternative tranquillizers, sedatives and hypnotics certainly makes it possible for the general practitioner to eliminate barbiturates from his range of drugs though even these new drugs are now causing anxiety about their addictive properties. Wells[1] has reported favourably on one such exercise in his own general practice.

Habituation refers entirely to psychological dependence. Habituation may occur with any drug: it is probably unrelated to its pharmacology but closely related to the relationship which the patient forms with the medication itself, and with what the medication represents. The dynamics of these relationships, so central to the so-called 'repeat prescriptions' of general practice (long-term prescribing of medication without proper clinical review), has been described in the monograph, *Treatment or Diagnosis* by Balint and his colleagues.[2]

Repeat prescription, often initiated months or years or decades before for a symptom or a disease long past, comes to represent a talisman for health or care for the patient which it is almost impossible for him to give up without a great deal of suffering. This is not quite the same thing as a placebo response: it is much more long term and it is characterized by the reappearance of fresh symptoms and complaints if the repeat prescription is withdrawn, or altered in any way. The study by Balint and his colleagues suggests that this form of treatment may, in fact, be quite appropriate for many of the patients receiving it, provided the drug prescribed is not itself causing physical harm. There is little doubt, however, that many of these repeat prescription regimes are established because the doctor has failed to review the situation. A sleeping tablet is prescribed for a patient who is disturbed during a bereavement, or following a surgical operation, and five years later the same drug is being issued on a repeat prescription. A bulk laxative is prescribed for a patient who has become constipated because of an inappropriate diet or a failure to set aside time for the regular evacuation of the bowel: the patient then settles down to a lifetime of medication in place of a simple change of behaviour.

Principles of prescribing

From the foregoing considerations there emerge a number of general principles. These are:

1. *The doctor should seek to prescribe from a limited number of useful drugs.* It is not important to know the characteristics of the majority of drugs in the pharmacopoeia. The doctor should familiarize himself well with one or two drugs in each of the major categories. He should resist the temptation to change frequently to newer preparations or variations of established drugs, on the grounds that small therapeutic benefits have been conferred on the new preparation. If he follows the policy of always changing to newer preparations, it is likely that the possible (often unproven) pharmacological benefits of the new drug will be more than offset by the fact that the doctor will never become really familiar with the characteristics of the drugs that he uses.

2. *Where no drug is positively indicated, no drug should be prescribed.* A great deal of minor illness, for example acute viral infections of the respiratory tract, requires no prescribed drugs. It will take longer to explain this to the patient, and to educate the patient about his condition, than it will to write a prescription. In the long term the doctor will save himself and his patient the problem of treating the unwanted effects of the drugs he prescribed, and the patient will become more self reliant in the management of his own minor problems. Judicious use of aspirin, including aspirin gargles for upper respiratory infections, the use of hot lemon drinks and postural drainage and percussion of the chest by a relative in the management of chronic bronchitis, the tolerance of and even the creative use of the shortened sleep pattern of old age are all to be encouraged.

3. *The treatment of cause has priority over the treatment of symptoms.* Most treatment in general practice is (quite appropriately) symptomatic. Wherever possible, however, treatment should be directed at the cause (for example a bacterial infection) and not the presenting symptom (for example pain). Thus the earache of otitis media and the dysuria of cystitis should be treated with appropriate anti-infective agents: the symptoms will

begin to diminish in twenty-four hours and self-medication with minor analgesics may be encouraged at this time.

4. *The fewer the drugs prescribed, the safer.* In the treatment of major and more chronic conditions, it is vital that whenever possible only one new drug should be introduced at a time. The patient seen initially with early congestive heart failure should not be treated at once with both digoxin and a diuretic. The patient whose benign hypertension is to be controlled should not be introduced to more than one drug at a time, and sufficient time should be given to observe the effect of this drug's action. For example, in the management of benign hypertension it would be quite wrong to begin by exhibiting both a beta blocker and a diuretic, and for this reason most proprietary combined preparations should be avoided in initial treatment. The same principle applies to the management of depressive illnesses with manifestations of anxiety: if drug treatment is thought appropriate, and it may not always be so, then it would be wrong to exhibit both a tranquillizer and an antidepressant in the initial trial of therapy.

5. *When a number of alternative treatments are available, choose the least toxic.* To quote the most obvious example, in terms of drug sensitivity, it might be argued that chloramphenicol is the drug of choice because of its effectiveness in controlling *H. influenzae:* the possibility that this drug may occasionally cause a fatal aplastic anaemia is sufficient to ban it from all use except one, where its specificity may be life saving (in the treatment of typhoid fever). Effectively, this means that chloramphenicol, except in the form of eye-drops, should not appear in the general practitioner's armamentarium. But there are other less dramatic examples. In the treatment of migraine-like headaches, simple analgesics or sedatives should precede the use of ergotamine, and the exhibition of methysergide, which is contraindicated in a large number of conditions and which may rarely cause retroperitoneal fibrosis, should be reserved for the most intractable and severe cases, in which other treatments have failed to bring relief.

6. *The cheapest effective medication should be preferred.* Whether, as in the vast majority of cases, the patient is being treated under the National Health Service, or whether the patient is being treated privately, the doctor should choose the cheapest possible effective medication. For the most part, though not always, this means that the doctor should prescribe a drug by using its approved name rather than a trade name. There are some exceptions to this rule: some proprietary preparations are cheaper, and in some instances the formulation or presentation of the proprietary drug may be

superior.

In many cases the doctor is faced with a choice of drugs whose actions are pharmacologically related, but whose costs vary greatly. Treatment with talampicillin is approximately twice as costly as treatment with ampicillin, although in general practice the latter drug will usually be found to be quite as effective as the former in the treatment of *E. coli* urinary tract infection. Large disparities of cost exist in the choices available in other categories of drugs whose specificity and effectiveness are far less certain than the antibiotics: for example, the psychotropic drugs. It is worth noting that when a drug company produces a new preparation, its cost is greatest; indeed the relative cost of a preparation within a particular category is often in inverse proportion to its established utility in general practice. On the grounds of cost therefore, as well as on the grounds of safety and utility, a conservative approach to new preparations should be the rule.

7. *The patient should be given the fullest information about his drugs.* Once a decision has been taken to prescribe a drug, time should be spent in explaining what the drug is intended to do, what likely symptoms the patient may experience (for example drowsiness, dryness of the mouth, alteration in bowel habit and so on) and the time sequences of the drug's action. These should all be carefully explained to the patient. It is of the utmost importance that the patient should understand that imipramine is unlikely to lift the feelings of depression for some ten days, although the unwanted side-effects of the drug may be experienced before then; that if the pain of otitis media has not receded after twenty-four hours' treatment with phenoxymethylpenicillin, the patient should return to the surgery in order to have the medication changed; that the five- or ten-day course of antibiotics must be completed even though the symptoms of the disease have receded; that the control of diabetes mellitus involves a fine balance between the ingestion of food and the injection of insulin, and that the patient must be aware of the dangers of missing a meal, or the effects of an intercurrent fever. Information about long-term steroids or insulin should be recorded on a Medic Alert bracelet.

8. *The cause of any new symptoms in an established illness should first be looked for in the drugs which have been prescribed for that illness.* In this way, the vast majority of drugs prescribed for drug-induced symptoms or signs can be avoided.

9. *The addition of any new drug in the treatment of an established illness should always be preceded by a review of the current drug regime.* When a new drug is added, the question should always be asked: 'Would it now be possible to withdraw some of the current

therapy?' The problem of the multiplication of drugs is particularly acute in the care of the elderly, and geriatricians have stressed that the stopping of all medication often results in marked improvement in the health of the patient.

10. *Repeat prescriptions should be reviewed.* While being sensitive to the psychological contract implied by the repeat prescription, as already noted, there should be a policy of monitoring all repeat prescriptions and the doctor should be aware of instituting such repeat prescriptions, particularly of drugs of known or marked or cumulative toxicity. For those patients who require some form of continuing medication whose basis is psychological rather than pharmacological, inert or harmless substances should always be preferred. Small doses of ascorbic acid, simple linctus B.P.C., or a mild tranquillizer offered as an hypnotic may be acceptable.

11. *Frequent reference to the literature and a readiness to consult the hospital information pharmacist should be the rule.*

Method of administration

The route and frequency of administration of drugs are subjects which are often inadequately considered. There is evidence that many drugs are not prescribed in adequate dosage, or at appropriate intervals of time to ensure adequate blood levels throughout the twenty-four hours. There are some drugs which are better absorbed on an empty stomach, such as ampicillin, and others whose absorption is interfered with if they are administered with certain foods, such as tetracycline, the absorption of which is impaired if taken with milk. Yet others are less likely to produce side-effects if given with food: for example indomethacin or ibuprofen. Every doctor should study carefully the drugs he uses frequently and make sure that he is prescribing them correctly.

In addition to attaining the optimal pharmacological effect, the doctor's choice of administration may be influenced by other factors. Penicillin may be given by injection because rapid action is required. It may also be given in this way because the patient cannot be depended upon to adhere to regular oral therapy, either because of an unstable personality, forgetfulness often associated with old age, or with the harassment of rearing a large family. Some children are particularly unwilling to take drugs by mouth, and, while giving unnecessary injections to children is to be deprecated, it may sometimes be the only safe treatment.

Some drugs are administered inappropriately through ignorance. This is particularly likely to occur in the application of topical preparations to the eye, ear and skin. Careful instructions should be given to patients using them for the first time, and if possible the method of administration should be demonstrated by the practice nurse. Incorrect use is not only ineffective, but also wasteful.

Compliance with drug therapy is known to be notoriously unreliable. In treating short-term illness, treatment is often terminated once the patient feels better. When symptomatic remedies are being used this is appropriate, but its occurrence in antibiotic therapy may lead to relapse, and may facilitate the development of resistant organisms. In the long-term management of such conditions as hypertension, diabetes mellitus or heart failure non-compliance can be highly dangerous.

Compliance cannot be expected unless the patient understands the doctor's instructions. These must be communicated in language the patient can comprehend, and where appropriate some explanation of the mode of action of the drug may be helpful. The patient, for instance, who expects tricyclic anti-depressants to relieve his symptoms in the same way as aspirin relieves pain, may well be disenchanted with his therapy when no benefit has occurred within forty-eight hours, and indeed he has only the unpleasant side-effects of the drug added to his original symptoms.

The elderly often have difficulties adhering to drug regimes. Many of them suffer from a variety of conditions, and they are sometimes expected to take four or five different types of medication. If their memory is failing, if they have difficulty in hearing the doctor's instructions, or in reading the pharmacist's instructions, it is not surprising that they may be unable to follow a regime. In all age-groups it has been shown that therapy taken once daily is more likely to be adhered to than multiple administrations throughout the day, and this should be given careful consideration, particularly in the elderly. In some cases it is appropriate for the nurse or a relative to lay out the patient's drug therapy for a week in advance. The plastic trays used for making ice cubes in a refrigerator can be easily adapted for this purpose and greatly facilitate drug taking in the elderly.

Personal pharmacopoeias

It should be possible for each doctor to construct his own limited pharmacopoeia, and to reduce a seemingly bewildering complexity of choice to a few well-known and well-tried remedies.

Antibiotics

If one considers the possible range of bacteria, the different ages at which infection may occur, and the number of possible sites of infection, it seems unlikely that a small number of drugs may suffice. Yet this is probably the case. In general practice, for instance, antibiotics are used in the following:

1. Infections of the upper respiratory tract
2. Infections of the lower respiratory tract
3. Infections of the genito-urinary tract
4. Infections of the skin.

1. *Upper respiratory infections* in general practice are largely made up of sore throats and associated conditions, otitis media and sinusitis. If an antibiotic is indicated, the drug of choice is probably phenoxymethylpenicillin. In initiating treatment of a sick child procaine penicillin by injection may be indicated, in order to deliver a reliable loading dose. If oral penicillin is contraindicated because of suspected allergy, erythromycin may be substituted: the estolate is said to give higher blood levels than the base. There is some evidence that *H. influenzae* may be an important causative organism in acute otitis media in children. If phenoxymethylpenicillin has failed to relieve the symptoms within twenty-four hours, a change to amoxycillin is recommended.

2. The same antibiotics may be chosen for *lower respiratory tract infections* in children. In the case of chronic bronchitis a broad-spectrum antibiotic, particularly one which will affect *H. influenzae,* should be used. Of all the tetracyclines, oxytetracycline is cheap and effective.

Amoxycillin is a useful alternative. The tetracyclines should never be used in pregnant women or in children under the age of seven, when amoxycyllin is to be preferred. Co-trimoxazole is useful and relatively safe.

3. *Urinary-tract infections*. Nine out of ten infections of the lower urinary tract caused by bacteria are caused by *E. coli*. If a broad-spectrum antibiotic is needed, or if an upper urinary-tract infection is to be treated, trimethroprim, cotrimoxazole or ampicillin are the drugs of choice. Unlike respiratory infections, urinary-tract infections in general practice are often investigated for antibiotic activity. The three drugs mentioned will cover almost all eventualities, except perhaps recurrent urinary-tract infection in the elderly.

4. *Skin infections*. There are only a small number of skin infections which require treatment with antibiotics. Topical antibiotics are a potent source of allergy, and wherever possible (for example in the treatment of secondarily infected eczema) an antiseptic preparation such as povidone-iodine (Betadine) is preferable. Impetigo is best treated topically using fucidic acid 2 per cent or framycetin 0.5 per cent cream. Unless the lesion is very small and

localized, a systemic antibiotic like erythromycin or penicillin should be used. Pustular comedones in acne have been successfully treated with daily doses of oxytetracycline over two or three months, but the mode of action is not fully understood. Cellulitis requires vigorous treatment, and penicillin or erythromycin are the drugs of choice. Rarely in general practice the problem of penicillin-resistant staphylococci may be dealt with by switching to flucloxacillin.

With these antibiotics alone the general practitioner should be able to deal with almost all the infections which he meets. Of course, many other antibiotics will be prescribed for his patients, but these will be for conditions whose treatment is initiated in the hospital.

Psychotropic drugs

There are three symptom groups for which the general practitioner prescribes: anxiety, depression, and psychotic behaviour. Anxiety and depression are both a part of the experience of normal life, and the translation of these symptoms into the language of psychiatric diseases has been a matter of debate among psychiatrists, philosophers and sociologists for many decades. Howie's work[3] on the relevance of the prescription of antibiotics to the perceived, as opposed to the stated, diagnosis, has relevance also for the treatment of patients with psychotropic drugs. When the general practitioner prescribes an anxiolytic or an antidepressant drug he makes the statement that there is a chemical as well as a psychological and social component in the patient's symptoms. Like most treatment in general practice the treatment with psychotropic drugs is symptomatic treatment, and this is wholly appropriate given the present state of the art.

There is no reason why the general practitioner should require more than one minor tranquillizer, one or two major tranquillizers and three different antidepressants in his personal pharmacopoeia for the treatment of anxiety and depression.

The symptoms of anxiety, when they are not thought to be the manifestations of an underlying depression, can be well controlled with either diazepam or chlordiazepoxide. It is important however to bear in mind the fact that in some patients benzodiazepines may cause depression and may release aggression. It makes no sense to change from one of these drugs to another when there is a poor response, or to have recourse to other benzodiazepines, meprobamate, the barbiturates or any of the other miscellaneous tranquillizers. Anxiety is never simply a manifestation of chemical upset in the patient, and too much should not be expected from an anxiolytic drug. The enormous proliferation of these drugs in our society, proliferation both in the range of drugs and in the numbers prescribed, suggests a therapeutic desperation rather than a growth of the symptom to epidemic proportions. All anxiolytic drugs cause some side-effects — for example, drowsiness, faintness, palpitations, dry mouth, weakness and extrapyramidal effects — which may be misinterpreted by the clinician as further symptoms of anxiety. When the anxiety is thought to be a manifestation of an underlying depression, or when depression of mood is the major symptom, an antidepressant may be thought appropriate. It is a mistake to initiate treatment with both an anxiolytic and an antidepressant drug, or one of the proprietary combined preparations. Basically, the general practitioner will require only three antidepressant drugs: a non-sedative tricyclic, a sedative tricyclic and an M.A.O. inhibitor. In the first category imipramine is the drug of choice: in the second amitriptyline. Tricyclic antidepressants may cause a number of autonomic nervous symptoms, many of which mirror the symptoms of depression itself. In addition there is a particular problem with dosage. There is some evidence that metabolism of these drugs is genetically determined, since a ten-fold difference in blood levels can be found in different patients receiving the same dose. Very occasionally the patients with a clear history of depressive illness who do not respond to therapy need to have their blood levels monitored: this is unlikely to be practical in general practice and may require supervision from an appropriate psychiatric unit. The sedative tricyclics should normally be given in a single dose on retiring to bed, when they will have the additional benefit of acting as a mild hypnotic. The antidepressant effects of a tricyclic drug do not begin to manifest themselves until after the 10th to 14th day of treatment. If treatment with tricyclics fails, it may be worth exhibiting an M.A.O. inhibitor. Despite attempts to suggest that the symptomatology of a depression can be a reasonable guide to the choice of a drug between the two main groups, it is probably safer to suggest that in general practice the indication for an M.A.O. inhibitor is the failure of a tricyclic. Again one drug will suffice: for example phenelzine dihydrogen sulphate (Nardil). The two groups must never be given in combination, and strict instructions should be given to the patient about avoiding tyramine-containing foods during the ingestion of M.A.O. inhibitor drugs, and for some two weeks after the drug has been withdrawn. Patients taking M.A.O. inhibitors should carry a card stating that they are on the drug. The control of psychotic behaviour with the major tranquillizers will usually be initiated by a psychiatrist, and the general practitioner is likely to meet a wide variety of new drugs, often in combination. From the point of view of general practice chlorpromazine hydrochloride, whether by injection or orally, is perhaps the most useful preparation. An alternative, which has the advantage of causing less drowsiness but the disadvantage of sometimes causing marked extrapyramidal reactions, is trifluoperazine (Stelazine). In the treatment of senile agitation, promazine (Sparine) is said to have particular advantages. In the management of schizophrenia, depot injections of fluphenazine decanoate (Modecate) or flupenthixol decanoate (Depixol) are particularly valuable.

Because the symptoms of anxiety and depression and of psychotic behaviour are still so poorly understood in relation to the patient's physiology, the number of remedies developed is large and their actions uncertain. The overprescribing of psychoactive drugs is a major feature of modern therapeutics, both inside and outside hospital practice. The general practitioner should be slow to prescribe the psychotropic drug and should constantly be alerted to the need for a review of the patient's therapy. The offer of a psychotropic drug is often far less effective than the acceptance by the doctor of another person's human suffering, and often all that is offered to the patient are the unwanted effects of an inappropriate medication. The habit of reacting to the patient's persisting symptoms by hunting from one drug to another and experimenting with the use of combinations of drugs has nothing to commend it.

Steroid preparations

Of the three main pharmacological actions of corticosteroids — replacement therapy, pituitary suppression, and anti-inflammatory and immunosuppression — the general practitioner will normally be concerned only in initiating therapy with a view to the third action: that is the anti-inflammatory/immunosuppressive action. Among the diseases for which the corticosteroids may be prescribed by the general practitioner are allergic phenomena such as asthma (the most important instance of the use of systemic steroids in general practice), hay fever and acute urticaria; the collagen diseases: for example, rheumatoid arthritis (though the use of the steroids in rheumatoid arthritis is now frowned upon by most authorities) and ulcerative colitis.

Hydrocortisone is the naturally occurring corticosteroid, and is the drug of choice in replacement therapy. The anti-inflammatory and immunosuppressive action of the steroids is simply a gross exaggeration of the normal physiological action, and so these drugs must be given in many times the physiological dose. At therapeutic levels therefore there is always a danger of Cushingoid effects: oedema, hypertension, sometimes overt diabetes mellitus, muscle wasting, osteoporosis, atresia of the skin, with bruising, striae and major skin damage from minor injury, centripetal distribution of body fat, psychoses and sometimes epilepsy, peptic ulcer and glaucoma. The synthetic steroids have been developed in order to maximize the anti-inflammatory response and minimize the unwanted effects.

Many advantages are claimed for the fluorinated steroids in terms of the ratio of anti-inflammatory response to unwanted effects. Because the distribution of all the glucocorticoid and mineralocorticoid actions is different in each preparation, it is impossible to give simple dose equivalents between one and another. The general practitioner would do well to restrict himself to the use of prednisolone which has approximately five times the anti-inflammatory effect of hydrocortisone. The indications for systemic corticosteroids are dealt with in the relevant symptom chapters. The patient suffering from severe rheumatoid arthritis or ulcerative colitis may receive moderate doses of prednisolone (say 2.5 to 10 mg a day) for long periods of time. The general practitioner should exercise the greatest caution in initiating such a regime, and may well wish to have the advice of a specialist before taking such action. In monitoring the care of these patients, it is worth remembering that the normal defence mechanisms against infection are suppressed: at the same time the occurrence of some intercurrent infection will require an increase in the basal dose. Patients on long-term steroid therapy should be seen regularly, and the drug should not be prescribed for months on end by repeat prescription without consultation. Oedema, high blood pressure and the appearance of sugar in the urine should be watched for, and in patients on very long-term treatment an annual X-ray of chest and spine should be taken to exclude tuberculosis and osteoporosis. The patient should always carry a card which details the steroid prescribed, and the current dose, and should wear a Medic Alert bracelet.

One of the most important uses of corticosteroids in general practice is for the control of severe asthma and status asthmaticus. In this condition intermittent doses may be given when the attack becomes severe. On the first day an adult may receive 40 mg of prednisolone taken as one dose, and this may then be reduced by 5 mg a day over the succeeding week. In status asthmaticus much higher doses are needed, and a loading dose of 200 mg of hydrocortisone may be given intravenously. The use of betamethasone valerate in an aerosol is a most significant advance in longer-term treatment of severe asthma combining good control of asthmatic symptoms with freedom from steroid side-effects.

The use of intra-articular injections of corticosteroids is discussed in the relevant chapters. Intra-articular hydrocortisone is the drug of first choice, but on the rare occasions when repeated injections may be required a change of preparation to one of the newer fluorinated steroids may be useful when the effects of the intra-articular hydrocortisone wane.

Corticosteroids and the skin. – The use of steroids in topical applications to the skin has been one of the major advances in the treatment of eczema. Corticosteroid applications are also used, with more variable success, in the suppression of the active phase of psoriasis. In the latter condition there is often a 'rebound', so that the short-term gain is completely negated by an exacerbation of the condition.

For most purposes hydrocortisone ointment or cream with a concentration of 1 to 0.25 per cent is useful in eczema. Fluorinated corticosteroids are much more powerful and useful in the treatment of thick or dry lesions. Because of their liability to cause atrophy with striae and telangiectases fluorinated steroids should rarely be used for children, or on the face or flexures. In widespread eczema, particularly in children, fluorinated corticosteroids may be absorbed, with consequent damage from the systemic effects. Betamethasone cream or ointment made up in a concentration of 0.1 per cent may be used when a fluorinated steroid is required, but these concentrations may be further diluted by using buffered cream, B.P.C. for the cream, and white soft paraffin, B.P.C. for the ointment. When response to steroid cream is poor, there is nothing to be said for changing constantly from one to another of the many fluorinated steroid preparations. The so-called differences in response which dictate the preferences of doctors and patients alike is probably due to nothing more than a misinterpretation of the natural history of the condition in terms of response to a particular preparation.

In the treatment of inflammatory diseases of the eye corticosteroid eye-drops have only a limited use. There are so many dangers, for example exacerbating dendritic ulcers, herpes simplex or other viral infections, the precipitation of glaucoma and so on, that these drugs are best prescribed only on specialist advice. The use of eye-drops containing both a corticosteroid and an anti-infective agent has little to commend it, and these preparations should be avoided.

Corticosteroids are a group of drugs which dramatically illustrate the problems of modern pharmacology: they are powerful drugs, sometimes life-saving, sometimes life-enhancing, but their unwanted effects may be crippling or indeed fatal. Except when they may be vital to the preservation of life, and in general practice this situation is usually confined to the management of severe asthma, they should be a treatment of last resort. In systemic treatment, for example the treatment of rheumatoid arthritis in which aspirin is the drug of choice, they should be used only if no effective alternative can be found. In topical treatment, where the steroids have been an important advance in the management of eczema, hydrocortisone is to be preferred, in the first instance, to fluorinated preparations.

In summary, corticosteroids should only be prescribed with reluctance, and only a small number of preparations need to be used. In particular, because the different formulations of fluorinated corticosteroids differ in the distribution of their steroid action, it is impossible to give dose equivalents between one drug and another. For this reason it is positively dangerous for the general practitioner to use a number of different preparations, or to switch from one preparation to another without extreme caution. The smaller the range of drugs in this group used by the doctor, the less the danger that he will precipitate serious iatrogenic disease.

Conclusion

It should be possible for the general practitioner to construct a limited personal pharmacopoeia in relation to all the major drug groups. The doctor will always be under considerable pressure from the pharmaceutical industry to experiment with new preparations, and to use as wide a range of drugs as possible. He will be persuaded that to use a wide range of drugs is to have a flexible approach to the individual problems of his patients, and that to use the latest preparations is synonymous with being 'up to date'. The price that is paid for this sort of 'flexibility' and 'up to dateness' can only be a proliferation of the negative effects of valuable medicines. The optimum use of powerful therapeutic agents with a minimum of harm to the patient is the major challenge of modern therapy. This can best be accomplished by an economy of the number and the amount of drugs which the doctor habitually uses.

The management of the patient in general practice requires a response to all three aspects of the doctor's diagnosis – the physical, the psychological and the social. Indeed the only reason for making a balanced diagnosis is that the management should reflect such a balance.

References

[1]Wells, F.O. (1973): Prescribing barbiturates: drug substitution in general practice. *Journal of the Royal College of General Practitioners, 23,* 164.

[2]Balint, M., Hunt, J., Joyce, D., Marinker, M. and Woodcock, J. (1970): *Treatment or Diagnosis.* London: Tavistock Publications

[3]Howie, J.G.R. (1973); A new look at respiratory illnesses in general practice. *Journal of the Royal College of General Practitioners*, *23*, 895.

2.2 Immunizations and prophylaxis for overseas travel

J. J. C. Cormack

Vaccines and immunization procedures

The following are commonly used vaccines which may be administered by the general practitioner or his team, or about which he may be consulted:

Toxoids and killed vaccines	*Live vaccines*
Diphtheria	Measles
Tetanus	Polio (oral)
Pertussis	Rubella
Influenza	Yellow fever
Typhoid	BCG
Cholera	

The following points should be noted:
1. It should be routine practice, whenever vaccination procedures are to be undertaken, to have a supply of adrenaline 1:1,000 available for immediate intramuscular administration if (as very rarely happens) there is an immediate hypersensitivity or anaphylactic reaction.
2. An interval of at least three weeks should be allowed to elapse between the administration of any two live vaccines. If for any reason this is not possible, it is preferable to give the two vaccines simultaneously at different sites; if the vaccines are administered separately at a shorter interval there is a risk of immunological interference.

Contraindications

A. General contraindication to all immunizations:
Acute febrile illnesses, until fully recovered (afebrile upper respiratory tract infections without systemic upset are *not* contraindications)

Vaccine	*History or family history in a first degree relative of fits or epilepsy*	*Eczema*	*Hypersensitivity to:* *Eggs*[1]	*Rabbits*	*Penicillin*[2]	*Neomycin*[2]	*Streptomycin*[2]	*Polymyxin*[2]
Pertussis	×							
Measles			×			×		×
BCG		×						
Polio (oral)[2]					×	×	×	×
Influenza			×					
Rubella								
(Almevax and Meruvax)						×		×
(Cendevax)				×		×		×
Yellow fever			×			×		×

Notes

[1] Only a history of severe hypersensitivity to eggs (generalized urticaria or angioneurotic oedema) needs to be considered as a contraindication.

[2] Only extreme cases of hypersensitivity to these antibiotics need to be considered as contraindications.

Table I. — Specific contraindications to vaccines

B. Contraindications to live vaccines:

1. Pregnancy (except when significant exposure to serious conditions such as polio may outweigh possible risks to the foetus)
2. Malignant conditions such as leukaemia or Hodgkin's disease
3. Hypogammaglobulinaemia or other immunological deficiency states
4. Corticosteroid or immunosuppressive therapy

C. Specific contraindications:

Noted under specific vaccines, and in Table I.

Routine immunizations

First year of life (Three months, five months, nine months — six to eight weeks between first and second doses; four to six months between second and third doses)	Diphtheria, tetanus and pertussis (triple vaccine) Oral polio vaccine (Offer unimmunized parents course of polio vaccine)
Second year of life 13–18 months	Measles vaccine
School entry	Diphtheria and tetanus (double vaccine) Oral polio vaccine
10–13 years	BCG
11–13 years (girls)	Rubella vaccine
School leaving	Tetanus toxoid Oral polio vaccine

Table II. — The recommended timetable for routine immunizations

Although the suggested intervals between doses of the basic courses of DPT and polio vaccines are the optimum ones, if for some reason the basic course has been interrupted immunity will still be established by giving these omitted dose(s) at a later stage. In other words if a basic course is interrupted it can be completed without repeating the earlier doses.

Vaccine	*Specific contraindications*
Diphtheria	Standard diphtheria vaccine should not be administered to individuals over the age of 10 years: such individuals should be given

adult-type low dose vaccine. The Schick test, previously recommended for individuals exposed to a case of diphtheria, is now only recommended as a test of immunity in those likely to be exposed in the course of their work.

Tetanus	No specific contraindications. (*Note* Reinforcing doses of tetanus vaccine should not be given to individuals known to have received a booster dose within a year. For advice on the use of tetanus toxoid in patients with open wounds see the chapter 'The injured patient' — 3.76.) Apart from cases of injury boosters are only necessary at 10 year intervals.
Pertussis	History of convulsions or cerebral irritation; children with developmental neurological defects; a history of fits or epilepsy in parents or siblings; any severe local or general reaction to a preceding dose; parental objection after informed discussion. Pertussis vaccine should not be given during any febrile illness until the patient has fully recovered. Vaccine containing a pertussis component should not normally be offered after the age of 6 years. (*Note* Because of the serious morbidity and mortality which whooping-cough may cause in young infants, it is currently recommended that routine immunization should begin at the age of about three months. It is felt that this factor outweighs the theoretical advantage of a more fully developed antibody-forming system in the older infant.)
Polio (oral)	General contraindications to live vaccines (B. 1-4 above); gastro-intestinal disturbances including diarrhoea; individuals known to be strongly hypersensitive to penicillin, streptomycin, neomycin or polymyxin. (*Note* Advisable for travellers to areas outside Northern Europe, Canada, USA, Australia or New Zealand.) Adults requiring primary immunization should have a basic course of 3 doses at intervals of 4

weeks. Reinforcing doses are necessary every 10 years to maintain protection.
It is now recommended that when infants are given oral polio vaccine it should also be offered to the parents if they are unimmunized, in order to protect them from the risk (albeit a very small one) of contracting vaccine-associated poliomyelitis.

Measles	General contraindications to live vaccines (B. 1-4 above); individuals known to be severely hypersensitive to egg products, neomycin or polymyxin. A history or family history of convulsions or epilepsy is now considered *not* to be a contraindication to immunization; in such cases human immunoglobulin for use with measles vaccine should be administered simultaneously in a separate intramuscular site from that used for the measles vaccination.
Rubella	Pregnancy is an absolute contraindication to rubella vaccination and must be avoided for 12 weeks after vaccination. General contraindications to live vaccines (B. 1-4 above); 'Cendevax' contraindicated in individuals known to be hypersensitive to rabbits, polymyxin or neomycin; 'Almevax' and 'Meruvax' contraindicated in individuals known to be hypersensitive to neomycin or polymyxin.
BCG	General contraindications to live vaccines (B. 1-4 above); individuals with positive tuberculin reactions; local septic conditions and chronic skin conditions such as eczema. BCG vaccine must be administered intradermally and not (as with other vaccines) subcutaneously.

Non-routine immunizations

Vaccine	*Specific contraindications*
Influenza	Individuals known to be hypersensitive to egg products.

Yellow fever	(normally administered only at special centres) General contraindications to live vaccines (B. 1-4 above), individuals known to be hypersensitive to egg products, neomycin or polymyxin; infants under the age of 9 months. (*Note* Yellow fever vaccine is mandatory for travellers to certain areas in Africa and South America.) Re-vaccination is required at 10-yearly intervals.
Typhoid	Chronic illness. (*Note* Indicated for travellers to areas outside Northern Europe, Canada, USA, Australia and New Zealand. Two doses at 4 to 6 weeks' interval (minimum interval 10 days). Reinforcing dose if required at 3-yearly intervals.) A single dose of typhoid vaccine confers a useful degree of immunity, lasting up to one year.
Cholera	Chronic illness or severe reaction to previous cholera vaccination. (*Note* Indicated for travellers to sub-tropical and tropical Africa and Asia and the Mediterranean coast. Two doses at 4 to 6 weeks' interval (minimum interval 7 days). Reinforcing dose if required after 6 months.)

Less commonly used immunizations

Hepatitis A (HNIg)	Human normal immunoglobulin (HNIg) affords protection against hepatitis A (infectious hepatitis) and is indicated for travellers who intend to live or work in rural areas of poor sanitation in certain developing countries. Individuals who have hepatitis A antibodies do not require immunoglobulin. It is advisable to administer any required live vaccines (e.g. polio, yellow fever) at least three weeks before giving the immunoglobulin, which can interfere with the development of active immunity to live virus vaccines.
Rabies	Pre-exposure immunization with human diploid cell vaccine is recommended for

	certain laboratory and veterinary workers but *not* for routine prophylaxis for travellers abroad. General practitioners consulted about rabies prophylaxis should refer to a communicable diseases unit.
Hepatitis B	The vaccine for hepatitis B (serum hepatitis) is an inactivated preparation, and a course of three injections is recommended. It is indicated for certain health care and laboratory personnel involved with the handling of potentially infectious material, and renal dialysis patients travelling abroad. As there is an increased incidence of hepatitis B carriers among intravenous drug abusers certain police and ambulance personnel may request hepatitis B immunization. Decisions about recommending this extremely expensive vaccine are probably best arrived at after first checking that the patient requesting it does not already have hepatitis B surface antibody (or antigen) — if he does the vaccine is not necessary — and then consulting local colleagues before making the final decision.

Malaria prophylaxis

Malaria is widely prevalent in many parts of Asia, Africa and Central and South America. Travellers to malarial areas should be advised to take prophylactic tablets one week before departure, during their time abroad and for 6 weeks on return. At present it is recommended that chloroquine ('Avloclor', 'Malaviron', 'Nivaquine') 300 mg of base (i.e. 2 tablets) should be taken weekly. Problems are increasingly being caused by the emergence of resistance by *plasmodium falciparum* strains to chloroquine, particularly in India, South-East Asia, East Africa and South America. As the position is constantly changing it is advisable to consult the local Community Health Department in each individual case. Travellers to such areas are recommended to take Fansidar (pyrimethamine and sulfadoxine) one tablet weekly in addition to their chloroquine. Fansidar is contraindicated in pregnancy because of its sulphonamide content, and if a pregnant patient seeks advice prior to travel to a resistant area reference should be made to the Community Health Department or the local Infectious Diseases unit.

References

Department of Health and Social Security (1982): *Immunization Against Infectious Disease*. HMSO

Scottish Home and Health Department (1977): *Immunization Against Communicable Diseases*. Letter from CMO. SHHD/CAMO 77, 17

Lothian Health Board (1983): *Communicable Disease Newsletter*. Issue 9

3
The Complaint

3.1 The patient complaining of tiredness

Marshall Marinker and C.A.H. Watts

Fatigue is often presented to the doctor as an important symptom, but it is difficult to arrive with any confidence at a statement about its frequency. Dunnell and Cartwright[1] found that 16 per cent of adults reported having experienced 'undue tiredness' in a two-week period, women reporting this symptom twice as often as men. The 1981–82 Morbidity Statistics from General Practice[2] listed 'debility and undue fatigue' with a frequency of 12 persons per 1,000. This compares with 69 persons per 1,000 of the population who were labelled as suffering from some psychiatric disorder. As with most of the psychoneurotic illnesses, there were almost twice as many women as men. In most medical dictionaries tiredness is not even defined. To record it as the definitive diagnosis, or at least as the definitive statement of the problem, is to admit that the diagnostic process has led nowhere. The modest figure of 12 per 1,000 of the population represents the reach of such diagnostic honesty among the recording doctors in 1981–82.

Presentation

Precisely because fatigue is so much a part of everyday life, patients are often shy of making this their presenting complaint. The symptom is more likely to be hidden in the request for a tonic, or a wish to have a physical check-up. Because the word depression has been so much used by doctors in recent years, patients complain of depression when they mean that they feel tired, or tense, or unhappy, or suffering from any uncomfortable change in their mood or energy level. Because depression (see Chapter 3.3) may sometimes be amenable to dramatic improvement with drug treatment, the temptation to convert the symptom of tiredness to one of a depressed mood is great for both doctor and patient alike.

Causes

The basis for the symptom of tiredness can be sought under three main headings.

Physiological.– Tiredness following any form of exertion, be it mental or physical, is normal. Only the complaint to the doctor about such tiredness is abnormal. Indeed a state of exhaustion after a hard day's work, or the exertions of sport, or the absorption of watching a dramatic play or film can be deeply pleasurable. It is unusual for patients to complain of tiredness after such activities, but such a complaint may suggest unrealistic expectations of life in many of its aspects, and may hide more fundamental disappointments to which the doctor must remain sensitive. For the most part, however, the sense of fatigue is an unpleasant feeling. The uninhibited reaction of small children to tiredness, as they whine in their misery, demonstrates how uncomfortable it is. The popular conviction that if a child becomes 'overtired', he will be unable to sleep, perhaps reflects a recognition that his condition represents a considerable constitutional disturbance.

Tiredness can be caused by too much or too little stimulation. It can be brought on by 'burning the candle at both ends', and if this is the case the doctor may wish to look for the cause of this overactivity. Sometimes there may be a physical cause to account for it or a hypomanic temperament, but hypomanic patients rarely complain about their tiredness. Sometimes the overactivity is a defence mechanism, a way of coping with painful areas of personal experience. Often the overactivity can be explained by the mores of our competitive society. Certain categories are particularly vulnerable: the small shopkeeper; the self-employed craftsman; the single-handed farmer; the business executive and so on. A number of patients will be found to be 'moon-lighting'. That is to say they are holding down two jobs, one during the day and another during the evening or night. They may do this in order to overcome a temporary financial problem, or in order to save money for a holiday or a house. Such patients are not so much concerned with the complaint of tiredness as with the request for some sort of stimulant to help them continue their self-destructive struggle with the need to sleep. In the experience of most doctors it is the patient with some sort of executive responsibility rather than the heavy manual worker who complains of tiredness. For the factory worker, particularly one involved in repetitive manipulations, or long periods of inactivity, fatigue is the product of boredom.

The young adult and the elderly seem to need less sleep than those in the middle period of life. The whole picture is made much more complicated by the considerable differences between individuals in their expectations of work, their perceptions of fatigue and their beliefs about the right to complain to the doctor.

Energy output is also related to diet. In the long run dietary fads, both in relation to the quantity of food eaten and the type, may result in pathological changes such as anaemia or cachexia, but the general practitioner is more likely to encounter morning fatigue suffered by people who go to work without having eaten breakfast, or the diabetic patient who becomes hypoglycaemic.

Just as boredom can cause fatigue, so can a sudden upset in routine. Many people have noted the disappointing lack of vigour during the first few days of a holiday or, for that matter, immediately after it. A change in family routine can have a similar effect, as when grandparents take charge of grandchildren for a few days and are exhausted by the sudden change in the tempo of life.

Pathological.– Any physical illness lowers one's feelings of vitality. With diseases of insidious onset tiredness may precede other more tell-tale symptoms and signs like the thirst of diabetes mellitus, the pallor of pernicious anaemia, or the obvious stigmata (once the disease has been thought of) of myxoedema. Cancer in particular, often so slow to reveal itself until the damage is great, may present with fatigue alone. Yet precisely because fatigue is so common a human experience, and the search for an unidentified cancer so costly in time, money and anxiety, a knowledge that cancer can cause tiredness before any other symptom is more of a hindrance than a help in the diagnostic process.

Psychological.– Fatigue often accompanies feelings both of anxiety and of depression. The diagnosis and management of these conditions are dealt with in chapters 3.2 and 3.3. Sometimes it will be the presenting symptom of an emotional upset, of disturbed interpersonal family relationships, or of fears which cannot yet be expressed concerning the possibility of physical illness, future life events and so on. Occasionally, the process of ageing may be experienced as fatigue. Here the patient's expectations may not keep pace with the physical, psychological and social changes of human development. The middle-aged man who strives for the athletic achievements or the social patterns of his youth may in this way express an anxiety about sexual potency, physical disability – or dying. There are many ways in which the doctor is asked to supply the elixir of life and much skill is needed in bringing the patient to an acceptance of the realities of life, and the limited possibilities of medical intervention.

History and examination

Because fatigue can point in so many different diagnostic directions, the first consultation on account of fatigue may be prolonged. The nature of the tiredness should be defined. Is it pervasive, or does it vary at different times of day or in relation to different activities? Is the tiredness predominantly a mental symptom, a feeling of ennui, or is there marked physical fatigue? If there is muscular weakness, is this general, or confined to a particular group?

While the patient is talking, the doctor is observing the non-verbal cues, such as movement and facial expression. The search for causes concentrates first on the possibility of demonstrable disease, such as diabetes mellitus, myxoedema, pernicious anaemia, depression. Particularly in the elderly, there may be a multiplicity of physical conditions, giving rise to the tiredness. Important, in this connection, is the careful taking of a drug history. Much of the fatigue of which patients complain is the price that they pay for their previous medication, or over-medication.

Whether or not a physical cause of tiredness presents itself, the doctor should enquire about the life-style and habits of the patient, in order to determine to what extent these either cause or exacerbate the fatigue. The doctor must remain sensitive to any offers which the patient makes about disturbances of relationships, problems at work or at home, or anxieties about health, vigour, and death. This part of the history cannot be usefully taken by the catechism of direct questions. Michael Balint expressed the problem as 'the doctor who asks questions will only get answers'. To obtain this sort of history the doctor must create a permissive atmosphere in which the patient, if he so wishes, can begin to express feelings which he has previously hidden, perhaps even from himself.

A physical examination is most likely to be of help when in the course of the history the doctor has already picked up clues about the possibility of a disease process. Many doctors would include a routine examination of the blood to determine the erythrocyte sedimentation rate (E.S.R.), the haemoglobin and an analysis of the urine for protein, blood and sugar. There are many pitfalls. The finding of a moderately raised E.S.R. may be of no diagnostic help whatsoever, but may initiate in the pathology laboratory or the radiology unit a further fruitless search for diseases. Weight loss and tiredness suggest a physical disease. Weight gain and tiredness suggest boredom as a cause. Tiredness in the absence of weight loss, and in the presence of a normal ESR is unlikely to be caused by physical disease. The finding of a low haemoglobin may be important in itself, but research has shown a poor correlation between feelings of tiredness and the level of haemoglobin. Elwood and his colleagues[3] showed that there was no evidence to suggest that haemoglobin levels in the range 10 to 12.0 g per 100 ml were related to fatigue, nor for that matter to any of the other commonly regarded symptoms of anaemia. The finding of a low serum iron may be much more significant in explaining the cause of tiredness.

Precisely because fatigue can point in so many different directions, it is important not to jump to diagnostic conclusions. The finding of a physical disease process should not preclude a further search for other causes of tiredness. Nor should the complaint of an exacerbation of fatigue in a patient who is known to have a chronic marital problem preclude the search for a new and super-added physical cause. The commonness of the symptom and its peculiarly undifferentiated nature make perhaps the greatest demands on the diagnostic skills of the doctor.

Management

The management of the many disease processes which may be found is dealt with in other appropriate chapters of this work, and we will deal here briefly with just one relatively uncommon but nevertheless important condition, hypothyroidism or myxoedema. It is important in treating myxoedema, particularly in the elderly, to proceed cautiously, starting with a low dose of thyroxine in order to avoid precipitating angina, myocardial infarction or cardiac failure. An appropriate regime is to start with 0.05 mg thyroxine daily, increasing at monthly intervals by additional 0.05 mg doses up to a maximum total dose of 0.4 mg. The clinical features (sense of well-being, weight, pulse rate) and the biochemical response should be monitored monthly until the patient has become euthyroid, after which follow-up at infrequent (perhaps annual) intervals should be sufficient. If a patient should develop symptoms or signs of either angina or cardiac failure the dose of thyroxine should be reduced; clinical well-being is of far greater importance than biochemical euthyroidism.

Whether or not the disease processes causing tiredness can be diagnosed and treated, for the vast majority of patients who complain of fatigue there will be a need to readjust the life-style to changing events. Fatigue which accompanies the process of ageing, or which follows in the wake of major life events like the birth of a new baby, a sudden bereavement, the tiredness of chronic diseases, or the exhaustion which follows a severe acute illness, will require of the patient a readjustment of expectations and a change in behaviour. These changes will best be achieved if doctor and patient can successfully negotiate an agreement about the cause of the problem, and if the doctor can demonstrate that the advice which he gives actually does help. The process may be a prolonged one, and many consultations may be required (Chapter 4.1).

Finally, something should be said about the place of drugs. We know that so-called tonics have a negligible pharmacological effect, but they continue to exert a strong psychological effect on the patient, and it is interesting that, more than any other, this group of drugs continues to be supplied in the form of medicines whose taste, smell and consistency have a part to play. Provided that the doctor is aware of certain long-term dangers, for example the patient habituated to a tonic which may eventually cause bromism, the prescription of tonic medicines has a role in modern therapeutics. It is no longer timely to consider the possible uses of amphetamines. There has been so much adverse publicity about the unwanted effects of these drugs and about their social abuse that they are no longer considered a proper remedy for the relief of chronic tiredness. They belong with cannabis to Class B in the 1971 Misuse of Drugs Act, and are not now listed in the current *British National Formulary*. Nonetheless, the exhibition of small doses of amphetamine to a small minority of patients who were resistant to any other form of help, was once an important adjunct to the management of such patients in general practice. In the management of fatigue which results from sleeplessness the reader is referred to Chapter 3.16, and in the diagnosing of fatigue associated with depression to Chapter 3.3.

References

[1] Dunnell, K. and Cartwright, A. (1972): *Medicine Takers, Prescribers and Hoarders*. London: Routledge & Kegan Paul

[2] Royal College of General Practitioners, Office of Population Censuses and Surveys, Department of Health and Social Security (1986): *Morbidity Statistics from General Practice 1981–82*. HMSO Series MB5 No. 1

[3] Elwood, T.C., Waters, W.E., Greene, W.J.W., Sweetman, T. and Wood, M.M. (1959): Symptoms and circulating haemoglobin level. *Journal of Chronic Diseases*, *21*, 615

3.2
The anxious patient

Marshall Marinker

Feelings of anxiety are common in everyday life. Most often the cause of the anxiety is apparent: there is some sort of threat to the integrity of the individual, real or imagined. The young man about to take an examination or date a girl for the first time experiences this sort of anxiety, or it may be the patient presenting to the general practitioner with a lump in the breast. Sometimes the anxiety is free-floating; it seems to have no focus in a threat which the individual can recognize. What all anxieties have in common are a combination of: a rapid pulse, tense muscles, dilated pupils, sweating, often diuresis and increased gut motility. Physiologically, these symptoms are part of an adrenergic response to threat and prepare the body for either fight or flight.

Perhaps because anxiety is so much a part of living, it is particularly difficult to arrive at figures concerning incidence. Hodgkin[1] suggests a range of 56 to 120 persons per 1,000 NHS patients per year. The Third National Morbidity Survey[2] suggests 19 per 1,000 persons, with women affected twice as often as men. Because classically anxiety can present to the general practitioner with any variety of somatic symptoms, little reliability can be placed on any of these figures. They represent the sensitivity and perception of the doctor and not the validated incidence of presented disease.

Presentation

The acute anxiety state is a terrifying experience for the patient. Usually it is a brief, self-limiting condition, the patient having recovered by the time the doctor is called for. The sense of terror seems to be almost infectious, and members of the family may be very shaken by the episode.

More commonly, anxiety presents in a variety of somatic guises. It may mimic organic diseases like thyrotoxicosis and diabetes mellitus, or it may present with any of the symptoms of organic medicine. When the patient shows manifest anxiety, and the symptoms do not fit any recognizable physiological pattern, the diagnosis of anxiety state suggests itself early but, with the growth of medical sophistication in the lay public, the symptoms may closely counterfeit those of known somatic diseases like cardiac ischaemia. Indeed, if the mimicry is close and consistent, the diagnosis may permanently be left in doubt. 'I cannot find a physical cause for your symptoms. Perhaps we have to look elsewhere for an explanation . . .' is both less censorious and more honest than 'You do not have a disease. It must be your nerves . . .'

Anxiety must be looked for in every presentation to the doctor, who then makes a judgment about the appropriateness or otherwise of this anxiety. The anxiety of a woman with a lump in her breast or of a man with central chest pain is to be expected, and dealt with in the course of the consultation. This is a different sort of anxiety from that of the woman who palpates her breasts daily and creates a feeling of lumpiness by palpating the breast tissue between finger and thumb, or the man whose central chest pain is but the latest episode in a long series of somatic complaints organized around his fear of disease. It is one of the challenges of general practice that each new episode, however it is surrounded or motivated by anxiety, may also include a new and serious physical disease.

The general practitioner will come to recognize that certain body functions are particular targets for anxiety: for example, swallowing, defaecating and having sexual intercourse. Human relationships are often invested with a great deal of anxiety. Mothers may present their children time and again with complaints of minor fevers, or disturbances of behaviour, or sleeplessness, as an expression of their own anxiety about the maternal role. Marital difficulties and the problems of adolescence often present with the symptoms of free-floating anxiety. Sometimes the patient is aware only of a general feeling of dread, or simply uneasiness. Here the request for help may be non-specific – for a tonic or a check up or a few days off work because of tiredness.

Causes

There is still much controversy over the nature of anxiety. Although the physiological response is well recognized, there is disagreement about whether the feelings of anxiety cause the behaviours of anxiety, or whether the behaviours engender the feelings. Such theoretical problems have implications for behavioural therapy, but are not of immediate interest to the general practitioner. From the point of view of general practice, the classification of anxiety into the following three types[3] has clinical significance:

1. *External or objective anxiety.* Here the stimulus for the anxiety is recognizable in the real world. The individual may be threatened with loss of a job, or with some hazardous enterprise like a surgical operation. This is often a manifest sort of anxiety, and the stimulus can be identified without too much difficulty. If the external threat, however, is very frightening for the patient, there may be more resistance to facing the nature of the problem, and consequently much more diagnostic work will be required.
2. *Internal or impulse anxiety.* Most people are aware of hidden impulses, often angry or destructive feelings which it would be harmful or dangerous to express. As long as the individual feels confident that he can control these feelings there is no anxiety, but such may arise because the patient fears that he cannot control these, or other similar feelings. It can also arise because the individual fears that if he expresses his hostile feelings there will be some sort of painful retaliation. Impulse anxiety represents a fear of loss of control and a fear of retaliation. It is this type of anxiety which is presented by the mother who fears the destructive impulses she feels towards her own child, or her husband; by the young man, unhappy at work, who hates his boss but dare not show it.
3. *Moral anxiety.* Freud coined the term 'superego' to describe those functions of the mind that have to do with observation and judgment, and with reward and punishment. The superego 'punishes' by creating a sense of disapproval, a feeling that the individual has done something wrong. Moral or superego anxiety is a form of anticipatory guilt; it is experienced when the individual believes that he may do something, or may be tempted to do something, of which he thinks society will disapprove. Of course these so-called moral precepts by which the individual judges his own actions or impulses are not always rational. In psychoanalytical theory the superego is an internalized form of parental judgment, and stems from the earliest experiences of childhood. The strategies which the patient employs in order to deal with these anxious feelings manifest themselves as obsessional behaviour and the phobias.

Anxiety is concerned with two basic forms of fear. The first is separation anxiety, which in psychoanalytical theory is believed to have its origin in the experience of birth, in the physiological responses which result from the physical separation of the foetus from the mother. This sort of fear is concerned with helplessness, loneliness, loss of security, the danger of novelty. A classic example is so-called school phobia. Time and again the general practitioner may find that the problem of the absenting child is not a difficulty in the schoolroom, but intense anxiety at leaving the parental home, even for a few hours each day. The second sort of anxiety concerns fear of injury. In psychoanalytical theory, much concerned with sexual development, this is thought to have its prototype in the so-called castration anxiety of the child's oedipal experience. But one does not need to subscribe to any of these particular mythologies about human development in order to recognize that fear of injury is basic to many anxiety states.

In practice many of these modes of anxiety may appear at the same time in the same patient. A number of competing theories may approximately fit the clinical picture. A familiarity with biochemical changes, learning theory and pyschodynamic models allows the general practitioner a fairly flexible response to some of the most demanding clinical situations which he is likely to meet.

The history of an anxiety state is part and parcel of the therapy. The search for causes, the attempt to find a model for the patient's experience which explains what is happening, and allows him or her to come to terms with the symptoms, is intrinsic to the pyschotherapy of general practice. Particularly when the symptoms mimic organic disease, careful attention will be paid in the history and examination to those features which differentiate the anxiety from other diseases. For example, in the patient with thyrotoxicosis the tremor of the hands will be finer than that observed in anxiety. The hands will be warm and pink from the hyperkinetic circulation, not cold, pale and clammy as in anxiety. Even so, there will be many instances when doubt must remain, and here response to treatment may be a useful guide. History and examination, including electrocardiography, may alone not be sufficient to rule out the possibility of ischaemic heart disease in a chronically anxious patient. Failure to respond to the usual medication for these symptoms may, however, reinforce the diagnosis of anxiety, and later a positive response to anxiolytics may further reinforce it. But the doctor can never be altogether certain.

Management

The management of patients presenting with anxiety and its many somatic manifestations will be dealt with under four main headings: the doctor/patient relationship; psychotherapy; drug treatment; referral to psychiatrists, clinical psychologists or other colleagues.

The doctor/patient relationship. – A patient whose illness is rooted in feelings of fear or guilt will not be able to present his story, or to confess his feelings, unless the doctor is able to create an atmosphere of acceptance and support. There is much in medical education which has taught doctors to regard the patient with organic disease as a first class citizen, and the patient with an anxiety state as a third class one. There are many ways of transmitting this message to the patient: words like 'neurotic' are as much terms of abuse as they are diagnostic formulations, and it is painfully easy to wound the patient with an inflection of the voice or a dismissive gesture. The failure to identify an organic cause of the patient's symptoms, or a specific event or fear to account for the patient's anxiety, represents neither professional failure for the doctor, nor moral failure for the patient. The doctor who makes it clear to his patient that he has no time to listen to his feelings, or to discuss his fears, will not only fail to help the patient, but may spend many fruitless hours in the future chasing the illusions of somatic diseases. Even within the confines of a relatively fraught general practice consultation, the doctor should be able to allow the patient to express himself, to look for the words that he needs and the courage to utter them.

Psychotherapy. – William James said: 'We may philosophize well or ill but philosophize we must'. The same is true of psychotherapy. Only a minority of general practitioners will have had sufficient training to allow them to undertake psychotherapy in any depth. But to a certain extent all general practitioners are involved in psychotherapy, whether they do it well or ill. The object of psychotherapy, whatever its theoretical basis, is to give the patient some understanding of the strategies, particularly the inappropriate strategies, which he employs in order to cope with his anxiety. If he is able to understand something of the nature of his anxiety, then the level of his anxiety may go down. If he is able to understand something about the inappropriateness of his responses to it, then he may be able to change his behaviour so that it becomes less destructive or painful to him.

For the newcomer to general practice it is sometimes hard to see how so time consuming a process as psychotherapy can be adapted to 'the six-minute consultation'. In fact, because the short consultation in general practice is not an isolated event but part of a continuum, much good work can be done with these techniques. The reader is referred to chapter 4.1 and a number of useful texts.[4,5,6,7] There are several components of this so-called 'talking treatment' (although this is a misnomer because listening is more important than talking both for doctor and patient, and because the non-verbal communication in the consultation may be of greater importance than the words that are spoken).

First, there has to be an explicit *acceptance* of the patient's problem. The doctor must make it clear that he accepts the patient's illness, at least for the time being, on the patient's terms. The object is not simply to dissuade the anxious patient that he has a cancer of the bowel, or that it is stupid to be frightened to leave the house. The doctor must show that even if he has no belief in the reality of the cancer or the fear, he accepts the reality of the patient's feelings.

Next there must be a mutual *exploration* of the causes of the anxiety. The task of the doctor is to allow the patient to talk freely, but also to direct the attention of the patient to those matters which he or she seems unwilling to examine, or to point out obvious omissions. For example, a young man living at home may describe his relationship with a number of significant people in his life, but consistently omit any reference to his father. If the doctor notices this, then he may ask the patient to comment on it. Is there, for example, any reason why the patient finds it difficult to talk about his father? In this sort of treatment the patient is asked to do a great deal of work, and much of it may be painful. The object of the therapy is in part to discover something new about the self, and for the most part discovering something new about oneself means discovering something unpleasant.

It is now, when the work of exploration is under way, that the doctor may occasionally wish to make an *interpretation* of what the patient is telling him. The doctor must be cautious in making such interpretations, because they invariably increase the anxiety of the patient, and may accelerate the process of self-awareness. For this reason the doctor must be fairly confident of the interpretation which he offers, but extremely diffident in the way in which he offers it. In the case of the young man who does not mention his father, already quoted, there may be evidence from the patient's story that, although he feels very strong love for his father, he is also terrified of him and frightened of never being able to live up to his expectations. The probing of this sort of area must be very gentle. Something like 'You make him (your father) sound rather a formidable man', might be an appropriate sort of observation and the non-verbal response of the patient may tell the doctor much more than the words that he uses in replying, or avoiding making a reply.

Very occasionally tentative interpretation may need to give way to something stronger. The doctor may need to attempt a *confrontation* when the consultation gets stuck. Confrontation must always be firm, but should never be accusatory. For example, still using the model of the young man who does not mention his father, the doctor may say: 'Several times this morning I have invited you to say something about your father, but I notice that you do not like talking about him. Would you like to tell me why?'

When the patient's feelings about someone, or something, can only be approached after this sort of confrontation, the doctor must expect a great deal of strong and often distressing emotion to be released. If the doctor is to open this sort of Pandora's box he must be prepared for the consequences. It is also important to stress that if the patient continues to defend himself and refuses to explore further, the doctor must respect the patient's autonomy. but he must also make his acceptance of this explicit: 'I have to accept that you don't want to talk to me about this. Let's move on . . .'

Psychotherapy must never be destructive. It is only too easy to discover the fears, the weaknesses, the fragile defences of the patient. What must be looked for assiduously are the strengths of the individual, his or her creativity and potential for growth. Basic to the tenets of counselling is the idea of *beginning again*.

The method outlined is based on psychodynamic theories of human behaviour. Other treatments based on learning theory have been outstandingly successful for certain sorts of problems, in particular some of the phobias and obsessional behaviours of the anxious patients. There are two basic techniques. The first is concerned with rewarding 'good' behaviour, that is the sort of behaviour which the patient wishes to or needs to achieve, and withholding reward or approval of the patient when he or she exhibits the unwanted behaviour. The second technique is described as desensitization. Here the patient is introduced in a gradual and non-threatening manner to increasing doses of whatever situation induces anxiety. In a manner analogous to the desensitization of the patient to allergens, the patient is gradually taught to tolerate what was formerly intolerable. Most often, these techniques will be more appropriately used by other colleagues, for example psychiatrists or clinical psychologists, and appropriate referral will need to be made.

Drugs. – Anxiolytics can be an important adjunct in the treatment of anxiety, and are sometimes needed as a prerequisite to a psychotherapeutic approach. If there is too much anxiety learning cannot take place. If, however, the patient is too tranquillized, if the doctor is too assiduous in chemically annihilating moderately or mildly anxious feelings, there will be no motivation on the patient's part to co-operate with the doctor in changing things. There is a wide choice of so-called minor tranquillizers, but it is recommended that each doctor should prescribe from a limited range of drugs with which he has become familiar: the reader is directed to the section on psychotropic drugs in chapter 2.1. If the anxiety is a manifestation of an underlying depression, then it is recommended that a sedative tricyclic preparation, such as amitriptyline be used, rather than a combination of tricyclic drug and anxiolytic. For the drug treatment of insomnia the reader is referred to Chapter 3.16.

It is best if the minor anxiolytics are regarded both by doctor and patient alike as neither a cure nor a maintenance therapy, but rather as an aid to management. Inevitably there will be a number of instances when the patient becomes habituated to these drugs. For some, whether the mechanism is pharmacological or psychological, life without tranquillizers is simply intolerable. When this happens, and the patient is established on a long-term repeat prescription, the doctor and his staff should be at pains not to punish the patient for the profession's bad conscience. Long-term dependence on minor tranquillizers is not necessarily either a sign of moral laxity on the part of the patient, or a sign of professional incompetence on the part of the general practitioner. Nonetheless, on most occasions, the minor tranquillizers should be prescribed for short periods of time, and ideally some sort of 'contract' should be entered into with the patient. The patient is given to understand that the prescription is for a limited period, and is only a part of the doctor's management of the problem.

Referral. – If the condition is severe, or fails to respond to the doctor's management, the doctor may wish to refer to a consultant colleague. Every referral carries with it some message of rejection of the patient. Occasionally the general practitioner will wish the psychiatrist to deal with the problem, not because it is necessarily outside his competence, but because he can no longer stand the strain or distress of looking after a particularly trying individual. This is a legitimate reason for referral, provided that the general practitioner makes clear in his letter the nature of the problem – not only the patient's but his own.

Although most general practitioners believe that they can identify a small group – the most often quoted figure is 10 per cent – of patients who are frequent attenders and give rise to an inordinate amount of work, consulting rates are in fact continuously distributed within a practice population, and the identity of frequent attenders changes over the years. That is to say that the frequent attender of this year is not likely to be a frequent attender in five years' time. But over long periods of time, perhaps two or three years, the anxious patient can make considerable and apparently unreasonable demands on the doctor's time. In the real world there is always a limit to how much time a particular general practitioner can devote to a particular patient. When a patient's demands become inordinate, the doctor has to ask himself whether there has been a serious attempt to tackle the underlying cause of the patient's anxiety. Even when such serious attempts have been made, it is not uncommon to get stuck, to have little more to offer than support, drugs and time. In such circumstances the doctor must make it clear to the patient that there are limits to what is reasonable, and some sort of contract must be entered into. The doctor will promise to give a certain amount of time, and a certain amount of support, *but no more.* It is a serious disservice to the patient to promise more than can reasonably be given.

References

[1] Hodgkin, K. (1973): *Towards Earlier Diagnosis.* Edinburgh: Churchill Livingstone.

[2] Royal College of General Practitioners, Office of Population Censuses and Surveys, Department of Health and Social Security (1986): *Morbidity Statistics from General Practice 1981–82.* HMSO Series MB5 No. 1

[3] Hodge, J.R. (1975): *Practical Psychiatry for the Primary Physician.* Chicago: Nelson Hall

[4] Balint, M. (1964): *The Doctor, His Patient and the Illness.* London: Pitman

[5] Balint, M. and Balint, E. (1961): *Psychotherapeutics in Medicine.* London: Tavistock

[6] Balint, E. and Norell, J.S. (1973): *Six Minutes for the Patient.* London: Tavistock

[7] Browne, K. and Freeling, P. (1976): *The Doctor-Patient Relationship.* 2nd Ed. Edinburgh: Churchill Livingstone

3.3 The depressed patient

Marshall Marinker and C.A.H. Watts

Depression is a relatively common diagnosis in general practice. In the Third National Morbidity Survey[1] the total number of depressive disorders reported was 17 persons per 1,000, of whom only 0.8 persons per 1,000 were regarded as having an affective psychosis. Reactive depression, that is to say a lowering of mood in response to some life event, is a relatively common human experience. Dunnell and Cartwright[2] noted that 21 per cent of adults recording symptoms over a two-week period reported feelings of 'nerves, depression or irritability'. Women recorded these symptoms twice as often as men and the Morbidity Survey shows that women patients have consulting-rates for depressive neuroses more than three times higher than men patients. Even so, it is clear that only a small proportion of individuals who experience a lowering of mood actually report this to the doctor.

One of the difficulties in arriving at any firm conclusion about incidence or prevalence is the wide range of diagnostic criteria which doctors use in diagnosing depression. for example, Watts[3] suggests a rate of 12 to 15 per 1,000 persons suffering from depression. Hodgkin[4] reports some 19 persons per 1,000 suffering from endogenous depression and 20 per 1,000 suffering from reactive depression. Such figures must be interpreted in the light of the findings of Kessel and Shepherd[5] that psychiatric morbidity rates reported from a number of general-practice surveys showed vast differences in the rates recorded. For example there were three-fold differences in studies of the percentage of patients at risk, ten-fold differences in studies of the percentage of patients consulting and fifteen-fold differences in studies of the percentage of complaints or episodes. Although these studies were carried out in different general practices, and the criteria for diagnosis varied from one study to another, the large differences in rates suggests that what we are looking at are differences in the perceptions and beliefs of doctors, rather than differences in the morbidity of populations.

Presentation

For the general practitioner diagnosis is important only in relation to judgments about the prognosis and decisions about management. From this point of view arguments about whether the biochemical changes in depression are the cause or the consequence of altered mood are not of great consequence. In relation to each patient who is diagnosed as being depressed, however, the doctor has to decide whether some form of psychotherapy or counselling alone is sufficient, whether to prescribe an antidepressant drug, whether or not there is a risk of suicide, or whether the help of a consultant psychiatrist is needed either urgently, or in the near future.

It has become almost a shibboleth of modern psychiatry to assert that mental illness must not be diagnosed by the exclusion of physical illness alone. Yet the exclusion of physical illness in a patient who presents with a depressed mood remains of great importance. As with so many other problems in general practice, the difficulty is to decide how far the doctor ought to go in his exclusion. If, however, a patient presents with a depressed mood, and there is little else in the history or appearance of the patient to suggest a concurrent disease, the diagnostic process will be aimed at the discriminating features of depressive illness.

A major difficulty is presented to the doctor by the wide variety of symptoms which psychiatrists believe to belong to the criteria for depression. For example, W. Parry-Jones[6] describes the following classical psychological changes in depression: lowered mood; difficulty in thinking; loss of interest; delusional ideas; hallucination and depersonalization. He describes the following classical physical changes: sleep disorders; weight loss; constipation; reduced libido or sexual potency; disturbance of menstrual function. Indeed, writing about the concept of a masked depression, he suggests that depression may be looked for whenever the patient presents with somatic complaints for which there are no demonstrable physical signs, or when there are atypical features in established physical illness, or when the patient presents with what he describes as neurotic reactions or changed patterns of behaviour. In a series of 486 cases, Watts[3] listed some 71 presenting symptoms. It is of interest to note that pain occurred in 35 per cent of the cases. Depression can sometimes present with intractable and unexplained pain and this clears up dramatically when the depression itself is treated.

Psychotic depression.– Classical psychotic depression is a rare disease these days. Once psychotic levels have been reached, the illness is unmistakable. The patient may be retarded, slow in speech and movement, or he may be agitated, pacing the room like a caged animal, muttering his anguish. Often when depression has reached this stage, the patient is beyond tears. Some have frank delusions: they may claim to have committed some unforgivable sin and are full of self-denigration. More difficult to detect is the patient who is convinced that he has a cancer or some other lethal disease. In such instances early diagnosis is crucially important since such patients may be suicidal.

Non-psychotic depression.– The patient may present overtly with depressed mood, or with the symptoms of anxiety, or with a variety of somatic complaints. There is no easy guide to the differentiation of the patient with an organic disease who feels depressed, and the depressed patient with the symptoms of organic disease. Indeed enquiry about the mood of the patient, and the emergence of a classical picture of depressed mood, early morning wakening, constipation or general retardation, do not exclude the possibility of other concomitant diseases. If the somatic symptoms are ominous, for example altered bowel habit or persistent pain, further investigation of the patient is indicated. On the other hand, if the symptoms remain vague, if there is no other support for an alternative diagnosis and the patient is responding to treatment for depression, it is unwise and unkind to subject the patient to an exhaustive search for alternative (somatic) diagnoses.

Most often acute observation of the patient is the key. The doctor who wastes the precious few minutes of the general-practice consultation in writing the medical record or the prescription without observing the patient's face and gestures while the history is being related will inevitably miss many cases of quite florid depression. Sometimes the depression which the patient is feeling, and the tears which may go with it, will only be elicited if the atmosphere of the consulting-room permits it.

Anxiety is by far the most common disguise of a depressive state. Watts[3] suggests that the patient over 30 years of age who presents with anxiety for the first time is probably depressed, and the patient who presents over the age of 50 years is almost certainly depressed. Severe anxiety amounting to agitation is almost certainly a masked depression.

The physical changes of depression may themselves suggest organic disease. Loss of appetite and weight, bowel sluggishness and distention, a rapid pulse and sweating may thus mimic an intestinal obstruction or thyrotoxicosis.

A number of behavioural changes should alert the doctor. A persisting debility, or unwillingness to return to work after a viral infection such as influenza or hepatitis should suggest the possibility of a depressive illness. Depression after childbirth is well recognized, and can reach psychotic levels. More

commonly the mother who becomes agitated because she cannot establish successful breast feeding, or the woman who presents with frequent anxieties about the health of her infant, or who avoids the postnatal examination, may well be masking a depressed mood. The outrageous behaviour of the manic patient is easily recognized; but depressed patients can also present with disorders of behaviour. The patient who suddenly presents with heavy bouts of drinking, or shoplifting or unusual sexual behaviour may well have an underlying depression.
Finally, it is worth remembering that the insidious onset of forgetfulness and physical slowness in old people may not always be accounted for by senile dementia alone. Often there is also a basic depression, and this may well respond to psychotropic drugs.

Causes

Terms like endogenous and exogenous depression are so imprecise, that a taxonomy based on cause is still not possible. Indeed many causes may be present in the same case. It is, however, important to recognize the wide variety of causes which may be present, and for that matter know something about the theoretical models of depression, so that in the management of the depressed patient, the doctor may be able to address himself to the physical, psychological and social factors involved.

Diseases.– Almost any significant disease can cause a concomitant depression. The most commonly recognized is influenza, which can cause a quite severe disturbance long after the viral infection has itself resolved. Myxoedema and carcinoma are other important causes.

Drugs.– Depression is a not uncommon iatrogenic symptom. The most notorious among the drugs which cause depression are reserpine and methyldopa: these drugs act by altering the metabolism of serotonin and the catecholamines, but many drugs, including some of the tranquillizer group, can retard the patient and make him feel depressed.

Constitution.– There is some evidence that a predisposition to depression is genetically determined. Depression is commoner in people with a pyknic body build and also in obsessional self-critical and self-driving persons. In practice the doctor may be aware of a family pattern of depressive illness but it is difficult to determine what is due to nature and what to nurture. Certainly there are many individuals whose natural response to life is a pessimistic one, and whose disposition is gloomy even when they are not clinically depressed. Such patients can be recognized by the marked depression which the doctor experiences while they are consulting him.

Psychological models.— There are several theoretical models of depression deriving from psychoanalytical literature. The most important concepts are those of loss of self-esteem, and the internalization of guilt feelings. Freud describes depression as an introjection of anger which the patient cannot otherwise express: at its most extreme the experience of this introjected aggression results in suicide.

Social models.— Depression may be potentiated by any one of a number of life crises, or significant life events. Most often these events involve either loss or change. Puerperal depression, and the depression of the menopause and of old age are obvious examples: the fact that there may be, indeed probably are, concurrent biochemical changes does not invalidate the social model. Bereavement, resulting either from death or separation, can lead to a profound depression. Browne[7] has provided one of the most convincing social models. Looking at psychiatric disturbance among women he suggests that there are certain vulnerable groups including women of low social class who are at the stage of life when there are children living at home. Depression is potentiated by some severe life event or major difficulty, and this is amplified by having no full-time or part-time employment, or having three or more children under the age of 14. The early loss of the mother is thought also to be such an amplifying factor. These social factors are thought to precipitate depressive episodes. Of particular interest is the finding of a protective factor: this is an intimate and caring relationship, a confidante relationship, rather than a sexual one, with either a husband or friend.

Management

The wide variety of causes of depression gives some clue about management. The patient suffering from depression, no less than the patient suffering from a fractured femur, must be treated in a way which recognizes the physical, psychological and social components of his condition.

This short chapter cannot encompass the theory and practice of counselling and psychotherapy. It is, however, important to point out that whether or not the general practitioner decides to employ drugs, or to refer the patient to a consultant psychiatrist, an appropriate handling of the psychological aspects of the problem is essential. This means that he must be prepared to accept the patient's expression of misery, and, if it is appropriate and the patient allows it, must be prepared tactfully and sympathetically to explore the painful areas of the patient's life.

It is important to establish whether the patient has had ideas about suicide, or an intention to commit suicide, both to gauge the depth of the depression and to help to release some of the guilt the patient may feel about having such ideas or intentions. Such questions as 'do you ever feel when you go to bed that you wouldn't care if you didn't wake up?' or 'are there times when you feel like ending it all?' or 'have you ever tried to end your life?' are worth asking.

The reader is referred to Chapter 3.2. This sort of approach should never be of a probing confronting kind; neither is it necessary for the general practitioner, if he has not had the appropriate training, to employ an interpretative psychotherapeutic role. Indeed, questions of training aside, an interpretative or probing therapy can be very destructive for some depressed patients and may lead to an exacerbation of the situation.

In most cases, when the depression is clearly established, or when there is no response to a non-pharmacological approach, the doctor may decide to prescribe antidepressants. Drugs of the tricyclic group should be tried first (see pp. 92–94). Imipramine is a non-sedative and amitriptyline a sedative tricyclic drug: the choice must depend on the amount of agitation present, and the desirability of sedating the patient. The sedative action of the tricyclics appears in the first day or two, while the antidepressant activity is not noticeable until about the tenth day. The most common mistake in prescribing is to opt for inadequate doses for an inadequate period of time. A major problem, too, is that of non-compliance. The tricyclic drugs may cause a number of unpleasant symptoms: for example drowsiness and dryness of the mouth. The depressed patient whose self-esteem is low is unlikely to be highly motivated to stick to his treatment. He will therefore need to be encouraged, and perhaps to be seen fairly often early on in the treatment. Most authorities suggest that the drug treatment should continue for at least six weeks and probably for three months — even though the symptoms may have resolved much earlier.

Monoamine-oxidase inhibitors (M.A.O.I.) have recently become unpopular because of the severity of unwanted effects: high blood pressure with occasional cerebrovascular accidents. This hazard can be avoided if the patient is given careful instructions concerning dangerous foods and other drugs including self-medication. If tricyclic antidepressants fail, then it is certainly worth trying the patient with an M.A.O.I. (see pp. 93–94).

There is little to be said for the prescription of anxiolytics: although they may control the symptoms of anxiety which overlie the depression, they are themselves depressing. They should be exhibited only when anxiety is the major feature, and is distressing the patient.

Early referral for a consultant opinion may sometimes be urgent. The following categories of patients should probably be seen by a consultant psychiatrist: the severely psychotic depressed patient; the suicidal patient; the patient who has failed to respond to therapy; the depressed patient who is living alone, and, of course, those patients who may be suffering from a depressive illness, where the diagnosis is still in doubt. Decisions about electroconvulsive therapy and the long-term administration of lithium will be taken by the psychiatrist.

It should be remembered that, even though the mortality from this illness is small, the general practitioner with an average size list can expect that within a period of four years one of his patients will successfully commit suicide. Perhaps more significantly, a great deal of morbidity can be caused in other members of the family by the depressed patient. The working-class mother of children under 14 years is particularly at risk, and so are her children. Referral to the social worker early on in the management may therefore be crucial.

References

[1] Royal College of General Practitioners, Office of Population Censuses and Surveys, Department of Health and Social Security (1986): *Morbidity Statistics from General Practice 1981–82*. HMSO Series MB5 No. 1

[2] Dunnell, K. and Cartwright, A. (1972): *Medicine Takers, Prescribers and Hoarders.* London: Routledge & Kegan Paul

[3] Watts, C.A.H. (1966): *Depressive Disorders in the Community.* Bristol: John Wright

[4] Hodgkin, K. (1973): *Towards Earlier Diagnosis.* 3rd ed. Edinburgh: Churchill Livingstone

[5] Kessel, N. and Shepherd, M. (1962): Neurosis in Hospital and General Practice, *Journal of Mental Science*, *108*, 159

[6] Parry-Jones, W.Ll. (1973): 'Masked' depressive illness. *Update*, *6*, 491

[7] Browne, G.W. (1976): Social Class and Psychiatric Disturbance Among Women. Seminars in Community Medicine, Vol. I, p. 49. London: Oxford University Press

3.4 The mad patient

Michael Courtenay

Madness, like anaemia, is a concept open to such diversity of interpretation that any attempt at definition may not only be unhelpful, but positively restricting. Psychiatrists are no better at definitions and setting limits than the medically unqualified.[1] There is a willingness in society to accept unusual behaviour as normal. The less privileged members of our society may be prepared to accept quite eccentric behaviour as being normal, but once these limits are over-stepped the person concerned will be rejected, even though he is seen to be 'sick'. More educated people tend to notice psychiatric disturbance earlier, but reject the sick person less. These attitudes are important as it is often the relatives or neighbours of the 'mad' patient who complain to the general practitioner, rather than the patient himself. With this in mind the general practitioner must be very circumspect about labelling patients as mad, since by so doing he may not only be unhelpful but may be putting the therapeutic prospects in jeopardy. The admission of a patient to a mental hospital confers on the patient the clearest label, and, although this may be acceptable to doctors, the patient's peer group may not share this acceptance.[2] With regard to social class Hare[3] has shown that the incidence of schizophrenia rises as the social class declines, while the incidence of manic-depressive psychosis increases proportionately to the rateable value of the house in which the patient lives.

It may seem therefore that we have total chaos, surrounded as we are by lack of definitions, difficulties in diagnosis and pressures from society. This situation is, of course, the normal one for a general practitioner in any context. There is, however, one advantage in having few formulae for diagnosis and treatment with regard to the mentally disturbed, and that is the necessity of examining each person as an individual in relation to his own body, thoughts, feelings, family, background and community. It is a most fruitful field of patient-oriented medicine.

This lack of definitions has not altogether inhibited attempts at studying the epidemiology of mental illness. Admissions to mental hospitals have continued to rise. Estimates based on the admission data for 1964 to 1969 suggest that one-in-nine men and one-in-six women were likely to be admitted to a mental hospital at some point during their lifetime.[4] The only major comprehensive study in this country of mental disorder in general practice was made in 1960–61 by Shepherd and his colleagues.[5]

Presentation

It must be emphasized that there is no 'global' description of a psychotic illness which can apply to, say, schizophrenia, mania, and organic psychosis. The distinguishing features of these divisions will be considered in the next section, but in general a psychotic condition is a measure of the degree of disturbance rather than an entity in itself. We know this from our common speech when people are considered 'mad with rage' or 'madly in love'. So even in florid cases the distinction between sanity and madness is not always as simple as it might seem, and the context may be crucial.

A man may be diagnosed as psychotic when he kicks the television tube in because of a disagreement with his father as to which programme to have on, but only in the event that this incident brought to light that the family had kept this man at home a year without consulting the doctor, after he had given up his good job, stayed in bed half the day and collected rubbish for a continuous bonfire in the back-yard. On the other hand, the diagnosis may be inappropriate in a woman who breaks every window in her house and throws her husband's things out of them, even though she had been admitted to hospital for a puerperal psychosis years before, because this behaviour was not particularly outrageous in the context of a marital row, and of the couple's subculture of which this incident formed a part.

Classically, the distinction has rested on how much insight the patient has into his condition, but even this ground is treacherous as patients with developing schizophrenia (and rarely in developed cases) have a curious 'double insight' into their condition.

The complaint which is difficult to evaluate provides the main challenge to the general practitioner and can be fascinating as well as challenging. A patient may, for instance, attend to have his ears syringed. He may go on to describe that on a recent business trip abroad he had found his personal effects in his hotel room had been disturbed, and he was suspicious that he had been the target of industrial espionage. The story may be entirely coherent and plausible as told in the context of our cloak and dagger world. It may become apparent, however, when pursuing the conversation that the network of suspicion ranges far and wide and finally it emerges that the crucial piece of evidence in the hotel bedroom had been his discovery of a soiled handkerchief which had confirmed his suspicions. The diagnosis may only be confirmed as a conversation occurring at an apparently banal consultation reveals serious thought disorder and paranoia.

Causes

The causes of the psychoses remain obscure. The incidence world-wide is pretty uniform, though there are a few local names for types which do not seem reported elsewhere.

There is some disagreement about the criteria for the diagnosis of *schizophrenia*, which seems more common in the USA and the USSR, probably because of the disagreements. The debate continues between those who consider it to be due to biochemical factors based on a genetic predisposition, and those who consider environmental factors, albeit dating back to infancy, as of crucial importance. Clearly organic factors can produce a psychotic illness. Recent research suggests that abnormal dopamine metabolism in the brain is associated with schizophrenia, while other biochemical changes have been observed in depressed patients.

Manic-depressive illness seems to have a hereditary factor, and it is not uncommon to find more than one schizophrenic patient in a family, but the variables are so great that the essential factor, if there is one, is elusive. In recent years the exponents of the environmental theory have studied the effect of mothering and even of the effect of the fabric of society. Whether the attitudes of schizophrenics are causes or results of the illness in the child seems difficult to determine.

From the standpoint of the family doctor it is perhaps only necessary to be aware of the familial aspects of psychotic breakdown until further research throws more definite light on the etiology of the more common varieties.

History and examination

Because psychotic conditions vary with the type of illness, the history and examination are largely determined by the initial clues which are brought to the doctor's attention; inevitably this will involve a further study of the complaint in a more specialized way.

A new case of *schizophrenia* will only be seen by a general practitioner on average about once every three years. There has been a lot of discussion about premonitory symptoms, and the concept of pre-psychotic schizophrenia has been postulated.[6] The occurrence of non-specific symptoms in the early stages is well recognized, and can include almost any psychiatric disturbance. Particularly common are irritability and restlessness, but the picture can be confusing with the appearance of depressed mood, hypochondriasis and withdrawal, suggesting a depressive illness, often associated with a reduction in the patient's usual performance at work and leisure.

The difficulty is to detect the specific symptoms among the non-specific. Intense withdrawal, lack of emotional involvement with others and a preoccupation with self are suspicious, but not pathognomonic. Such behaviour is often due to an impairment in perception and concentration which puzzles and bewilders the patient. Some general remarks that make it clear the doctor is aware that the patient is in difficulties and has some understanding of them may encourage the patient to talk about his experiences which he may then report in delusional terms. Alternatively the patient may think that the interference in his concentration is that others are deliberately altering or putting thoughts into his mind by artificial means (e.g. through the television set), while his perceptual disturbance may lead him to think that people are not what they seem or are really other people in disguise. It is at this point that the characteristic 'double-insight' of schizophrenia is common. The explanations of his experiences take on a variation both in type and degree of certainty, and he constantly wavers in his choice of what is real.

A definite diagnosis must be based on positive evidence of abnormal perception and thinking, as judged by the patient's own account and the reports of relatives and friends. It must never depend on vague concepts such as 'the quality of rapport' or 'blunting of affect' as these are too subjective to be reliable, and easily give rise to false positives and false negatives. The difficulties of diagnosing schizophrenia are so great, and the implications so far-reaching for the patient, that a psychiatric opinion in a suspected case is virtually obligatory at some stage, the urgency being the subject of the practical decision.

Full-blooded *mania* reactions seem rare in Britain today according to Anderson and Trethowan.[7] Hypomania is fairly common, and sometimes follows treatment of a depressive illness with antidepressant drugs. It is often difficult to evaluate whether a patient is well or 'better than well', as, after coming out of his depressive episode, he will say that he has never felt so well in his life.

The diagnosis may be masked by a disturbance of behaviour which on the surface appears acceptable but, if his previous personality is known, it may be realized that the patient is more active and over-talkative than usual. Elation is not invariably evident, however, and the patient may be sulky and uncommunicative, and it may be inappropriate behaviour that gives the signal, like the girl who came into the surgery knitting two sweaters at once. Or like the civil servant who walked about the consulting-room in an agitated fashion, name-dropped ministers of state throughout the conversation and spread his official papers all over the desk from his brief case in the course of requesting help to set the country to rights. His wife had previously telephoned to say he was coming and described the difficulties with which she was coping at home.

Depressive illness is common. The high incidence and prevalence as seen in general practice pose problems in themselves, because the severity is sometimes difficult to assess. In a culture where suicidal attempts are increasingly common, the patients who are quietly and determinedly preparing suicide can easily be missed. Even if a grossly retarded patient is now a rarity, the capacity of a depressed patient to hoodwink the doctor and closest friends and associates in preparing to end his or her life is well known to general practitioners and psychiatrists.

The wide spectrum of depressive illness presents perhaps the greatest single diagnostic challenge in the general-practice setting. Although mood change is common, all the classic depressive symptoms of sleep disturbance and diurnal energy variation with loss of performance may be present without any subjective feeling of sadness, let alone despair. There may be some difficulty in thinking, particularly with regard to making decisions, and the thoughts are often painful, involving loss of self-esteem, and deprecatory ruminations over past actions.

On the other hand, depressed patients often become very self-centred, and tend to dwell on their symptoms and problems. They appear to feel that they are entitled to as much of the doctor's time as they want, regardless of the needs of his other patients or his other responsibilities. In spite of the obvious distress that the depressed patient feels, and the hopelessness about the future which pervades his whole outlook, the very intensity of the distress and the self-centredness together may place too great an emotional burden on relatives, friends and the doctor. Difficulty in coping with everyday tasks is perhaps the most characteristic feature. Everything becomes a burden, from dressing in the morning to making the simplest decisions or undertaking the easiest tasks. Anxiety may mask the underlying depression at first contact and is a potent cause of diagnostic error. The patient may complain of irritability with others and also express a loss of interest in almost everything.

Physical symptoms are also prominent and still contribute to the substantial under-diagnosis of depressive illness in practice. Fatigue and bodily pains, with changes of appetite and digestive functions, as well as menstrual and sexual difficulties, can all occur in depression. On the other hand, it is probably wise to do an erythrocyte sedimentation rate on all patients in whom a diagnosis of depression is made, as many organic conditions may present with an apparently depressive picture.

Recurrent mood swings in a patient, with hypomanic episodes, will alert the doctor to recognizing that manic behaviour may lead to a breakdown in the patient's social context, which may in turn lead to the necessity of urgent admission, whilst on the other hand the swing towards the depressive pole may be sudden and severe, and so increase the risk of suicide.

Organic psychosis is less common, but in young people manic, aggressive states may be due to drug abuse, usually with amphetamines or LSD, or rarely with marijuana. In elderly people nutritional deficiencies, (mostly of the vitamin B group), degenerative brain disease or cerebral neoplasm, or even infection may lead to psychotic states. These can present with minor forgetfulness, such as leaving spectacles on items of furniture and then not being able to find them, progressing to a belief that someone is hiding the spectacles deliberately. There may also be a tendency to repeat the same stories incessantly and to mutter to themselves while going about household tasks, and finally becoming confused with disorientation for time and place. Alternatively, there may be progressive withdrawal, accompanied by irritability when help is offered, and finally unusual behaviour such as going out into the street in night-clothes.

These people are to be distinguished from that curious group who appear to be unclassifiable, though they may develop paranoid states. They have been called 'God's oddies': a label which will have meaning to most general practitioners. They are generally well accepted by their neighbours, though seen to be eccentric, and walk along the street talking to the air. They do not seem to be depressed, cope fairly competently with the ordinary business of living and seek no medication apart from simple remedies for constipation and the like. They often seem to want to see the doctor frequently for a while, and then disappear from the surgery for years at a time.

Childhood psychosis should very rarely be diagnosed in general practice and any very disturbed child should be referred for a specialist opinion.

Autism is now widely recognized as a congenital disorder affecting certain aspects of brain function. It is normally first diagnosed at about two years of age because it usually presents as a disorder in speech development. The essential characteristic of the abnormality is, however, a lack of response to other individuals. The affected child becomes cut off from its environment. Such children are often thought initially to be blind or deaf. Some lie for hours in the cot or pram without taking any notice of their environment and are thought by their parents to be 'good babies'. Others, however, are constantly grizzling or whining but quite unresponsive to what goes on around them. Most autistic children are mentally retarded but a few are of above average intelligence.

Schizophrenia can present in teenage children. They often appear isolated from their friends and may fail to achieve their educational potential.

Depression is relatively common in children. This disorder is often missed by school teachers because the depressed child is usually undemanding. In contrast, the anxious child may seek attention and consume a great deal of the teacher's energy. It is important to recognize depression in childhood because it will not only interfere with the child's education but in some cases may lead to suicide attempts. In Japan, child suicides have reached almost epidemic proportions. This is particularly due to the very competitive educational system, but should be a warning to Western societies where teenagers are often exposed to enormous educational pressures as a result of parental ambition.

Management

If, as happens occasionally, a patient, owing to confusion, delirium, paranoid panic, or some other acute psychotic state, is wildly unco-operative then nothing short of force may be required. Here the golden rule is to have a sufficient number of persons to hand to deal adequately with the situation. Otherwise an unduly severe or prolonged struggle may bring harm both to the patient and to those who attempt to control him. It should not be forgotten that most mentally disturbed patients tend to use force only when frightened. In this respect they differ little from normal people. Initially therefore there should be no suggestion of force, and with due regard for safety the patient should be interviewed alone or in the presence of one other person, preferably a trusted relative. If,

following this, forcible action has to be taken, an attempt should always be made to explain clearly and simply what course of action is proposed and why. Deception is to be avoided at all costs, even in the case of those who are so disturbed as to appear unable to comprehend what is going on.
Apart from force, sedation will often be needed. If so, sufficient should be given, for too small a dose may do no more than make a bad situation worse. On the whole barbiturates and paraldehyde are best avoided. The latter, though relatively safe, is unpleasant and it should be remembered that, although given by injection, it cannot be sterilized and also dissolves plastic syringes unless used immediately after drawing up. Drugs which are safe and effective are chlorpromazine (100 to 300 mg) injected intramuscularly, or haloperidol (5 mg) given intramuscularly or intravenously. In older people parenteral chlorpromazine may produce a fall in blood pressure and should be used with caution on this account.
Compulsory admission to hospital can be affected only under the provisions of the Mental Health Act, 1959. Except in dire emergencies, a psychiatrist should be asked for a domiciliary consultation, and in any case agreement by a hospital to admit the patient under Section 26 or 29 should be sought: if there is time for the consultation then admission will proceed under Section 26 with the assistance of a social worker (usually with special training and experience), an ambulance and crew and the police if a struggle is thought likely. Often, however, the doctor and social worker with the help of a relative are all that are needed in the event. Urgent admission can be effected under Section 29 (Section 24 of the 1984 Act in Scotland) which obviates the need for a second doctor (psychiatrist or approved medical practitioner with special experience in the diagnosis and treatment of mental disorder). Administrative convenience should not be the reason why this Section is invoked, especially as experience shows that, given tactful handling, many of those admitted under this Section could have been persuaded to accept informal admission. It has been said, however, that those on the receiving end may sometimes doubt the need for urgency unless the patient is admitted under some form of compulsion, and also because some patients discharge themselves after informal admission because of the initial shock of entering a mental hospital.

Conclusion

The incidence of psychotic breakdown is low, although recurrences in a given patient may be common. The diagnosis can be obvious in a florid case but may be difficult in the early stages, especially in schizophrenia. There should be a low threshold of referral. Urgent action to achieve admission is necessary in a high proportion of cases, and this needs skill as well as community resources, in addition to help from the patient's family.

References

[1] Mechanic, D. (1969): *Mental Health and Social Policy*. Englewood Cliffs, New Jersey: Prentice Hall

[2] Dohrewend, B.P. and Kolo, L. (1969): *Urban Challenges to Psychiatry.* Boston: Little, Brown

[3] Hare, E.H. (1956): Mental illness and social conditions in Bristol. *Journal of Mental Science*, *102*, 349

[4] Hill, G.B. (1972): *The Expectation of Being Admitted to a Mental Hospital. Psychiatric Hospitals and Units in England and Wales*. (Department of Health and Social Security, Statistical and Research Report No. 4). HMSO

[5] Shepherd, M., Cooper, B., Brown, A.C. and Kalton, G.W. (1966): *Psychiatric Illness in General Practice*. London: Oxford University Press

[6] Mears, A. (1959): The diagnosis of prepsychotic schizophrenia. *Lancet*, *i*, 55

[7] Anderson, E.W. and Trethowan, W.H. (1973): *Psychiatry*. 3rd ed. London: Baillière Tindall

3.5
The confused patient

Cyril Josephs

Mental confusion is difficult to define, even though most people know what it means. In a fairly loose context, it implies a state of mind in which those notions persons ordinarily have of their relations with time, place and their own personalities become less clear. The degree of confusion may be such that the inhibitory effects of higher cerebral centres are removed and the person so affected displays varying degrees of agitation and excitement, and true insight may be diminished or lost. Hallucinations and delusions may occur.

It is important to differentiate between confusion and dementia: the two words are all too often regarded as synonyms. Apart from the woolliness of thought implied in the assumption, there is a greater and more practical danger. *Dementia* implies the mental deterioration which occurs with advancing years. There is usually chronic diffuse structural damage and atrophy of brain tissue: such organic changes may be hastened by concurrent disease such as advanced arteriosclerosis. Dementia is usually slow in onset, likely to be static or progressive and to be unaffected by treatment. The demented patient is often apathetic, fatuous or euphoric. *Confusion,* on the other hand, is often of rapid onset and short history; it tends to fluctuate and the patient is often fearful, apprehensive or bewildered. It may be eminently responsive to treatment, and recovery may be complete, depending on the cause.

Either condition can and does occur separately; both can and do occur together. The demented person will often be confused: the confused person will often not be demented, or may have a degree of dementia which is so slight that he is able to 'get by' when not under too much pressure. Failure to recognize this difference in diagnosis is a common reason why a confused person may be given sedatives and hypnotics with a subsequent worsening of the condition. Treatment may easily be diverted from that of the cause to how best to dispose of a seemingly hopeless mental case.

It is necessary only to think how grossly confused a person can be when very drunk, even to the point of being hallucinated.

with complete recovery after the alcohol has been eliminated, to appreciate the reversibility of such confusion. Despite the foregoing, deciding whether a patient is suffering from dementia or confusion is often difficult or impossible, particularly when dealing with an elderly person. The diagnosis may only be made with hindsight. Nevertheless it is important to keep an open mind, to understand some of the causative factors affecting each condition, and to be prepared to change the diagnosis as the picture unfolds. By applying these precepts, the practitioner can often improve the state of mind of a patient to an unexpected degree: a most gratifying result.

The commoner causes

It is useful to differentiate between those causes which operate in the younger age-groups and in the old. Whilst there can be no hard-and-fast dividing line between these groups, and some of the causes must necessarily be common to both, the management by the family doctor is likely to differ between them. He is more likely to seek specialist help and advice earlier when dealing with a young patient. Old people easily become confused: indeed any illness in an old person is likely to cause confusion which can be so marked as to mask the underlying cause.

Causes in the younger age-groups

Toxic confusional states may occur when the cells of the cerebral cortex receive some physical injury. This may be due to anoxia, electrolyte disturbances, hormonal imbalance, or hypoglycaemia. It may be due to an accumulation of drugs, notably the amphetamines, sedatives, tranquillizers, and steroids. Hallucinogenic drugs (such as LSD) and alcohol are examples of drugs taken for pleasure which commonly cause confusion. In children, confusion may be due to acute infections, particularly if hyperpyrexia occurs. Such causes as lobar pneumonia, particularly if apical, and acute pyelitis, should be borne in mind. Direct involvement of the brain tissues by an infective process such as occurs in encephalitis, meningitis, abscess, or by a tumour may present with confusion. Concussion after head injury and the confused state following a major epileptic fit may present diagnostic problems if the preceding insult is not known. Psychotic syndromes, particularly those of schizophrenia and mania, often cause confusion.

The diagnosis of these conditions depends largely on obtaining as full a history as possible and carrying out a careful physical examination. The treatment is, in the main, directed at the cause, though occasionally sedatives may be needed during the acute phase. In many of these cases, specialist help will be obtained and often the patient will be treated in hospital as an emergency.

Causes in old people

There are several important causative factors of a general nature which contribute to confusion: an understanding of these will stress why confusion so often occurs in old people.

The brain as a vulnerable organ.–

(a) The brain is particularly vulnerable to anoxia. A sufficient supply of oxygen to the brain depends on heart function, an adequate amount of haemoglobin in the blood, efficient pulmonary function and the integrity of the sinoaortic and spinal baroceptor reflexes. The rigidity of the arteries tends to increase with age, so causing decreasing efficiency in those reflex mechanisms which respond to stretch of the arterial wall. It is common to have more than one factor existing simultaneously.

(b) Minor disorders of cerebral function are more likely to cause apparent functional disturbance than would such a degree of impairment in other organs.

(c) Even minor chemical changes in brain cells are likely to produce marked changes in function.

(d) With advancing years it is likely that relatively frequent episodes of ill health will occur: these will give shorter intervals for recovery of damaged brain cells.

Inadequate external stimulation.– Even a perfectly healthy young person needs stimulation from outside sources to preserve his orientation. Removal from external stimuli will inevitably cause confusion sooner or later. Experiments have shown that an individual suspended in a motionless, sound- and light-proof tank becomes disorientated. Similarly, everyone is familiar with the difficulty of remembering the day of the week when on holiday, when the normal daily routine is broken. Without newspapers, radio and the like, relative confusion is common.

A lady, aged 83, lived alone in a flat overlooking a main road. From her dining-room window she could see children crossing the road each morning before nine o'clock to go to school. There was a greengrocer's stall near where the children crossed.
When the greengrocer was shut and no schoolchildren appeared she knew it was Sunday. A bank holiday always caused confusion and when the greengrocer closed his stall down for good, the old lady became severely muddled.

Particularly important in this context are the senses of sight and hearing. With increasing age the field of vision may become more restricted. Familiar objects, situations and people become less obvious, and mistaken identities with consequent incorrect conclusions occur with increasing frequency. Complete blindness presents a considerable hazard, particularly if of relatively sudden onset.

> A man of 90 years had a mature cataract in one eye and developed sudden blindness in the other eye due to a thrombosis involving the retina. This left him blind, and he became severely confused and could not walk. It was decided to risk removing the lens with the cataract. This was done successfully, and the man was returned to his home soon after the operation. He was able to see with one eye and appropriate spectacles. Within twenty-four hours of regaining vision he became rational and walked with the aid of a stick.

A more potent source of confusion is impaired hearing. The need for external sounds is not always appreciated until they are removed. Everyday sounds experienced while going about the daily routine are of great importance for orientation. Deafness is probably a greater handicap than blindness. One of the cardinal differences between human beings and animals is their ability to communicate by direct speech. Thus deafness easily produces confusion: particularly does it ostracize the sufferer and cause paranoid feelings. He tends to become garrulous because he hears his own voice best. He tends to become antisocial, limiting his contacts to those he can hear more comfortably. As outside noises diminish, auditory hallucinations replace them adding greatly to the degree of confusion. Fortunately, complete deafness is relatively rare in those who have been born with hearing.

Limitation of physical activity. — As infirmity increases, less activity is undertaken and the whole pattern of life becomes restricted. What used to be a commonplace situation may become a relative rarity; and an unfamiliar situation may produce unusual responses.

Changes in routine and in surroundings. — An old tree does not like to be uprooted and transplanted. Neither does an old person. It is remarkable how often confusion follows the move from home to hospital or to a residential home.

> A man in his eighties was admitted to a large residential home to give his family an opportunity to go on holiday. The man suffered from mild Parkinsonism but seemed otherwise lucid and cheerful. Within a few days of his admission he became very confused and wandered about aimlessly by day and by night. He gradually improved and was back to his normal self just before his return home. Within days of joining his family he again became confused, settling down again as he grew familiar with his surroundings.

If the intellectual reserves are poor, even a simple change such as a change of bedroom or furniture can confuse.

Loneliness. — Being left alone for long periods, particularly if the life pattern is somewhat restricted, may cause confusion. This is especially liable to happen if the loneliness is produced suddenly, as occurs with the death of a spouse. This is a common hazard made worse by the normal depression which accompanies grief. The death of a dear friend, particularly when frequent meetings were the rule, can have a devastating effect as can the death of a beloved pet.

Hypothermia. — Isolation in the elderly exposes them to the risk of hypothermia during periods of cold weather. This frequently causes confusion which in turn may lead them to respond inappropriately to the cold so that rather than turning on further heating they sit inertly in an armchair and may ultimately die in this situation.

Drugs. — Old people tend to have multiple diseases and it is common to find them taking many drugs. There is probably no drug which cannot confuse the elderly, unless perhaps it is completely inert. The list of common offenders is long and the danger is that it is all too easy to add yet another drug to treat confusion not realizing it is iatrogenic in origin. The barbiturates, at one time a common cause of confusion have been superseded by the benzodiazepines of which the longer acting ones e.g. diazepam and nitrazepam are the worst offenders. If these drugs are needed in the elderly, lorazepam or temazepam are safer alternatives. Diuretics, by causing potassium deficiency, hypotensive drugs by causing cerebral ischaemia, and benzhexol used in treating Parkinsonism may all cause confusion. The phenothiazine group of drugs may interfere with temperature regulation and contribute to hypothermia. A special word of caution regarding the danger of digitalis seems appropriate. It is a most useful drug and is often needed. It tends, however, to accumulate in the blood, particularly if renal function is impaired, as is so often the case in the elderly. Over-dosage commonly causes confusion. The doctor may be misled if he relies on the pulse rate as an indication of toxicity, because, while it is true that digitalis initially slows the heart, toxic levels may cause tachycardia.

> An old lady with chronic heart failure for which she had had digitalis for years became confused and the heart rate increased. The dose of digitalis was increased and the heart rate carefully checked at frequent intervals. As the rate increased, so was the digitalis. Finally, when all else failed the drug was stopped. After several days the heart rate returned to normal and the lady recovered physically and mentally.

The toxic effect of digitalis is increased when the potassium in the blood is low: e.g. due to diuretics or diarrhoea, or in the presence of a low plasma calcium.

Old people may need several drugs given concurrently but the drug regime should be regularly revised and drugs discontinued when no longer needed. It is surprising how often the physical and mental state is improved by stopping all drugs.

Finally, it is important to remember that alcohol is a drug which is a powerful confusing agent. Over-indulgence is not the prerogative of the young or of the male. The elderly, prim lady living alone and becoming more confused may have a drinking problem.

> An old lady living alone in a downstairs flat became increasingly garrulous, confused, querulous and ataxic. Extensive investigation in hospital suggested the diagnosis of cerebral tumour but as she improved in hospital she was returned to her home with the original diagnosis in doubt. Recurrence of the original state of weakness and confusion prompted a further search for a cause. The diagnosis was finally made when the upstairs neighbour suggested looking in the dustbins, where numerous red wine bottles were found — all empty.

Physical illness. — It is true to say that any physical illness can cause confusion in old people: this may be the presenting symptom and mask an underlying extracerebral cause. It is useful to consider an old person's mode of life as akin to living in a house built from a pack of cards. The structure may appear sound from the outside, but take one card away and the whole edifice begins to totter, showing weaknesses on all sides. Thus an old man may have managed reasonably well to cope with a fairly humdrum sort of life until some traumatic experience occurs which upsets every aspect of his existence. The effects are out of all proportion to the magnitude of the physical or mental disturbance and certainly in no way comparable to the effects likely to occur when a like abuse attacks a young and robust person.

Among the commoner physical causes of confusion are:

(a) *Strokes.* The diagnosis is relatively easy if paralysis occurs, but the mild stroke may not be so obvious.

(b) *Infections*, particularly those of the respiratory and the urinary tracts. Without fever, the diagnosis may be missed and it is common enough for pneumonia to be unsuspected until well advanced, the presenting symptom being mental confusion. Just as fever, from whatever cause, can precipitate a fit in a young child, so it may cause confusion in an old person.

(c) *Coronary thrombosis.* The sudden fall in systolic blood pressure may lead to confusion in the absence of the characteristic symptoms.

(d) *Deteriorating cardiac failure.*

(e) *Cerebral tumour* and other intracranial space-occupying lesions. Confusion in these cases may be of gradual onset and variable intensity over a period of time.

(f) *Respiratory failure.* This is a profound cause of cerebral anoxia.

(g) *Myxoedema.* Usually this presents with slowing of the thought processes and general sluggishness, but occasionally it presents as confusion varying from mild to severe degree.

An old lady became gradually confused. This was thought to be due to an underlying dementia until it was noted that she was unusually quiet and apathetic. The diagnosis of hypothyroidism was suggested by the slow relaxation phase of her deep tendon reflexes (a particularly useful sign in old people). Thyroid function tests confirmed the diagnosis and soon after receiving thyroxine she recovered remarkably, becoming active and quite lucid.

(h) *Diabetes mellitus.* Diabetic hypoglycaemia or ketosis may cause confusion. Even though the capillary blood sugar is relatively high, the patient may have hypoglycaemic confusion. This is probably because the brain has got used to a high level of sugar. Thus, long-acting hypoglycaemic agents, such as chlorpropamide, must be used with caution in old people. The shorter-acting glibenclimide is safer. Mild diabetes is probably best treated by diet alone.

(i) *Anaemia.* Whatever the cause or type, anaemia may cause mental confusion.

An old man, hitherto of lucid nature, was found wandering about at night and behaving most oddly by day being both muddled and agitated. When he passed black stools the diagnosis of intestinal haemorrhage was made. The most likely cause was ingestion of aspirin. Correction of the resultant anaemia produced rapid improvement in his mental state.

A striking example of cause and effect was afforded by a lady with aplastic anaemia who received transfusions at intervals. The degree of confusion was a good guide as to the need for transfusion.

(j) *Vitamin deficiency.* Low levels of vitamin B_{12} or of folate may cause confusion, even without anaemia or spinal cord degeneration.

(k) *Tissue necrosis.* Large haematomata, gangrene of the extremities, bedsores, and fractures of large bones may cause confusion in an old person: probably due in part to absorption of toxins and to worsening of physical disabilities.

It can thus be seen that it will often not be possible to pinpoint a single cause for confusion in an old person. Multiple factors will often be at work and it needs perspicacity, experience, and some ingenuity to elucidate the cause.

Alzheimer's disease. — This is now thought to be one of the

commonest causes of dementia, especially in the elderly.
By definition (and in the International Classification of Diseases), dementia beginning before the age of 65 is termed presenile; after 65 it is termed senile. To differentiate Alzheimer's dementia in those over 65 from other senile dementias it is now commonly called senile dementia of the Alzheimer type (SDAT).
The history is of an insidious onset with early loss of insight and a steadily progressive deterioration, which is particularly rapid in the presenile form. The brain shows a pathological shrunken appearance with widespread loss of nerve cells particularly in the cortex.
Interest in Alzheimer's disease has been stimulated by the recent discovery that there occurs a reduction of choline acetyltransferase and acetylcholinesterase in the cortex, particularly in the hippocampus. Since cholinergic systems are linked with learning and memory it seems logical to treat Alzheimer's disease by replacing the deficient acetylcholine in some way, very similar to replacing dopamine in Parkinsonism. Indeed, there may be a link between the two pathologies since many old people exhibit both conditions. Unfortunately, the position is further complicated by the fact that treatment of Parkinsonism is often with dopaminergic or anticholinergic drugs which themselves may produce confusion. Confident diagnosis of Alzheimer's disease is not easy, during life, but its importance lies in the implication that the dementia may be treatable to a degree, as is Parkinsonism. Preliminary attempts at increasing the acetylcholine by giving choline and lecithin have so far produced impressive improvement in only relatively few cases. Likewise, trials designed to activate directly the muscarine receptors e.g. acetylcholine and physostigmine, have improved test scores in only a few patients. It seems likely that more molecular research is needed to fully understand the pathogenesis of this disorder and lead to a real therapeutic breakthrough.

History and examination

It is important to realize at the outset that 'confusion' is not a diagnosis in the sense that it refers to a specific pathological process: it is but a 'symptom of illness'. As full a history as possible should be taken from the patient, and his relatives and friends. Particular note should be taken of the onset of the symptoms and whether or not there have been similar episodes in the past, and, if so, under what circumstances A worth-while history may be difficult or impossible to obtain where no close contacts are available. Such recent hazards as moving house, bereavement, illness, accident – anything which has caused a change in circumstances – may signpost the cause. The enquiry must take note of drugs and drink. Particularly any new drug therapy should be suspect.

Since diagnosis really embraces the whole field of medicine, the physical examination is most important. In the elderly confused patient a good case may be made for routine blood examinations including estimations of urea, folate and vitamin B_{12}. An examination of the urine should always be done: without this, late-onset diabetes mellitus may be missed.

Sometimes it may be useful to enlist the help of a consultant geriatrician or psychiatrist. Should the patient be so confused as to be unmanageable at home, or where insufficient support is available in the house, admission to hospital will be necessary, though this should not be lightly advised because a confused patient may be made worse by removal to strange surroundings. It may be a justifiable risk, however, if the intention is to elucidate the cause of the confusion by further intensive investigation.

Treatment and management

Treatment is largely that of the cause. Management will depend on the severity of the confusion and the facilities available. Thus a relatively mild degree of confusion in an old man living alone in poor circumstances and in poor general health with no family or neighbours to help may call for immediate admission to hospital, whilst a more severely confused old man surrounded by a devoted family and living in a cosy house may be manageable in his home. It is important, however, to be aware of the real extra strain that confusion brings to the attendants: it can be an intolerable burden to the most loving spouse and relatives and the devotion normally afforded by the family group may suddenly give way to rejection, particularly if the confused state is prolonged or the behaviour is particularly objectionable or embarrassing.

On occasions the onset of confusion in an old person may constitute an emergency in general practice. A visit is requested, often at night, to an old person who has suddenly begun to behave in a highly irregular and possibly reprehensible manner. He may suddenly become a danger, usually to himself rather than to others, and be found wandering aimlessly at large. Prompt action by the practitioner may appropriately be requested. The choice of action usually lies between immediate sedation or admission to hospital, depending on such circumstances as have been described earlier.

Drug treatment of confusion. — There is undoubtedly a place for drugs in the treatment of confusion: the cardinal rule is to use the smallest amount necessary to produce the desired effect and for the shortest time practicable. There are many drugs available. The practitioner is well advised to limit his selection to a few with which he is familiar rather than to try every new one as it comes on the market.

When restlessness is the prominent feature, the phenothiazine group seems best. Thioridazine, which is available in various strengths from 10 mg to 100 mg in tablets, and in syrup containing 25 mg in 5 ml, is a most useful drug with a relatively low incidence of side-effects. The dose for a restless, confused patient would be 25 mg three times daily, though a larger dose may be needed at first to produce the desired calming effect. For the acute emergency, when a rapid effect is required, as when confronted with a severely confused, agitated and aggressive patient, an intramuscular injection of 50 mg of chlorpromazine will usually be effective. In the very frail patient promazine may be preferred. An injection of phenothiazine should not be repeated unless the agitation has not been successfully controlled.

Hypnotics will often be required since restlessness is apt to be much worse during the dark hours. Short-acting drugs are best and 5 mg to 10 mg of temazepam (Euhypnos, Normison) at night is very useful. Dichloralphenazone (Welldorm) seems a relatively safe hypnotic in the elderly and has the advantages of mildness in action with little hangover the next day. A usual dose would be 1,300 mg at night. It is available in tablet form, each tablet containing 650 mg of dichloralphenazone B.P.; and a syrup, containing 225 mg in 5 ml. Barbiturates should not be used in elderly confused patients. As well as being relatively long acting, they have undesirable side-effects, not the least of which is a tendency to increase confusion after the sedative effect has worn off and to cause unsteadiness and falls, possibly due to postural hypotension.

It is important to remember that the apathetic, confused patient may be suffering from depression amenable to treatment by drugs. Caution should be used in instituting treatment because the drugs used may themselves cause confusion. A trial dose of a tricyclic drug should be closely monitored and the regime only continued beyond three weeks if there is evidence of improvement. The unwanted side-effects of such drugs, e.g. retention of urine or glaucoma, should be watched for. In some patients dramatic improvement may occur.

General management. — Drug treatment forms a small part of the overall treatment and should be discontinued as soon as possible. Of great importance are the general care and attention, much of which will be related to the cause of the confusional state. Every effort must be made to seek the cause and treat it, where possible. A careful watching brief by the practitioner, aided by the district nurse, the health visitor and social worker, is rewarding. The confused patient having devoted relatives is fortunate. These must be given as much support as is feasible, and their stresses and strains anticipated. An optimistic attitude on the part of the doctor is essential and will often be justified.

Particular attention must be given to faulty vision or hearing. To see a confused old person 'return' to his family soon after being given correct spectacles or a hearing aid is a most gratifying reward. With a hearing aid, in particular, a degree of perseverance on the part of the attendants is required which is sometimes daunting as the old person often resists wearing one, and the relatives often refuse to admit he or she is deaf.

An old lady who was almost completely blind had severe deafness and eventually all communication became impossible. A special hearing apparatus combining headphones and an amplifying box was bought for her by her children as a last hope. Although cumbersome, it worked and to see the old lady conversing with her children after months of silence was a most moving experience, and she was to be found listening to the radio with renewed enthusiasm.

Concluding guidelines

1. The treatment of confusion is essentially that of the cause.
2. When confusion appears suddenly in a hitherto lucid individual, look for focal neurological signs. In their absence, suspect some acute, recent disease which is potentially reversible.
3. Sudden onset of confusion occurring soon after a change in medication has been made may well be due to the medicines.
4. Resist the temptation to give sedatives without making a diagnosis, and never do so without carrying out a physical examination.
5. The more clear-cut the cause, the less likely is there to be coexistent dementia.
6. Drug therapy is relatively easy to initiate but less important and helpful than the other aspects of the treatment.
7. Always have an optimistic attitude. This is often justified.
8. Attention to defects of vision and hearing is of great importance.
9. Keep the patient at home if at all possible during the confused state.

3.6
The unconscious patient

Chris Watkins

The presentation of an unconscious patient to the general practitioner is a rare event, but the correct assessment and management of the situation by the doctor of first contact are critical. It may mean the difference between life and death, or a difference in degree of cerebral function of the patient after recovery of consciousness has taken place.

In general practice the three most probable causes of unconsciousness are syncope, concussion and cerebral haemorrhage and thrombosis. In a study of the incidence of disease in general practice, syncope was thought to be the cause of consultations of 4 per 1,000 patients in one year, concussion provoked four consultations per 1,000 patients in one year, whilst a firm diagnosis of cerebral thrombosis or haemorrhage was made in 2.4 in every 1,000 patients per year. Although these are the commonest causes of unconsciousness that the general practitioner may encounter, his prompt and adequate handling of the less common causes is vital.

Presentation of the complaint

This is abrupt and dramatic and will prompt the doctor to attend forthwith. The relative or friend of the patient who has requested medical attention will often be overwrought and unable to give a coherent history, apart from saying that the patient has 'passed out' or 'collapsed'. The best advice the doctor can give in this situation is to advise the patient's attendants to lay the patient on a horizontal surface in the semi-prone position with the neck extended and clothing loosened. If the doctor can obtain the patient's medical records before attending, this may provide information as to the cause of the loss of consciousness.

History

The doctor should be aware of the variety of the different sources of information which are available to him in the assessment of the unconscious patient.

First, the medical record is invaluable. Does the patient suffer from diabetes mellitus, heart disease, hypertension or chronic psychiatric illness? Has the patient attempted suicide in the past? Does the patient take any major tranquillizers or sedatives, in particular barbiturates? Has the patient a previous history of stroke? All this information can be extracted rapidly from a medical record, if there is a separate sheet on which are prominently displayed those chronic illnesses from which the patient suffers.

Secondly, neighbours or relatives may provide information about the way in which the patient lost consciousness. Did the patient fall unconscious after standing up, and lie on the ground without shaking? Such an attack would suggest syncope. Did the patient fall to the ground, shake, bite his tongue and was he incontinent of urine? This would suggest grand mal epilepsy. The onset of unconsciousness in a patient who has a cerebral arterial occlusion may also be abrupt, but may occur during the night, so that relatives cannot rouse the patient in the morning. Concussion may be difficult to differentiate from drop attacks in the elderly, and indeed the elderly patient may be concussed due to a head injury sustained as a result of a drop attack.

Thirdly, the patient's home may give clues to the cause. The presence of a large number of empty beer, spirits, or methylated spirits bottles will suggest alcoholic intoxication. Gas and carbon monoxide poisoning may be self evident, but does not preclude the additional ingestion of tablets or alcohol to induce unconsciousness. Bottles of tablets should be examined and if they can be identified the information should be supplied in the referral letter to the hospital doctor. If they cannot be identified, samples of the tablets can be enclosed with the letter for identification by the hospital pharmacist. Syringes with their residual contents may also be of value in the same way.

Finally, information may be obtained from the patient. The breath of the patient will be ketotic in a diabetic (hyperglycaemic) coma, and smell of alcohol when unconsciousness is due to alcohol ingestion. Venepuncture marks suggest the injection of drugs, while bruises on the head may suggest injuries inflicted by an assailant.

Assessment and management

The doctor's first task, when confronted by an unconscious patient, is to assess the state of the respiratory and cardiovascular systems and the level of consciousness.

The doctor will observe the patient's colour, if the patient is breathing, and if the carotid pulses are present. If the patient is blue, carotid or femoral pulses are absent and the patient is not breathing, then cardiac arrest can be assumed to have taken place. Provided the patient is young, and is not suffering from terminal illness, resuscitation should be attempted. The object of this is to restore adequate cerebral circulation by a combination of pulmonary ventilation and external cardiac compression.

Expired air ventilation is performed with the patient lying in the supine position, with the neck well extended to maintain a patent airway. The operator expires directly into the mouth of the patient, while the nasal airway is compressed, and the chest should be checked to ensure that adequate expansion of the lungs has occurred. A Brook or double-ended Guedel airway can make this manoeuvre more effective as well as more aesthetic.

External cardiac compression is maintained at the same time. The patient should be on the floor, or some similar rigid surface. The legs are elevated to an angle of 30° to 40° to facilitate venous return to the heart. Pressure is applied to the lower sternum about sixty times a minute. When effective a carotid pulse should be felt and the patient's colour improve. External cardiac compression is the simpler manoeuvre and can be performed by one operator, perhaps a member of the family or friend, while a doctor performs the more difficult task of expired air ventilation. External cardiac compression should be performed in a ratio of three to one to expired air ventilation. An ambulance should be summoned immediately and resuscitation continued until the patient is in the hands of the specialist resuscitation team in the hospital.

The concussed patient should be allowed to lie on a horizontal surface with clothing loosened to allow easy breathing. Blood clots and vomitus should be removed from the mouth and pharynx to improve the patency of the airway, and in a profoundly unconscious patient an artificial airway may be of value. The concussed patient may also suffer from other injuries, most important of which for immediate attention by the doctor are spinal injuries, flail chest, and haemorrhage. If there is any suggestion of injury to the spine, the patient should be moved with great care, to allow as little movement of the spine as possible. Flail chest renders physiological ventilatory exchange impossible as some degree of paradoxical respiration occurs. For some such patients, expired air ventilation may be necessary. Arrest of haemorrhage may be performed by occluding the arterial supply of the bleeding limb, by digital compression or a tourniquet. Admission to hospital for all concussed patients for a period of observation is advisable.

The patient who is unconscious as a result of cerebral infarction or haemorrhage requires similar attention to the patency of the airway and preservation of vital functions. Most patients who are unconscious due to cerebrovascular accidents will need to be admitted to hospital, chiefly for the expert nursing care that the hospital provides. Some authorities recommend first aid treatment with steroid and acetazolamide in an attempt to reduce cerebral oedema. It is suggested that dexamethazone (Decadron, Oradexon) should be administered intravenously or intramuscularly in a dose of 10 mg, followed by 4 mg every six hours, along with acetazolamide (Diamox) 500 mg intramuscularly and then 250 mg every six hours. From time to time the general practitioner will find himself caring for the unconscious patient at home, for a few days prior to death. He will rely heavily on the nursing skills of the district nurse and close relatives.

The epileptic patient requires little more from the doctor than observation that he does not injure himself and that pulmonary ventilation is adequate. Occasionally the general practitioner may encounter a patient with major status epilepticus. This is defined as the occurrence of repeated fits between which the patient fails to regain consciousness. It is a grave medical emergency with a mortality of about 10 per cent. For many years paraldehyde was advocated as the initial treatment of major status epilepticus in a dose of 5 ml by deep intramuscular injection in each buttock. Although effective and unlikely to depress respiration, local reactions at the site of the injections may produce sterile abcesses. In recent years, diazepam has been gaining favour as an alternative drug for the treatment of major status epilepticus, and is given in a dose of 10 mg by intravenous injection over about one minute.

Hypoglycaemic coma is diagnosed in the unconscious diabetic patient whose loss of consciousness was of abrupt onset and associated with sweating. The diagnosis can be confirmed by the use of Dextrostix. It is treated by the injection of 20 ml of 50 per cent dextrose intravenously, or, alternatively, 0.5 to 1 mg of glucagon intramuscularly.

Attempted suicide is one of the common causes of unconsciousness in general practice. Having ensured that the patient has an adequate airway, the doctor should arrange immediate admission to hospital and should provide as much information as possible about the probable cause of unconsciousness.

Conclusion

The list of causes of unconsciousness presenting to the general practitioner is long, but most unconscious patients will be treated in hospital. This chapter has therefore concentrated on those

conditions which the general practitioner should recognize and for which immediate effective treatment is of vital importance.

Reference

[1] Royal College of General Practitioners, Office of Population Censuses and Surveys, Department of Health and Social Security (1986): *Morbidity Statistics from General Practice 1981–82*. HMSO Series MB5 No. 1

3.7
Fits and faints

Chris Watkins

In a study of new symptoms provoking consultation with the general practitioner, disturbances of consciousness were presented at 1.9 times per 1,000 consultations. Twice as many women as men presented with the symptom.[1]

In another study,[2] the most common cause for a patient consulting for loss of consciousness of short duration was the simple faint. Of every 1,000 patients who consulted in the course of a year, this diagnosis was suspected in 4, occurring most commonly in patients in early pregnancy and in young girls. Epilepsy was suspected in 1.1 per 1,000 patients consulting. Febrile convulsions – 0.4 per 1,000 patients consulting – were found to occur most commonly in children under the age of 7 years. Breath-holding attacks occurred most commonly in children under the age of 3. Other less common causes for consultations for fits and faints were Stokes–Adams attacks and vertebro-basilar insufficiency due to arteriosclerosis in old age. Hysteria and the hysterical manifestations of depression were also causes of consultation for this symptom.

The occurrence of a single seizure in an individual during his lifetime is very common. One person in 20 will have an epileptic fit at some time during his life. Of those people who have one seizure, one in 8 will go on to develop epilepsy. Thus the estimates of the prevalence of all varieties of epilepsy in the general population in the United Kingdom are about 5 per 1,000. Incidence varies by age-group, being higher in children and the elderly. In children of school age it has been estimated that between 6 and 8 per 1,000 suffer from epilepsy.

Presentation of the complaint

In assessing the patient who presents with 'fits' or 'faints' it is important to establish what events the patient is describing. The word 'fit' may be used to describe an explosive outburst of anger (a fit of rage), a prolonged episode of coughing or a grand mal epileptic fit. Both the words 'fit' and 'faint' carry with them a diagnostic significance which is emotionally highly charged for the patient and the doctor. Uppermost in the mind of the patient who has had a fit will be the possibility of grand mal epilepsy. The person who has fainted may also suspect serious illness, such as heart disease or a stroke.

The doctor may be presented with this symptom as a reason for an urgent home visit. The request will often be made by telephone by a distraught relative or friend, who may be unable to give an accurate description of the events which have taken place. In such circumstances the doctor should tell the attendant to lay the patient on one side on a horizontal surface, usually the floor, and to keep the neck well extended. The collar should be loosened and false teeth removed if this can be easily accomplished. The attendant should be told not to attempt to insert any object, such as the handle of a spoon, in the mouth of the unconscious patient. In the hands of an inexperienced lay person, such action can cause trauma and bleeding,which does not improve the patency of the airway. By the time the doctor arrives the patient will usually have recovered consciousness. Those patients who report at the surgery with a history of fits or faints are commonly accompanied by friends or relatives. In establishing an accurate record of what has occurred the latter may prove to be invaluable. The management of the situation requires a certain dexterity if consultation time is to be used effectively.

Causes

From birth to 3 months, fits are often due to birth injury or hypoglycaemia. Attacks occurring several days after birth but within the first month may be due to hypocalcaemia if the infant is being bottle-fed. Metabolic disturbances secondary to pneumonia or gastroenteritis may also provoke fits. In the first year of life meningitis may be a cause of fits and can be very difficult to diagnose. Other causes of fits in this age-group are epilepsy due to prenatal or neonatal brain damage, and febrile convulsions. Febrile convulsions are the commonest cause of fits in children between the ages of 1 and 3 years. Breath-holding attacks also occur in this age-group. They are characterized by cessation of respiratory movements, cyanosis and unconsciousness, and the attack is often preceded by an emotional outburst. Families whose members suffer these attacks often demonstrate disturbed relationships between parents and children.

Over the age of 3 years the types of epilepsy that a child may develop are similar to those found in adults. The international classification of epilepsy describes two main seizure types and is useful as the allocation of a seizure to one or other of these categories is of prognostic importance. The first category is primary generalized epilepsy or ideopathic epilepsy. Here the seizure activity is generalized from the start of an attack. It may take the form of petit mal epilepsy with minor brief absences lasting only seconds, difficult for observers to notice, although fluttering of the eyelids is common. It may also start with a full-blown grand mal attack without any warning. The grand mal seizure starts with an immediate loss of consciousness, the patient falling to the ground. The tonic stage follows with stiffening of the body and change of the colour of the face to red or blue. The clonic stage or rhythmic jerking gradually supervenes and continues from one to three minutes. It is in this stage that generalized muscle-twitching and tongue-biting occurs. A stage of flaccid coma follows and may last between five and thirty minutes. As consciousness returns the patient remains drowsy and frequently goes to sleep. He may remain confused from one to two hours after the attack, being disorientated and aggressive if disturbed. In primary generalized epilepsy there is often a positive family history, neurological examination is normal and the prognosis is good. In secondary generalized epilepsy the attacks are again generalized from the start but follow some insult to the central nervous system. There is no family history and the prognosis is variable. The second category is focal or partial epilepsy. Here the attacks are usually preceded by a warning or aura. The aura lasts several seconds and may be abdominal, visual, olfactory or psychological in temporal-lobe epilepsy. In Jacksonian epilepsy the aura may start with twitching of the thumb if motor areas of the brain are affected, or with sensory or visual aura when lesions are in those areas of the brain. The aura may end or it may extend and develop into a grand mal or partial seizure. Focal epilepsy always indicates a localized area of damage in the central nervous system and unless amenable to surgery presents a more serious prognosis.

The simple faint, which occurs most commonly in early pregnancy and in young girls, is characterized by severe pallor and unconsciousness. It may follow acute blood loss, either external or internal, or be provoked by psychological factors. It may also be due to postural hypotension, due to sudden assumption of an upright position after lying down, due to prolonged standing, or following over-treatment of hypertension. Acute hypoglycaemic attacks in diabetes mellitus may present as fainting. The attack is of sudden onset and may be preceded by abnormal behaviour. Sweating is profuse during the attack. Rarely, spontaneous hypoglycaemia may present in a previously normal individual and may be related to a long interval since the last meal followed by

vigorous exercise. Hysterical fits or faints occur most commonly in girls and young women who have been observed to have immature personalities. They often occur in company and excite attention in those around. The attacks do not follow the pattern of any of the other causes of unconsciousness in this age-group. There is often a previous history of psychological upset.
In the older patient fits or faints may arise through inadequate arterial perfusion of the brain. This may be due to cardiac causes, such as complete or incomplete heart block, Stokes–Adams attacks, or aortic stenosis. Intermittent obstruction of the arterial supply as a result of arteriosclerosis, or constriction of the vertebral arteries due to narrowing of the vertebral foramina, can also cause fainting in the elderly. A grand mal epileptic fit occurring in the elderly for the first time suggests cerebral arterial occlusion or secondary neoplasm. Focal neurological signs may be present after the attack is over.

History

A description of the events leading to the fit or faint is best obtained in two stages. If the patient is an adult, the doctor will want to hear from the patient himself a description of the events leading to the attack. If an infant, the same history should be obtained from the mother or most immediate attendant. This initial interview is best handled by excluding all other observers and allowing the patient to describe in as unhurried a fashion as possible what he has experienced. This can be followed by direct questions about past or family history of fits, and of any illnesses for which the patient is at present receiving drug treatment, with particular reference to diabetes mellitus, hypertension or cardiac arrhythmia.
A detailed account of the minutes and seconds before the onset of loss of consciousness can be very helpful in establishing the diagnosis of epilepsy. Minutes before the attack, was the patient feeling well? Was he going about his normal daily routine? Was he involved in any psychologically stressful task? Had there been a family row? Did he feel as though something was going to happen, but could not say exactly what? Seconds before the onset of loss of consciousness, did he experience any unusual feelings in any part of his body? Did he feel his limbs move automatically? Did his thoughts become jumbled or confused? Could he speak prior to the onset of the loss of consciousness? Was his hearing or vision changed in any way at this time? When the patient recovers consciousness it is important to find out how long the duration of the period of unconsciousness was. What was the recovery phase like? Did consciousness return quickly or slowly? Was there a period of confusion as consciousness returned? Did the patient

have any difficulty in speaking after the attack? Did he notice any weakness of his limbs? Were his muscles stiff or aching? Had he got a headache, and did he go to sleep? It is also important to establish whether he had bitten his tongue during the attack, hurt himself, or been incontinent of urine. If a child, was he unwell or feverish before the attack? If an infant, did he have a normal delivery and is he breast- or bottle-fed?

Outside observers may then be asked to provide information about the nature of the fit. Did the patient fall to the floor, and lie there motionless until consciousness returned? Such an event would suggest a syncopal episode. Did the patient shake after losing consciousness? Did the patient turn blue? Had the patient been well before the attack? Information may also be obtained from relatives or friends about past medical history. The patient's emotional state preceding the attack should be established. Behaviour following an attack is important to establish as it can contribute important information to the diagnosis. Confusional states following the attack suggests the possibility of an organic episode and a possible seizure. Attacks of loss of consciousness in which postural tone is retained and during and following which a period of automatic behaviour occurs, sometimes associated with difficulty in speaking, suggest the possibility of temporal-lobe epilepsy.

Examination

In a child, the presence or absence of fever will be noted. If present, the chest, ears and throat will be examined for signs of localized infection. In an older child, meningitis can commonly be excluded in the absence of signs of meningism, but these signs may be absent in an infant below the age of 1 year who has meningitis. The examination of the adolescent or young adult who has what is described as a simple faint will include measurement of pulse and blood pressure. It is important to exclude the possibility of acute hidden blood loss, in particular as a result of ruptured ectopic pregnancy. Viral illnesses affecting the respiratory or gastro-intestinal tract may cause syncope in this age-group. Not infrequently the cause is found to be emotional, the patient being acutely distressed at some unpleasant experience.

The young adult who shook during the attack, hurt himself or was incontinent of urine or bit his tongue should be examined neurologically to identify any localized neurological signs. Occasionally syncope causes such severe anoxia of the brain that a fit occurs. This is more likely if friends support a person who is fainting, rather than lying him down.

In the child who has short transient episodes of loss of

consciousness without grand mal fits, the diagnosis of petit mal or temporal-lobe epilepsy should be considered. Episodes of loss of awareness, whether or not associated with behavioural disorders, or postictal automatism can suggest focal epilepsy, possibly temporal-lobe epilepsy.

In the middle-aged and elderly person who experiences a fit, idiopathic epilepsy is a less likely diagnosis as the probability of the fit being caused by a neoplasm or vascular disease increases in this age-group. Patients of this age who faint should be suspected of interruption of blood supply to the brain, either due to cardiac arrhythmia, hypotension from a variety of causes, e.g. drugs, coronary thrombosis or haemorrhage, or insufficiency of the vertebro-basilar system. In the diabetic patient who suffers transient loss of consciousness, a blood-sugar estimation (Dextrostix, Ames) is helpful in identifying hypoglycaemia as a cause.

Management

As the diagnosis of meningitis is difficult to make on clinical examination alone in the first year of life, all children of this age presenting with fits should be admitted under the care of a specialist paediatrician, to exclude meningitis by lumbar puncture.

In the older child presenting with febrile convulsions, where there is a clear relationship between the fit and the fever and there is no evidence of meningitis, special investigations are not needed. The mother should be instructed that if the fever recurs, the child should be cooled, by sponging with tepid water. Paracetamol 60 to 120 mg, should be given as soon as a fever starts and continued every six hours until there has been no fever for two days. If in spite of this treatment the child has another attack, then anticonvulsants should be given. Under the age of 4, diazepam, 2 to 5 mg, should be given initially, then 2 mg every six to eight hours depending on the child's tolerance. Diazepam should be given until at least two days after the child is well. Phenobarbitone is contraindicated because of the risk of withdrawal seizures. In older children diazepam, 2 to 5 mg, or sodium valproate, 200 to 600 mg, may be used.

There is evidence that prolonged seizures in children may cause anoxic brain damage and continuing epilepsy. The emergency treatment of prolonged convulsions in this age-group is therefore important and the general practitioner should take action pending hospital admission. If the child is still convulsing when the doctor arrives, he should if possible inject diazepam intravenously in a dose of 0.2 mg/kg body weight. In a chubby toddler this may however be difficult. In these cases, paraldehyde in a dose of 1 ml/year of age should be injected intramuscularly. Plastic syringes, contrary to common belief, can be used for injecting paraldehyde as long as the injection is made within 30 minutes of drawing up the drug. Alternatively, diazepam (at a dose of 1 mg per year of age + 1 mg) may be administered rectally, using a 2 ml syringe with the needle removed.

Breath-holding attacks in children require reassurance of the parents by the doctor that the child is not epileptic. In some cases this will be strengthened by referral for specialist opinion. Repeated breath-holding attacks suggest major psychological upheaval in the family. The family should be told that dramatic resuscitation of the child who has an attack is unnecessary. If allowed to lie prone the child will soon recover consciousness.

Some children may use breath-holding attacks as a means to manipulate parents to their own ends. Parents should be told to be on their guard about this, and to establish consistent policies of management.

In most cases in which the diagnosis of epilepsy is suspected, specialist referral is desirable. The diagnosis will affect the patient's job prospects; it may affect his ability to obtain life insurance, and may bar him from driving a car or riding a bicycle. Petit mal epilepsy occurring during childhood may interfere with schooling; treatment should be instituted with capsules of ethosuximide, 200 mg, once a day initially, but gradually increasing to a maximum of four times daily. It may be given as tablets or a syrup.

The control of grand mal epileptic attacks requires the general practitioner to identify those factors which may precipitate an attack. In individuals who are photosensitive a flashing light or television set is one of the most common precipitating factors. The patient should never switch on the television set or adjust it without covering one eye and should sit well back when viewing in a room which should have good background lighting. Premenstrual retention of fluid may lead to increased frequency of fits in epileptics. A diuretic given during the premenstrual phase may reduce the number of attacks. If the patient is taking an oral contraceptive and experiences fits in the premenstrual phase, a change of contraceptive to one containing a higher dose of progestogen may be helpful. Sleep loss and alcohol withdrawal after evenings of drinking are potent precipitating factors in epilepsy, and should be carefully avoided.

Phenytoin and phenobarbitone were formerly the most commonly used drugs for the prevention of grand mal attacks. Phenytoin is given in a dose of 100 to 600 mg a day and need only be administered twice daily. Carbamazepine is now the alternative first drug of choice in a dose of 200 to 800 mg daily. It is considerably more expensive than phenytoin. When these drugs are unacceptable or unsuccessful in controlling fits sodium valproate in doses of 600 to 1200 mg daily should be tried. Neither primidone, because of its conversion to phenobarbitone in the body, nor sulthiame, because of its very weak anticonvulsant effects, should be used. Most general hospitals now run a service to measure the serum anticonvulsant levels and epileptics whose seizures are not easily controlled should have their anticonvulsant dose adjusted until the serum levels are in the therapeutic range. Any patient on long-term anticonvulsant therapy should have at least a yearly blood picture, serum folate and serum anticonvulsant estimation.

All anticonvulsants have been shown to be teratogenic to some degree. However, the present feeling is that the risks to the fetus are probably greater from the mother having uncontrolled seizures than they are from the drugs. The present policy is thus to leave the anticonvulsant regime unchanged during pregnancy. During a grand mal attack those present should place the patient in a semi-prone position which allows easy breathing. No restraint should be used and the patient should be in a position where he is unable to hurt himself.

Normal activities such as sport including swimming should be allowed wherever possible, as it is better to take some risks if it allows the patient a more normal life. A patient who has been free from attacks (or had them only while asleep) for three years, whether on drugs or not, may have a licence to drive a car. If, however, the drug regime is withdrawn or changed the patient should be told that he is required to inform the driving licence authorities at Swansea. Further information concerning driving for the epileptic can be obtained from the British Epilepsy Association, New Wokingham Road, Wokingham, Berks., RG11 3AY (Tel: Crowthorne 3122) which provides an advisory service for epileptics and their relatives, general practitioners and social workers.

The management of the simple faint, provided that the doctor is confident that the cause is not acute haemorrhage, requires little more of the general practitioner than reassurance that the attack is not of serious consequence, and a short period of rest. Repeated attacks require the elimination of anaemia and psychosocial factors as causes. The pregnant patient who faints on rising should be advised against standing up suddenly or sudden activity after lying or sitting for some time. Similar attacks occurring in patients on treatment for hypertension may require modification of dosage or schedule of medication.

Acute hypoglycaemic attacks in the diabetic require the injection of 30 ml of 50 per cent glucose intravenously or 0.5 to 1.0 mg of glucagon intramuscularly. If the patient recovers consciousness sufficiently to swallow, then a cup of tea sweetened with four teaspoonfuls of sugar will suffice.

Hysterical fits or faints require identification of the emotional conflict which has caused them. Management may include treatment of underlying depression and modification of interpersonal pressures by simple counselling. A patient with frequent (epileptic) fits which do not respond to changes of medication may be having hysterical attacks. The patient who experiences frequent attacks is often an individual of limited emotional development. There is a danger that such patients will develop a dependent relationship with the doctor which will take up time and energy out of all proportion to the therapeutic effect.

Management of the elderly patient with loss of consciousness due to cardiac arrhythmias requires treatment of the arrhythmia. Digitalis toxicity may lead to complete or partial heart block, and on stopping the drug, the pulse will often return to normal. Heart block due to damage to the conducting fibres of the heart by infarction may require treatment with sympathomimetic agents (such as isoprenaline slow tablets, 30 mg, which are effective for about eight hours). If frequent Stokes–Adams attacks occur the patient may be referred to a cardiologist for a pacemaker.

A cervical collar may help the patient who faints on rotation of the head. It restricts the movement of the neck and lessens the likelihood of compression of the vertebral arteries by the narrowed vertebral foramina.

A grand mal epileptic fit occurring in the middle-aged or the elderly for the first time suggests a neoplasm (often a secondary deposit) or infarction. The most common sites of primary tumours causing cerebral secondary neoplasms are the bronchus, the breast and the prostate. The history and physical examination should be directed towards identifying the presence of a primary tumour. Any recent changes in memory, mood, or sensation, or development of muscular weakness, associated with focal neurological signs should be noted. In many cases it is not possible to distinguish between fits caused through infarction or a neoplasm. In the very elderly, further investigation is usually unwarranted. In the younger patient, referral for full neurological assessment is desirable, as radical treatment or radiotherapy may be possible. The management of fits due to secondary neoplasms or infarctions is identical to the management of idiopathic grand mal epilepsy.

The occurrence of an epileptic fit always causes anxiety to the patient and relatives. The general practitioner has an important role in trying to interpret the physical events in a way which they can comprehend. A helpful approach may be to talk about the brain as an area of continuous electrical activity. A small short circuit in the brain as might occur with a tiny, frayed fibre in a cable causing a short circuit is one way which may be readily understood. It may be explained to the patient that many factors can lead to this short circuit, such as fever, and that this tendency may be suppressed by drugs. It is important to stress that as normal a life as possible should be encouraged and a guarded optimistic prognosis should be given, particularly in the young suffering from an isolated fit.

References

[1] Morrell, D. C., Gage, H. G., and Robinson, N. A. (1971): Symptoms in General Practice *Journal of the Royal College of General Practitioners, 21*, 32
[2] Royal College of General Practitioners, Office of Population Censuses and Surveys, Department of Health and Social Security (1986): *Morbidity Statistics from General Practice 1981–82*. HMSO Series MB5 No. 1

Acknowledgement

It is a pleasure to acknowledge the helpful advice received from Dr Peter Fenwick, Consultant Physician to St. Thomas's Hospital, London, in updating this chapter.

3.8 The patient complaining of dizziness

Chris Watkins

Of a random sample of adults in the United Kingdom who were asked if they had suffered faintness or dizziness in the preceding two weeks, 10 per cent of women and 6 per cent of men had experienced the symptom. Those over the age of 65 admitted to the symptom almost twice as often as those below that age.[1] In a study of new symptoms presented to the general practitioner, disturbances of balance were presented at 1·3 per 1,000 consultations in one year. Twice as many women as men presented with the symptom.[2] Dizziness is a common symptom and its interpretation may cause some anxiety to the doctor. Although the underlying cause may be trivial, it can be a symptom of serious disease, which requires early diagnosis.

Presentation of the complaint

It is difficult for the patient suffering from giddiness to explain to the doctor the sensation that he experiences. According to the geographical situation of the practice and local idiom, patients may say that they feel dizzy when they have a sensation of faintness, a headache or sinus congestion. Usually the patient will be referring to a subjective sensation of instability. For the purposes of history taking and examination it is helpful to distinguish two types of sensation: (i) a feeling of unsteadiness in the head or more vaguely a feeling of 'light-headedness', (ii) a sensation of rotation, that either the patient or his surroundings are spinning round. This sensation of 'rotation' is what is meant by 'vertigo' and in its severest form may be accompanied by nausea, vomiting, pallor and sweating. Vertigo may also be associated with a disturbed sense of balance and may be accompanied by unsteadiness of gait.

Causes

Dizziness is most often presented by patients suffering from psychiatric illness and time needs to be given to identify this. The commonest cause of the symptom, after psychiatric illness, is probably acute infection, usually viral in origin. It may occur in epidemics and be associated with other symptoms such as gastric or bowel disturbance and aches and pains in the limbs or body. The diagnosis is usually made in the light of the doctor's knowledge of the infectious diseases prevalent in his own practice population.

In the elderly patient dizziness is often due to inadequate perfusion of the vertebro-basilar system, either due to arteriosclerotic narrowing of the blood vessels or narrowing of the intervertebral foramina due to osteoarthrosis. In the young woman who is otherwise fit, it may suggest postural hypotension in the earlier stages of pregnancy. Postural hypotension in the known hypertensive on treatment may also be a cause of dizziness, whilst the known diabetic may suffer from attacks of dizziness, associated with sweating and hunger, when hypoglycaemic.

True vertigo presented to the general practitioner can be caused by middle-ear disease such as otitis media. It is a symptom of serious import as it suggests fistula formation from the middle to inner ear. Attacks of Menière's disease usually start after the age of 50 and cause true vertigo which may last for hours. Malaise or instability may persist for a day or two, and there is always associated deafness, which may be unilateral. Long periods of freedom between attacks are common.

Vestibular neuronitis is characterized by the acute onset of rotatory vertigo, with systemic disturbance. The vertigo may subside spontaneously after a day or a few hours, although it may recur on sudden head movement or on postural change during the following few weeks. Though self limiting, the illness may occasionally recur. A viral infection of the labyrinth has been held responsible but there is little direct evidence for this.

Rarer causes of vertigo include multiple sclerosis, which may be suspected in a young patient with a history of vertigo lasting several weeks, epilepsy and an acoustic neuroma.

History

When the patient presents with 'light-headedness', not associated with rotation, the history and examination will be directed towards identifying a non-vestibular complaint. This symptom is often presented by those patients suffering from anxiety states, or depression. Other probable causes include the malaise of fever, syncope, postural hypotension, anaemia and hypoglycaemia. The history will be directed towards identifying the cause of the symptom. Are there any circumstances in the patient's life which are causing anxiety? What is the patient's pattern of sleeping? Is the patient depressed? Are there any viral illnesses, such as influenza, prevalent among the doctor's practice population, which might cause fever and malaise? Does the patient experience the symptom after rising rapidly from the sitting position? Is the patient receiving treatment for hypertension or diabetes mellitus? Does the patient sweat or feel hungry during an attack, and is it relieved by eating food?

True vertigo is caused by a lesion of the labyrinth or its central connections. Since the cochlea forms part of the labyrinth, the patient with vertigo may suffer from ringing noises in the ear and impaired hearing. A patient complaining of such symptoms should be asked if he has suffered any head injury in the recent past, or about ingestion of drugs with known toxic effects on the inner ear (such as salicylates, quinine and streptomycin). The addition of headache to these symptoms suggests the possibility of raised intracranial tension.

Examination

The patient who suffers from 'light-headedness' unaccompanied by rotation is not suffering from any disease of the labyrinth. According to the history, the clinical examination will be directed towards identifying the cause. It will include recording of the pulse, temperature, and blood pressure on lying and standing. If an infective cause for the symptom is suggested by raised pulse and fever, then a general examination of throat, sinuses, ears, chest and abdomen will be conducted to identify the site of the infection.

The young woman who is in the early stages of pregnancy and the patient who is taking hypotensive agents are both likely to suffer from postural hypotension. The known diabetic requires measurement of his blood-sugar level using Dextrostix to identify hypoglycaemia as a cause of his symptoms. The patient whose history strongly suggests mental illness may require a simple examination of blood pressure, heart and lungs, to reassure him that his physical health is good. This will put the doctor in a stronger position to manage the patient's psychiatric problems.

True vertigo requires detailed examination of the ears and the function of the labyrinth. Conductive deafness (bone conduction better than air conduction in Rinne's test) will suggest a local middle-ear cause for vertiginous symptoms. Perceptive deafness (air conduction greater than bone conduction) will suggest the possibilities of disease of the eighth nerve or cochlear end organ. Those doctors who possess their own audiometer will find that deafness caused by a lesion of the cochlear end organ (e.g. Menière's disease) shows the characteristic known as loudness recruitment: as the sound intensity is increased, the subjective loudness in the affected ear progressively approximates that of the good ear.

Nystagmus is caused by interruption of visual fixation. Jerk nystagmus consists of a slow drift of the eyes away from the attempted fixation point followed by a quick corrective movement. It may be caused by disease of the labyrinth or its central connections, but may occur in normal subjects on extreme lateral gaze, or if the test object is held too close. If the patient is asked to sit on a couch and is then laid down so that his head, turned to one side, is over the end of the couch, a rotatory nystagmus may be seen. If this develops only after an interval of time, abates as the position is maintained and fatigues with repetition it can be attributed to a lesion of the peripheral vestibular apparatus, probably the utricle. The nystagmus occurs when the affected ear is undermost in the test. Further information about the site of the lesion may be obtained by caloric stimulation, but this is probably best performed by the specialist, who is experienced in conducting the test and interpreting the results.

Management

If the dizziness is caused by psychiatric illness, this may require appropriate management by psychotherapeutic means, tranquillizers or antidepressants. If due to infection of self-limiting viral etiology, treatment with rest in bed, aspirin and fluids is all that is needed. If the site of the infection is identified and the organism amenable to antibacterials, then appropriate antibiotics may also be required.

The elderly patient with dizzy attacks may benefit from the wearing of a cervical collar which will restrain the movement of the cervical spine. The advice to rise slowly from the sitting position and to avoid movements which will provoke the attack is also of help. Prochlorperazine tablets, 5 mg twice daily, will often reduce the intensity of the attacks.

The hypertensive patient with postural hypotension will require readjustment of the dose or schedule of hypotensive agents. The hypoglycaemic attacks occurring in the known diabetic require similar reassessment of his regime of treatment.

Vertigo in the presence of middle-ear infection requires an urgent opinion from an ear specialist.

The medical treatment of Menière's disease is at presesnt symptomatic. Low-salt diets and diuretics may be employed with variable degrees of succees. Betahistine has had some success in a dose of 8 mg thrice daily. Vestibular sedatives are helpful and of these cinnarizine has been recommended. Vestibular neuronitis is also treated with symptomatic remedies, such as cinnarizine or prochlorperazine.

References

[1] Morrell, D.C., Gage, H.G. and Robinson, N.A. (1971): Symptoms in General Practice. *Journal of the Royal College of General Practitioners*, *21*, 32

[2] Hodgkin, K. (1937): *Towards Earlier Diagnosis.* 3rd ed. Edinburgh: Churchill Livingstone

3.9
Clumsiness, weakness and palsy

Judith Millac

This group of symptoms indicates a lesion within the nervous system.

Morrell and his colleagues[1] found that 2.75 per cent of total consultations in one year in general practice, and 1.90 per cent of new patient-initiated consultations were due to diseases of the nervous system. Multiple sclerosis and Parkinsonism together are likely to affect two people in every thousand,[2] and in the community, at any one time, about six patients per thousand of the population have experienced a cerebrovascular accident.[3]

In an analysis of 5,325 new symptoms, six involved disturbance of movement in the upper limb, and nine involved disturbance of movement in the lower limb.[1]

These symptoms often represent a disease of serious prognostic significance. They are frightening to the patient because they affect his activity in the present as well as threatening his ability to function in a fully active way in the future.

Presentation

Palsy may present with a dramatic telephone call for help from a relative with the story that the patient has 'lost the use down one side'. Lesser degrees of paralysis may be revealed in a more roundabout fashion during a surgery consultation. The complaint may be of dropping small things, of difficulty in opening jars, turning taps, or turning the key in the front door. If the weakness is above the knee the leg may drag when walking any distance and cause problems mounting bus platforms or stairs. The knee may disconcertingly give way without warning. Below the knee weakness may cause foot-drop and a history of tripping.

Common causes

Stroke.— Cerebrovascular disease is the third most common cause of death in the developed countries. The annual incidence of new cases has varied between 1.3 and 1.9 per 1,000 population.[3] Predisposing factors include hypertension, diabetes mellitus, polycythaemia and smoking.

In its apoplectic presentation stroke is not difficult to diagnose. The patient is unconscious with a flaccid paralysis of one side, the opposite to the lesion, with the head and eyes turned to the side of the lesion. A clinical paradox not always appreciated is that the smaller the stroke the greater the urgency in its management, since it is the small stroke, the transient ischaemic attack (TIA), which is the harbinger of the catastrophe of a complete stroke. The practitioner who hears a carotid bruit in the neck of a patient whose 'arm went lifeless for an hour the other day' may reduce his risk of hemiplegia by prompt referral. An attack of palpitations before the episode may indicate embolism from atrial fibrillation, and anticoagulants may be life-saving.

Tumours.– These will cause similar weakness but the onset will be gradual, progressive and perhaps accompanied by morning headache with vomiting. An occasional stroke may do badly because the underlying lesion is neoplastic. Unfortunately, most will be malignant as benign intracranial tumours comprise only 15 per cent of the total.

Multiple Sclerosis[4].– In Great Britain, the prevalence of multiple sclerosis is around 50:100,000 population, approximately one patient on each practitioner's list.[5] It is a disease which affects women more than men in the ratio of 3:2 but is more severe in men. It is almost unique in selecting the age-group 15 to 55.

The diagnosis is a clinical one with the evidence of dissemination of lesions in time and space as the keystone. Charcot's triad of dysarthria, nystagmus and intention tremor emphasizes how often the cerebellar pathways are involved in the later stages. Optic neuritis, past or present, with weakness of a limb is a most suggestive combination. There may be bizarre sensory disturbances such as tight bands around digits, joints or the body, or the sense of water running down a limb.

Multiple sclerosis is a disease of remissions and relapses, which may be precipitated by emotional disturbances, trauma, cold, or the puerperium. In practice, the patient may present with no more than a transient limb weakness or diplopia of short duration. At this stage signs in the nervous system may be few or absent and the optic disc is unlikely to show pallor. The general practitioner is wise to show not only therapeutic discretion (there is no specific treatment) but also not to rush the diagnosis. It may be months or years before new symptoms present. Eventually, of course, the disease may become established with spasticity, micturition problems, speech difficulties, and ataxia. The average duration of life from the onset of the disease is over 20 years.

Parkinsonism.–This condition affects 1:1,000 of the total population and possibly as many as 1 per cent of all individuals over 50.[6] It is usually idiopathic, rarely post-encephalitic, but can be produced by certain drugs such as the phenothiazines.
It is a disease to suspect when a patient complains bitterly of being unable to use a limb, yet objectively there is little to find. The handwriting may become smaller and voice less easy to hear. The three basic features of the disease, which are tremor, akinesia and rigidity, are not always present together, and sometimes the symptoms remain entirely on one side for years: 'hemiplegic Parkinsonism'. If the diagnosis is not suspected it is easily missed. The classic picture is of a patient with cog-wheel rigidity, 'pill-rolling' tremor and passive unblinking facies, who sits in a fixed flexed posture, has dysarthria and walks with a typical shuffling gait.

Cervical spondylosis.– This common condition occurs in middle age. There may or may not be a history of neck stiffness. It is often present without neurological involvement, but occasionally compression of the spinal cord or pressure on nerve roots may occur. Pain may be a prominent feature, weakness develops gradually and there may be sensory symptoms in the hands. There are increased reflexes in the lower limbs, while in the upper limbs the biceps jerk may be absent or greatly reduced. Rotation of the neck may appear adequate, but lateral flexion is always reduced.

Motor neurone disease.– This progressive, fatal disease most commonly affects middle-aged men. There is insidious weakness of groups of muscles. It can be difficult to distinguish from cervical spondylosis, but there is usually little diagnostic doubt if the patient has widespread wasting and fasciculation with brisk reflexes and extensor plantar responses. Bulbar symptoms include dysphagia, and slurred nasal speech. It is the bulbar involvement that eventually leads to death.

Less common causes

Subacute combined degeneration of the cord.– This rare condition which affects both motor and sensory tracts is so eminently treatable that it assumes diagnostic importance. There will usually be striking sensory changes with loss of position and vibration sense accompanied by pyramidal weakness. Anaemia need not be present as the symptoms may precede it. Serum B_{12} levels should be estimated to confirm the diagnosis.

Peripheral nerve palsies and spinal cord lesions.– A weak wasted hand may be due to a Pancoast tumour in the lung, an ulnar nerve lesion at the elbow, or disease within the spinal cord such as a tumour or syringomyelia. This latter condition produces a characteristic 'cape' sensory loss in which pain and temperature sense are lost, but joint and position sense are preserved. The abrupt onset of painless weakness of the wrist and finger extensors, the so-called 'Saturday night palsy', is due to radial nerve palsy. In the lower limb, foot-drop of sudden onset may be due to root compression by a disc lesion, or to damage to the common peroneal nerve as it winds round the fibula and can be injured by pressure from, for instance, leg plasters or operating tables.

Neuropathies.– A mononeuropathy may be the presenting feature in diabetes mellitus and collagen diseases. Uraemia, myxoedema, alcohol, lead poisoning, virus infections (Guillain-Barré syndrome) and poliomyelitis may all produce a neuropathy with muscle weakness, wasting, and severe sensory symptoms.

Myopathies.– These rare conditions are due to disease within the muscles. They may be genetically determined as in muscular dystrophy, or acquired as in polymyositis or metabolic disorders. The muscles are weak and may be atrophied or hypertrophied. *Duchenne dystrophy* begins in early life, usually in boys before the age of 4, and presents as weakness of the pelvic girdle and back. *Facio-scapulohumeral dystrophy* presents in the second or third decade in both sexes, and involves weakness of the muscles of the face, shoulders and arms. *Limb girdle dystrophy* presents between adolescence and middle life and involves the shoulder girdle or pelvic girdle. *Polymyositis* can occur at any age, and usually involves proximal limb muscles. The muscles are tender, and the patient may be ill and febrile. When skin changes predominate *dermatomyositis* is likely which in the young is usually benign but in the older patient is often associated with carcinoma.

Myasthenia gravis.– This rare disease of young women is eminently treatable in many instances. The eyes are often implicated with ptosis, but any group of muscles may be involved. It is usually a symmetrical weakness with undue fatiguability as the outstanding feature. Intravenous edrophonium may reverse the weakness dramatically and can be safely administered in the surgery provided the patient is lying down and a test dose of 1 mg is given before the remaining 9 mg.

History taking

A careful history from a patient with clumsiness, weakness or palsy, can be of more use to a general practitioner than a neurological examination. Judicious questioning will help in assessing the remainder of the nervous system. The patient may be confused or have a speech disorder, and it may be necessary to involve another member of the family in the history-taking.

The mode of onset is of prime importance. Was it sudden or gradual? Has the weakness increased since it was first observed, improved, or remained unchanged? Is it generalized or localized, proximal or distal? Are there associated sensory changes or pain?

The severity of the symptoms can be assessed by relating the complaints to the activities of daily living. How far can the patient walk? Can he get out of the chair easily? Can he get out of the bath unaided? Has his writing changed? The intelligent patient may notice wasting and sometimes fasciculation. Other questions may reveal a history of headache, visual symptoms, or speech difficulties. A past history of a previous neurological dysfunction may lead to a suspicion of multiple sclerosis. The family history is relevant in the younger patient.

General medical disorders may present with neurological features and inquiry should be made into a history of recent weight loss, cough, polyuria or polydipsia.

At this stage it is useful to assess the social situation. What is the patient's job and how will this symptom affect his ability to work? What are his home conditions like? Is there a satisfactory family background with relatives able and willing to help during a difficult and possibly prolonged period of the patient's life?

The patient will be anxious and feel threatened by his symptoms. He may be at the beginning of his career in the 'sick role', and be resentful of his new position of dependence on relatives, doctors, and other helpers. He will be most helped by a doctor who is honest, and calm, and able to assure him that every action is being taken to help him.

Examination

These symptoms are rare but if the presentation suggests neurological disease a full neurological examination is desirable and with practice can be carried out expeditiously.

The patient who comes to the surgery.– How does the patient perform in the surgery? Does he walk with the high-stepping gait of foot-drop, or with the waddle of a proximal myopathy? Does he walk with the laborious stiffness of spasticity? Does he have to push himself up from the chair with his arms? Can he undo his buttons easily? Can he stand on one leg to remove his trousers without leaning on some support?

The paralysed patient at home. – The acute paralysis presenting at home will usually be due to a stroke. The patient may be unconscious with a flaccid paralysis, or fully conscious with a suddenly weak limb. Neurological examination should include assessment of the level of consciousness, the extent and locality of the weakness, and changes in muscle tone and reflexes. It is important to examine the heart for atrial fibrillation or murmurs, the neck for the presence of a carotid bruit, and the peripheral pulses for the presence of generalized vascular disease.

Examination and interpretation of findings. – Examination may reveal that the joints are stiff to move, the reflexes are brisk, and the plantar responses are extensor, suggesting a lesion of the upper motor neurone. A well-known adage in diagnosing multiple sclerosis is 'symptoms in one leg, signs in two'. In the older age-group, the commonest cause of spastic weakness in both lower limbs is cervical spondylosis; limitation of neck movement may therefore be apparent.

The observation of wasting and twitching of weak muscles indicates denervation. If there is marked tendency to fatigue, myasthenia gravis may be suspected. Cog-wheel rigidity, a sign of extrapyramidal weakness as in Parkinsonism, is strikingly shown if the patient is asked to clench and unclench the hand of the arm not being examined. Pill-rolling tremor may give the diagnosis away. Cerebellar clumsiness may be accompanied by nystagmus, slurred speech, and shakiness when the patient brings the index finger to the tip of the nose. He is unlikely to be able to walk in a straight line heel-to-toe. The posture in hemiplegia is characteristic. The arm is held flexed, adducted, with 'clasp knife' rigidity, and is more severely affected than the leg which is stiff, straight, and with a spastic inverted foot-drop. As the patient walks, he circumducts the leg to clear the foot from the ground.

General examination should include blood-pressure estimation, examination of the urine for sugar and protein, and ophthalmoscopic examination of the fundi. This latter examination will show if there is papilloedema indicating raised intracranial pressure, pallor of the disc as in multiple sclerosis, or abnormality of the blood vessels as in arteriosclerosis. The heart should be examined for the presence of murmurs or arrhythmias.

General management

Many of the diseases causing these symptoms have a poor prognosis. There is the possibility of long-term disablement and patients often become anxious, dependent and frustrated. There may be severe depression.

The correct diagnosis is imperative, particularly in predicting the likely course of events. Often there will be doubt about the diagnosis and the practitioner may need help from a specialist colleague. The condition involved is nearly always chronic, and continuity of care in a situation which must inevitably deteriorate over the years as in multiple sclerosis, will tax the skills of all members of the primary care team. The practitioner will need to have full support from relatives, nurses, social workers, physiotherapists and occupational therapists, with the result that the patient may be surrounded by a large group of helpers of which the doctor must act as co-ordinator.

The patient may wish to discuss the illness in detail; such discussion will tax the sensitivity, courage and communication skills of the doctor. Truth is often the best medicine and evading the issue may cause tension between doctor and patient which will prove a barrier to successful management. Patience will be required, and consistency in maintaining a regular commitment of care for the patient and his relatives.

Rehabilitation.— This must be started as soon as possible and the aim should be to improve the patient's functional capacity. For example, a drop-foot splint may make walking easier simply because it is no longer necessary to swing the foot outwards to obtain clearance. Modern foot splints will fit over most walking shoes and are scarcely discernible if worn with slacks or trousers. Provision of a light wrist splint to correct wrist-drop will enable the fingers to grasp again having been useless in the dropped position. With more severe degrees of weakness in the legs, a stick, tripod, elbow crutch or frame may give additional support while walking. Gripping devices and page-turners may render a weak hand more useful. For severe paralysis, 'Possum' electronic devices are available. Transport problems can be solved using automatic transmission or having the car converted to hand controls when only one good limb is necessary.

It is often best to be selective with aids, perhaps initially hiring for a trial period. Advice regarding special aids, including bathroom equipment and cutlery, can be obtained from the social services department occupational therapist. Under the Chronically Sick and Disabled Persons Act 1970, patients may be entitled to meals on wheels, home helps, and telephones which can be provided by the social services department.

Specific treatment

Stroke.— Treatment of the underlying hypertension, diabetes mellitus, anaemia or polycythaemia is obviously a priority. Anticoagulants are indicated when the cause is likely to be an embolus from atrial fibrillation or a mural thrombus, as is possible when there is a history of a transient ischaemic attack. Recent reports suggest that aspirin in doses of 300 mg daily may be useful in preventing further strokes following transient ischaemic attacks.

Multiple sclerosis.— In this condition particularly, the patient's confidence and trust in the doctor may depend more on a realistic attitude to improvements and exacerbations than to a superficial and constantly disappointed optimism. In the acute phase, injections of 40 units of corticotrophin (Acthar) twice daily may be used for one week, decreasing to daily for a week, then on alternate days for a week, and finally to twice weekly for a further three weeks. The value of this is still uncertain. Ephedrine, 15 mg three times daily, may be used for the treatment of urgency of micturition. Baclofen (Lioresal) or dantrolene (Dantrium) can sometimes usefully improve function by relieving spasticity.

Parkinsonism.— A combination of levodopa and carbidopa has been shown to produce the best response and the least side-effects.[7] This is available in tablets (Sinemet), each containing 250 mg of levodopa and 25 mg of carbidopa. The initial dose is ½ tablet three times daily, increasing by ½ tablet every two or three days until adverse reactions develop. These adverse reactions include the appearance of involuntary athetoid movements, vomiting, hypotension and restlessness. The dose can then be reduced by ½ tablet.

Cervical spondylosis.— If this is causing spastic weakness of the lower limbs a laminectomy may well be necessary and hospital management indicated.

Many of the other diseases mentioned in the causation of this group of symptoms will require hospital management.

Conclusion

Table I illustrates a problem-solving pathway. Clumsiness, weakness and palsy can be alarming symptoms which may affect young age-groups, and which often indicate a disease process with a grave outlook. Care and long-term management have to be planned on the basis of a correct diagnosis, and a realistic attitude towards the complaint and its prognosis.

Table I.— Problem-solving summary

UNILATERAL PALSY OF SUDDEN ONSET

Minor stroke in younger patient with carotid bruit. T.I.A.	May herald a major stroke	Refer urgently for anti-coagulants or surgery
With rheumatic heart disease, murmur and atrial fibrillation	Embolism	Refer urgently for anti-coagulants or surgery
With history of recent chest pain	Embolism from mural thrombus	Refer urgently for anti-coagulants or surgery
Completed stroke. Elderly patient	Cerebrovascular disease	Manage at home if circumstances permit
Previous neurological incident. Multiple lesions	Multiple sclerosis	Observe or refer if diagnostic help required

UNILATERAL PALSY OF GRADUAL ONSET

Progressive weakness with symptoms of raised intracranial pressure	Cerebral tumour	Refer for further investigation
In older patient with few obvious signs / rigidity and tremor	Parkinsonism	Treat with a form of levodopa

BILATERAL PALSY WITH SENSORY SYMPTOMS

Weakness, wasting associated with sensory symptoms	Neuropathy	exclude diabetes	Refer for investigation

(continued overleaf)

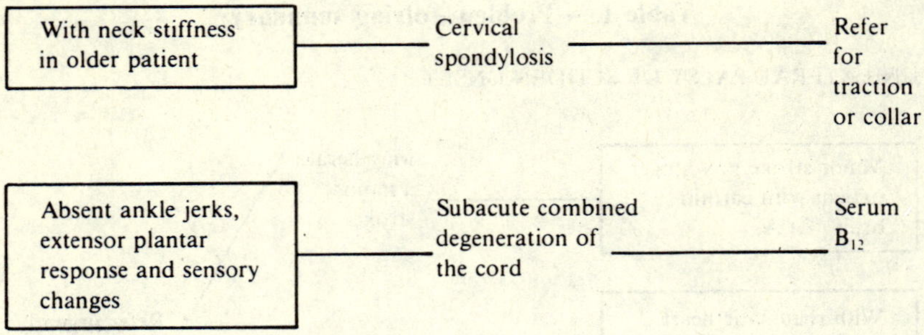

BILATERAL PALSY WITHOUT SENSORY SYMPTOMS

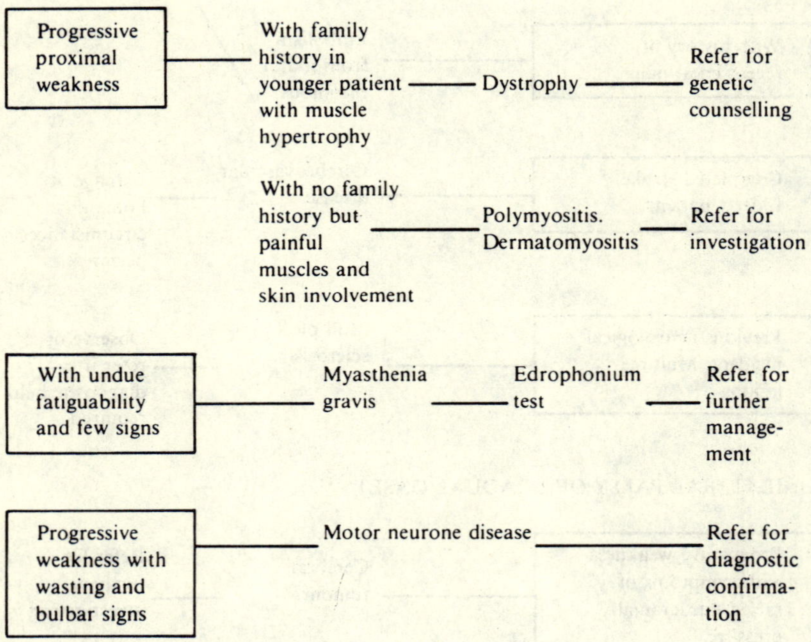

References

[1] Morrell, D.C., Gage, H.G. and Robinson, N.A. (1971): Symptoms in General Practice. *Journal of Royal College of General Practitioners*, *21*, 32

[2] Gilliatt, R.W. (1974): Preface. *Medicine*, *31*, 1800

[3] Marshall, J. (1974): Management of strokes. *Medicine*, *31*, 1838

[4] Matthews, B. (1974): Multiple sclerosis. *Medicine*, *33*, 1914

[5] Acheson, E.D. (1972): Epidemiology of Multiple Sclerosis. In *Multiple Sclerosis.* Ed. D. McAlpine, C.E. Lumsden and E.D. Acheson. 2nd ed. Edinburgh: Churchill Livingstone

[6] Brewis, M., Poikanzer, D.C., Rolland, C. and Miller, H. (1966): Neurological disease in an English City. *Acta Neurol. Scand.*, *42*, supp 24.1

[7] Calne, C.B. and Pallis, C. (1974): Parkinsonism. *Medicine*, *32*, 1895

3.10 The patient with numbness and pins and needles

Judith Millac

In an analysis of 5,345 symptoms presenting in general practice, there was a total of fifteen disturbances of sensation other than specific complaints of pain: four in males and eleven in females.[1] Although transient numbness with pins and needles is an almost universal experience, only rarely will this be the harbinger of a lesion of the nervous system or lead to a consultation. The general practitioner has the task of distinguishing the banal from the sinister, and a basic grasp of the organization of the sensory pathways will assist considerably in the assessment of these symptoms.

Presentation

There may be difficulty in describing sensory symptoms. Although pain is a symptom that most patients understand and can easily describe, numbness and paraesthesiae are sensations more difficult to express in words. Patients may say that a limb or part of the body feels cold, hot, numb or heavy. Other descriptions include tingling, pins and needles, feeling that a limb is swollen, sensations such as tight bands around parts of the body or of water trickling over the skin. They may notice 'electric shocks' on moving the neck which radiate rapidly to the head or feet. The complaint may be of difficulty in performing normal tasks: for example, if the hand is affected there may be inability to thread a needle. If the lower limb is affected, the patient is unsteady and feels as if he were walking on cotton wool. Occasionally, the problem of using the correct descriptive term leads the patient to use the expression 'numbness' to describe paralysis. Numbness may be produced by excessive cold particularly if there is vascular insufficiency, and pins and needles can occur on warming a cold extremity.

As the sensory system mediates our perception of the environment, so in emotional disturbances normal sensibilities can be heightened to the extent of producing sensory symptoms without disease. Conversely, the human mind cannot bear total deprivation.

Causes

These are considered in terms of the level at which the sensory pathways are involved.

Peripheral nerve lesions.– The commonest cause of pain and paraesthesiae in the distal part of the upper limb is entrapment of the median nerve at the wrist giving rise to the *carpal tunnel syndrome.*[2] The patient, usually a woman in pregnancy or early middle age, complains of burning pain or tingling and pins and needles in the first three fingers of the hand, which wakes her at night. On waking the hand feels numb, swollen and painful. The right hand is most commonly involved, and the symptoms are aggravated by manual activities. This syndrome may be symptomatic of myxoedema or rheumatoid arthritis.

Certain occupations involving active use of the arm, and injuries and deformities at the elbow, can produce an *ulnar nerve lesion.* The numbness involves the fourth and fifth fingers and the adjacent border of the hand. There is often wasting of the small muscles of the hand.

Entrapment of the *lateral cutaneous nerve* of the thigh as it passes under the inguinal ligament produces pain in the thigh: the syndrome known as *meralgia paraesthetica.* This occurs in obese, middle-aged people often after recent weight gain and presents initially as pain and pins and needles over the outer aspect of the thigh precipitated by standing and relieved by recumbency. It is a benign condition, which nevertheless can be distressing.

Compression or trauma to the *lateral popliteal nerve* as it winds round the neck of the fibula causes a foot-drop with numbness of the outer border of the foot extending some way up the leg. It can be caused by a tight bandage or plaster.

Generalized disease of peripheral nerves (neuropathies).– Diabetes mellitus, renal disease, drug intoxication (for example with nitrofurantoin, isoniazid and vincristine), alcoholism, vitamin B_{12} deficiency, the collagen diseases and virus infections can produce a clinical picture of 'glove and stocking' sensory loss to all sensations and may be accompanied by distal weakness and absent reflexes.

Ten to twelve per cent of *diabetics*[3] develop a significant neuropathy but an even larger proportion have a mild symmetrical sensory polyneuropathy. This presents as numbness and pins and needles in the feet, less commonly in the fingers. Aching or stabbing pains in the legs, particularly at night, may also be a feature. On examination there will be diminished ankle jerks and loss of vibration sense in the feet.

In *alcoholic* neuropathy, the symptoms are distal sensorimotor with spontaneous aching pain in the extremities, cutaneous hyperaesthesia and tenderness of the soles of the feet and calf muscles.

In the *Guillain-Barré syndrome,* the presentation is usually of weakness, but distal paraesthesiae in the limbs are common. There is either acute or subacute onset over a few days and an antecedent viral infection is identifiable in over 50 per cent of the cases.[4]

Those who work in immigrant areas need to realize that discrete patches of sensory loss over trunk or limbs, particularly with pigmentary changes or erythema, may signify *leprosy.*

Nerve plexus lesions.– Damage to the lower roots of the *brachial plexus* will produce sensory changes similar to those of an ulnar nerve lesion with extension to involve the median aspect of the arm. The possibility of cervical rib, which may sometimes be palpated in the neck, or an apical pulmonary tumour has to be considered.

The lumbosacral plexus is rarely damaged and then usually by malignant disease in the pelvis in an advanced stage.

Nerve root lesions.– The sensory disturbance due to 'root' lesions is often less prominent than the complaint of pain.

The commonest lesion of the nerve roots is *herpes zoster,* typically affecting a thoracic segment, but no level of the nervous system is immune. The characteristic rash, which may appear up to ten days after the hyperaesthesia, is diagnostic.

Cervical spondylosis may interfere with nerve roots, causing tingling and numbness in the upper limb, involving both the fingers and outer aspect of the arm. It sometimes occurs after an attack of neck stiffness and pain. Lateral movement of the neck may be limited and there may be diminution of the biceps or triceps jerk.

The *lumbar root syndrome* is most commonly due to a prolapsed intervertebral disc compressing the fifth lumbar and first sacral roots. Other less common causes are intraspinal tumours, neurofibromas or secondary neoplasms. The sensory disturbance is in the form of pins and needles and subjective numbness passing down the back of the thigh on to the lateral aspect of the leg and foot, but pain is the predominant symptom. Rarely a central disc protrusion may cause extensive perineal sensory loss, often with sphincter upset as well.

Diseases involving damage within the spinal cord.– These conditions are relatively uncommon, except *multiple sclerosis* which often presents with sensory symptoms, some of which may sound so bizarre as to suggest hysteria. For example, the patient may complain of tight bands around the rib cage and limbs, crawling sensations on the skin (formication) and even the illusion of water running down the leg. The symptoms hardly ever persist, but recurrent attacks are common. 'Electric shock' sensation down the back and legs may be induced by neck flexion (Lhermitte's sign).

Rare, but eminently treatable, is *subacute combined degeneration of the cord* due to vitamin B_{12} deficiency. The cause may be pernicious anaemia, but it can also follow gastrectomy or ileal resection, in gluten enteropathy, or in individuals on a strictly vegetarian diet. There is often a distal sensory neuropathy giving rise to glove and stocking sensory disturbances, as well as extensor plantar responses: a highly distinctive clinical picture.

The main features of the unmistakable but rare syndrome of *syringomyelia* are a dissociated sensory loss to pain and temperature accompanied by weakness.[5] The sensory loss which usually occurs first along the ulnar border of the hand extends upwards to the face with relative sparing of the snout area, and downwards to the chest: the so-called 'half-cape' distribution. The patient may present with painless burns or injuries of the hands.

Syphilis of the central nervous system is now uncommon but in *tabes dorsalis* damage to the posterior columns causes loss of joint position sense and hence loss of balance. There may be the so-called 'lightning' pains. The patient will exhibit a Romberg's sign. The typical irregular unequal pupils unresponsive to light should be sought.

Brain stem lesions.– The presentation may be circumoral pins and needles, and tingling in the limbs of both sides. Another presentation may be sensory loss on one side of the face and the opposite of the body. Diplopia and vertigo are also likely to be present.

Damage to the sensory cortex.– This produces a more sophisticated sensory impairment with loss of the finer discriminative aspects of sensibility which are difficult to assess. The hand may be unable to distinguish shapes and textures and numbers drawn upon it, and there may be loss of two-point discrimination. Gross sensation, however, is intact. Occasionally epilepsy may manifest as focal sensory attacks.

History

Salient points for enquiry include mode of onset and duration of symptoms, as well as their character and distribution.
Does the sensory loss involve all types of sensation, or is it dissociated? In other words, are pain and temperature disturbed but not touch and vibration?
Are the symptoms persistent, intermittent or more pronounced by day or by night? Are they brought on by changes in posture, or movements of the neck or back?
Is the distribution that of a peripheral nerve, a spinal segment, cord pathways, thalamic or cortical? If the sensory manifestations do not conform with any of these, either a generalized metabolic disturbance or neurosis is a possibility. Other relevant symptoms therefore, such as those suggesting diabetes mellitus, myxoedema, acromegaly, or pernicious anaemia must be excluded.
Finally, does the patient describe the sensory disturbance in realistic terms or with lurid elaboration suggesting a strong emotional content in the disability.

Examination

This is used to confirm the distribution of symptoms, and a knowledge of the anatomical distribution of the sensory spinal roots is helpful (figure 1). Light touch is tested with cotton-wool with the patient's eyes closed. Superficial pain is tested by pin-prick, and deep pain by squeezing a muscle between thumb and finger. Temperature sense is tested by using two tubes, one filled with ice and the other with water at 45°C, and postural sense by placing a segment of the limb in a certain position, and asking the patient to describe the position with his eyes closed. Vibration sense is tested with a tuning fork and tactile discrimination by a two-point compass. Stereognosis, or the appreciation of form, is tested by asking the patient to recognize a common object placed in his hand. Other observations include examination for wasting, and noticing if there is a high-stepping gait indicating sensory ataxia. Increased unsteadiness when the patient is asked to stand with the eyes closed (Romberg's sign) demonstrates loss of proprioceptive sense.
The general examination should indicate whether pernicious anaemia, myxoedema, acromegaly or diabetes mellitus is present.

Investigation

Immediate investigation must include examination of the urine to

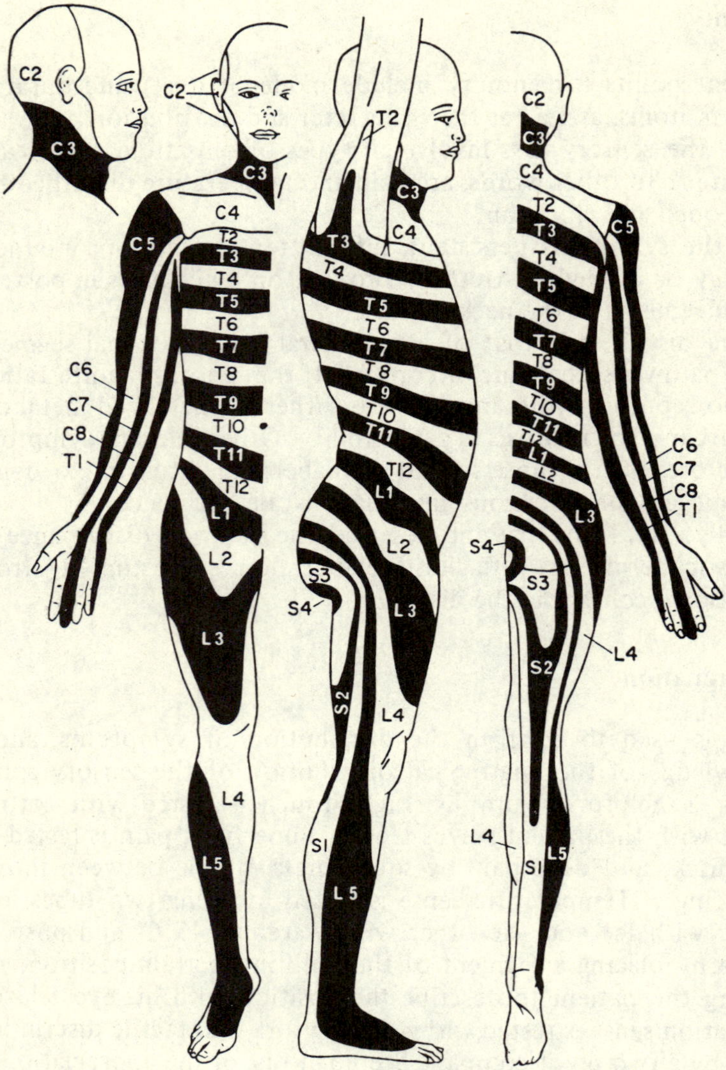

Figure 1. A diagram of the distribution of the sensory spinal roots on the surface of the body

(From Holmes, G. (1968): *An Introduction to Clinical Neurology*. 3rd ed. Edinburgh: Churchill Livingstone)

exclude diabetes mellitus. A full blood count will help to exclude pernicious anaemia, although serum vitamin B_{12} estimation is also important as this may well be low before the blood picture changes. A Wassermann reaction (WR) must also be considered as a possible investigation.

Interpretation of signs

Loss of cutaneous sensation with wasting indicates a peripheral nerve lesion, and the area involved will correlate with the distribution of that nerve. Where this distribution is in the so-called 'glove and stocking' area, a polyneuropathy is likely. Individual sensory modalities may be lost where there is a lesion within the spinal cord. This is the dissociated sensory loss, typified by syringomyelia where loss of pain and temperature sensation indicates a lesion involving the spinothalamic tract.

Diminished vibration and position senses occur where there is posterior column damage, and in the case of subacute combined degeneration of the cord this is often associated with a lesion of the pyramidal tract, thus the finding of extensor plantar responses. Loss of position sense and associated touch and tactile sense occurs in a lesion known as the Brown-Séquard syndrome. Here, half the spinal cord is damaged by trauma or malignancy, or occasionally multiple sclerosis. Impaired two-point discrimination and stereognosis indicate a lesion within the sensory cortex.

The practitioner needs to be aware that hysteria may present as loss of all sensory modalities in a pattern which does not conform to any anatomical boundaries: e.g., the description of total numbness involving the whole of one side of the body, or in a distribution not unlike the 'glove and stocking' effect in neuropathy but ending in a sharp border instead of fading away.

Management

Diagnosis in cases of neuropathy is important in order to treat the underlying cause, although in over half there will be no obvious cause. Hospital referral for specialist advice is needed for these patients. In others, in whom the underlying cause for the symptoms is benign, as in meralgia, reassurance is all that is required. Similarly, when there are transitory symptoms, which are not disabling, a 'wait and see' policy can be adopted. Even in the lumbar disc syndrome there is no necessity for rapid intervention, and unless the sphincters are involved, a conservative policy can be adopted.

Carpal tunnel syndrome can often be successfully managed in general practice, by the use of night splints, analgesics and diuretics. Injection of the carpal tunnel with hydrocortisone can be helpful. The injection is made at the medial side of the palmaris longus muscle at the site of the distal skin crease using 1 to 2 ml of an intra-articular steroid preparation. In severe

cases referral for decompression surgery may be necessary.
In *meralgia paraesthetica* when pain is severe injection of local anaesthetic around the nerve may give relief.
A cervical collar in patients with *cervical spondylosis* can give rapid and effective relief of symptoms, although more severe cases may need bed rest, and analgesics, or traction and even decompression.
Subacute combined degeneration of the cord due to vitamin B_{12} deficiency should be treated with hydroxocobalamin 1,000 micrograms daily at first, reducing to 500 micrograms twice weekly, until maximum benefit is reached when a maintenance dose of 1 mgm every three months is sufficient.

Conclusion

Table I illustrates a problem-solving pathway. In many cases of localized numbness and pins and needles, a relatively minor condition is involved and local treatment or reassurance is all that is required. Reassurance and time are useful forms of therapy. Awareness of the more serious presentations, however, an example of which is the glove and stocking sensory loss accompanied by weakness characteristic of peripheral neuropathy, is essential.

Table I.— Problem-solving summary

Peripheral nerve lesions

Pain and tingling in the hand, mainly the first three fingers, worst at night	Carpal tunnel syndrome	Exclude pregnancy, myxoedema, rheumatoid arthritis	Inject or refer for decompression
Pain or tingling in little finger and median aspect of hand with wasting of small muscles of hand	Ulnar nerve lesion	Exclude injury or deformity at elbow	Refer if progressive
Pain or tingling in outer aspect of thigh after recent weight gain, worse on standing	Meralgia paraesthetica		Usually no treatment necessary

Numbness of outer border of foot with foot-drop and history of injury or pressure at knee	Lesion of lateral popliteal nerve		Usually no treatment necessary

Neuropathy

Glove and stocking sensory loss, distal weakness, wasting	Peripheral neuropathy	Exclude diabetes mellitus	Refer for urgent diagnostic help

Nerve root lesions

Hyperaesthesia followed by a rash	Herpes zoster		Treat with idoxuridine
Tingling and numbness in upper limb with neck stiffness: C 5,6	Cervical spondylosis	Confirm by neck x-ray	Refer for collar or traction
Pain, pins and needles, sometimes numbness down back of thigh, lateral aspect of leg and foot/suggestive history	Lumbar disc lesion		Bed rest and analgesics initially

Spinal cord lesions

Bizarre intermittent sensory symptoms, with 'electric shocks' induced by neck flexion, and other signs such as optic neuritis or cerebellar ataxia	Multiple sclerosis		Observe, or refer for diagnostic help
Glove and stocking sensory loss with extensor plantars	Subacute combined degeneration of the cord	Confirm with full blood count and serum B_{12}	Treat with B_{12}

Signs	Diagnosis	Action
Painless burns, loss of reflexes in limbs/ loss of pain and temperature sense/ weakness	Syringomyelia	No known treatment
Lightning pains/ unequal pupils/ Rombergism	Tabes dorsalis	Confirm with WR

Brain stem lesion

Signs	Action
Circumoral parasthesiae, sensorimotor signs all limbs/vertigo and diplopia	Refer for further investigation

Cortical lesion

Signs	Action
Astereognosis/loss of two-point discrimination/gross sensation intact	Refer for further investigation

References

[1] Morrell, D.C., Gage, H.G. and Robinson, N.A. (1971): Symptoms in General Practice. *Journal of the Royal College of General Practitioners*, *21*, 32

[2] Gilliat, R.W. (1970): Spinal root and peripheral nerve lesions. *Medicine*, *33*, 1940

[3] Annotation (1972): Diabetic Neuropathy. *British Medical Journal*, *4*, 5

[4] Thomas, P.K., Lascelles, R.G., Hallpike, J.F. and Hewer, R.I. (1969): Recurrent and chronic relapsing Guillain-Barré polyneuritis, *Brain*, *92*, 589

[5] Barrett, H.J.M., Foster, J.B. and Hudgson, P. (1973): Syringomyelia. *Major Problems in Neurology*, Vol. 1. London: W.B. Saunders

3.11 The patient with difficulty in speaking

Marshall Marinker

Broadly speaking the general practitioner meets disorders of speech in three situations. The first, and by far the commonest, is the difficulty in phonation experienced by people suffering from acute or recurrent laryngitis. The second, and perhaps the most important, is the presentation by parents of speech disorders, real or imagined, in their children. Last, a relatively rare group, come the speech disorders which are part of general systemic upsets such as myxoedema, multiple sclerosis, Parkinsonism, cerebrovascular accidents and so on. In this last group the presentation of speech disorder as the primary symptom is rare.

Presentation

The patient who presents with a hoarse voice needs no describing. In the acute attack there is almost invariably a recent history of a coryza-like illness. Sometimes the hoarseness is recurrent, and may be precipitated by excessive use of the voice, or sometimes overuse or faulty voice production. In the 1981–82 National Study of Morbidity[1] there was an average of 15 episodes of acute laryngitis or acute tracheitis per 1,000 of the population at risk; 40 per cent of these patients were under the age of 5.

Complaints made by parents about their children's speech may concern the quality of the speech: for example hoarseness or huskiness. There may be a complaint that the tone is unusual: for example, the so-called hypernasality in children with a short or cleft palate, or with profound perceptive deafness. Or there may be the hyponasality of children with large adenoid pads or sometimes with conductive deafness.[2] There may be disorders of fluency, the most common of which is stammering. One survey suggests that three to four per cent of school children stammer for a period, although only 1 per cent of children have a stammer which persists into adult life.[3] Dysarthria, that is a neurologically determined motor disorder of articulation, may present as a failure of communication, often with words which are intelligible only to the parents. Usually this is part of a larger picture of

motor handicap and mental retardation. Sometimes the complaint is simply one of delayed speech in a child whose general friendliness and sociability appear quite normal. Two-thirds of children say their first words by twelve months and approximately the same proportion begin to use phrases by twenty-four months. Many otherwise normal children remain more or less mute for some time after this, and it becomes important to distinguish between serious physical or psychological disturbance and the tail end of a normal distribution of speech development.
The changes in speech associated with major systemic upsets are often typical of the disease which they represent: for example, the lalling or baby speech, sometimes including words of the patient's own invention, which results from congenital auditory interception. Once heard the 'scanning speech' of multiple sclerosis is unmistakable, as is the thin monotonous voice of Parkinsonism. These diagnoses, however, rarely depend on a recognition of voice change, nor is the first complaint likely to be one of alteration in the ability to speak. Similarly the low gruff voice of myxoedema is only part of a clinical picture and rarely the presentation of the disease. Occasionally, particularly in the elderly, a small cerebrovascular accident may present simply as a disturbance of speech, paralysis of an arm or leg being only partial and perhaps not even appreciated by the patient or the relatives.

Causes

The physiological causes of speech disorders associated with the major systemic upsets mentioned are not relevant to the management of the problem, which is usually the management of the disease process itself. This section is mainly concerned with the causes of language disorders in childhood.
Hoarseness, when it is not caused by an acute laryngitis or tracheitis, is associated with small benign tumours on the vocal cords. These are said to occur either as a result of recurrent attacks of laryngitis or often misuse of the voice. Hypernasality occurs as a result of cleft palate. Hyponasality is characteristic of enlarged adenoids and sometimes is associated with conductive deafness.
Stammering or stuttering occurs as a result of faulty learning, and is thought to be associated with inappropriate reception of the child's speech by others, most commonly the parents.
In children slurred speech, as well as delayed speech, may occur because of the disruption of muscular coordination consequent on cerebral palsy. This problem may be much more important

than a concurrent mental retardation in that improvements may be looked for from speech therapy.

Mental retardation is the disorder most often associated with delayed speech. Great care, however, must be exercised before reaching this diagnosis, since children with normal intelligence may delay for some time and the premature incorrect labelling of a child as mentally retarded can have a devastating effect on family and child alike. It is reported[4] that Lord Macaulay did not speak until the age of 4, when he replied to a lady who had trodden on his toe with his first uttered sentence: 'Thank you, Madam, the agony is abated'.

Next to mental retardation, deafness is the commonest cause of delayed speech. The faculty of speech is delayed because the child does not receive an adequate sensory input.

Psychiatric causes of speech disorder and delay are rare. Occasionally, as part of a larger condition affecting the personality of the developing child, speech is delayed or distorted as part of a general problem with communication. The grossest disturbance occurs in autism. Here a delay in speech and the development of language is accompanied by a failure to develop interpersonal relationships, and ritualistic and compulsive phenomena.

It is not only in autism that failures in relationships and communication in the home adversely affects the development of speech. Stevenson[2] lists such factors as institutionalization, large families, deaf parents, mothers with depression or other mental illness, and poor child-minding arrangements. She points out that the middle-class child in the care of a succession of au pair girls may be more handicapped than poor children. She also makes the important point that in children of the poor, there is not only an increased likelihood of adverse environmental factors, but also an increased incidence of biologically based speech and language disorders, because of the increased risk of perinatal morbidity in this group.

Lastly, it should be remembered that changes in phonation caused by adenoidal hypertrophy in recurrent upper respiratory-tract infections, or a period of stuttering or slowness to develop the facility of speech and language may all be part of normal growing up.

History and examination

In the case of hoarseness or the changes in voice or speech associated with major systemic upsets, the presentation will suggest the line of enquiry and the extent of the examination. For example, in hoarseness of recent origin, (almost certainly an acute laryngitis) laryngoscopy is totally unnecessary. In chronic or recurrent hoarseness, laryngoscopy may be considered in order to exclude the rare neoplasm, or the benign wart-like growths on the cord; but this manoeuvre will usually be performed by an ear, nose and throat surgeon. A history of voice misuse, or identifying a precipitating factor to which the patient is peculiarly sensitive, may sometimes help in preventing future attacks.

Hysterical aphonia may be difficult to diagnose and the clue is often given by what is known of the patient's personality and reaction to stress. Even in such circumstances, the diagnosis is often made by the failure to establish physical causes for the aphonia.

Rarely, damage to one of the recurrent laryngeal nerves, either in the course of thyroid surgery, or as a result of invasion from carcinoma of bronchus, may give rise to hoarseness, as may the still more rare carcinoma of larynx.

The changes in voice or speech associated with systemic conditions will lead simply to a search for further stigmata of these conditions. They will not be dealt with in this chapter.

It is in elucidating the speech problems of children that the general practitioner requires a systematic approach to history and examination.

The history should be directed at possible causes of deafness in the child: for example, rubella in the mother during pregnancy, or the taking of ototoxic drugs. The history of the delivery, when this is available, should be scanned. Was there any accident or trauma to the infant? Were any defects of ear, nose or throat noted? Was the baby premature by dates or weight? Was there a history of anoxia or a low Apgar score? From the history of the post-natal period and early infancy, symptoms and signs suggesting motor disturbance, hyperactivity, abnormalities of the reflexes, recurrent ear infection, a history of mumps, meningitis or measles or the use of ototoxic drugs will all give clues as to a possible physical cause.

Socio-cultural deprivation is an important cause of speech delay. Not so much from the past history, which can be misleading, but from an observation of the interaction between mother and child in the consultation, much can be learned about the quality of the relationship, the degree of intimacy, the way in which the mother listens to the child and responds to it. For a more detailed account of developmental assessment in infancy and childhood the reader is referred to Chapter 4.2.

Chapter 3.20 deals with the measurement of hearing loss, appropriate to the general practitioner's consulting-room. However, even when such measurement fails to give positive results, particularly when the measurement is made not with an audiometer but with more crude measures such as rattles, voice and tuning fork tests, early referral is important in order to rule out limited hearing defects which may interfere with adequate development of speech and language. In skilled hands such defects can be detected as early as six months. Indeed, high risk babies should be referred for assessment in the first two months of life.

The physical examination may be directed to a search for the stigmata of such conditions as cerebral palsy, or cleft palate, or serous otitis media suggested by the history. In particular the doctor will be at pains to assess the milestones of development and to compare these with the child's age (see Chapter 4.2). An exploration of the child's capacity to learn the names of things, or of the child's semantic system and use of syntactic structures, is generally left to the clinical psychologist.

Management

Acute laryngitis is best treated by resting the voice, by encouraging hot drinks and the use of steam inhalation to which compound benzoin tincture B.P.C. may be added. Recurrent hoarseness, even when vocal nodules have been demonstrated, is treated in the same way. The surgical removal of these nodules is often followed by their return. As in the rare hoarseness which results from damage to one of the recurrent laryngeal nerves following thyroid surgery, there is no alternative to acceptance of the disability. The management of speech disorders caused by local structural lesions is self-evident; the referral of the child with cleft palate, or the child with grossly hypertrophid adenoids, for surgery. So-called 'tongue-tie' almost never gives rise to a speech disorder, although parents often incriminate a short or thickened frenulum. If the tip of the tongue can be protruded beyond the teeth, the parents can be reassured that the frenulum presents no structural impediment to the normal development of speech.

In those disorders of speech which accompany major systemic upsets in the adult, such as a cerebrovascular accident, Parkinsonism, multiple sclerosis and so on, there may be some limited help from speech therapy, but this will almost always be initiated by the neurologist who has been consulted. Except in the case of a stroke, where recovery of speech may sometimes be much more marked than recovery of the paralysed arm, the doctor should be cautious not to promise too much.

Stammering in the child is most often a short self-limiting episode. There will often be a great deal of parental anxiety accompanying the common speech variants of childhood, stuttering, lisping, a regression to infantile speech patterns and so on. An explanation to the parent that this is within the normal range of human behaviour in the development of the child may be enough, but often the parents need considerable support from the general practitioner, and in particular they need guidance on how to react to the child. They should be encouraged not to show their anxiety to the child, nor to be over 'helpful', by correcting him whenever he stutters, or suggesting that he talk 'more slowly'. The elements of learning theory may be explained to the parents, who are then told to encourage and reward the child when the speech patterns are normal, but to make no adverse comment, either in the way of scolding or in the way of patient correction, when the child stutters. If the problem persists for more than three months a speech therapist should be consulted.

In childhood, any speech disorder which may be associated with deafness, or mental retardation, or a neurologically based motor disorder should be referred for specialist assessment. By and large, referral to a speech therapist is via a paediatric specialist, and as a general rule referral cannot be too early.[2]

For the toddler with late speech development, attendance at a nursery school is often recommended: the child most likely to benefit, that is the child who comes from a deprived environment, is the one least likely to attend regularly. As in so many serious diseases of childhood, there is a vicious cycle of deprivation, biological and social. The breaking of this cycle, and the attempt to give the child a new beginning, is a major challenge to the quality of primary medical care.

References

[1] Royal College of General Practitioners, Office of Population Censuses and Surveys, Department of Health and Social Security (1986): *Morbidity Statistics from General Practice 1981–82*. HMSO Series MB5 No. 1

[2] Stevenson, P. (1976): Problems of Childhood: Speech Problems. *British Medical Journal, 1,* 635

[3] Andrews, G. and Harris, M. (1964): *Clinics in Developmental Medicine,* No. 17. London: Heinemann

[4] Sir George Otto Trevelyan (1932): *Life and Letters of Lord Macaulay.* London: Oxford University Press

3.12 The patient complaining of headache

H. R. Patterson

Presentation

Headache is a common symptom, and for the most part patients who suffer from headache do not consult their doctors on this account. In one survey[1] 38 per cent of adults who kept health diaries recorded at least one episode of headache during a two week period. In that same survey 41 per cent of those taking medicines took analgesics, and of those who took analgesics, two-fifths said that they took it in order to relieve 'migraine'.

Fry (1966) noted that headache was reported as a symptom in only 12 per cent of general practitioner consultations, and the diagnostic rate for specific headaches is much smaller than this. It is difficult to have much confidence in the epidemiology of headache because for the most part what is being measured is a symptom, whose severity and significance are related to such uncontrollable variables as culture and personality. None the less it is claimed that about 20 per cent of the population suffer from 'migraine'.

The commonest headaches are so-called tension headaches. Typically the tension headache is described as a feeling of pressure or a band around the head. Although there may be a diurnal variation, these headaches often last all day and may occur daily. Many people who have tension headaches are labelled as migraine sufferers by themselves, by their relatives and sometimes by their doctors. Here the term migraine is used as an expression of severity, and not as a description of a separate and specific disease entity. Headaches which occur daily, apart from cluster headaches, are never due to migraine.

Migraine is often a familial disorder; the headaches, which are sometimes unilateral, are throbbing and vary in intensity, frequency and duration. They may be cyclical, for example occurring on the same day of the week or in relation to the menstrual cycle, and they may remit for long periods of time. The headaches may be preceded by visual symptoms, nausea and vomiting, and other neurological disturbances. The following classification is useful:

1. Classical migraine — headache preceded by transient focal neurological symptoms.
2. Common migraine — similar headache without the prodromal symptoms.
3. Cluster headaches — more commonly occurring in men than women and starting with severe pain in one eye which then spreads over the face. They occur in bouts lasting from two to 12 weeks at intervals of three months to three years.
4. Hemiplegic and ophthalmoplegic migraine in which the neurological signs follow the headache.

There are a small number of serious, damaging and comparatively rare causes of headache: temporal arteritis, meningitis, glaucoma. The rarity of these events should not dissuade the doctor from trying to elicit a palpable tortuous temporal artery, or neck stiffness, or a raised intraocular tension.

Headache is often a component of other generalized illnesses, in particular of acute infections which cause a fever.

Causes

The causes of tension headache defy listing, and the reader is referred to Chapter 3.2 (The anxious patient). The causes of migraine include a familial vulnerability to the condition, dietary factors, hormonal factors, environmental factors like heat, light and sound, sleep (both too little and too much), the occurrence of emotional stress and also the release from it. Migraine often occurs after a period of intense activity or strain.

History

In coming to a decision about the nature of a headache, the history is all important. In contrast, the physical examination plays a minor role, and is often conducted more for the comfort of the patient than for the elucidation of the problem. The strategy of a history should be aimed to answer the following questions:

1. Why has the patient come *now*?
2. What does the patient believe to be wrong, or what does he fear?
3. Are there sufficient features of migraine to warrant an exhibition of the more specific remedies? (see below)
4. If this is a tension headache, what are the sources of tension?
5. Can I be reasonably certain that none of the very rare but potentially dangerous causes of headache is likely to be present?

At some stage in the consultation, doctors should find out why the patient has chosen to come at this particular time. The headache may have been recurrent over months or years, and the reason for consulting now may shed light on an underlying fear. A relative may have had a stroke, a colleague may have developed a cerebral tumour, there may have been a family crisis or the patient may have been invited to take on new responsibilities which are proving too much. Linked to these questions is the issue of the patient's own diagnosis. The patient may say, 'It's really the tension rather than the headache. I'm worried about my blood pressure . . .'. Although hypertension is very rarely a sufficient cause for headache, no such consultation should end without the patient's blood pressure having been checked — whatever else transpires between doctor and patient.

As with any pain, it is important to ask detailed questions under the following headings:

1. *Time.* When did the headaches first occur? What is their duration? How frequently do they occur, and is the frequency changing?
2. *Site.* Where is the pain? Over what area does it extend? Is there any referral?
3. *Character.* A vascular headache is always throbbing: the description of a tension headache may vary according to the degree of anxiety present, or the patient's flair for rhetoric; but a throbbing headache is usually migrainous.
4. *Precipitating factors.* Tension, domestic or work stress, other causes of emotional upset, may be involved both in migraine and in tension headache. Migraine, however, is more usually precipitated by specific 'triggers'. Dietary factors include fasting, alcohol (particularly red wine) and chocolate. There may be hormonal factors, presenting as headache around the time of menstruation or made worse (sometimes better) by taking the contraceptive pill, or pregnancy, during which the headaches often remit. Physical factors like heat, light, certain sounds and even certain smells can trigger an attack of migraine. As to the psychological factors, so many are described that it is unlikely that any one can be specifically incriminated. However the so-called 'release from tension' headache manifesting as an attack of migraine at the weekend, or at the beginning of a holiday, is often a feature of the history.
5. *Relieving factors.* Migraine usually responds to a number of simple remedies: in particular, patients may learn to take analgesics early in an attack, to lie in a quiet, darkened room, and sometimes to use a cold compress on the head. A headache which does not respond at all to analgesic tablets is unlikely to have a physical cause.

   In the case of children, it is particularly important with a recent headache to elicit a history of pyrexia or of head injury.

Associated symptoms

Tension headache may often be accompanied by other symptoms of tension: a tachycardia, sweating and a subjective feeling of general anxiety. Patients often complain of 'pain behind the eyes', though the doctor should bear in mind that anxious patients also get glaucoma.

There is a wide variety of neurological symptoms associated with migraine. The doctor should enquire about disturbances of vision, for example fortification spectra, scotomata, diplopia, or difficulty in focusing. There may be speech disturbance, clumsiness, vertigo or paraesthesiae. Most of these phenomena occur before the onset of the headache, during the phase of vasoconstriction, and are in effect a migrainous transient ischaemic attack. In hemiplegic and ophthalmoplegic migraine, the symptoms may follow the headache and can be alarming, not only for the patient but for the doctor also.

Finally, attention should be paid to the early past history and the family history. Patients with migraine may give a history of cyclical vomiting in childhood or so-called abdominal migraine. There may be a strong family history, and this has to be differentiated from a family tradition of headache, which may simply reflect the way in which the patient and his relatives take on the role of sick person.

Physical examination

Physical examination rarely leads to a further differentiation between migraine headaches and tension headaches. If there are neurological symptoms, or a change in mood or personality, the physical examination will be necessary to eliminate the likelihood of some other form of neurological damage. If there are focal signs, particularly some hours following the headache, the opinion of a neurologist should be sought. In a child with persistent headache of recent onset, the presence of neck stiffness is almost always sufficient evidence to require hospital admission.

In the adult the possibility of glaucoma should be checked by testing the visual fields, inspection of the pupils and depth of the anterior chamber, some estimation of intra-ocular tension by palpating over the closed lids, and inspecting the optic discs with an ophthalmoscope.

Most patients with migraine will exhibit only a few of the classical symptoms. Most persuasive are the presence of a family history, the periodicity of the headaches, and the fact that they are throbbing in character. A headache which occurs daily is very unlikely to be migraine. The exception is cluster headaches, described earlier.

Management

There are three important aims in the management of headache. The first is the relief of anxiety. But because headache is such a common human experience, the fact that a patient consults a doctor because of his symptoms may suggest a considerable heightening of anxiety, and this may be associated with fears about the cause. Wherever possible, therefore, the doctor should be at pains to explain to his patient the nature of the headache, its natural history and the fact that the course of the illness, although often disturbing, is also usually benign. Patients with migraine, particularly those who experience focal neurological symptoms, may well fear that they are about to have a stroke.
The second aim is the relief of pain. In the case of migraine, it is also important to relieve any associated vertigo, nausea or vomiting. The third aim is to minimize the frequency and severity of subsequent attacks. The natural history of most headaches is that they recur at unpredictable and varying intervals (though some cases of migraine are in fact regular and predictable) over many years.

1. *The relief of anxiety*

Drugs are the least important component of this aspect of management. The exclusion of the rare serious causes of headaches, and a sensitive explanation of the nature of the symptoms to the patient, are of prime importance. When anxiolytics are required, small doses of minor tranquillizers will usually suffice. A suitable choice is diazepam 2 mg twice or three times a day. This is not only used for the treatment of anxiety consequent upon headache but also prophylactically in the management of tension headache and migraine.

2. *The relief of pain, nausea and vomiting*

The distinction between tension headaches and migraine is important here as classical migraine has certain specific treatment. For an established headache of any kind simple measures may have been neglected by the patient, but are an important adjunct to drug treatment. The patient may gain relief by lying still in a quiet darkened room. The application of a cold compress to the head may relieve the pain and if the patient can sleep this will usually relieve an attack of migraine.
Simple analgesics should be tried first in all types of headache. In the adult, soluble aspirin in doses of 600 mg three hourly, or paracetamol 1g three hourly, can be useful. Absorption is delayed especially once headache and nausea have developed so it is very

important to take the analgesic early. In treating migraine 900 mgm of aspirin may be combined with 10 mgm of metoclopramide to facilitate absorption. For tension headache the addition of diazepam 5 mg can prove helpful.

Specific treatment for classical migraine. Although the aetiology of migraine is unknown the mechanism has been shown to be the abnormal behaviour of blood vessels inside and outside the skull. The pain will often respond to simple analgesics if given early enough and in big enough doses. However, the prodromal symptoms that occur in classical migraine provide an opportunity to intervene and sometimes abort the subsequent headache and vomiting with ergotamine tartrate.

1. The earlier it is given the smaller the required dose will be.
2. Tolerance does not occur but habituation does. There is no place for the prophylactic use of ergotamine, which can be dangerous.
3. Ergotamine causes vomiting in 10 per cent of people when given orally and 20 per cent when given by injection. This may aggravate the nausea that accompanies migraine so ergotamine is often usefully combined with an anti-emetic. Nausea and vomiting may respond to prochlorperazine (Stemetil) by suppository or injection.
4. Side-effects include nausea, muscle pain and weakness and paraesthesiae. Paraesthesiae may indicate vascular disturbance and the drug should be stopped. Ergotamine is contraindicated in pregnancy and in patients with arterial insufficiency.
5. The dose frequency should be strictly observed.

Ergotamine may be administered by injection, by suppository, orally or by inhalation.

— *Injection*. Dihydroergotamine injection (Dihydergot) is the drug of choice as it causes less vomiting than ergotamine tartrate. It is given subcutaneously or intramuscularly and may be effective in 15 minutes. The dose is 1 to 2 mg and it may be repeated in half an hour.

— *Suppository*. Ergotamine compound suppositories (Cafergot) contain ergotamine, caffeine, belladonna and butalbital. Absorption is rapid and reliable. Further suppositories can be used one and two hours after the first if necessary and in later attacks the total required dose can be given at one time. Not more than six should be taken in one week. The caffeine is said to enhance the action of ergotamine.

— *Tablets*. The dose of ergotamine is 1 to 2 mg repeated if necessary in half an hour. Not more than 8 mg should be given in one day and 12 mg in one week.

Sublingual tablets are available but have no particular advantage.

— *Inhalation*. Medihaler ergotamine contains 360 mg per dose. Absorption is rapid but uncertain, particularly in patients with bronchospasm. It is sometimes difficult for patients to recall how many doses they have taken. Not more than six inhalations a day or 15 a week should be taken.

Specific treatment for cluster headaches. Ergotamine tartrate injection (0.25 mg) or suppository is the treatment of choice. It can be given at bedtime in those who have attacks at night or even three times a day for five days each week for those with more frequent attacks. Stopping treatment for two days a week allows the patient to know if the attack has stopped and minimizes any risk from treatment. Pizotifen (Sanomigran) tablets 0.5 mg, three to 12 daily, are an alternative treatment.

3. *Minimizing subsequent attacks*

Tension headaches and migraine may well be significantly influenced by the patient's life-style. Most often such life-styles cannot easily be changed, nor would the patients themselves wish to institute such changes. But headaches may often be a presenting symptom of a chronic or relapsing crisis in the patient's life, and the chance of exploring this with the doctor or social worker may be helpful. There may be more specific provocative stimuli in the patient's diet or environment that can be identified in the case of migraine. Some of these may be avoided. Examples are periods of hunger or overeating, tyramine-containing foods, including dairy produce and fish, alcohol and chocolate. A patient's symptoms may be triggered by heat, intense artificial light, particular sounds or even smells. The patient should be encouraged to look for likely triggers to his symptoms and take steps to avoid them. In the search for trigger factors it can be helpful to encourage the patient to keep a diary to note the timing of his attacks in an effort to work out possible relationships with specific foods or activities.

Occasionally severe migraine may be associated with an underlying depression. The treatment of this depression with tricyclic anti-depressants may produce a marked change in the pattern of symptoms.

Specific prophylaxis for migraine. Ergotamine is not a safe prophylactic. Methysergide is the most effective. However, there is a considerable risk of symptoms similar to ergotism, and a small minority of patients develop retroperitoneal fibrosis. For this reason it is advised only in patients with severe and frequent attacks and should be withdrawn for a period of two months every six months.

Other drugs worth trying include:

clonidine 25 mg, 2 to 6 daily
pizotifen 0.5 mg, 3 to 12 daily
propranolol 30 to 120 mg, daily

Particularly in patients whose migraine is associated with premenstrual tension, the exhibition of diuretics in the week prior to the menstrual period may abort or abate attacks.

Migraine and the oral contraceptive. The effect of the combined pill on migraine is varied. It may appear to initiate attacks, to exacerbate previously present migraine, to change its character or even to abolish it. Those whose attacks are aggravated by the pill may find that changing to a more progestogenic variety will help, but those whose attacks change to a more focal pattern must discontinue as there is real danger of provoking cerebrovascular occlusive episodes.

Conclusion

The wide variety of drugs and classes of drugs available for the treatment of headache and migraine bears testimony to the unsatisfactory nature of our understanding of the condition and of our specific responses. Because of the natural history of the condition and the fact that it is given to spontaneous remissions and exacerbations, it is difficult to judge the effectiveness of a particular treatment. Nonetheless trial and error are necessary to establish a useful regime, and the participation of patients in the planning of their own treatment is crucial.

Reference

[1] Dunnell K. and Cartwright A. (1972): *Medicine Takers, Prescribers and Hoarders.* London: Routledge and Kegan Paul

Appendix
A practice policy for the management of migraine

This appendix describes the policy which was developed by a general practitioner, who was asked by his partners to establish guidelines for the treatment of migraine.
In developing this policy, he searched through recent publications on this subject and decided to use the paper by J.N. Blau, published in the *British Medical Journal*[1]. He selected this paper because:
— It defines the disorder.
— It describes the many factors which may provoke an attack of migraine and how these may be identified.
— It draws on information from randomized controlled trials of treatment.
This paper was, however, taken in conjunction with a paper by Bass[2], which was reported in the proceedings of the International Meeting of WONCA 1983. Bass described the findings in 272 patients newly presenting with headaches in general practice. Only 4.5% of these patients could be diagnosed as suffering from classical migraine. This clearly demonstrates that the problems of evaluating treatment for migraine are closely concerned with the problems of diagnosing this condition, and from his work in general practice, Bass puts this into perspective. Blau defined migraine as 'episodic headache accompanied by visual or gastrointestinal disturbance, or both, attacks lasting hours with total freedom between attacks'.

The practice policy

(1) From the history, and if necessary use of a symptom diary, attempt to identify trigger factors for attacks of migraine. These may be dietary, hormonal, environmental, psychological or allergic.
(2) If triggers cannot be identified and attacks prevented, the first line of treatment should be the use of metoclopramide 10 mg followed 10 minutes later by the administration of 3 tablets of paracetamol or soluble aspirin.
(3) If this fails, the second line of treatment should be the use of ergotamine. This may be administered by mouth, suppository or inhalation. Absorption is rapid when it is administered as an aerosol ergotamine (Medihaler), sublingually (Lingraine) or

by suppository and this avoids the problem of vomiting during an attack. Doses of 6–8 mg per attack, or 10–12 mg per week, should not be exceeded.

(4) With frequent attacks, preventive treatment may be required. The drugs available are clonidine (Dixarit) 50 mg twice daily, pizotifen 1.5 mg at night or prochlorperazine 5 mg 3 times daily.

In view of the relative infrequency of administration of these drugs for acute attacks, cost factors are not important. It is, however, cheaper to prescribe metoclopramide and aspirin separately than to use a combined preparation such as Migravess. For interval treatment, pizotifen is more expensive than either clonidine or prochlorperazine.

References

[1] Blau, J.N. (1982): The plain man's guide to the management of migraine. *British Medical Journal, 284*, 1095.

[2] Bass (1983): Proceedings of the International Conference of the World Organisation of National Colleges and Academies of General Practice.

3.13
The patient complaining of pain in the face

John Bennison

There is no reliable record of the incidence of facial pain. Each general practitioner in the United Kingdom may expect in the course of one year to see some fifty patients with such complaint. In the majority of cases the cause will be easily discovered.[1]

You may *see* the diagnosis, though perhaps not at first glance. Injuries, bruises, abrasions will show, though a scalp haematoma may track in the facial subcutaneous tissues, causing pain and tenderness whose origin may not be obvious to the patient. Small furuncles in the nostrils and ears may cause a lot of pain in the area, and may not be obvious unless sought. A small pre-auricular gland can be extremely painful.

You may *hear* the diagnosis, notably nasal sinus block. The characteristic lack of vocal resonance is diagnostic; more apparent when the previous quality of the patient's voice is known. The nasal airway may be clear, particularly in the cases of vacuum pain, where there is no true sinusitis but only a pressure difference. This is usually associated with some degree of allergic rhinitis, causing an intermittent closing off of the sinus ostia. The pain is variable, with no clear temporal pattern, and usually affects the antrum rather than the frontal sinus. The face is sometimes tender over it, but the sinus is clear on transillumination, and on X-ray. Treatment should be symptomatic, and a sparing use of local decongestants may help. There is usually an underlying anxiety.

An acute sinusitis will declare itself as part of a general upper respiratory disturbance. There will be pain on moving the head, stooping, and anything which raises the venous pressure in the face. The pain is often worse as the day wears on, and sometimes remarkably constant in timing. The sinuses will be tender and dull to transillumination. There may be overlying oedema of the face, and also of the floor of the antrum, which will produce the 'proud tooth', usually the upper 3, 4 or 5, noticed by the patient on closing the bite, and occasionally presenting, therefore, as toothache.

The general practitioner with an average sized list may expect some twenty-five cases each year. The incidence will vary with the season. Sinusitis accounts for approximately half of the cases of facial pain that he meets. Treatment is with antibiotics, erythromycin being the first choice of drug. Drainage should be encouraged, with an inhalation of steam containing menthol, and the use of local decongestant drops (xylometazoline hydrochloride) or a systemic decongestant such as pseudoephedrine hydrochloride.

Sometimes – perhaps in one in ten cases – the condition may not respond to this regime, even after a change to another broad-spectrum antibiotic, and become subacute or even chronic, and may necessitate surgical intervention in the form of washouts or other drainage operations.

The patient who presents in this phase will exhibit much less tenderness, though there will be dullness, and X-ray examinations will confirm the replacement of air by fluid.

If every child were taught to sniff and swallow, or hawk up sputum instead of pressurizing the upper nasopharynx in a paroxysm of nose blowing, the incidence of sinusitis, both acute and chronic, as well as of otitis media, would fall. The opportunity for this kind of simple health education for mothers is constantly presented to doctors and nurses in the primary health care team.

The other common, and usually fairly obvious, cause of facial pain is that arising from the upper or lower jaw – where a tap on the crown will often identify the offending tooth whose apical abscess may not be easily visible. Less common causes of dental pain will not be discussed, but caution is sometimes necessary to prevent wholesale extractions on inadequate grounds.

If these common causes are eliminated, the practitioner must look further afield, and try from the history and description of the pain to localize the diagnosis. Where is it? How long has it been present? Why consult now? Is the pain constant, or is there any pattern to it? What character has it: throbbing, lancinating, superficial, deep? Has the patient noticed any precipitating factor?

There can be no clear path to the solution here, because the site of the pain, its character and its timing will suggest different diagnoses, which will be confirmed or not by appropriate leading questions and, occasionally, examinations.

From the answers to these leading questions and our observations of the patient, his age, sex and personality, it is possible to identify some of the following.

Children, and adults, often experience pain around the angle of the jaw and in front of the ear before the swelling of mumps appears. Tenderness behind the jaw, and a red duct opening are helpful in reaching a diagnosis. So is the presence of an epidemic. For some reason, the submandibular glands are rarely painful in mumps. A blocked parotid duct usually presents as swelling – sometimes intermittent – rather than pain.

Pain about the upper mandible, sometimes throbbing, but usually steady may be due to unerupted lower molars; impacted, sometimes infected. A painful temporomandibular joint may often result from an acute strain, an unusual bite or yawn, and is self-limiting. The diagnosis is usually easy if it is looked for. Sometimes a disordered bite is responsible for a more chronic pain and the help of the dental surgeon may be sought. Rarely, it may be part of a general rheumatoid process.

Migraine is sometimes facial, and may be difficult to diagnose, but the history is often helpful. The deep, boring constant pain with a throbbing element which lasts a few hours only, sometimes following a visual aura, sometimes with vomiting, is characteristic. Complete freedom between attacks virtually clinches the diagnosis. The site may be temporal, or peri-orbital, and may vary in the individual patient. The management is the same as that for other migrainous headaches (the reader is referred to Chapter 3.12, The patient complaining of headache). Any pain of this sort which lasts for more than 48 hours should bring into question the possibility of more sinister but very rare causes like cerebral tumours and abscesses.

A related condition is ciliary neuralgia, or cluster headache, where the pain is behind the eye. Unlike other forms of migraine, the pain seems to encourage the sufferer to move about rather than lie still, and often occurs in the early hours of the morning. The affected eye reddens and weeps, and the face may flush. The attack is usually over in an hour or two, and characteristically occurs in bouts or clusters over several weeks (hence the name), with long periods of remission: hence prophylaxis is not very effective. A night-time ergotamine suppository in those for whom the nights are to be dreaded is valuable, and there is probably still a place for phenobarbitone rather than a benzodiazepine.

The throbbing 'vascular' headache, so-called tension headache, and the pain of temporal arteritis should be borne in mind. The reader is referred to Chapter 3.12 (The patient complaining of headache).

Most other causes are related to the sensory nerve supply to the face: the three divisions of the fifth nerve, and the second and third cervical roots which supply the angle of the jaw.

Foremost among the diagnoses here is herpes zoster, which affects the fifth nerve in almost one case in ten. It is more common in the elderly, but may occur at any age when infection with varicella has occurred. The characteristic pre-rash stage may sometimes be recognized by the well-defined distribution of hyperaesthesia, and the malaise, which is common. Opinion is divided as to whether corticosteroids, for example corticotrophin (ACTH), are worth while at this stage but, unless there are other contraindications, they may be prescribed: for example as tetracosactrin acetate (Synacthen Depot) 1 mg daily for three days. When the rash has appeared, local treatment will consist of drying applications (for example aluminium acetate lotion); idoxuridine (Herpid) has been shown to lessen scarring and post-herpetic pain. Herpes zoster affecting the eye requires careful supervision for corneal ulceration and keratitis. It is probably wise to consult an ophthalmologist early in the disease. The pain from all these may be severe, and require much more than aspirin, paracetamol and codeine. Pentazocine may be useful; methadone may be required. Post-herpetic pain, or more properly dysaesthesia since it includes anaesthesia of the scars and many other sensations besides pain, is much more common in the elderly. Treatment, when possible, is prophylactic and psychotherapeutic.

More rarely occurs zoster of C2 and C3 over the angle of the jaw, and of the facial ganglion – giving facial and buccal pain with eventually a few spots in the ear or on the drum and buccal ulcers. This latter may lead to a facial palsy, but rarely.

Trigeminal neuralgia, or tic douloureux, declares itself by the characteristics of the history. It is paroxysmal, each attack lasting a few seconds only, though occasionally there may be a run of paroxysms lasting up to half-an-hour. These may be initiated by sensory stimulation within the affected area – chewing, shaving, a draught. Sometimes the stimulant will not be apparent. Carbamazepine has proved of great value in treatment, and denervation of the sensory ganglion is now rarely needed.

The cervical roots may refer pain from the cervical spine to the lower face, as well as indirectly over the scalp to the forehead. Clearly the cause, if the pain is severe and prolonged, must be established, but the finding of a painful cervical articulation associated with this pain may encourage the enthusiast to practise manipulation; often with excellent results. These are probably variants of tension headaches.

These cervical roots may also refer the pain of angina pectoris to the jaw. The history should be sufficient, again if the possibility is borne in mind. It may rarely occur as the only site of pain, and for this reason pain in the lower jaw or gums should always be regarded as a possible covert symptom of ischaemic heart disease.

Hysterical patients may have pain in the face as anywhere else, but even in the established 'hysterical' patient diagnosis will proceed by exclusion of likely physical causes.

There remains a group of persistent atypical pains which do not fit clearly into any of these categories. These are described by various authors as 'psychogenic facial pain' or 'atypical facial neuralgia'; and opinions differ as to the pathogenesis. The sufferers are almost always depressed, but apparently successful treatment of the depression will not always remove the pain; nevertheless this syndrome should be regarded as depressive in origin and treated as such. It is this group which must be protected from unnecessary dental extractions.

It should be possible for the general practitioner to elucidate all but the most uncommon causes of facial pain from the history, and simple examination.

Reference

[1] Royal College of General Practitioners, Office of Population Censuses and Surveys, Department of Health and Social Security (1986): *Morbidity Statistics from General Practice 1981–82*. HMSO Series MB5 No. 1

3.14
Changes in facial appearance

John Bennison and Marshall Marinker

We know our patients best by their faces. In the consultation, even before the patient has stated the complaint, or uttered a first greeting, much of the problem to be presented may be predicted by the discerning doctor who looks his patient in the face. The doctor who greets his patient with his own head down, eyes scanning the clinical notes, is guilty not simply of a discourtesy, but of a grossly deficient clinical method.

Presentation

Sometimes changes in the face are part of the general appearance of the disease process, the so-called facies. The flat, puffy eyed, dry coarse-skinned appearance of myxoedema is instantly recognizable although the changes may be so slow to appear in the individual patient, that neither patient nor doctor is aware of the march of events. Similarly, the so-called moon face and oily complexion of the patient who is taking large doses of steroids is easily recognized. Here the recognition depends on the conjunction of a number of changes, the sum of which, in one patient, suggests the underlying disease. Beyond these few typical facies, however, the doctor should train himself to observe the patient's face not only as a whole, but also in a systematic way. He should observe the expression, the contour, the muscle tone, the colour and the state of the skin.

Expression.– The doctor must learn to read the patient's changing mood in the changes of facial expression. It is inappropriate in this chapter to specify the typical changes of anxiety or depression, but the appearance of the face in these situations is commonly unmistakable. The more the patient tries to control an expression of agitation or fear or melancholy, the more dramatically the expression will portray the feelings. Much more rarely, the doctor may encounter *la belle indifférence* of true hysteria. Hysterical dissociation, so common in the literature of neurology and psychology at the beginning of this century, is now a rarity – and except as a subject for dramatic clinical presentations, it may always have been.

Observation of the patient's face during the process of the consultation is of the greatest importance. Expressions of anxiety and depression may be provoked by a particular topic, or even a particular name. The doctor must learn to value such changes in the same way as he values other important clinical signs. Just as important, the doctor should learn to watch the patient's face for signs of pain. Pain will often be betrayed by expression long before the patient is prepared to utter a sound. Palpation of the abdomen is often a fruitless procedure unless the doctor is closely observing the patient's face at the same time. In chronic disease, for example in chronic arthritis, the facial expression will often betray the pain of the uncomplaining patient.

Contour.– The general contour may change with weight gain or loss due to changes in diet, or in relation to some disease process: for example, the weight changes in anxiety or depression, or hyper- and hypo-thyroidism. Changes in facial appearance may suggest those general changes in body weight, which otherwise may not be immediately apparent to the doctor at the beginning of the consultation.

There may be a generalized swelling due to angioneurotic oedema, or there may be a puffiness around the eyes typically seen in the nephrotic syndrome, or in myxoedema. Particularly in children, observation of the face may give the first clue that the patient is dehydrated: there is a general sharpness of the features and the eyes are often markedly sunken because of the loss of extracellular fluid.

The patient himself is much more likely to complain of localized swelling. During a local outbreak the parotid swellings of mumps may be self-evident when fully blown, but it should be borne in mind that the condition is often unilateral, particularly in its initial presentation. Sometimes the pain precedes the palpable swelling by a day or two. Submandibular mumps may cause quite marked swellings and there may well be an absence of parotid enlargement. When the swellings are unilateral, particularly in the adult, the differential diagnosis of salivary duct obstruction should be entertained. Enlargement of lymph nodes is a further important differential diagnosis. Enlargement of the superficial parotid, the submandibular or submental nodes may all mimic mumps. Infection of the antrum or around a tooth may cause quite a pronounced unilateral and painful swelling.

Muscle tone.– Facial appearance may be considerably altered by changes in muscle tone. Perhaps the commonest sign is that of unilateral paresis which occurs in Bell's palsy. In this condition both the upper and lower parts of the face are equally involved. When paresis occurs because of a supranuclear paralysis (as in a cerebrovascular accident) the lower part of the face is chiefly affected. Many diseases affecting nerve/muscle may result in changes in facial appearance. Some of the rarer changes, for example the weakness of the eyelid and lip muscles which occurs in one form of muscular dystrophy, will present so rarely to the general practitioner that he is unlikely to recognize the disease from the facial change alone. Other conditions, even though their incidence may be small, are so well known that they may be instantly recognized. Examples are the bilateral ptosis found in myasthenia gravis and lid retraction seen in thyrotoxicosis. In Parkinsonism, the face assumes a fixed unblinking staring expression: the so-called Parkinsonian mask, sometimes the sign of the unwanted effects of the phenothiazine group of drugs.

Colour.– Changes in facial colour are usually of gradual onset, and will rarely be presented by the patient. The doctor may notice the changes of jaundice in the skin of the face, while the patient is still explaining symptoms of fatigue or gastro-intestinal upset. In pernicious anaemia the skin colour is described as being lemon yellow and this may be very faint. Even in obstructive jaundice, skin changes may be slight at first, and may easily be missed in artificial light. The brown pigmentation which occurs in Addison's disease may easily be dismissed as the affect of sunlight. In congestive heart failure cyanosis, particularly of the lips, nose and cheeks, will be self-evident. A facial flush may reflect the hormonal imbalance of the menopause or where the flush is largely malar, the increasingly rare case of mitral valve disease. Other changes in colour are rare. The patient, however, may confuse pallor with anaemia, and more commonly a high colour with a high blood pressure. The doctor must be at pains to educate the patient about the significance of these changes.

The light brown pigmentation of the cheeks, chloasma, was at one time most often seen during pregnancy. In the past few years this skin change has been seen in association with oral contraception. Occasionally, the patches may be quite marked and dark, and may constitute a reason for discontinuing oral contraception. Often the patches persist, though they may fade in intensity.

The state of the skin.– Many skin diseases have first been noted by the patient on the face. Some, like acne, may be largely restricted to the face. Rosacea is restricted to the nose and cheeks. Typically the rash of lupus erythematosus begins as an eruption over the cheeks and the bridge of the nose. Erysipelas may present as a progressive redness and thickening of the skin of the face, usually with a sharp advancing margin.

For a detailed discussion of rashes and spots which may affect the face of the skin the reader is referred to Chapters 3.37 and

3.38. Chapter 3.39 considers basal cell carcinoma (rodent ulcer). The subcutaneous yellow or more deeply pigmented nodules, round, discrete, and often occurring in small clusters around the inner canthus of the eyes, of xanthelasma are often associated with a high serum cholesterol. The condition is usually familial.

History and examination

Changes in facial appearance are often part of more widespread physical stigmata of disease. Many of the conditions mentioned are considered in more detail in other chapters of this book, to which reference has been made. This section is concerned only with the differential diagnosis of facial palsy and of swellings.

Facial paralysis.– Paralysis of the facial, or seventh cranial, nerve is usually unilateral, and the patient may give a history either of altered appearance, or of difficulty of feeding: food may be collecting between the teeth and gums and saliva or fluids may dribble from the paralysed angle of the mouth. Often the affected side seems to have lost its expression.
The function of the seventh nerve is tested by asking the patient to shut the eyes tightly: the affected eye will either fail to close, with an upward rotation of the eyeball, or the closure will be incomplete. If the paresis is only partial, and the eye appears to close normally, the following test will reveal any neuromuscular deficiency. The patient is asked to keep the eyes tightly closed, while the doctor attempts to open the eye using his fingers. In the absence of any lesion, it is almost impossible to open the forcefully closed eye. Even in quite partial damage to the seventh nerve, however, it is relatively easy to prise the eye open. The lower part of the face is tested by asking the patient to smile or to attempt to whistle. Sometimes, there is a history of exposure to cold. In one series diabetes mellitus was present in 11.4 per cent of those with the complaint, a rate 4.5 times greater than that to be expected. In those patients with bilateral Bell's palsy the incidence of diabetes was 28.4 per cent.[1]

Swellings.– Apart from soft tissue swellings due to infection or haematoma, the doctor must decide whether the swelling is due to enlargement of the lymph nodes or hypertrophy of the salivary glands.
Enlargement of the lymph nodes results in smaller, firmer and often acutely tender swellings. In the case of the parotid nodes, these must be differentiated from parotitis. If the parotid lymph nodes are implicated, infective lesions should be sought over the anterior two-thirds of the scalp, the upper half of the cheek,

including the lateral half of the eyelids and the anterior part of the pinna. The submandibular lymph nodes, enlargement of which may mimic submandibular mumps, drain the rest of the face with the exception of the anterior aspect of the chin, which is drained by the submental lymph node.

Enlargement of the salivary gland produces a much more brawny swelling than that caused by enlargement of the lymph nodes. Particularly in adults, it may be difficult to differentiate between salivary gland enlargement caused by mumps, and that caused by some form of stasis in the salivary duct – most often due to a calculus. A history of contact with mumps can usually be elicited, but the incubation period is a long one (14 to 21 days); it may therefore be difficult to establish contact. In the case of children during a local outbreak, there is no such problem.

Inflammatory enlargement of the salivary glands due to obstruction of the duct is usually unilateral (although of course mumps often presents as a unilateral swelling). Pain, however, is more acute than that experienced in mumps and the pain and swelling affect the glands most commonly during and after meals, the swelling gradually subsiding until the next meal time. A careful history of the relationship of the pain to mealtimes can sometimes be useful. Symptoms are also confined to the gland involved, in contrast to the general systemic upset of mumps. It is, however, difficult to differentiate between the two in some cases, because both the severity of the pain and occasionally a secondary infection of the gland can both give rise to a systemic upset. A painless swelling in the region of the parotid, increasing slowly in size over a period of years, suggests a mixed parotid tumour. Even when these swellings cause no discomfort, the patient should be referred for a surgical opinion, because occasionally the tumour may increase rapidly in size and malignant changes may occur.

There will be little difficulty in differentiating between the more commonly seen forms of oedema of the face. The oedema of hypothyroidism occurs under the eyes and is easily recognized as part of the typical facies. The oedema of nephritis is also periorbital but it will be unusual for this serious condition to *present* with such swelling. Angioneurotic oedema of the face presents with a dramatic history. The onset is sudden, the swelling may be unilateral or bilateral and if the tongue or throat is affected it will be accompanied by a severe (and realistic) anxiety. The swellings are usually single, often several centimetres in diameter, there is no sharp margin, the overlying skin appears normal, the temperature of the skin is rarely raised, and there is no pain. A provoking agent is rarely identified from the history even though the attacks may be recurrent.

Swellings of the face caused either by an apical tooth abscess or an infected antrum are usually evident from the history. Sinusitis is often preceded by a feverish cold, and in the case of apical abscess there is often, though by no means always, a history of toothache. If the antrum is infected, in addition to general systemic upset and fever, there will be severe throbbing pain over the antrum with referred pain along the second division of the trigeminal nerve. The cheek will be acutely tender. Confirmation of the diagnosis by transillumination or x-rays is rarely necessary. In the case of an apical abscess, diagnosis may be confirmed by lightly tapping the crown of the tooth, to determine which one is affected.

Management

Only the management of those conditions not discussed elsewhere in this book, are considered here. These are the management of Bell's palsy; certain swellings of the face (lymphadenitis, mumps, salivary duct stasis and calculus, angio-neurotic oedema, antrum infection and apical abscess); and three skin conditions: erysipelas, rosacea and the skin manifestations of systemic lupus erythematosus. The reader is referred to Chapters 3.9 and 3.10 for discussion of the management of other neurological conditions, to Chapter 3.34 for a discussion of the treatment of anaemia and 3.49 for a discussion of the treatment of the commoner causes of jaundice. Chapter 3.33 deals with the management of the commoner disorders giving rise to cyanosis. The management of the commoner skin conditions which alter facial appearance is given in Chapters 3.37 and 3.38.

Bell's palsy.– Many cases resolve spontaneously within six weeks, recovery beginning within a week of the onset of paralysis, but in cases of full paralysis complete recovery may occur in only 60 per cent of cases. Hence in addition to the general principles of management, in this case strict oral hygiene and the gentle massage of the affected muscles (which the patient can be taught to do for himself), there is some argument for a more active intervention. Unfortunately there is as yet no firm evidence for the effectiveness of these managements. The evidence of benefit resulting from 'decompression' of the facial nerve within the temporal bone is very weak, and surgeons are increasingly opposed to this sort of intervention. There seems to be a better case for treatment with corticosteroids. This must be initiated at an early stage of the illness and continued for some ten days. Treatment with prednisolone may be initiated with as much as 60 mg in divided doses on the first day and reduced by 5 mg each day. Alternatively corticotrophin gel may be used, starting with 80 mg on the first day. Early referral to a neurologist may facilitate better monitoring of muscular recovery, and make early physiotherapy available to the patient, but it is doubtful if either of these benefits will influence the prognosis.

Mumps.– The pain in the salivary glands is best treated with aspirin. Local applications of heat and cold, in the form of heated flannels or ice packs, both have their advocates and may occasionally give relief. Orchitis is best managed with scrotal support and analgesics. Corticosteroids given for three or four days may reduce the pain of orchitis but do not influence the course of subsequent atrophy.

Angioneurotic oedema.– This can be most resistant to treatment. Occasionally when the tongue, pharynx or larynx is involved immediate attempts must be made to reduce the swelling. In extreme cases tracheotomy may be required, but this is excessively rare. A description of this procedure is given in Chapter 3.29. Adrenaline may be given as a slow subcutaneous injection in doses of 0.5 ml of the 1:1,000 aqueous solution. Antihistamines, if they are to be of any benefit, will be required in large doses: for example chlorpheniramine 8 mg 4 to 6 hourly. In these doses, antihistamines have a profoundly sedative effect which may in itself be of considerable value. If the swelling is large, or has been resistant to treatment in the past, corticosteroids are indicated: 15 mg of prednisolone may be given at 6-hourly intervals until the swelling goes down.

Infection of the antrum and apical abscess.– The key to the management of sinusitis is to re-establish drainage. This is best achieved by the short-term use of decongestant drops: xylometazoline hydrochloride being preferred because this preparation does not cause rebound congestion. If infection of the antrum is severe enough to cause a change in facial appearance, antibiotics are indicated and erythromycin is the drug of choice.
Apical abscess is best treated in the short term with analgesics such as aspirin, and a five-day course of phenoxymethylpenicillin, 250 mg four times a day. The pain is often exacerbated when the patient lies down, and this is thought to be a pressure effect. If the patient is encouraged to sleep propped up the usual increase in pain which the patient experiences on going to bed can be alleviated. The patient should be referred for dental treatment as soon as possible.

Skin conditions

For the treatment of most of the skin conditions causing a change in facial appearance the reader is referred to Chapters 3.37, 3.38 and 3.39. Three conditions not dealt with elsewhere in this book are here considered.

Erysipelas.– This is a group A streptococcal skin infection which can cause considerable systemic upset. Bed rest while the patient still has a fever, and analgesics such as aspirin will help. The antibiotic of choice is phenoxymethylpenicillin: for the adult a dose of 500 mg every six hours is appropriate. Treatment should be maintained for at least five days.

Systemic lupus erythematosus.– This is a systemic upset of unknown aetiology. It runs a chronic course and affects many organs and systems. There is almost always an arthritis or arthralgia and there may be widespread skin manifestations, with involvement of the kidney, the gastro-intestinal tract, the lungs, the heart and so on. About half the patients suffering from this rare condition present with a 'butterfly rash' of the face. This is an acute erythematous maculopapular rash affecting both cheeks and meeting over the bridge of the nose. The rash is best managed by avoiding sunlight, the local application of corticosteroid cream and the occasional use of antimalarials like chloroquine.

Rosacea.– The etiology of this condition is unknown. The onset usually occurs in middle life and the condition is exacerbated by hot drinks and spicy foods, both of which the patient should be counselled to avoid. Topical corticosteroids should not be used because they make the condition worse. A soothing lotion can be of some help, and exacerbations are best treated with oxytetracycline, 250 mg twice daily for some six to eight weeks.

Conclusion

The face of the patient is not simply his visiting card, it is the mirror of his body, his mind and the relationships that he makes with others. The clinician who does not search the face of his patient ignores perhaps the most important statement of the problem which the patient can make, and deprives himself of the answers which he may otherwise ineffectively seek in a battery of questions.

Reference

[1] Adour, K.K. (1975): The bell tolls for decompression. *New England Journal of Medicine*, *292*, 748

3.15 The patient complaining of pain in the neck

Donald Irvine

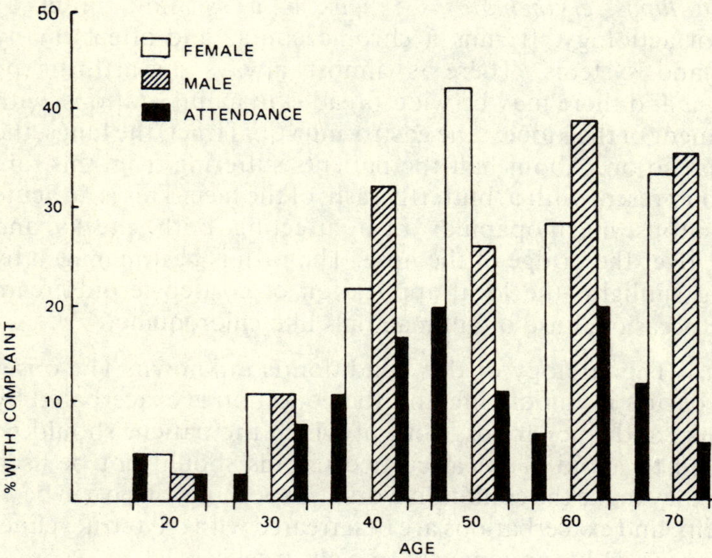

Figure 1.– Incidence of cervico-brachial pain in a 10-year period

Patients complaining of pain in the neck go to their general practitioner less often than one might expect, bearing in mind that such complaints are common in the population. This is probably because many episodes are minor, a nuisance for a day or two, and are normally relieved by an analgesic bought at the chemist.

There have been relatively few population studies of neck pain. A study of rheumatic complaints in a representative sample of the people in the town of Leigh[1] showed that pain in the 'neck-shoulder-brachial' region was second only in frequency to pain in the 'back-hip-sciatic' area. A similar picture of cervicobrachial pain emerged from a representative sample of 500 adults who were examined in the population of a coal-mining practice in Ashington:[2] symptoms recalled in the previous ten years were recorded and the over-all incidence in this period was 24 per cent; here, too, there were no significant sex or occupational differences. Complaints rose between the third and fifth decades and then remained fairly constant (figure 1).

Presentation

In a topographical classification of symptoms in the Ashington study three groups were recognized: those patients with pain in the neck and arm together (41 per cent); those with neck pain alone (38 per cent); and a smaller group with pain in the arm alone (21 per cent). Many complaints in the middle-aged and elderly were regarded as trivial or 'rheumatic', and so were not usually brought to the general practitioner (figure 1). Morrell,[3] reporting on 5,325 patient-initiated new consultations in one year, found that 54 were for pain in the neck, but he did not indicate whether there were associated symptoms.

Among patients attending the general practitioner, those with cervicobrachial radicular syndromes are probably the most important. In the Third National Morbidity Study,[4] the incidence of syndromes related to the cervical spine was 9.4 per thousand patients, a figure higher than the 5.4 per thousand recorded in Ashington[5] for all new cases of cervical spondylosis with radicular symptoms presenting in a year in that study practice.

Brain and Wilkinson[6] have classified the symptoms of cervical spondylosis into five main groups:

1. Those due to involvement of nerve roots – radicular symptoms
2. Those due to involvement of the spinal cord – cervical myelopathy
3. Pain in the neck
4. Headache
5. Symptoms of vertebrobasilar insufficiency.

Any of these symptoms may occur singly, or any combination of them may be present. Neck pain may therefore be present in all groups.

Causes

Cervical spondylosis

It is generally accepted that cervical spondylosis is essentially a degenerative process affecting the intervertebral discs and vertebral bodies. The primary factor appears to be a chemical disturbance within the disc associated with ageing: there is dessication of the nuclear material, and distortion and weakening of the annulus. It seems probable that trauma is significant in the etiology of the skeletal lesion as well as in the precipitation of symptoms in patients with previously asymptomatic radiological spondylosis. Cervical spondylosis, which may cause involvement of one or more cervical roots, or the cord, or both, is really a radiological diagnosis. The diagnosis may be made when:

(a) there is reduction in the disc space at any level;
(b) when osteophytes are present around the circumference of a vertebral body or are encroaching upon an intervertebral foramen from the neurocentral joints at any level.

Osteoarthrosis of the zygapophyseal joints is almost as common as disc degeneration and so is associated osteophytosis although it tends to occur at a higher level in the cervical spine than cervical spondylosis. From a practical point of view, despite their differing etiologies, it is useful to consider the effects of these two conditions together since the symptoms are invariably indistinguishable.

Radiological investigation.– For most patients who present at the surgery with a stiff neck, radiological investigation is not indicated since at that stage it will serve no useful purpose. When associated symptoms are present, or when it becomes clear that the condition is progressive, or when there is positive evidence or suspicion of nerve root or cord involvement, the general practitioner will probably want to order the following plain radiographs: antero-posterior views; lateral films in flexion and extension (for evidence of spondylolisthesis); and right and left oblique films to demonstrate the foramina. Disc narrowing, reflecting loss in the volume of disc material, is a virtually constant feature of cervical spondylosis. Narrowing of the disc may occur alone but it is usually followed by the formation of osteophytes. Lesions are commonest at the C5/6 and C6/7 levels. It is posterior osteophytes encroaching upon the cervical canal, and more laterally placed lesions intruding on a foraminal space which have most diagnostic significance.

Many general practitioners work some distance from their hospital radiology department and this can make a personal examination of the films difficult; hence they usually rely on the radiologist's report alone. When possible, however, it is helpful for the practitioner to examine the films himself. Not only is it useful to be familiar with the radiological diagnosis of a common condition, it is not practical for the radiologist to report on what may be extensive changes in detail. In minor degrees of spondylosis the diagnosis may not be easy, and observer variations have been widely reported.

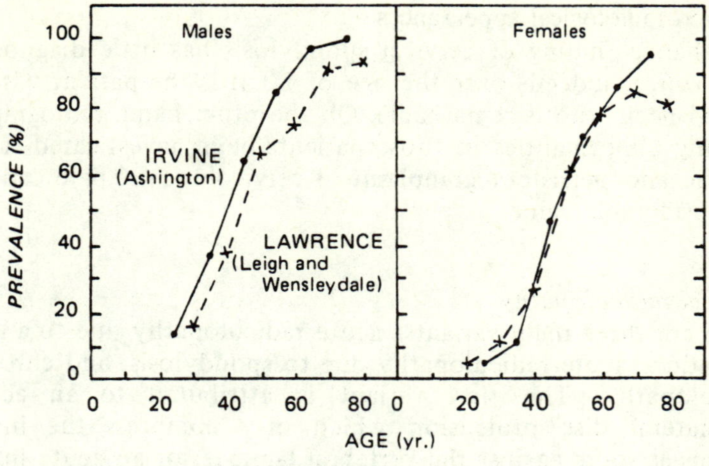

Figure 2.– Prevalence of spondylosis; comparison of Leigh and Wensleydale with Ashington

The films, taken in conjunction with the clinical findings, will determine whether further investigations such as tomography, myelography, or vertebral angiography, are indicated as the clinical situation develops. Patients with severe unexplained symptoms and normal plain films will need specialist investigation. In those patients with severe symptoms and positive radiological findings the decision will depend on the nature of the radiological abnormalities encountered taken in conjunction with the unfolding picture of the complaint.

Radiological prevalence of cervical spondylosis.– The age-specific prevalence of cervical spondylosis is similar in both sexes though spondylotic changes tend to be less severe in women. The results of two large series[1, 5] are shown in figure 2. In both studies no significant sex differences were noted in over-all prevalence; indeed the prevalence was remarkably similar, with the sole exception of a higher rate in Ashington males in the fourth decade (possibly due to the excessive repetitive trauma to which this group, containing a high proportion of underground mine-workers, was exposed).

Correlation between radiological findings and symptoms.– It is well known that there may be wide discrepancies between the site and level of radiological spondylosis and the segmental level of symptoms and signs. To some extent these discrepancies reflect the multiple mechanisms which may be operating. For example, disc material arising from an uncinate process and irritating a nerve root will not show on a plain film. Root sleeve fibrosis may produce a multiradicular picture despite evidently localized radiological appearances.

The chance finding of cervical spondylosis has little diagnostic significance; indeed, over the age of 50 it is the patient with a normal neck who is remarkable. On the other hand, radiographs showing abnormalities in those patients being investigated for a specific and persistent complaint of cervicobrachial pain can be of considerable value.

Cervical radiculopathy

There are three main variants: acute radiculopathy due to a soft herniation, acute radiculopathy due to spondylosis, and chronic radiculopathy. The first variant is attributed to an acute dorsolateral disc protrusion which may compress the intrameningeal roots against the vertebral laminae, or an acute intraforaminal protrusion arising from the uncinate part of the disc and compressing the radicular nerve against the articular process. This type of protrusion is particularly common in young individuals and not infrequently is associated with trauma. Here symptoms are normally acute in onset, the pain coming on suddenly and reaching a peak within a day or two. The pain is usually a severe ache or is shooting in character; moreover, it is invariably radicular in distribution, the fifth, sixth and seventh roots being most commonly involved. The pain may be related to the position of the neck, which is tender and given to muscular spasm. Movements can make the pain worse: whether by active or passive rotation, tilting, flexion or extension of the head, or by lying on the affected side. Very often patients are most comfortable when lying face downwards. Pain is the predominant feature, and other sensory symptoms are less prominent.

The other acute variant more closely resembles the commonly described 'brachial neuritis'. Here, by contrast with the first, neck pain and spasm tend to be less prominent whilst arm pain and other sensory symptoms predominate in a radicular distribution. The patient may have had silent spondylotic changes in the neck for some years.

Chronic neck pain may persist after an acute attack and may be accompanied by minor radicular symptoms. Patients with a history of a previous acute attack are more likely to report subsequent minor episodes to their family doctor.[2]

Cervical myelopathy

Cervical spondylosis involving the cord is less common than isolated radicular lesions but can be more significant for those patients who suffer from it because of its more disabling potential. The presenting picture is protean, but pain in the neck is relatively unusual compared with bilateral radicular pain and sensory symptoms in both arms and legs. The differential diagnosis can be difficult; and if in doubt referral may be indicated. It is important to avoid another common diagnostic pitfall: that is to ascribe to radiological cervical spondylosis symptoms and signs which are actually due to another cause such as multiple sclerosis, motor neurone disease, spinal tumour or subacute combined degeneration of the cord.

Cervical spondylosis may cause occipital headache though why is not clear. It may also be responsible for symptoms of vertebrobasilar insufficiency, presumably due to a combination of factors which include atheroma of the vertebral vessels and intermittent compression of one or both arteries by osteophytes arising from the neurocentral or apophyseal joints. Symptoms are typically of sudden onset, precipitated by head movement laterally or in extension. They may be confined to an episode of unsteadiness, may lead to profound giddiness, or may result in a drop attack.

Infections and haemorrhage

Pain in the neck may also be due to an infection or less commonly may be the presenting symptom of a small subarachnoid bleed. The main diagnostic possibilities to consider include aseptic, purulent and tuberculous meningitis. Meningism resulting from a systemic infection is another related cause of neck pain. When the onset is sudden and the effect severe, and when there are general supportive findings pointing to the presence of infection, the steps to be taken in establishing a diagnosis become self-evident. Problems arise mainly when there has been an insidious onset of neck pain, perhaps with headache and an intermittent low fever, such as may occur with tuberculous meningitis or a small subarachnoid haemorrhage. In helping him to come to a conclusion about the possibility of infection, the general practitioner must look for evidence of true neck rigidity rather than a 'stiff neck'. The presence of Kernig's sign may help to differentiate these two conditions.

Causes of spinal cord compression

Spinal cord compression may occur at any level and the cervical region is no exception. Cord compression in the neck may cause considerable pain in this area and in the related occipital region, and it is normally made worse by movements of the cervical spine. Severe and especially progressive pain in the neck should always alert the family doctor to the possibility of a space-occupying or bone-destroying lesion. These cases should always be referred for a second opinion.

Other causes of neck pain

Other, less common, causes of neck pain always to be borne in mind are rheumatoid arthritis, ankylosing spondylitis, Paget's disease, steroid arthropathy, gout and osteomyelitis, all of which can produce pain and radiological changes in the neck.

Spasmodic torticollis, a painful condition of unknown etiology usually presenting in young adults and in middle-age, produces its own characteristic picture. Most cases are said to be organic in origin, a few hysterical. In developed cases the head is almost permanently on one side. Muscle contractions, not always confined to the sternocleidomastoid muscle, may be painful, and patients often become depressed or anxious because they may think they look stupid or ridiculous.

Undiagnosable pain

Minor complaints of pain in the neck in which no precise diagnosis can be made have already been mentioned. These conditions attract such labels as 'fibrositis', 'stiff neck', 'cricked neck', 'draughty neck' and 'rheumatism'. It is arguable whether it is worth while attaching a label when it obviously does not give any indication of the pathogenesis. There is a common assumption that patients require a diagnosis from their family doctor; on the other hand, many experienced practitioners have found it perfectly feasible, and highly desirable, to leave the situation at the level of a description of symptoms and a clear explanation to the patient of what further steps will be taken to elucidate their cause if there is no improvement in a reasonable time. The merit of this method is that misleading labels are not attached to undiagnosed conditions, so avoiding the creation of a false sense of security for both patient and doctor alike. Moreover, the label is not committed to the patient's record, there possibly to mislead a partner or trainee assistant who may become involved.

History and examination

Since the history will give the main clues to diagnosis, it is important to enquire into the nature of the neck pain and to elicit related symptoms which may help by pointing to the most likely cause. An antecedent history of twinges of pain in the neck is common in cervical spondylosis. A history of injury may be significant in several conditions. For example, the sudden onset of pain following injury in a young person may suggest an acute, soft herniation of a cervical disc. Whiplash injury is well documented, and severe injuries following a blow or fall may cause a fracture. Less often recognized is the repetitive minor trauma characteristic of some occupations; coal miners, for example, are subject to frequent minor head injuries as they bump their heads against roof supports, and there is evidence to suggest that this may be of etiological significance in cervical spondylosis.[2]

The mode of onset of the pain can also be helpful. Many patients awake with pain in the neck, and ascribe their condition to lying awkwardly, whilst others will observe that the pain came on quite soon after sitting in a draught. The cause of sudden attacks of stiff neck, especially if unaccompanied by other symptoms, may be impossible to determine initially. It is usually necessary to watch the unfolding picture over several days, and even then one may never reach a definitive diagnosis, especially if the pain goes away. Neck pain associated with chronic cervical spondylosis is not always as uncomfortable as one might expect and can come on gradually, even though there may be considerable pain in one or both arms accompanied by unpleasant 'pins and needles'. This pain is characteristically worse on wakening in the morning and is normally aggravated by head movement.

Specific enquiry should be made about associated pain and other sensory symptoms in the shoulders, arms and legs. Nerve-root pain has well recognized characteristics but there is a group of patients who may have pain in the neck, shoulder and upper arm which conforms more to a muscle group than a nerve root distribution, and which may be related to cervical spondylosis through a mechanism which is not clear. Quite mild neck pain may be associated with upper and lower limb symptoms of cervical myelopathy; indeed it is not unusual for the patient to present with limb symptoms, the antecedent history of neck pain being mentioned only on specific questioning.

The general health of the patient is also important. For example, neck pain exacerbated by flexion will alert the doctor to look further for evidence of meningitis, remembering especially tuberculous meningitis, and to bear in mind the possibility of a subarachnoid haemorrhage. Any evidence of loss of weight or of a steadily progressive disability will direct questioning towards the major causes of cervical cord compression, especially metastases and tumours arising within the spinal cord or its coverings.

In the clinical examination particular attention should be given to the neck and the nervous system. General inspection may be informative; in the painful spasm of torticollis, for example, the neck is usually held in a characteristically inclined position. There may be tenderness with deep pressure in the cervical muscles or over one or several spinous processes. Neck movements are usually limited especially in flexion and lateral rotation, and with cervical spondylosis and acute soft herniation pain may be induced by head turning under pressure. Examination of the nervous system will be directed to finding signs of nerve-root irritation or the more general evidence of cervical myelopathy or other cause of cord compression. A general examination is an essential preliminary in the search for a neoplasm, especially if an admittedly uncommon cervical secondary deposit is suspected.

Two common pitfalls are worth mentioning. First, there may be a temptation to treat all cases of pain in the neck symptomatically, even for quite long periods, on the assumption that cervical spondylosis is the most probable cause. This uncritical approach is easy to adopt when the doctor knows that more serious conditions are unusual, but it can lead to delays in establishing other diagnoses. Secondly, in busy surgeries there is a tendency to confine the examination to the neck region even when symptoms persist and indeed may be worsening. Regional examinations alone can lead the unwary to overlook important diagnostic signs elsewhere, especially in the nervous system. For example, characteristic changes in the reflexes are usually present at an early stage in the development of cervical myelopathy, even when symptoms are apparently of little trouble or significance.

Are these diagnostic enquiries consistent with a five-minute consultation? In theory, perhaps not, but in fact, as with many other clinical situations in general practice, time is available when needed to observe the unfolding natural history of the condition through the use of 'extended consultation', or for general examination provided the doctor is flexible in the use of his appointment system. In most cases in which there are no related symptoms, a regional examination and expectant policy of wait and see, over a short period, is perfectly adequate. Major injuries, which are extremely uncommon in the average practice population in any one year, will need to be referred to hospital immediately, but the other important group of patients, those with severe neck and arm pain in whom a diagnosis cannot be reached, should have time set aside to develop the history thoroughly and to complete a full physical examination. Patients are perfectly willing to come back a day or so after their initial consultations for a more thorough examination if the practitioner explains why it is necessary to do so. Indeed most appreciate the time and trouble taken.

Management

In the first instance it is a matter of explaining the likely cause or of stating the possibilities, of indicating what is to be done, and of making the patient comfortable. Particular attention should be paid to the positioning of the stiff and painful neck, including the use of a neck pillow, and to adequate analgesia. Specific treatment will be determined by the underlying cause. In the case of infections the management plan will be clear and needs no elaboration here. Similarly, in patients for whom there are grounds to indicate further investigation of unrecognized symptoms, appropriate referral should be arranged.

Several methods of treatment are used for cervical spondylosis. It is perhaps not surprising therefore that the only major multi-centre trial[1] comparing various methods with placebo revealed that placebo was as effective as others. The immobilization of the neck in a cervical collar, made of felt, plastic, or more substantial material, is one method. Another is to apply intermittent traction with or without the use of short-wave diathermy. Manipulation of the neck is practised by some family doctors and orthopaedic surgeons, whilst other patients refer themselves for osteopathic help. Whilst gentle extension of the neck may be helpful, especially in affording temporary relief from muscle spasm, the dangers of manipulating a grossly spondylotic neck must be appreciated. The spinal canal in the cervical region is narrow, and there is consequently little room between it and the cord which lies within. A spastic quadriplegia induced by injudicious manipulation can profoundly shatter the confidence of the doctor who recommended or did it; and the results for the patient are self-evidently disastrous.

Whatever the approach, in all except a small proportion of cases, the outcome will be determined by the natural tendency of acute exacerbations of cervical spondylosis to remit after a period varying from a few days to several weeks. Even with cervical myelopathy, the untreated prognosis is far better than was once thought. It is perhaps for this reason that in cervical spondylosis surgery plays so much less a part in management in the United Kingdom than it has done in the United States. Over-active treatment, like over-enthusiastic investigation at the wrong time, can have long-term effects which may be harmful. Some patients can become morbidly preoccupied with chronically recurring cervical spondylotic pain, and so tend to excessive and unnecessary requests for analgesics and time off work. A few will use their complaint to gain and legitimize their annual 'entitlement' to sickness absence. Experienced family doctors will soon distinguish these people by the pattern of surgery attendance which begins to emerge with time.

Episodes of spasmodic torticollis can be treated with two or three applications of ethyl chloride or similar spray on the affected side of the neck, almost invariably with gratifying and immediate successful response.

Conclusion

Pain in the neck is a common complaint, often not precisely diagnosable and rarely of long-term practical consequence. The much smaller proportion of patients with persistent or progressive pain in the neck, especially when they have other symptoms and signs, should always be the subject of careful observation, investigation and management. Cervical spondylosis is the commonest diagnosis made.

References

[1] Lawrence, J.S., de Graff, R. and Haine, V.A.I. (1963): *The Epidemiology of Chronic Rheumatism*, Volume 1. Edited under the direction of J.H. Kellgren by M.R. Jeffrey and J. Ball. Oxford: Blackwell Scientific Publications

[2] Irvine, D.H. (1964): *Cervical Spondylosis in General Practice*. M.D. Thesis, University of Newcastle

[3] Morrell, D.C., Gage, H.G. and Robinson, N.A. (1971): Symptoms in General Practice. *Journal of the Royal College of General Practitioners*, *21*, 32

[4] Royal College of General Practitioners, Office of Population Censuses and Surveys, Department of Health and Social Security (1986): *Morbidity Statistics from General Practice 1981–82*. HMSO Series MB5 No. 1

[5] Irvine, D.H., Foster, J.B., Newell, D.J. and Klukvin, B.N. (1965): Prevalence of cervical spondylosis in a general practice. *Lancet*, *i*, 1089

[6] Brain, Lord and Wilkinson, Marcia (1976): *Cervical Spondylosis and other disorders of the cervical spine*. London: Heinemann

Further reading

British Association of Physical Medicine (1966): Pain in the Neck and Arm: a Multicentre Trial of the Effects of Physiotherapy. *British Medical Journal*, *1*, 253

3.16
The patient who cannot sleep

Luke Zander

The complaint of disordered sleep is common. It has been estimated that from one-sixth to one-quarter of the adult population is affected by sleep problems[1] and in psychiatric conditions the incidence is as high as 45 per cent.[2] According to Oswald,[3] there is no normal sleep time which is necessary for adequate physical and psychological functioning, the definition of insomnia depending on subjective criteria, and relating to a condition in which the individual sleeps less than he feels is adequate. A fundamental question concerns the accuracy of an individual's self-assessment of his own sleep pattern. A study attempting to assess this found that a group of self-reported poor sleepers had a more disturbed sleep pattern than a matched group of good sleepers, indicating a considerable degree of subject reliability, although various studies have shown that an individual will usually over-estimate the amount of time spent in wakefulness. The complaint of poor sleep increases significantly with age. That of morning tiredness, however, is less often complained of as age advances. This would suggest that the elderly require less sleep, but neither the individuals concerned, nor their medical advisers, accept this proposition: in one large study 45 per cent of women over 75 years old were taking hypnotics.[4]

In order to make an assessment of the significance of this common complaint, and then to select the appropriate therapeutic approach it is essential to understand the characteristics of sleep.

Nature and function of sleep

Following birth a baby sleeps for most of the twenty-four hours, but rapidly develops a diurnal rhythm of sleeping and wakefulness. By the age of 5 years a child has established a sleep pattern similar to that of his parents. The amount of sleep an individual requires usually decreases with age, so that, whereas a baby will sleep approximately 16 hours, at 40 years an individual sleeps 7.4 hours, and by 70 this is further reduced to 6 hours. Nevertheless, there is clearly marked individual variation and some people appear to function perfectly adequately on only three to four hours, a condition which has been termed healthy insomnia.

It is clear that sleep, far from being a time of general inactivity, is a state in which complex and essential processes are being actively undertaken, although the exact function of these is still poorly understood. There are two quite distinct sleep patterns or phases.

(a) *Orthodox sleep.*– This appears to be especially necessary for the restoration of body processes. It is markedly increased following sleep deprivation. It is increased following physical exercise and is more marked at the beginning of a night's sleep, thus giving some truth to the statement that the hours of sleep before midnight are worth twice those afterwards.

(b) *Paradoxical or rapid eye movement (R.E.M.) sleep.*– During this phase the blood supply to the brain far exceeds that in wakefulness. It occurs for about 20 minutes every 1½ to 2 hours and it has been found to be particularly related to dream fantasies. If a subject is woken repeatedly during this phase he will become increasingly irritable and when asleep will show an increase in the time spent in the paradoxical phase, thus suggesting that the body has a real need for this type of sleep.

When studying the effects of drugs on sleep patterns, it has been found that quite small quantities of a barbiturate or amphetamine largely suppressed the paradoxical sleep, as well as the accompanying eye movements and the vividness of the associated dreams. When the drugs were then discontinued there was a significant rebound effect with a marked increase in paradoxical sleep, vivid dreams, nightmares and associated insomnia. It is this rebound effect which makes it difficult for individuals to discontinue their use of hypnotics once they have started. It will take up to two months before the normal pattern of paradoxical sleep is re-established after cessation of drug therapy, even when the hypnotics have only been prescribed for a short period of time.

Causes

Although it is well recognized that insomnia is part of the symptom complex of certain mental illnesses, especially depression, the majority of people who complain of sleep disturbance cannot be said to suffer from mental illness as such. Anxieties and worries, often related to the stresses and pressures of everyday living, appear to be the main cause for the high frequency of this complaint. Clearly, physical factors, such as pain and coughing, can and will affect sleep, but there is evidence to show that these are much less significant as aetiological factors than psychological problems.

History taking and diagnosis

The complaint 'I can't sleep, doctor' is one of the most common with which the general practitioner has to deal, and it is of critical importance to establish accurately what is meant by this expression. The following grouping of questions is suggested as a suitable schema to approach this complex problem.

(a) *Specific characteristics of the patient's sleep pattern.* — What time does he go to bed? Does he have difficulty in getting off to sleep, or does he wake early? Is the sleep broken by intermittent periods of wakefulness? Does he wake feeling tired?

(b) *General state of patient's health with special regard to particular factors which may affect his sleep pattern.* — What is the state of his general mood? Is there evidence of any depression? Does he complain of any other symptoms, such as pain, cough or pruritus? Does he suffer from nocturnal dyspnoea, or frequency of micturition?

(c) *External factors which may affect his sleep.* — Is the bedroom subject to excessive noise or light? Is the bed comfortable? Is the patient disturbed by his sleeping partner?

(d) *Significance of complaint.* — It is important to try to assess the patient's attitude to his sleep and whether it really is the insomnia that is the cause for the consultation. The symptom may be another example of the commonly appearing signposts to other problems perhaps less readily presented, such as psychosexual difficulties.

Management

In spite of what is known about the disadvantages and dangers of drug therapy for insomnia the prescription of hypnotic drugs is widespread. In 1973, over 16.5 million of these prescriptions were dispensed[5] and Dunlop has estimated that one night in ten of British sleep is induced by such therapy.[6] Most of the authorities on sleep problems unite in their condemnation of the indiscriminate prescription of hypnotics, but such advice often comes from those not faced with the problem in their consulting-room, and if these drugs are to be prescribed less often some other effective approach must be available.

Despite the social and medical importance of insomnia, there is little published research on alternative methods of treatment. It has been shown that a drink of Horlicks and milk before retiring has improved the quality of sleep.[7] Subjects who take regular exercise sleep more deeply following such activity than on other days. Muscular relaxation is a normal accompaniment of sleep onset and a number of studies have demonstrated the value of inducing relaxation as an aid to sleep.[8] There are therefore a number of important and helpful steps that an individual can take in preparing for sleep. These include taking some physical exercise during the day, stopping any excessive mental effort at least half-an-hour before going to bed, and then spending a little while just pottering about as a means of unwinding. It is often helpful to take a hot bath and a warm milky drink before retiring and when in bed to take up some light reading material, perhaps against a background of relaxing music. The bedroom should be well blacked out, the bed well warmed, and if necessary wax ear-plugs used to minimize noise disturbance. Some old people find bed socks help to keep their extremities warm. The possible addition of a rather more structured method of relaxation such as a form of yoga might be worth considering in certain suitable cases. If a patient wakes during the night, rather than tossing and turning, restless to get back to sleep, he might with benefit have a further warm drink and read until ready for sleep again.

In spite of the disadvantages of hypnotics, in certain instances drug therapy is clearly the treatment of choice. It is important, however, to consider carefully both the drug itself and the way it is prescribed. It has been shown that one of the most important factors in the prevention of drug dependence appears to be frequent review by the doctor after the first prescription and his cautionary advice to the patient at the time of starting drug treatment.[9]

In considering the drugs of choice it is now widely recognized that most hypnotics, like the barbiturates, produce an abnormal sleep, with a suppression of the R.E.M. phase, followed by a rebound effect, when drug therapy is discontinued. This tends to encourage habituation. Certain of these drugs, such as the barbiturates and methaqualone (Mandrax) also cause psychological addiction and are therefore prone to misuse. The benzodiazepines have a hypnotic action of rapid onset but both nitrazepam and diazepam have been shown to have a prolonged action which makes them unsuitable for use when skilled tasks such as driving have to be undertaken within 24 hours. The shorter acting benzodiazepines, temazepam 10 to 20 mg, triazolam 125 to 250 micrograms or lormetazepam 0.5 to 1 mg do not produce hangover effects and are suitable for use as occasional hypnotics. Patients can be advised to leave one or two sleeping tablets by the bedside, to be taken if sleep has not supervened an hour after going to bed. One of the added advantages of the benzodiazepines is that they are comparatively safe when taken in overdosage.

In considering individual groups of patients, the management of the elderly insomniac requires special care. Older patients are particularly likely to suffer from drug toxicity and side-effects; attention to drug dosage is therefore especially important. The elderly often waken frequently at night, and may need to do so for micturition. Barbiturates should be avoided as they may cause confusion and increase the incidence of nocturnal falls.

Temazepam, and chlormethiazole (Heminevrin) have been shown to be suitable for use in the elderly, not only because hangover effects are avoided, but these hypnotics allow sleep to be interrupted safely.[10] The chloral hydrate derivative dichlorphenazone (Welldorm) is a useful alternative especially when mild pain or discomfort is present, as it appears to have an analgesic effect in addition to its hypnotic property.

In the case of children, hypnotics are rarely required and their long-term use should be strongly discouraged. Chloral hydrate elixir, 200 mg in 5 ml, is effective and safe, as is a sedative antihistamine, e.g. promethazine hydrochloride, 5 to 10 mg (Phenergan). For patients suffering from terminal illness the aim should be to ensure their maximal comfort, using when necessary powerful analgesics with or without hypnotics.

References

[1] Dunnell, K. and Cartwright, A. (1972): *Medicine Takers, Prescribers and Hoarders*. London: Routledge and Kegan Paul

[2] Sheppard, M., Brown, A.C., Cooper, B., Kalton, A.W. (1966): *Psychiatric Illness in General Practice*. London: Oxford University Press

[3] Oswald, I. (1966): *Sleep*. 1st ed. Harmondsworth, Middlesex: Penguin Books

[4] McGhie, A. and Russell, S.M. (1962): The subjective assessment of normal sleep patterns. *Journal of Mental Science*, *108*, 642

[5] Health and Personal Social Services Statistics for England (1974) HMSO

[6] Dunlop, D. (1970): Abuse of drugs by the public and by doctors. *British Medical Bulletin*, *26*, 236

[7] Southwell, P.R., Evans, C.R. and Hunt, J.N. (1972): The effect of a hot milk drink on movements during sleep. *British Medical Journal*, *2*, 429

[8] Clift, A.D. (1972): Factors leading to dependence on hypnotic drugs. *British Medical Journal*, *3*, 614

[9] Rachman, S.J. and Philips, Clare. (1972): *Physiology and Medicine*. London: Temple Smith

[10] Briggs, R.S., Castleden, C.M. and Kraft, C.A. (1980) Improved hypnotic treatment using chlormethiazole and temazepam. *British Medical Journal*, *1*, 601

3.17 The patient with difficulty in seeing

J.J.C. Cormack

Out of a sample of 1,410 adults asked to report on any symptoms experienced in a two-week period, 14 (i.e. 1 in 100) reported 'eye strain or other eye trouble'. In the National Morbidity Survey, 1.3 consultations per 1,000 patients were accounted for by refractive errors, with a further 6 consultations per 1,000 patients for conditions which might affect eyesight. Extrapolating to an average practice of 2,000 patients, one could expect 2.6 consultations per annum for refractive errors and a further 12 consultations for eyesight problems (compared with 60 consultations for conjunctivitis, 10 for styes and 10 for blepharitis). 'Eyestrain' is a lay term which may simply denote ocular headaches (often due to underlying emotional tension), or difficulties in seeing due to refractive errors, or partial loss of visual fields or haziness of vision from more serious causes. In fact, although patients do not often complain to their general practitioners of 'eyestrain' as such, they do complain of difficulties in seeing (which will be the subject of this chapter) or of painful eyes or red eyes (which will be dealt with in subsequent chapters).

Presentation

Difficulties in seeing may be presented in a number of different ways which give clues to their causation. A convenient scheme is to divide symptoms into painless and painful visual symptoms. Painful symptoms are dealt with in Chapter 3.18. Painless visual symptoms comprise:

- Gradual loss of vision
- Sudden loss of vision
  - Unilateral
    - Total
    - Partial
  - Bilateral
- Fleeting loss of vision
- Floaters
- Haloes
- Flashing lights
- Double vision.

Causes

Gradual loss of vision. — The commonest cause of gradual loss of vision (which may be unilateral or bilateral) is refractive error. The other major causes are:
— Senile cataract
— Chronic glaucoma
— Diabetic retinopathy
— Hypertensive retinopathy
— Senile macular degeneration
— Pituitary adenoma
— Choroiditis.
The ophthalmic findings in these conditions are set out in Table I.

	Visual acuity	Peripheral visual fields	Ophthalmoscopy
Refractive errors	Diminished	Normal	Normal
Senile cataract	Diminished	Normal	Hazy because of grey reflex in the pupil
Chronic glaucoma	Usually normal	Variable loss	Cupped discs
Diabetic retinopathy	Impaired as the condition progresses	Normal	Haemorrhages and exudates
Hypertensive retinopathy	Variable (depending on involvement of macula)	Normal	Vessel changes Haemorrhages and exudates Papilloedema in extreme cases
Senile macular degeneration	Central vision lost	Normal	Variable pigmentary change at the macula
Pituitary adenoma	Usually normal	Bitemporal or irregular field changes	Pallor of discs
Choroiditis	Diminished	Normal	Vitreous haze, with darkened red reflex

Table I. — Gradual loss of vision

It should be noted that a normal pupil reflex is maintained in all the above conditions giving rise to gradual loss of vision.

Sudden loss of vision. — Bilateral sudden partial loss of vision is usually due to a homonymous field defect which may appear to the patient to be a sudden total loss of vision in one eye — a genuine optical illusion. Visual field testing will reveal an equal defect on the same side in each eye. The cause is usually an embolus or other vascular accident behind the midbrain.

Unilateral sudden total loss of vision is most commonly due to occlusion of the central retinal artery or one of its branches. Visual acuity is totally lost in the affected eye along with an absent pupillary reflex on the affected side. The fundus may be white (apart from a cherry red spot at the macula) and the disc may be swollen.

Unilateral sudden partial loss of vision may be due to:
— Occlusion of the central retinal vein or one of its branches
— Optic neuritis
— Retrobulbar neuritis
— Retinal detachment
— Vitreous haemorrhage.

The findings related to these conditions are set out in Table II.

	Visual acuity	Visual fields	Pupils	Ophthalmoscopy
Occlusion of central retinal vein or branch	Considerably diminished	Some distortion	Normal	'Stormy sunset' pattern
Optic neuritis[1]	Considerably diminished	Normal	Sluggish direct reflex	Swollen disc
Retrobulbar neuritis[1]	Considerably diminished	Normal	Sluggish direct reflex	Normal disc
Retinal detachment	Variable, depending on area involved	Complete field loss in area of detachment	Normal	Greyish rippling appearance in place of red reflex
Vitreous haemorrhage	Considerably diminished	Variable	Normal	A black reflex obscures the normal red reflex

[1] Optic neuritis and retrobulbar neuritis are in fact the same condition, occurring at different parts of the optic nerve.

Table II. — Unilateral sudden partial loss of vision

Fleeting loss of vision. — Fleeting visual loss may be caused by emboli, aneurysms, migraine, hypertension or hypotension.

Floaters. — Floaters are experienced as fine black filaments which float with eye movements and are most noticeable when looking at a white or clear background. They are caused by fine vitreous opacities.

Haloes. — Haloes are classically the early warning of angle closure glaucoma. The pupil dilates to accommodate poor light and produces a partial angle block which causes the intra-ocular pressure to rise. The oedematous cornea then splits the light into rainbow-coloured rings and gives the subjective appearance of haloes.

Flashing lights. — Flashing lights imply irritation of either the retina or of the visual cortex. Bilateral, vague flashing lights may be due to disturbances in cerebral blood flow, a cerebral tumour or migraine. Persistent unilateral flashing lights are usually caused by a developing retinal detachment.

Double vision. — A child with a squint rarely complains of double vision because the image in the squinting eye is readily suppressed. The presentation of squint in children depends on the observation of relatives or of the doctor. Intermittent or small angled squints are easily overlooked, but are still very significant.
In adults a complaint of double vision may in fact simply imply blurred vision and the distinction must be elicited by careful history taking.
There are three cranial nerve palsies which cause squints and diplopia in adults: third, fourth and sixth nerve palsies. Third nerve palsy limits ocular movements on the affected side except lateral and inward and downward movement. A third nerve palsy will also cause a dilated pupil and ptosis on the affected side. The causes of third nerve palsy include cerebral aneurysm, pituitary tumour, multiple sclerosis and myasthenia gravis. Fourth nerve palsy limits downward and inward movement of the affected eye, and is almost always caused by trauma. Sixth nerve palsy which limits lateral eye movements may occur in cerebrovascular disease, diabetes mellitus, head injury or increased intracranial pressure.

History and examination

The history taken from a patient complaining of loss of vision or visual difficulties should seek answers to the following points:

1. Was the loss of vision or difficulty in seeing gradual or sudden?
2. Is the visual loss total or partial?

3. Are both eyes affected or only one?
4. Does the side vision appear to be normal?

A simple but comprehensive routine regime for examining the eyes consists of the following sequence:

1. Visual acuity (central vision)
2. Fields of vision
3. State of pupils and pupillary reflexes
4. State of cornea
5. Depth of anterior chamber
6. Finger tension
7. Examination of the fundus.

Two additional general points complete the examination:

8. Blood pressure
9. Urine for sugar.

Visual acuity is conventionally tested by means of test types, but accurate assessment is best left to ophthalmologists and opticians. For simple diagnostic purposes fixation on any convenient object about 6 metres (18 feet) away — such as a television set or bookcase — will serve to assess whether vision is normal, impaired or grossly impaired. Visual fields, similarly, can only be accurately mapped out with the use of special instruments, but can be roughly assessed by the confrontation test using hand movements.
The state of the pupils and pupillary reflexes can easily be observed with a simple torch.
The state of the cornea can likewise be examined by the light of the torch and observed as clear or cloudy, but if there is any suspicion of injury or corneal infection fluorescein must be used in addition.
The depth of the anterior chamber is assessed by shining in the torch beam from the side of the eye; the 'eclipse' effect where the light does not penetrate through to the medial half of the anterior chamber indicates a narrow drainage angle which predisposes to acute glaucoma. Finger tension or 'digital tonometry' consists of palpating the eyeball with light pressure from the examiner's middle and index fingers on the top of the closed upper eyelid (above the tarsal plate); a tense hard eyeball indicates glaucoma and calls for urgent referral.
Examination of the fundus should ideally be conducted with the pupil dilated with tropicamide drops. In general practice it is rarely practicable to arrange this and a moderately good view, at least of the optic disc and retinal vessels, can usually be obtained with an ophthalmoscope in a darkened room. It is useful to have some specific fixed point on which the patient can focus and keep his eye still when sitting in the consulting-room chair. If the patient is examined lying on an examination couch it is helpful to have a

picture fixed to the ceiling above the head end of the couch for the purpose (this can also help the more apprehensive patient to relax when other examinations are being carried out).

Management

The one preventive measure which can check the insidious and symptomless development of chronic glaucoma is routine effective examination (including visual fields and inspection of the optic discs) of middle-aged and elderly patients at two to three yearly intervals. Such examinations are usually carried out by opticians but general practitioners can certainly remind and encourage their patients to undergo them, and should themselves carry out the examination routine described above whenever patients present with complaints of visual difficulties.

The importance of vision to the maintenance of normal function in an individual of any age is so great that the general practitioner's role when faced with a patient complaining of visual difficulties is in many instances to secure specialist referral for full assessment. In the case of apparent refractive errors the appropriate specialist is the ophthalmic optician; in all but a few of the other conditions listed in this chapter referral to an ophthalmologist is indicated. The degree of urgency with which such referrals should be initiated and the action expected from ophthalmological specialist colleagues is set out in Table III.

It is for consideration in the individual case whether patients presenting with diabetic or hypertensive retinopathy should be referred in the first instance to the ophthalmologist or to the physician concerned. In these fields close inter-specialist co-operation is obviously of the greatest importance. The only condition referred to in the table which is amenable to non-specialist first-aid intervention is retinal artery occlusion, when the immediate institution of steroid therapy (prednisolone 40 mg a day) is indicated. Retinal circulation may return if the patient lies supine and massages the eye.

Haloes. — This subject is dealt with in Chapter 3.18, The Patient with Pain in the Eye.

Flashing lights. — Unilateral light flashing, which may possibly herald a developing retinal detachment, calls for urgent referral to an ophthalmologist. Vague bilateral light flashing may be indicative of migraine, which should be appropriately treated. If the additional history or examination raises suspicions of disturbed cerebral blood flow or of the development of a cerebral tumour, a neurological opinion should be sought.

	Immediate	Soon	Non-urgent	Action expected
Senile cataract			X	Possible eventual surgery
Chronic glaucoma		X		Advice on meiotic treatment, timolol or surgery
Diabetic retinopathy		X		Assessment, then co-operation with diabetic physician Consideration of light coagulation
Hypertensive retinopathy		X		Assessment, then co-operation with cardiologist
Senile macular degeneration			X	Assessment and explanation (no treatment possible)
Choroiditis	X			Possible systemic steroids
Homonymous field defect		X		Assessment of possible treatable causes: embolus, hypertension, diabetes
Retinal artery occlusion	X			Systemic steroids and assessment for possible temporal arteritis
Retinal vein occlusion	X			Assessment for possible development of chronic glaucoma
Optic or retrobulbar neuritis		X		Assessment, reassurance and lookout for development of multiple sclerosis
Retinal detachment	X			Surgery (cryo-surgery or laser)
Vitreous haemorrhage			X	Assessment and co-operation with physician

Table III. — Degree of urgency of referral and expected action

Fleeting loss of vision. — If a single episode of fleeting visual loss is reported, further history and examination should attempt to elicit migraine, hypertension, hypotension, or a source for an embolus. In the absence of findings indicating these, reassurance and an injunction to report any further episodes are probably sufficient. If further episodes are reported an aneurysm may be suspected and the help of a neurologist should be sought.

Floaters. — The description of the symptoms and (sometimes) the visualization of fine vitreous threads are sufficient to establish the diagnosis; simple reassurance is all that is required; the floaters absorb and disappear with time.

Double vision. — Any suspicion of squint in children from the age of 6 months onwards should indicate referral for assessment. A neglected squint can lead to permanent loss of vision in one eye. Likewise adults with double vision and/or squint require to be referred for assessment.

Conclusion

While it is clear that the general practitioner's primary role in dealing with visual disturbances is to assess the underlying pathological lesion and in many cases to arrange appropriate referral, his responsibility does not end there. As with all referrals he needs to give his patient an explanation of the probable procedures which the specialist will undertake, to give an indication if possible of the prognosis and most importantly to supervise follow-up, especially if partial or total blindness is the outcome. There are many services available for the blind and partially sighted and ideally each practice should maintain a register of its patients in these categories so that checks can be made from time to time to ensure that all appropriate means are being harnessed to alleviate the distress and disability of those condemned to a world of darkness or diminished light.

Further reading

Royal College of General Practitioners, Office of Population Censuses and Surveys, Department of Health and Social Security (1986): *Morbidity Statistics from General Practice 1981–82.* HMSO Series MB5 No. 1

Bedford, M.A. (1971): *A Colour Atlas of Ophthalmological Diagnosis.* London: Wolfe Medical Books

Chawla, H.B. (1981): *Essential Ophthalmology.* Edinburgh: Churchill Livingstone

Jackson, C.R.S. (1975): *The Eye in General Practice.* 7th ed. Edinburgh: Churchill Livingstone

3.18 The patient with pain in the eye

J.J.C. Cormack

The painful eye is usually red, but the conditions in which redness is the predominant sign (conjunctivitis and episcleritis) are considered in Chapter 3.19 on The Red Eye. No figures are available for the incidence of trauma to the eye or periorbital structures, but there can be little doubt that trauma (including foreign bodies) is the commonest single cause of the painful red eye. Similarly figures are not easily available for the incidence of corneal ulcers, but these, too, are important, if less common, causes of eye pain. Acute glaucoma and acute iritis are both rare conditions, accounting in each case for less than one patient per 1,000 consulting per annum in general practice, but because of their importance they must be considered. When pain in the eye is complained of and the eye is white, further inquiry will usually reveal that the pain is not in fact in the eye, but around it.

Presentation

The patient with a painful red eye will usually present as an emergency, either asking for an immediate appointment or a home visit. In the case of a foreign body (the usual form of trauma) there is often a clear history of getting a speck of dust or grit in the eye, although the actual incident may pass unnoticed. With other forms of trauma (direct blows or chemical burns) the history is obvious. Corneal abrasions and ulcers, acute glaucoma and acute iritis all cause fairly sudden and very acute pain in the eye – so severe in acute glaucoma that it can be accompanied by vomiting.

Flash burns in welders who expose their unprotected eyes to oxyacetylene torch light ('arc eye') presents, often at night, as acute pain and blepharospasm some hours after the exposure. When the presentation of pain in the eye is less acute it is likely that the cause is either conjunctivitis or that the pain is round or near the eye rather than in it.

Causes

Foreign bodies are obvious primary causes of painful eyes: the cornea especially becomes acutely painful if injured. Corneal abrasions can be caused by relatively trivial injuries or slight scratching. Corneal ulcers may result from the secondary infection of an abrasion. In the case of dendritic ulcers the herpes virus is implicated. 'Arc eye' is due to conjunctival irritation caused by unprotected exposure to ultra-violet light, as from an oxyacetylene torch flame.

Acute glaucoma is caused by dilatation of the pupil (e.g. in the dark or under sympathetic stimulation) in an eye predisposed by narrow drainage angles as present in hypermetropic (long-sighted) eyes and worsened by the gradual forward movement of the lens with the passage of the years. The description of the patient liable to acute glaucoma as hypermetropic, hyperanxious and highly unlikely to be menstruating still is no more (and no less) likely to be true than that of the patient liable to develop gall-stones as fat, fertile and forty. The dilatation of the pupil blocks the narrow angles and causes obstruction to the outflow of aqueous humour; it is the high pressure of the aqueous which causes it to permeate the cornea and produce the typical haziness (or, if the pressure rise is transient, cause corneal oedema which produces the 'coloured haloes' described in Chapter 3.17 on The Patient with Difficulty in Seeing).

Acute iritis can be found in conjunction with collagen disorders such as rheumatoid arthritis or ankylosing spondylitis, but it is more commonly an idiopathic condition. The inflammation of the iris produces a fine exudate which infiltrates the aqueous and may form adhesions, which bind down the pupil margins to the lens causing a characteristic irregular appearance, and which may agglutinate to form keratic precipitates.

History and examination

The history should concentrate on the circumstances and mode of onset of the pain; if a foreign body is involved especial care should be taken to enquire if it was travelling at speed (e.g. injury with a fragment of chisel). As the initial examination consists of observation of the colour of the eye, this will often precede the history. If the eye is red more detailed examination can proceed straight away after enquiring about onset and the likely presence of a foreign body.

The examination consists of:

1. Testing of the pupil's reflex to light

2. Inspection with a torch and magnifying glass to detect a foreign body, including a careful look in the fornices. In the case of the upper fornix, this involves asking the patient to look down and then everting the upper lid with the aid of gentle downwards pressure with a matchstick or similar instrument.
3. Instillation of fluorescein and careful inspection of the corneal surface. Abrasions and ulcers are shown by staining of the area of defective epithelium. Dendritic ulcers show up as characteristically branching stains. (Fluorescein eye-drops are liable to infection and impregnated strips in sterile packs are preferable).

The eye may be white if the patient is seen soon after the entry of a foreign body or if the cornea has been recently abraded (as with a twig or baby's finger-nail) but the history should establish the cause. If the eye is white and the history of the onset of pain is non-acute further enquiry may elicit features suggestive of any of the following:

1. Tension headache: a feeling of tightness or constriction, often also involving the occiput
2. Sinusitis, associated with other signs of upper respiratory infection, with nasal blockage or purulent discharge
3. Migraine: unilateral 'heavy' pain, sometimes preceded by an 'aura' and accompanied by nausea or vomiting
4. Post-herpetic neuralgia: a preceding unilateral rash will provide the clue
5. Trigeminal neuralgia: excrutiatingly severe lancinating pain of intermittent onset
6. Temporal arteritis: pain usually more specifically localized to the lateral side of the eye
7. Acute retrobulbar neuritis (rare, but important as early evidence of multiple sclerosis): dull pain on movement of the eyes accompanied by a central scotoma.

In this group of conditions further examination consists of palpation to elicit tenderness: over the frontal or maxillary sinuses in the case of sinusitis, or the temporal region with temporal arteritis, or over the eyeballs themselves in acute retrobulbar neuritis. Tension headaches, migraine, post-herpetic neuralgia and trigeminal neuralgia will be diagnosed mainly from the history and the exclusion of ocular foreign bodies or corneal damage.

In acute glaucoma and acute iritis (anterior uveitis or iridocyclitis) the findings on examination are characteristic: in both the redness is maximal near the limbus.

Acute glaucoma:– Hazy cornea (but not staining)

– Pupil dilated and fixed
– Eyeball hard and tender

Acute iritis: – Cornea clear
– Small spastic pupil (sometimes irregular due to the formation of adhesions)
– Eyeball tender (but not hard)
– Sometimes keratic precipitates (due to agglutination of the exudate) seen as small white dots on the back of the cornea.

Management

The removal of a foreign body from the conjunctiva in the fornices is usually easily effected with a wisp of cotton-wool. If, however, it is lodged on the cornea a local anaesthetic in the form of amethocaine drops is advisable before making the attempt. The foreign body should then be brushed off with a cotton-wool swab; if this fails a gentle attempt should be made to lift it off with a sterile injection needle (rather than the traditional corneal spud which is liable to cause a good deal of blunt damage in the hands of the inexperienced). If this, too, is unsuccessful it is better not to persist and risk causing further unnecessary trauma, but to instil antibiotic drops (e.g. chloramphenicol) and refer the patient immediately to an ophthalmologist. Immediate referral is also indicated if there is any likelihood that the foreign body was travelling fast: in these cases a tiny fragment can enter the substance of the globe with little or no apparent damage to the cornea, and only specialist procedures provide any hope of saving the eye.

After the foreign body is removed or when on fluorescein staining there appears to be a corneal abrasion or ulceration, the pupil should be dilated with 1 per cent atropine drops (in an effort to prevent secondary iritis) and the eye covered for twenty-four hours with a pad secured with Sellotape (in contrast to the treatment of conjunctivitis in which the eye should not be covered). The instillation of chloramphenicol drops every six hours should prevent secondary infection. Dendritic ulcers form a separate category; they are treated with idoxuridine drops but this is preferably done under specialist supervision.

Chemical burns with acid or alkaline caustics should be managed in the first instance by advice immediately the message is received to wash out the eyes with copious amounts of tap water, and the immediate arrangement of referral to an ophthalmologist.

The treatment of 'arc eye' consists of the instillation of local anaesthetic to allow inspection, followed by the use of pads and bandages to rest the eye for 12 to 18 hours and the prescription of analgesics. The condition usually settles within eighteen hours; if it does not, referral for specialist opinion and reassessment of the diagnosis is indicated.

Acute glaucoma is a true emergency and calls for immediate referral after first-aid treatment has been instituted. This consists in contracting the dilated pupil with 2 per cent pilocarpine drops (with similar treatment to the unaffected eye in an attempt to avert similar disaster on that side). To allay the pain and anxiety morphine sulphate, 15 mg (or if there is vomiting morphine with cyclizine – Cyclimorph) should be administered and by this time one hopes that the ambulance would be on its way.

Acute iritis is less urgent, but referral should be ensured within forty-eight hours. The first-aid treatment of acute iritis is to dilate the contracted pupil with 1 per cent atropine drops, and thereafter instil betamethasone drops hourly, provided the cornea does not stain with fluorescein.

Conclusion

The diagnosis and treatment of the painful eye in general practice are usually not difficult. Foreign bodies are the commonest culprits and the possibility of fragments travelling at speed must constantly be borne in mind. The possibility of the development of dendritic ulcers and their detection should have equal priority. In addition to these, the possession of a good torch and some fluorescein and a knowledge of the characteristic appearances of acute glaucoma and acute iritis will equip the practitioner to deal with the majority of patients with pain in the eye.

3.19
The red eye

J.J.C. Cormack

In practice patients with red eyes often also complain of pain or discomfort, and patients with painful or uncomfortable eyes often exhibit redness. In this chapter those conditions where the redness is the predominant sign will be considered; conditions in which pain or discomfort is the main symptom, with redness but an incidental finding, are covered in Chapter 3.18 on The Patient with Pain in the Eye.

In the National Morbidity Survey[1] the annual consultation rate for conjunctivitis was found to be in the region of 36 patients per 1,000 at risk, so that in a practice of 2,000 patients one might expect to see 72 patients a year with this, the commonest single eye condition presenting in practice. The only other cause of a red eye in which pain or discomfort is simply a subsidiary symptom is episcleritis, and this, along with spontaneous subconjunctival haemorrhage (where the eye is painless), is sufficiently uncommon for figures to be unavailable (being categorized in the National Morbidity Survey under 'other diseases of the eye'). If for practical purposes one excludes the painful eye which happens to be red, in the vast majority of cases the red eye will be due to conjunctivitis. Conditions affecting the eyelids are considered separately at the end of this chapter.

The majority of patients with conjunctivitis are babies (in whom the condition may be associated with blocked naso-lacrimal ducts) and pre-school children. The condition accounts for 143 consultations per annum for each 1,000 children in the 0–5 year age-group. Thereafter the incidence for older children and adults up to the age of 75 is fairly uniform, being rather less common in the over-75 age-group.

Presentation

In conjunctivitis, in addition to the redness of the eyes there is often a complaint of discharge or stickiness for a few days, especially after sleep: typically in the morning the baby's eyes are stuck together and they require to be swabbed with water before they will open. In infants with obstructed naso-lacrimal ducts the eyes water continually. Adults, although rarely complaining of actual pain, will often note a sensation of 'grittiness'.

The onset of episcleritis is usually much more insidious, and the red eye (for this is often a unilateral condition) may be accompanied by a dull ache. The appearance of a raised patch of dull redness overlying part of the sclera will be found to have been present (sometimes slowly growing) for some time.

Spontaneous subconjunctival haemorrhages are dramatic in onset; the patient suddenly notices a segmental patch of redness, usually in just one eye, with no sensation of pain at all. The crimson red appearance totally covering a segment of sclera from the limbus to the margin is usually diagnostic.

Causes

Conjunctivitis is caused by:

1. Bacterial or viral infection
2. Irritants (e.g. tobacco smoke, cosmetics)
3. Allergy.

The commonest pathogens are staphylococci and viruses; the incidence of bacterial as opposed to viral infections is not known, as swabbing is rarely called for clinically. The trachoma virus may be implicated in newly arrived immigrants from Africa or the Indian subcontinent, and this may proceed to keratitis and blindness. Congenital obstruction of the lower end of the naso-lacrimal duct causes stagnation followed by infection of the tears in the lacrimal sac. Episcleritis is a form of rheumatic nodule: a manifestation of collagen disorder which is often isolated but should lead to a search for other systemic manifestations such as rheumatoid arthritis or ankylosing spondylitis.

Subconjunctival haemorrhage is due to the rupture of a blood vessel under the conjunctiva. Although painless, haemorrhage is usually taken to be spontaneous or idiopathic (painful haemorrhage most often being due to direct trauma). A history of straining is sometimes obtained: indeed in certain parts of Africa subconjunctival haemorrhages in children can be almost pathognomonic of whooping-cough.

History and examination

In the diagnosis of those conditions in which the eye is red, and pain is either absent or of secondary importance, the salient features of the history consist quite simply of enquiry into the mode and length of onset, the presence or absence of discharge or stickiness and enquiry about possible irritants or allergens. If unilateral the possibility of a foreign body or inturned eyelash should be considered.

The examination consists of inspection with a good torch. In all these conditions the cornea is clear and the pupils of normal size, equal in diameter and reacting equally to light. Bilateral congestion, apparent at the back of the lids and on to the scleral conjunctiva, usually becoming less apparent towards the limbus, and often associated with discharge, confirms the presence of conjunctivitis. In infants with blocked naso-lacrimal ducts

Condition	Onset	Uni- or Bi-lateral	Pain	Other features
Conjunctivitis	Acute	Bilateral	Grittiness	Stickiness or discharge
Episcleritis	Insidious	Often unilateral	Ache	Nodule often slightly raised
Spontaneous subconjunctival haemorrhage	Sudden	Usually unilateral	Painless	Sector of sclera involved

Table I. – Characteristics of the red eye

(dacryocystitis) pressure over the lacrimal sac may produce a reflux of pus into the conjunctival sac. Small, raised, dull red nodules denote episcleritis. The segmental crimson red appearance of subconjunctival haemorrhages with their sharply defined margins is quite characteristic. Table I summarizes the features of these three conditions.

Management

The most important point in the management of conjunctivitis is a negative one: the avoidance of covering or irritating the eye. Covering with an eye-patch (which is still the first remedy some patients resort to) converts the conjunctival sac into a culture chamber with potentially disastrous results. Possible irritation of the eye by regular bathing – a practice which is quite common among some older patients – should, if discovered, be discouraged.

The natural history of conjunctivitis is for the condition to abate within a period of a few days, although a low-grade subacute conjunctivitis may remain for a matter of two to three weeks. In the first instance treatment with chloramphenicol eye-drops instilled every two to three hours, with chloramphenicol ointment at night will clear the majority of infections in about three days. This will deal with the likely bacterial pathogens, and in the case of viral conjunctivitis will limit the development of secondary infections.

If the conjunctivitis persists despite this treatment, it is reasonable to stop the antibiotic (which on occasions may itself act as an irritant and prolong the reaction) and use warm water to clear away any discharge for 24 to 48 hours and then, if signs of infection persist, to take a swab and institute treatment with a different preparation (such as framycetin eye ointment) while awaiting the result. If trachoma is suspected (that is, when there are signs of conjunctivitis in a recent arrival from the tropics) referral to an ophthalmologist is indicated.

In infantile dacryocystitis finger pressure over the lacrimal sac followed by instillation of the antibiotic drops will reduce the infection and help the obstruction to clear. If the watering persists after 6 months of age referral for washing out under general anaesthetic is indicated.

If the history is strongly suggestive of irritants or allergy zinc sulphate eye-drops should be used. Topical steroids may be instilled in persistent cases of allergic conjunctivitis but only if (and this is of vital importance) one can be completely satisfied that the cornea is unaffected: it usually is, but to use topical steroids in the presence of a dendritic ulcer, however small, can create disaster and amount to malpractice. It is therefore wise to check that the cornea does not stain with fluorescein before resorting to local steroids. There is no justification whatever for using combined antibiotic and steroid preparations, although these continue to be marketed.

Episcleritis responds rapidly to local steroids (e.g. betamethasone eye-drops or ointment) though again it is important to satisfy oneself that the cornea is non-staining.

The only treatment needed for spontaneous subconjunctival haemorrhage is explanation and reassurance.

Conditions affecting the eyelids

Conditions affecting the eyelids might properly be thought to be of dermatological rather than ophthalmological interest. Such demarcation disputes, however, are of purely academic interest in general practice; the patient with inflamed eyelids will complain of a red or irritated eye and in most instances be diagnosed and managed without need for specialist referral. The three commonest conditions affecting the eyelids are styes, blepharitis and meibomian cysts (also called tarsal cysts or chalazions). Using the figures reported in the National Morbidity Survey, a practitioner with a list of 2,000 patients could expect some 12 consultations annually for styes and 12 for blepharitis. There are no separate figures available for meibomian cysts.

Presentation.– The patient with a stye or with a meibomian abcess presents with a complaint of pain and swelling of one eye, or more accurately of an eyelid, of a few days' duration. Pain is not a prominent feature of blepharitis, but irritation or itchiness is described, which is diffuse and almost always bilateral. A simple (uninfected) meibomian cyst is neither painful nor red, but presented as an awareness of a small nodule on a lid.

Causes. – Styes are abscesses of the glands related to the eyelash follicles. The offending organism is usually the staphylococcus. A meibomian cyst is a granuloma of the meibomian gland in the tarsal plate; this may become infected to give rise to a meibomian abscess. Blepharitis is a subacute or chronic infection of the lid margins and lash follicles, often associated with dandruff (seborrhoea capitis), often with an allergic element in addition to the infection.

History and examination.– The history of a stye is that of the development over a period of a few days of a painful swelling on an eyelid, sometimes beginning to discharge by the time medical aid is sought. An infected meibomian cyst may give rise to an identical history, although in this case there may be an awareness over a longer preceding period of a small painless nodule in the lid. A longer history is usually given in the case of blepharitis; irritation and diffuse redness of the lids have often been present for some weeks or even months before the doctor is consulted.

The initial examination takes place simultaneously with listening to the history, as the patient is observed sitting in the consulting-room chair. An inflamed unilateral swelling on one eyelid is almost certainly either a stye or a meibomian abscess: which of the two can only be determined by closer inspection. A stye 'points', sometimes with some discharge present, on the lid margin; a meibomian abcess points at some distance from the lid margin. In blepharitis the lids are red and thickened and there is usually scaling along the lid margin. The condition is almost always bilateral. An uninfected meibomian cyst is simply a small nodule in the substance of the lid, usually single, but occasionally multiple.

Management.– The initial management of a stye or a meibomian abscess is identical. The abscess should be encouraged to point and discharge by hot bathing. The traditional technique is to cover the bowl of a domestic wooden spoon with cotton-wool secured by a strip of bandage and to immerse this in water as hot as the patient can bear and then apply repeatedly to the affected eye over a period of about ten minutes every two or three hours. An antibiotic ointment (such as chloramphenicol) should be used three or four times a day to prevent secondary conjunctivitis or infection of other follicles. Once the stye has pointed the offending eyelash should be removed. Styes tend to occur in crops and when this occurs a course of systemic penicillin may abort further spread. Some authorities also recommend the twice daily application of Naseptin (chlorhexidine and neomycin) cream to the anterior nares in an attempt to eradicate the presumed source of infection.

Once a meibomian abscess has discharged, the residual nodule is incised and curetted; incision and curettage are also the treatment of meibomian cysts presenting as uninfected nodules. This is a relatively simple minor operation usually performed on an outpatient basis by ophthalmologists using local anaesthesia.

Blepharitis may run a long chronic course and treatment is often tedious. The eyelids should be bathed night and morning to remove crusts and then sulphacetamide or chloramphenicol ointment should be firmly massaged into the roots of the lashes. It is equally important to attend at the same time to the seborrhoea capitis, which is often the predisposing cause, by the regular use of a selenium-containing shampoo and in refractory cases the use of steroid lotions or gels.

[1] Royal College of General Practitioners, Office of Population Censuses and Surveys, Department of Health and Social Security (1986): *Morbidity Statistics from General Practice 1981–82.* HMSO Series MB5 No. 1

I am grateful to Dr G.T. Millar (Consultant Ophthalmologist, The Royal Infirmary, Edinburgh) for helpful criticism and advice in the preparation of Chapters 3.17, 3.18 and 3.19.

3.20 The patient with difficulty in hearing

George Gomez

Many individuals, particularly with increasing age, have some hearing loss. It has been shown[1] that in testing hearing at three frequencies, 500, 1000 and 2000 cycles per second, socially significant hearing loss (i.e. difficulty with normal speech) occurred with a mean loss of 30 decibels or more. This may therefore be regarded as the level of deafness which interferes with normal communication.

The prevalence of deafness of this degree is not known precisely in the United Kingdom, but it has been estimated[2] to rise from 0.8 per cent in men aged 15 to 24 years to 18 per cent in men aged 75 to 79 years. The figures for women are slightly lower than those for men in almost all age-groups. In a recent study in general practice in which patients between the ages of 40 and 64 years were screened for deafness[3] a prevalence of hearing loss greater than 35 decibels was detected in 5.8 per cent. It was found that the prevalence increased with increasing age and was more common in the lower social classes. In middle-aged men more deafness than expected was found in the left ear, possibly related to the use of rifles in the army. In a study of the symptoms presented in general practice[4] defects of hearing were presented by 24 per 1,000 patients per year. The symptom was equally presented by males and females, and most commonly by those aged 45 to 64 years.

Presentation of the complaint

Patients tend to report with deafness when it interferes with their social life or occupation. In children deafness may not be detected until the defect is severe. Minor changes in hearing may lead parents to interpret their child's behaviour as naughtiness or their failure at school as lack of intelligence or attention. The routine testing of hearing in the first five years of life is one of the most rewarding screening tests in general practice and the general practitioner should always exclude hearing loss in children with behavioural disorders or problems at school.

Adults presenting with hearing loss should be closely questioned about the onset of their symptoms. Was this gradual or did it occur suddenly, following, for instance, a flight in an aeroplane or swimming? Are there any associated symptoms such as pain in the ear, discharge, itching, tinnitus or vertigo?

In the elderly hearing loss is an uncommon complaint although it is often present. Patients at these ages expect some deterioration in hearing and it is often a relative driven to distraction by shouting at grandma or grandpa who draws the doctor's attention to the problem. Nurses, health visitors and doctors themselves frequently intervene before the patient complains of deafness. It is indeed both fascinating and sad that patients who would complain vigorously about any defect in vision strenuously deny that they are deaf.

Causes

The commonest cause of deafness in all age-groups is wax in the ear. The most common cause in children is otitis media. Table I illustrates the age and sex distribution in 64 patients consecutively complaining of deafness in general practice over a period of six months. Table II illustrates the causes of deafness identified in these patients. Otitis media in the young and old tubotympanic disease and presbyacusis in the older age-groups were the most common conditions requiring audiometry in this practice. Two children were seen whose ears had been slapped resulting in a ruptured ear-drum. Unsuspected deafness was also found:–

> J.B., aged 8, was found to be erratic in his work at school. He was excellent in some classes and very poor in others. He was found to be suffering from unilateral, perceptive deafness. His school performance depended on where he sat in the classroom. He was good when his good ear was directed to the teacher, for he had given up listening with his bad one. His school record improved when his unsuspected deafness was appreciated, so that he could be properly seated in the classroom.

Age	Male	Female	Percentage of total
0-20	10	12	34.3
20-50	8	9	26.4
Over 50	12	13	39.1

Table I.– Age and sex of 64 patients complaining of deafness.

Disease	No. of Cases
Recent acute otitis media	20
Old tubotympanic disease	13
Presbyacusis	10
Recent trauma to tympanic membrane	3
Acoustic trauma	2
Secretory otitis	3
Mixed deafness	3
Otosclerosis	2
Cholesteatoma	2
Congenital	2
Nerve deafness after measles	2
Nerve deafness after aspirin poisoning	1
Malingering	1

Table II.– Causes of deafness in 64 patients

Examination

A patient's voice often gives a clue to the type of deafness he has. If it is conductive he can hear himself speak and he usually talks softly. The loud, harsh monotone of sensori-neural deafness, when the cochlea is dead, is familiar to all.

For accurate diagnosis an otoscope is needed. The modern small pocket type is handy for the general practitioner visiting a screaming child at home who so often is found to have acute otitis media. Wax and debris need to be removed as it may obscure the tympanic membrane. This can be done by syringing, or with a ring probe. If a head-mirror and spotlight are used, both hands are free to manipulate the probe and aural speculum. Alternatively, pus and debris (but not wax usually) may be sucked out, using a low-vacuum pump and cannula.

The sheep among the hard of hearing can be separated from the goats by using a 512 cycles per second tuning fork. This will distinguish conductive deafness (often curable) from sensori-neural deafness which can only be partially alleviated with a hearing aid. At present, surgery does not improve hearing in perceptive deafness, although it may be life saving when an acoustic neuroma is removed.

Rinne's test.– In conductive deafness the Rinne test is negative: that is, bone conduction is better than air conduction, the opposite of normal. To carry out this test the foot of the tuning fork should be pressed firmly on the mastoid, with counter pressure by the other hand on the opposite side of the patient's head. The vibrating ends of the fork should then be carefully placed exactly opposite the external auditory meatus.

Weber's test.– In conductive deafness, the tuning fork placed on the vertex is heard more loudly in the deafer ear, as ambient noise is not detected in the ear with poor hearing. In sensorineural deafness, such as is found in presbyacusis, Menière's disease, acoustic neuroma, and acoustic trauma, the sound of the tuning fork placed on the vertex is better heard in the good ear, for the cochlea of the deaf ear does not function.

The measurement of hearing loss

The Keeler Audio-Tester is a fairly inexpensive screening audiometer which measures deafness. Full audiometric assessment requires a silent room in which to perform the test, for background noise interferes with auditory acuity. Properly fitting earphones must be used and a full range of frequencies tested, using expensive and complicated apparatus. Such an accurate assessment is not needed for screening purposes if a fail-safe programme is carried out, and all doubtful patients are referred. The Audio-Tester is a pure tone audiometer which can detect deafness in the normal speech range at frequencies of 250, 1,000 and 4,000 Hz. The apparatus measures 7 x 6 x 3 inches (18 x 15 x 8 cm) and weighs 3 pounds (132 grams). It is calibrated to test hearing at threshold (0 decibels) and at 10, 15, 20, 25, 30 and 35 decibels above threshold. There is then a gap to 60 to 65 decibels above threshold which enables the patient to hear clearly the sound he is to listen to during the test. The audiometer, fully transistorized, and powered by a 9-volt battery that should last six months, is contained in a metal case. An indicator shows when the battery is run down, and the switch cannot be left on by mistake. The latter need only be touched very lightly: it does not click.

A convenient method of using the instrument with a child is to ask him to hold up his hand, palm towards the doctor. He is told he is a lighthouseman and the doctor is a ship with a magic box sending him signals. When he hears a sound the child must flex his fingers and straighten them out again quickly and decisively. Signals should be sent at irregular intervals. Needless to say the ears must be inspected and any wax removed before beginning the test. When testing a child there must be a close personal relationship. He should be talked to at first, and a guess made of his hearing loss. The audiometer is then used at a louder level than his estimated hearing threshold. Patience may be needed in children with secretory otitis for they may find it difficult to interpret the pure tone audiometer.

The first test is made at 1,000 Hz and 60 decibels. The sound is then reduced to 35, 30, 25, 20, 15, 10, 5 and 0 decibels. Threshold level is rarely heard in the relatively noisy conditions prevailing in an ordinary room. This procedure is then repeated at 4,000 Hz and 250 Hz. The other ear is tested in the same way, and the audiogram is recorded. In adults ability to hear such frequencies at 30 decibels or less is satisfactory. In the case of schoolchildren, persistent hearing loss of over 20 decibels should be investigated by an otologist before a final diagnosis is made.

This simple hearing test will show up the child who does not want to hear – there are none so deaf as those who will not hear – and his mother can be shown that the child has good hearing. Ideally every child who has had acute otitis media should be tested a month later – few fail; those who do should be referred to a specialist. Poor scholars and those with congenitally deaf siblings may also be tested.

If an audiometer is not available, Reed's pictures are useful when a child's hearing is to be tested. These consist of four pictures in a row, such as of a cup and a duck. The words are whispered by the doctor and the child is asked to point to the appropriate picture. The words are monosyllabic and have similar vowel sounds.

Children are sometimes shy in co-operating in the surgery and mothers may be taught how to use the whispered voice to test their child's hearing at 10 feet (3 metres), and report back to the doctor if it is defective. In some areas, direct-access audiometry services are available and should perhaps be more commonly provided.

Management

The management of deafness depends on the cause.

Wax in the external auditory meatus.– The most common method of removing wax from the ear is by syringing after the wax has been softened by drops of olive oil administered each night during the preceding week. There should be no acute ear infection or coryza and the tympanic membrane should be intact before syringing is attempted. This most commonly performed surgical procedure in family practice is not without danger. Ear syringe pistons sometimes stick and when freed suddenly cause a jet of water of such force as to perforate the tympanic membrane, unless the syringe is carefully directed to the roof of the external auditory meatus. After syringing, the meatus should be carefully wiped dry in order to avoid a subsequent otitis externa.

Otitis media.– If otitis media is severe prompt antibiotic treatment is desirable. Inefficient therapy may result in a serous otitis media (glue ear). Only careful follow-up will reveal this common cause of deafness which may need surgical intervention and the insertion of grommets into the tympanic membrane.

Otosclerosis.– This relatively common cause of deafness in middle-aged adults, in whom there is not uncommonly a family history, may today be treated most satisfactorily by surgery.

Perforated tympanic membrane.– Chronic perforation of the tympanic membrane may lead to a conductive form of deafness. This may be improved by surgical repair of the tympanic membrane.

Sensori-neural deafness.– This is the most common cause of deafness in the elderly. There may be not only hearing loss but also distortion of sound which may be accompanied by tinnitus. In these patients the main hope for relieving the situation lies in the use of a hearing aid. Not all, however, are helped by an aid. Switching on a hearing aid makes the hearer suddenly aware of the noise in the environment which may be distorted both electrically and by the patient's cochlear defect. This can be most disturbing and a serious problem for those who live alone with no relative to encourage them to persist with the use of the aid until they have become accustomed to it. Background noise and the inconvenience of manipulating the tiny controls are the most tiresome drawbacks of any electrical hearing aid. The amplification required to render speech intelligible may result in unbearable loudness of unwanted environmental sounds. The volume control must be set with great precision, and varied almost without thinking when acoustical conditions change. This requires both an agile mind and dexterous fingers often absent in octogenarians with arthritic hands. Easy manipulation is usually more successful with body-worn aids than on the miniature head-worn type. The noise reproduced by clothes on the aid in a pocket or clipped to a brassière can be prevented by surrounding the aid with pure chamois leather.

In some commercial hearing aids automatic volume compression (AVC) is provided when sound exceeds a pre-determined level. Others have 'peak clipping' when sound is flatly cut out at a certain degree of loudness. Neither of these facilities is provided by the National Health Service aid.

The hearing aid should always be fitted to the better hearing ear so avoiding unnecessary amplification. This is in contrast to surgery which is always performed on the ear with greater hearing loss. In fitting a hearing aid it is important that ear-pieces should

fit correctly, or loud squealing noises may be produced. The elderly often forget to change the battery, and if the aid is used continuously, the battery will need regular renewal.
Patients with an aural discharge can be provided with inserts for both ears, so that each ear can be given a rest.
A pick-up coil causing sound to be heard by electromagnetic induction when a hearing aid is held near a telephone, or to be used in a specially wired room for television, excludes background noise entirely, with enormous benefit to wearers of a hearing aid.

General management. — Deaf patients may suffer much inconvenience in normal day-to-day life. They are unable to hear doorbells, telephones, radio and television. British Telecom will provide loud bells, flashing signals and special receivers with adjustable amplified volume control which are available for the deaf. In addition the deaf are always at risk when walking in traffic for they may not hear approaching vehicles. They should be encouraged to wear light coloured clothing, particularly when walking the streets at night.

Tinnitus. — Tinnitus can be a gravely disabling symptom with an incompletely understood aetiology and unsatisfactory management. The symptom of hissing, singing, humming or even shrieking in one or both ears is most commonly first experienced in late middle age. There may be a history of acoustic trauma (working in a particularly noisy environment or wartime or National Service exposure to gunfire). Approximately 70 per cent of patients with tinnitus have a degree of sensori-neural deafness. An association is sometimes noticed with the 'dying off' of hearing at higher frequencies as part of the ageing process, and in this case the tinnitus is self-limiting. Drugs (such as aspirin in high dosage or streptomycin) can cause tinnitus and in these cases withdrawal of the offending drug can cure the symptom.
More intractable is the tinnitus which, along with vertigo and deafness, forms the classic triad of symptoms characterizing Menière's disease. Most difficult of all is the tinnitus sometimes associated with depression, where there is a vicious circle effect — the tinnitus making the depression worse and the depression causing greater awareness of the tinnitus.
The history should include a search for acoustic trauma, a careful account of drug ingestion (both of prescribed and self-purchased medicines) and an assessment of the patient's mood.
In most cases specialist referral is indicated for further assessment, especially to exclude the rare but important possibility of acoustic neuroma.
Treatment is often unsatisfactory. Patients should be reassured

that tinnitus does not herald a stroke or cancer. There is no drug treatment for this condition though antidepressants can play an important role if there is major associated depression. The use of hearing aids or of specially produced ear level 'masker' devices may help to drown the tinnitus or distract sufficiently to make the symptom bearable. Lip reading classes can help the hard of hearing.

In a condition which is often so incompletely understood and where treatment is rarely totally effective it is helpful for patients to know that they are not alone in their affliction and one of the most therapeutic actions may be to put them in touch with the British Tinnitus Association (105 Gower Street, London WC1E 6AH) which helps such patients keep in touch by means of a regular newsletter.

References

[1] Committee on Medical Rating of Physical Impairment (1961): *Journal of the American Medical Association*, *177*, 489

[2] Rawson, A.(1973): *Deafness — Report of a Departmental Enquiry into the promotion of research*. Report on Health and Social Subjects, No. 4. HMSO

[3] D'Souza, M.F. (1975): Deafness in middle age — how big is the problem? *Journal of the Royal College of General Practitioners*, *25*, 472

[4] Morrell, D.C., Gage, H.G., and Robinson, N.A. (1971): Symptoms in general practice. *Journal of the Royal College of General Practitioners*, *21*, 32

3.21
The patient with pain in the ear

John Bain

Introduction

Acute earache is most commonly due to acute otitis media and this is particularly true in children where the annual incidence has been estimated at between 10 and 15 per cent in those under the age of 10 years and the condition is most prevalent in pre-school and early school years.[1,2] Recurrent attacks of otitis media are more common in a child who has had an ear infection in the first 2 years of life and a child who has a first attack aged between 5 and 7 years is less likely to have frequent recurrences.[3] Children with recurrent otitis media are more likely to have parents or sibling with a history of otitis media. Details of the incidence of serous otitis media are less readily available but it is probably in the order of 3–4 per cent per annum in children aged between 5 and 8 years.

Other causes of earache are less common but include otitis externa where there is often itching and intermittent pain; a boil in the external ear canal; and foreign bodies in the ear canal which can cause discomfort. Swimming and flying can also lead to painful ears. In adults cholesteatoma or tumours of the middle ear are rare but can result in earache.

When the above causes can be excluded, the possibility of referred pain has to be considered and a wide range of conditions can result in a painful ear. Infection in the nasopharynx, oro-pharynx, teeth and gums, salivary glands, and paranasal sinuses can result in pain being referred to the ear, and the history of patients' presenting symptoms should lead to the source of the underlying problem. Other causes of referred pain include temporomandibular joint dysfunction, glossopharyngeal neuralgia and the prodromal stages of Bell's palsy and herpes zoster.

Presentation

The onset of earache is often rapid and distressing with medical advice being sought as a matter of urgency. The large majority of cases are due to acute middle ear infection and relief from pain is a priority. Earache and toothache have certain similarities. The pain is acute and relief is difficult to achieve with over-the-counter preparations. There is a commonly held belief that earache in children frequently presents at night but the evidence to support this is scanty. What *is* true is that persistent pain causes stress, and parents are naturally unsure of how best to comfort a screaming and fractious infant.

Responses to urgent requests for an appointment or a home visit will vary but if it is the first occasion a patient has complained of severe earache medical advice on what immediate steps to take is of benefit to all concerned. Patients with otitis media, furunculosis, impacted foreign body, or a sudden onset of a bloody discharge are both anxious and in pain. Knowledge of the patient and the family's responses to unexpected events is invaluable. Where that knowledge is lacking attempts at deflecting patients' requests for medical care or the use of telephone advice and request for home visits is often unsuccessful. In children with ear complaints and where the doctor has little background information available it is probably best to arrange a 'fit-in' appointment at the end of a surgery, or in the case of a night visit request to 'go and see the child'. One thing is certain — the problem will not go away! Less acute or intermittent pain, where the underlying problem is related to a condition other than middle ear infection, is less likely to require immediate attention.

Causes

Acute otitis media

In children the most common cause of acute earache is middle ear infection. In this condition the child who has a cold or a respiratory tract infection for several days suddenly develops earache. This is usually the result of extension of infection up the Eustachian tube. In young infants middle ear infection should be suspected if a baby has fever, irritability or is unwilling to feed. Pain is the presenting feature in 80–90 per cent of children presenting with acute otitis media. In many circumstances the child does not have any serious underlying infection and has a 'painful red eardrum' associated with an upper respiratory tract infection.

The general practitioner is frequently faced with a patient during the early stages of the disease process and precise diagnostic accuracy is, and has to be, less exacting than that outlined in some textbooks. The natural history is variable and often unpredictable. Diagnosis in younger age groups may be difficult resulting in either under- or over-diagnosis.

It would be a mistake to make hard and fast classifications in the general practice setting. However a distinction between acute suppurative and serous/secretory otitis media remains useful when considering what is the most logical sequence of treatment steps.
Acute suppurative otitis media is an acute condition where earache is usually present and there is a range of abnormal eardrum appearances. In younger children the diagnosis of acute otitis media often depends on its probability in the presence of upper respiratory tract infection or unexplained fever. Children with cleft palate or Down's syndrome should always be considered to be likely to suffer from acute middle ear infection.

Examination of the tympanic membrane reveals a hyperaemic, opaque and sometimes bulging drum which has poor mobility. Inflammation of the drum is often accompanied by middle ear effusion which shows as fluid levels or bubbles on the tympanic membrane. When a number of bullae are seen on the surface of the drum the appearance can be described as bullous myringitis. This is probably not a specific entity but merely acute otitis media with blisters on the drum and evidence of association with mycoplasma pneumoniae or specific viruses is weak or doubtful.

Two organisms, *Streptococcus pneumoniae* and *Haemophilus influenzae* have been established as the principal aetiological agents in bacterial otitis media. Irrespective of age *Streptococcus pneumoniae* is the most common and although *Haemophilus influenzae* is more likely in younger than in older subjects it is still consistently less common than *Streptococcus pneumoniae*. Other organisms less commonly associated with middle ear infection are *Beta haemolytic streptococcus*, *Neisseria catarrhalis*, *Staphylococcus aureus*, and various gram negative bacilli. Viruses have been isolated in middle ear infections but the essentially negative findings regarding the role of viruses may be attributable to the difficulties in isolating viruses or non-involvement of viruses in the disease.[4]

Serous otitis media

Serous otitis media is commonly known as glue ear and in the majority of children with this condition acute earache is not a symptom. Glue ear often occurs during the resolution phase of acute otitis media, or in association with an upper respiratory tract infection or nasal congestion. It usually presents with deafness and discomfort or a 'stuffy feeling' in the ear and has a peak incidence between the ages of 4 and 7 years. Examination reveals an eardrum which has lost its lustre and there is often a yellowish tinge of the tympanic membrane with evidence of retraction and scarring of the drum. A fluid level or air bubbles may be visible behind the membrane.

Persistent effusion is due to a variety of causes but the underlying problem is mainly one of Eustachian tube dysfunction. There is lack of agreement about the role of enlarged adenoids as a cause of obstruction of the Eustachian tube but in some children enlarged adenoids result in blockage of the tube and consequently middle ear problems.

Otitis externa

Otitis externa is an acute or chronic reaction of the lining of the external ear canal to a variety of agents which may be bacterial, fungal, viral or chemical. It may also be due to ezcema or seborrhoeic dermatitis. In children with ezcema water remaining in the ears after washing or swimming can predispose to infection.
Otitis externa is frequently seen during warm humid weather and swimming often predisposes to this condition. Patients present with itching and discomfort in the ear and it is not uncommon to discover that in attempts to relieve the itch, objects such as paper clips or cotton tipped buds have made things worse.
On examination the ear canal is inflamed and often oedematous and where there is accompanying discharge and debris the eardrum cannot be visualized. Organisms associated with otitis externa include *Pseudomonus aeruginosa* and *Staphylococcus aureus*, with streptococcus and proteus species less commonly associated.

Flying and swimming

When flying, problems in the ear occur most commonly on landing. During rapid descent atmospheric pressure rises but the air pressure in the middle ear cavity remains continuously lower. To ensure equalization of pressure on each side of the eardrum the Eustachian tube has to open. Beyond a certain pressure difference opening of this tube is not possible and air cannot enter the middle ear through the Eustachian tube. This results in loss of eardrum mobility and increasing deafness with pain in the ear. Inequality of pressure on both sides of the drum also occurs when diving under water.

Furunculosis

This is an infection of a hair follicle and usually due to staphylococcal infection with marked pain and occasional discharge from the ear canal. When the infection extends beyond the canal there is often tenderness and enlargement of cervical glands.

Foreign body

A foreign body in the external auditory meatus can result in discomfort and inflammatory reaction in the canal. All types of foreign bodies can be introduced into the external canal but the chief danger lies in clumsy attempts at removal.

Wax

If produced in large quantities wax may form an impacted mass causing deafness and irritation of the meatal lining.

History and examination

In addition to assessing the presenting symptoms time taken in the history allows the practitioner to gain the confidence of the patient, assess patient or parental attitudes, and at this stage a tentative diagnosis is usually formulated.

Important points to note include:

1. A previous medical history of earache or a family history of ear problems. In addition, a history of atopy either in the patient or member of the family can be important. There are some children with atopy who are found to be more prone to middle ear infections.
2. Ascertain the circumstances of onset, duration, intensity, character and associated symptoms. It is important to ask specifically about the following signs and symptoms — itching or bleeding, discharge, vertigo, and hearing.

The history will tell the general practitioner about the patient as well as the presenting complaint and examination should begin with general observation of the external ear and surrounding structures followed by palpation of the neck and face to detect any localized swelling of glands, sinus tenderness or dental problems. Any discharge from the ear or evidence of eczema around the external meatus will be helpful in making a preliminary diagnosis.

Examination of the external ear canal and eardrum requires adequate lighting. Three types of lighting are generally used: (1) the hand held battery-operated auriscope; (2) the head mirror with light source placed near the patient's head; and (3) the head light. The head mirror and head light are seldom used in general practice but skill in use of these instruments and a simple aural speculum can add considerably to the quality of ear examination. Attention should be given to ensuring that (a) the auriscope batteries are efficient and (b) a suitable range of specula are available. The largest that can be used without causing pain will give the best view of the eardrum. Failure to ensure that instruments are suitably prepared can lead to frustration in examining the ear.

When examining younger children it is advisable to have the child sitting on the parent's knee with the mother or father gently restricting the child's arm with one hand and with firm application of the other to the child's head. It is important that the hand restraining the head should not obscure the child's vision of what is going on. From a remarkably early age children can be attracted by the auriscope light and the examination turned into a game.

Examination can be performed by holding the body of the auriscope in one hand or alternatively holding the instrument like a pen between thumb and index and middle finger whilst steadying the auriscope against the patient's cheek with the examiner's little finger. Before examining the eardrum, the auricle should be drawn gently upwards and backwards. This should straighten the meatus and help to reveal the tympanic membrane. In infants it is often necessary to pull the auricle downwards and then backwards.

Management

Acute otitis media

The general practitioner is most frequently faced with a cluster of symptoms and signs which can be best summed up by the term 'painful red eardrum'. Many parents will have commenced the use of analgesics before consulting their doctor and the sensible use of paracetamol is to be encouraged because relief of pain is a priority.

As the majority of children are seen at an early stage of the disease process, the ear signs may be minimal and previous medical history and presenting symptoms will often determine the approach to treatment rather than the actual signs on the drum. With only a brief glimpse of the drum which may be difficult to visualize the general practitioner has to choose between a 'wait and see policy' with the use of analgesics only, or more active treatment with antibiotics.

Although it is reasonable to withhold antibiotics where there is no systemic upset or minimal changes on the drum, this policy will depend on the doctor's capacity to respond quickly to any deterioration in the child's condition. Since the general practitioner is rarely certain of the presence or absence of bacteria in the middle ear, the use of antibiotics in presumed middle ear infection is probably justified in the majority of cases. Fry[1] has suggested that only one quarter of cases require antibiotics and a recent study from Holland[5] provided some evidence that neither antibiotics nor myringotomy had any notable effect on outcome for children with acute middle ear infection. Before giving wholehearted support to a policy of withholding antibiotics, it is necessary to scrutinize the methods of analysis and outcome measurements in these reported studies.

The longer the duration of treatment the less likely the patient is to follow a prescribed regimen and the conventional dosage and length of treatment have to be questioned and further study of the efficacy of shorter (e.g. 2 to 3 days) courses of treatment is required.[6] The use of intramuscular antibiotics has gone out of fashion but may still have a place when compliance or the severity of a child's infection is a problem faced by the practising doctor. With *Streptococcus pneumoniae* and *Haemophilus influenzae* as the predominant organisms, broad spectrum antibiotics such as amoxycillin and ampicillin are the drugs of choice. Phenoxymethyl-penicillin can be used in older children and adults although the fear is that in the case of haemophilus infection the patient may not receive sufficient antibiotic cover. Erythromycin or cefaclor have been found to be useful alternatives where a broad spectrum antibiotic is being considered. Decongestant and antihistamine mixtures are often prescribed for children with otitis media but no group of drugs has enjoyed such widespread use in medical practice without demonstration of efficacy in the treatment of the various stages of otitis media. There is little or no evidence to support the belief that they relieve the associated symptoms of otitis media and the contention that they reduce middle ear effusion and improve Eustachian tube function has not been proved. [7,8]

Children with acute otitis media should be followed-up 2 to 3 weeks after the initial consultation to check the appearance of the eardrums and to assess the return of normal hearing. If hearing has not returned to a satisfactory level within 3 months after an acute episode specialist referral should be considered.

Otitis externa

In deciding treatment it may be helpful for the general practitioner to take an ear swab but this is not essential. The corner stone of effective treatment is aural toilet and successful outcome depends on careful and complete removal of all debris which is best effected by using a Jobson Horne probe with cotton wool on the tip. Mild infections will respond to cleaning and acidifying the ear canal with dilute acetic acid solution, but most infections require topical antibiotic or antifungal eardrops and the addition of hydrocortisone enhances the anti-inflammatory effect. In more severe cases a half-inch or quarter-inch gauze wick soaked in one of these solutions is inserted into the meatus with dressing forceps and left for 24 hours and in the initial stages of treatment further dressings are often required.

Preparations most commonly used in the treatment of otitis externa include (a) a combination of antibiotic and hydrocortisone, (b) aluminium acetate or (c) ichthammol and glycerine. If the patient fails to respond and crusting in the ear canal or adjacent skin persists allergy to neomycin should be suspected. Systemic antibiotics should be used when there is accompanying cellulitis. Where otitis externa is present it is advisable to keep water out of the ears and swimming should be avoided during the acute phase of the complaint.

Flying and swimming

Alleviation of the problems associated with flying can be achieved by sucking sweets which stimulates swallowing actions. Valsalva's manoeuvre where the nose is pinched and the cheeks blown out, can inflate the middle ear space and is often successful. The problem is likely to be worse if the patient has a current upper respiratory tract infection or hay fever. In these circumstances it is worthwhile using a decongestant nasal spray or drops in advance of anticipated descent in an aircraft. If the patient has had a recent bout of hay fever it is advisable to ensure that an oral antihistamine is given before a flight. In the case of swimming there is some controversy about its effect on children with ear problems, but it seems common sense to avoid swimming where an acute infection is present. Ear plugs are advisable in children with previous history of perforation or history of insertion of grommets in the eardrum.

Furunculosis

The treatment consists of application of an antibiotic ointment, e.g. Neosporin and an oral broad spectrum antibiotic e.g. flucloxacillin. Incision and drainage of the furnuncle may be required when symptoms and signs have persisted and spontaneous drainage has not occurred.

Foreign bodies

Foreign bodies should be removed to avoid infection and persistence of symptoms. It is important that removal should occur under optimal conditions using adequate illumination and instrumentation. In younger children where co-operation may be a problem a general anaesthetic may be required. Some small foreign bodies can often be removed by syringing but removal of vegetable matter by syringing is contraindicated because of the danger of the material absorbing water and swelling.

Wax

If wax has become impacted it may be removed by using a wax hook or a probe with cotton wool attached. Where pain has been a presenting feature attempts at syringing can be preceded by the use of preparations such as olive oil or sodium bicarbonate ear drops to soften the wax. The metal syringe is the traditional instrument and several nozzles should be available to allow continued use of the syringe while contaminated nozzles are being sterilized. Syringing should be carried out with water at 37°C and the nozzle of the syringe should be pointed upwards and slightly posteriorly to project the stream beyond the wax. The water-pik irrigator, originally designed for use in oral hygiene, has been found to be a useful alternative to the traditional syringe but has not yet been tested widely in clinical practice.

Referred pain

The treatment of earache due to referred pain will depend on the underlying cause and in the majority of these cases such as infections in the oropharynx, teeth, salivary glands or paranasal sinuses, treatment will often include the use of systemic broad spectrum antibiotics. There are few circumstances where the symptom of ear pain alone will require a specialist opinion although there are still situations where an acutely ill child with a bulging tympanic membrane may require myringotomy. Where conditions such as dental abscess, glosso-pharyngeal neuralgia or temporomandibular joint dysfunction are suspected referral for a specialist opinion is usually indicated.

References

[1] Fry J. (1961) *The Catarrhal Child.* London: Butterworths

[2] Paradise J.L. (1980) Otitis media in infants and children. *Pediatrics*, *65*, 917–943

[3] Howie J.M., Ploussard J.H., Sloyer J. (1975) The 'otis prone' condition. *American Journal of Diseases of Children*, *129*, 676–678

[4] Bluestone C.D. (1981) Recent advances in the pathogenesis, diagnosis and management of otitis media. *Pediatric Clinics of North America*, *28*, 727–755

[5] Van Buchem F.L., Dunk J.H.M., Van't Hof M.A. (1981) Therapy of acute otitis media: myringotomy, antibiotics, or neither? *Lancet*, 2, 883–887

[6] Chaput de Saintonge D.M., Levine D.F., Temple Savage I. et al. (1982) Trial of three day and ten day courses of Amoxycillin in otitis media. *British Medical Journal*, *284*, 1078–1081

[7] Cantekin E.I., Mandell E.M., Bluestone C.D. et al. (1983) Lack of efficacy of a decongestant-antihistamine combination for otitis media with effusion in children. *New England Journal of Medicine*, *308*, 297–301

[8] Bain J.D.G. (1983) Can the clinical course of acute otitis media be modified by systemic decongestant or antihistamine treatment? *British Medical Journal*, *287*, 645–65

3.22
The discharging ear

David F. Coulter

The epidemiology of the discharging ear is in part that of acute otitis media and the remarks made in the chapter on 'The Patient with Pain in the Ear' as to age and seasonal incidence and diagnostic relevance also apply to the discharging ear. The relatively high incidence of chronic otitis media in my practice may be related to the geographical location of the practice in South Wales.

Presentation

Discharge from the ear seldom gives rise to the same request for urgent attention as does pain, except when the discharge is blood-stained and/or follows trauma, or is accompanied by earache, when immediate attention is usually requested. Occasionally mothers will give a history of ear discharge in their children when in fact what is termed 'discharge' is found to be simply normal soft wax.

Causes

In children or adolescents new and acute episodes of discharging ear will usually be due to a variety of acute otitis media, while in older age-groups an acute otitis externa will be more likely. When the condition appears of long duration chronic otitis media or chronic otitis externa may be the cause. Occasionally they may co-exist and such a condition as keratosis obdurans often combines the two in association with a chronic paranasal sinusitis and/or bronchiectasis.
Direct trauma to the meatus and tympanic membrane is an occasional cause. Blast injury, sufficient to bowl the subject over, is another rare cause of membrane damage and subsequent discharge.
A foreign body in the meatus seldom presents as discharge but more often as discomfort, a degree of deafness and blockage. Small

children sometimes insert a roll of paper or other foreign body in the meatus and adults leave pledglets of wool; these are recognized during the examination.

History and examination

The complaint of discharge from the ear may be approached in a way similar to that of pain in the ear, but there is a greater need to establish the duration of the condition. This will vary from a first acute episode to one of lengthy chronicity. Associated features will often assist in suggesting the site of the underlying cause. Generally speaking this will lie either in the meatal skin or in the middle ear cleft. An enquiry should therefore be made about symptoms referrable to the nose and throat, skin and scalp, and the presence and character of any earache and associated features such as deafness, tinnitus, vertigo, meatal irritation or a history of trauma.

Beyond examining the external ear and the surrounding skin, the presence of any discharge prevents further progress in the local assessment and hence attention must be focused on the discharge itself and on obtaining its eventual gentle but complete removal. A Jobson Horne aural probe carrying a wisp of cotton-wool should be gently introduced into the canal under direct vision and some of the discharge withdrawn. Its physical properties – consistency, quantity, the presence of wax, epithelial debris, mucus, pus or blood and odour – should be noted and a swab taken for identification of micro-organisms. If the condition of the patient permits it, all discharge is now gently removed. Once cleansing is complete, inspection of the canal wall and tympanic membrane usually allows a presumptive diagnosis to be made. On occasions, however, especially in the more chronic states, difficulty arises both in achieving meatal cleansing and in interpreting the appearance of the drumhead. In such cases empirical treatment followed by a further attempt at cleansing in a few days' time may resolve the question.

When chronic otitis media is believed to be present, the site of any perforation must be accurately defined, remembering the association of marginal defects involving the annulus especially in the postero-superior segment, with an unsafe condition – attico-antral disease, and that of a central defect with a safer condition – eustachian naso-pharyngeal catarrh. The presence of granulation tissue, cholesteatoma or polyp formation is also important and their recognition depends on the care taken by the practitioner in achieving complete cleansing of meatus and drumhead.

Other investigations such as radiology and microscopic examination of the tympanic membrane and cavity may be required in cases of chronic middle-ear disease but are the province of the aural specialist.

Management

The management of a discharge from the ear is that of the underlying cause but several points deserve emphasis. Meatal cleansing is important not only in diagnosis but also in treatment. It will require repetition until the discharge has ceased; the frequency depends on progress. In acute otitis media persistence of the discharge beyond seven to ten days merits a further course of the appropriate antibiotic (judged by sensitivity studies) and daily aural toilet. Although it is now rare, mastoid disease should still be suspected, and failure to improve, as judged by cessation of discharge, a satisfactory improvement of hearing and normal appearances of the drumhead, warrants specialist referral.

In chronic disease the presence of mucus is an aid in differentiating middle-ear from meatal disease as its source must be from the mucus-secreting cells of the middle ear cleft. In chronic otitis media it is most important to distinguish the 'safe' from the 'unsafe' and here most help is obtained by identifying carefully the exact location of any perforation: those involving the postero-superior segment of the annulus are likely to be 'unsafe' while the central antero-inferior variety are usually 'safe'. The character of the discharge is also of assistance as in the 'unsafe' it is more likely to be scanty and smelly (in attico-antral disease) while in the 'safe' (tubo-tympanic) it is much more mucoid. An unpleasant smell to an aural discharge, in the absence of perforation, is most commonly due to seborrhoeic otitis externa. Granulations, cholesteatoma and polypi imply an 'unsafe' ear. All patients in whom an 'unsafe' category is suspected merit urgent referral for specialist assessment and care. The general practitioner may manage those conditions categorized as 'safe' provided follow-up is ensured but, if he cannot achieve a dry 'safe' ear, referral to a specialist should be sought.

Management for both the 'safe' chronic otitis media and subacute otitis externa consists of ongoing canal cleansing followed by the installation of appropriate topical agents as dictated by sensitivity results from a swab taken from the discharge. Provided the organisms are sensitive, framycetin sulphate ear-drops instilled four times a day are effective and relatively inexpensive. In patients with chronic perforation contamination of the meatus during washing and bathing should be prevented, by the use of a generous plug of cotton-wool.

Finally, where a dry 'safe' perforated drumhead exists referral for consideration of myringoplasty may be appropriate.

3.23 The stuffy, running nose

J.G.R. Howie

Consultations for this almost invariably benign symptom are often unsatisfactory. On the one hand the illness may appear so minor that the doctor is left wondering why the patient has really felt the necessity for a professional opinion. Alternatively the illness may be chronic or recurring and being managed to neither the patient's nor doctor's real satisfaction.

The statistics relating to consultation for this symptom are, like so much of the epidemiology of general practice, confused by different perceptions of illness by doctors and patients, different expectations of what the doctor will prescribe and how effective this will be (this often conditioned by past experience) and the ease or difficulty of obtaining a consultation during the early stages of this symptom. The doctor's personal experience may create, for example, a particular sympathy towards sinusitis or allergic rhinitis leading to high diagnostic rates for these conditions while even the partners in the same practice may be recording very low rates for the same disorder. Figures will also be influenced by the doctor's interpretation of the use of physical symptoms as a presentation of non-physical illness.

Wisely and significantly, Hodgkin[1] avoids committing himself to an incidence of the symptom. Wadsworth, Butterfield and Blaney[2] accept the category 'cough and colds' without further qualification on its components. Dunnell and Cartwright[3] put catarrh in a group which includes 'coughs and phlegm' and running nose along with 'cold and 'flu'. Morrell and his colleagues[4] find nasal discharge accounts for only some 2 per cent of consultations, while my own study of respiratory illness in North-East Scotland found nasal symptoms to be offered by patients or found present on enquiry in 20 to 25 per cent of all consultations for acute respiratory illness.

Presentation

A number of recognizably different presentations can be described. Moving through the age-groups, the first patients commonly troubled with nasal symptoms are babies and infants in their first year of life. The principal complaint is most often of difficulty with feeding and mothers of first children often seek advice about this. In older children brought because of cough, nasal catarrh, by this time often purulent, may be mentioned. In the child of pre-school age, the intra-nasal foreign body is a further occasional and important reason for consultation.

The next common presentation is the young to middle-aged adult, either with apparently low tolerance of the early stages of viral illness, or requiring a certificate or other legitimization of sickness. In this group of patients are some weighed down by psychological or social stress. Typical is the mother, perhaps consulting with several children, any or all of whom may be the original patient or be added as patients as the consultation proceeds (a potent cause of doctor irritation). The low morale of such patients is often a prominent feature helping their recognition.

A different group of patients, but in the same age-group, is the allergy/hay-fever group, often recognizable by the season of the year and the long history of similar, often annual, episodes. Non-infective and recurring illness is also seen in patients, perhaps somewhat older, in whom persistent catarrh or nasal obstruction is the sequel to long histories of any of the illnesses already mentioned or of nasal irritation at work or from tobacco. Two further important groups of patients who may complain of this symptom must be referred to. First, in a number of patients with acute headache, nasal symptoms may suggest a diagnosis of sinusitis. Secondly, nasal stuffiness is a side-effect of many drugs used in the treatment of hypertension or depression and although this presentation is uncommon and principally met with in older patients its significance in relation to the prescribing of treatment is high enough to warrant separate mention.

Causes

The commonest cause of stuffy and running noses is infection, as a rule initially viral (adenovirus predominating), later becoming secondarily infected by bacteria (pneumococci predominating). In acute sinusitis the relative contributions of obstruction and infection to the illness may be difficult to determine. The next cause of importance is allergy, with hay fever or pollen allergy the commonest problem but allergies to animals, plants and possibly foods also requiring to be considered. Thirdly, stuffy running noses may be due to the environment. Physical features such as extremes of temperature and humidity as well as chemical agents may cause acute and eventually chronic nasal symptoms. Occupational exposure to, for example, chrome compounds is worth bearing in mind. A fourth small but important group of patients have some form of nasal obstruction. When, as with polypi, this follows a long history of an allergic or irritative illness, recognition of this new abnormality may easily be overlooked. Acute causes of obstruction (foreign body and fracture) are relatively easy diagnoses to make given an adequate history.

Finally, reference must be made to nasal congestion occurring as a side-effect of drug therapy, most importantly with adrenergic neurone-blocking antihypertensive agents, such as guanethidine, bethanidine and debrisoquine. The risk to such patients is that medication with prescribed or proprietary decongestants containing phenylpropanolamine or other sympathomimetic agents may produce loss of antihypertensive control and dangerous elevation of blood pressure. A common cause of persistent nasal stuffiness is the prolonged (often self-prescribed) use of nasal decongestant drops, which can prolong the stuffiness of a common cold during weeks or months of misuse.

History taking and examination

History taking and physical examination for this symptom are relatively straightforward and substantially confined to localized features of illness. The principal aim is to decide whether the illness is infective, allergic or obstructive in nature; the second is to assess whether non-physical components of the illness may be of greater importance than the physical ones.

The baby with a stuffy nose almost always has a concurrent feeding problem. If the baby appears hungry the consultation will be devoted to confirming the absence of serious illness and providing mechanical relief to the obstructed airway. If, on the other hand, the baby appears not to be hungry a careful search for a reason must be undertaken. In this second situation a red throat or inflamed ear-drum will often be found but any of the causes of anorexia in babies may be present. Differentiation of these two groups of babies is aided by a history of episodes of crying or screaming, often associated with cough and occurring at night. Equally important is the general appearance of the child: a lively well-coloured child is less likely to be seriously unwell than a limp or fractious one.

There is little need to elaborate history taking and examination of the adult patient with minor illness, in whom understanding of motivation for consultation is the dominant problem. It is not the purpose of this chapter to discuss the verbal and non-verbal clues which assist this process and any realistic appreciation of general practice must concede that, especially during epidemics of winter respiratory illness, many more of these clues will be 'ignored' than accepted. Examination of such patients is usually minimal or omitted. Although justifiable this may be tactically misguided; patients like to feel they have been taken seriously and twenty seconds spent on some local examination of nose, throat and sinuses is probably a wise investment.

Although differentiation between infection and psychological stress may be difficult, the separation of either from allergic disease is often an equal problem. The time scale of the illness is frequently of great help and careful inquiry into past history, as well as recent exposure to cut grass and domestic and farm animals, may be useful. A family or personal history of allergy should be asked about and examination – generally not particularly helpful – should aim at recognizing other clues to allergy, such as conjunctival oedema, wheeze or urticaria. The nasal mucosa is said to have a typically swollen greyish appearance but this sign is often not present. A home visit may on occasions yield useful clues as to possible animal or plant allergens although few doctors will specifically wish to arrange this for its own sake. Although it is true that allergic symptoms usually start suddenly, patients with viral illness may develop symptoms with surprising rapidity. Similar confusion arises when patients with allergy complain of cough, rather than the usual symptoms of rhinitis or wheeze.

Other clues may be suggested by the patient. A history of sudden, intermittent or one-sided nasal obstruction raises the possibility of nasal polypi, particularly when a long history of nasal symptoms exists. Confirmation of this may require examination by techniques more appropriately carried out by a specialist in this field. Unilateral nasal obstruction or discharge in a child raises the possibility of a foreign body being present and this may or may not be visible on examination. In sinus infection pain is prominent and acute sinus tenderness will be present. Either complete nasal obstruction or infected nasal discharge may be noted. A history of recent or concurrent upper respiratory infection is usually elicited.

History taking should include noting the drugs being taken by the patient – either on prescription or through self-medication.

Treatment

In this section I propose to comment briefly on selected aspects of management of nasal symptoms focusing only on the main difficulties met within this field.

Babies with snuffles. — The baby unable to feed because of a stuffed nose is usually helped by the instillation of nasal drops 15 to 20 minutes before feeding, after clearing the nostrils with cotton-wool sticks. Ephedrine (0.5 per cent) in saline appears as effective as the many proprietary preparations available. Its continued use may itself, however, lead to congestion of the mucosa.

Treatment of coryza. — Prescribed medicine has little effect on the natural history of uncomplicated coryza but does legitimize a consultation and may encourage the patient to consult in the future with similar illness. On the other hand, the doctor who declines to prescribe may face an emotionally draining and time-consuming dispute with a patient annoyed or rejected by this approach. Sympathy with the patient for the symptoms being suffered should be expressed and the patient advised to use salicylates, hot drinks and steam inhalations until they pass. Delivered positively such advice appears acceptable and a doctor genuinely convinced of its appropriateness should have no difficulty in persuading the patient. If medication is thought necessary the choice will lie between vasoconstrictor nose drops and oral antihistamines. The risks of overuse of the first are low except in the presence of hypertension and oral antihistamine probably exerts its beneficial effect through its general sedative action — inappropriate for those working in many occupations.

Self-medication. — Patients should be encouraged to use physical methods of treatment (such as steam inhalation in this case) but discouraged from the use of chemical ones (such as sympathomimetic preparations for this symptom). Obvious exceptions to this exist and the self-use of salicylates or paracetamol should be encouraged when this seems appropriate, and the limited self-use of proprietary cough preparations for their sedative and supportive benefits when patients find them useful.

Sinusitis. — Perceptions of sinusitis by patients and doctors vary enormously. Management varies accordingly and the following comments relate to illnesses at the acute physical end of the spectrum. Retained infected secretions are equivalent to an abscess and treatment must be aimed at release of muco-pus rather than, or simultaneously with, anti-infective measures. Steam inhalation and the use of topical vasoconstrictor agents should be tried when nasal obstruction is significant. The antibiotic of choice will hopefully be capable of acting against pneumococci and streptococci and possibly haemophilus: of the simple antibiotics, erythromycin or cotrimoxazole will normally be a better choice than a tetracycline. Pain may be severe and an analgesic may be required pending the establishment of free drainage. Once drainage has been established recovery is normally straightforward and a patient consulting at this stage may be adequately managed without the use of antibiotics. Surgical drainage is rarely necessary. Nasal symptoms last longer in smokers than non-smokers and a consultation of this type may be a useful opportunity for the appropriate health education of a suitably motivated patient.

Hay fever. — Treatment of hay fever and allergic rhinitis is generally difficult. Apart from the sensible avoidance of excessive exposure to known allergens when this is feasible, three lines of therapy are available. The mainstay remains the oral antihistamine. Patients develop a preference for the particular preparation which appears to cause least drowsiness for most relief. Many preparations are now available in sustained-action formulation requiring to be taken only once or twice daily. Two new antihistamines terfenadine (Triludan) and astemizole (Hismanal) are largely free from the anticholinergic effects. They rarely cause sedation or psychomotor impairment and do not potentiate the effects of alcohol or benzodiazepines. Astemizole has the advantage of once daily dosage but may cause weight gain. Terfenadine is given in a dose of 60 mg twice daily.

The second approach to management is through specific desensitization. Based on the variably reliable results of skin testing, this treatment may be regarded by some patients as worse than the disease itself. The relief is relatively short lasting and may not remove the need for antihistamine. Many of the courses are expensive although this is only one consideration in deciding management. Patients requiring annual prolonged antihistamine treatment should be informed of this sometimes effective alternative treatment; on the other hand there is no convincing indication for its use in patients whose illness appears minor or who require little antihistamine and can tolerate the side-effects reasonably well. Such courses should be administered only where facilities for full cardiopulmonary resuscitation are immediately available and where patients can be kept under medical observation for at least two hours.

The introduction of cromoglycate for topical nasal use has offered a third fundamentally different means of attack on this problem. As in bronchial asthma the treatment is prophylactic and early results suggest it to be much less effective in hay fever than in asthma. The need to insufflate the drug six times daily may create unfortunate introspection about an inconveniencing rather than serious disorder, and this coupled with the high cost suggests that this treatment (prophylaxis) should not be the management of choice. The use of sodium cromoglycate as eye drops (Opticron) in the management of the allergic conjunctivitis of hay fever is of considerable benefit.

Steroid therapy may be considered for refractory cases of hay fever — either as insufflation of beclomethasone or as depot injections. A short course of oral prednisolone is an alternative which can be helpful in exceptional circumstances, such as the patient sitting a crucial examination during the hay fever season.

Referral. — Referral for this symptom may be indicated for reasons related to the illness or to provide support for the doctor or patient. It should be encouraged for any nasal foreign body which is not readily removable, as the risk and consequences of inhalation to the bronchi are serious. Using the regime described referral for drainage of the sinuses is rarely necessary. A history of intermittent obstruction, raising the possibility of the presence of nasal polypi, merits a specialist opinion and a patient with persistent nasal symptoms who appears dissatisfied with the progress of his illness may be helped physically and psychologically by a second opinion. Skin testing may be carried out by the general practitioner but most hospitals offer a specialist service for this.

Conclusions

Patients consulting with the stuffy running nose vary considerably. On the one hand are those with symptoms of such apparently minor significance that history taking and treatment must be aimed at the reason for consultation rather than illness, whereas at the other extreme symptoms may be a genuine cause of either persistent or recurrent annoyance or acute immediate distress. Of these, some may require active management, others a long-term plan which recognizes the frequently unsatisfactory nature of the treatment currently available.

References

[1] Hodgkin, K. (1973): *Towards Earlier Diagnosis*. 3rd ed. Edinburgh: Churchill Livingstone.

[2] Wadsworth, M.E.J., Butterfield, W.J.H and Blaney, R. (1971): *Health and Sickness: the Choice of Treatment*. London: Tavistock Publications.

[3] Dunnell, K. and Cartwright, A. (1972): *Medicine Takers, Prescribers and Hoarders*. London: Routledge and Kegan Paul.

[4] Morrell, D.C., Gage, H.G. and Robinson, N.A. (1971): Symptoms in General Practice. *Journal of the Royal College of General Practitioners*, *21*, 32.

3.24
The bleeding nose

J.J.C. Cormack

Nose bleeds come within the ambit of basic Boy Scout first aid and it is likely that only a small proportion of the total incidence of epistaxes in the community is brought to the notice of doctors.

The recorded incidence varies widely: Morrell and his colleagues[1] saw 19 patients per 1,000 in one year with nose bleeding as the presenting symptom; Hodgkin[2] gives an incidence of 6 patients per 1,000 in one year, while the annual incidence per 1,000 patients in the National Morbidity Survey[3] is 3.3. Extrapolating from these figures, a general practitioner with 20,000 patients might expect to be consulted by from eight to 48 patients a year with a complaint of nose bleeds.

While males and females are approximately equally affected the condition is predominantly seen in children and young adults and in the over-65's.

Presentation

Nose bleeds are probably most commonly presented as telephone requests for advice or requests (often at night) for a home visit. The onset is usually sudden and precipitated by trauma either in the form of a blow to the nose or vigorous blowing of the nose, although apparently spontaneous onset (especially in the elderly) is quite common.

Causes

The commonest cause of epistaxis is trauma: either direct trauma caused by a blow to or fall on the nose, or trauma to the nasal mucosa by vigorous blowing or picking, especially if the mucosa is hyperaemic as the result of an upper respiratory infection, or there is crusting due to infection or if the vessels are markedly sclerotic. The site of the bleeding is usually the leash of veins draining the anastamosis of vessels at Little's area on the antero-inferior aspect of the septum. Less commonly the bleeding may be from higher up, as for instance in the ethmoid region.

It is often alleged that epistaxes may be associated with hypertension, although the epidemiological evidence for this is not clear. It is probable that in many instances where a nose bleed has drawn attention to raised blood pressure both the bleed and the pressure are secondary to arteriosclerosis and in such circumstances it is at least questionable whether treatment aimed at lowering the blood pressure is likely to be effective in preventing further bleeding. The associations between epistaxes and blood dyscrasias (especially leukaemia), and anaemia (which may be the effect rather than the cause of the bleeding), point to the relevance of a full blood count as a sensible initial investigation when nose bleeds are recurrent.

Other causes of epistaxes include foreign bodies pushed into the nose by small children, anticoagulant therapy and, rarely, malignant lesions of the nose and sinuses.

History and examination

In the majority of cases little in the way of either history or examination is indicated. Indeed this is one of the few conditions where advice on management may often be given without necessarily seeing the patient. An enquiry should be made about the circumstances of the onset of the bleed, the patient's general condition and what measures, if any, have already been employed to stop the bleeding. The practitioner may then, if he is satisfied that it is reasonable to do so, give advice on simple pressure techniques, with the proviso that if these fail to stop the bleeding he should be contacted again.

If simple measures fail, the patient must be seen. After the bleeding has been controlled, if the patient is elderly the pulse and blood pressure should be checked. Detailed examination of the nose should be deferred to a later consultation, which may be required if there is a history of recurrent or persistent bleeds. The anterior nares should then be inspected using either a nasal speculum and a torch or with a suitable aural speculum on an auriscope. If there is a history of recurrent bleeding or if the patient appears to be unwell blood should be taken for a full blood count, especially if the patient is between the ages of 20 and 50 – a group in which simple primary epistaxis is uncommon.

Management

Haemorrhage from the nose as from other external sites is

managed by direct pressure. Folk remedies such as keys down the back of the neck or cold compresses applied to the bridge of the nose are singularly ineffective. The patient should be instructed to sit leaning forward (unless feeling faint, when he should be lying down) and told to concentrate on breathing through his mouth. Pressure should be firmly applied either with the ball of the thumb pressed hard on the affected side or by pinching the nose tightly between finger and thumb. If the pressure is maintained consistently for a full five minutes the bleeding will stop in the vast majority of instances. Thereafter the patient should be warned not to blow his nose for twelve hours, and subsequently when blowing his nose to do so gently. If the bleeding settles with this regime and does not recur, no further action is necessary.

If this technique is not successful, the next step should be an attempt to pack the nose. This is not an entirely simple procedure, especially in the poor lighting that may be all that is available in a patient's house, but it is often worth a trial. While preparations are being made for packing the nose it is useful to give the patient an injection of diazepam or other suitable sedative. The equipment needed for nasal packing is a nasal speculum, a pair of angled forceps, a roll of ribbon gauze, a tube of bismuth iodoform paraffin paste (BIPP) or a bottle of Terra-Cortril suspension, a bottle of 5 per cent cocaine (or Minims Amethocaine 1 per cent), a vial of 1:1,000 adrenaline, a clean cup, a dressing pack and a plentiful supply of cold water.

The patient should be placed in the best light available and instructed to blow his nose gently to clear away any clot that has collected. A pledglet of cotton-wool, soaked in a solution of local anaesthetic and adrenaline (made up of approximately equal parts of each), is then inserted into the nostril from which the bleeding is coming and left in place for some 5 to 10 minutes. Meanwhile a strip of about two yards (2 metres) of the ribbon gauze should be cut off and impregnated with the BIPP or Terra-Cortril using the cup as a mixing bowl and then removing any excess with the blades of the forceps, laying the strip on a dressing towel as a working surface.

The cotton-wool should now be gently removed and the speculum inserted and a loop, made up of the first twelve inches (30 cm) or so of the gauze, pushed along the floor of the nose with the angled forceps, securing the end of the loop behind one of the blades of the speculum. Successive loops are then fed in until the nose is tightly packed and finally the speculum is gently withdrawn. The pack can be held in place by layering overlapping strips of Micropore on the nose and securing the final strip in 'U' fashion over the nostrils (see figure 1) so that it adheres to the tape on either side of the nose.

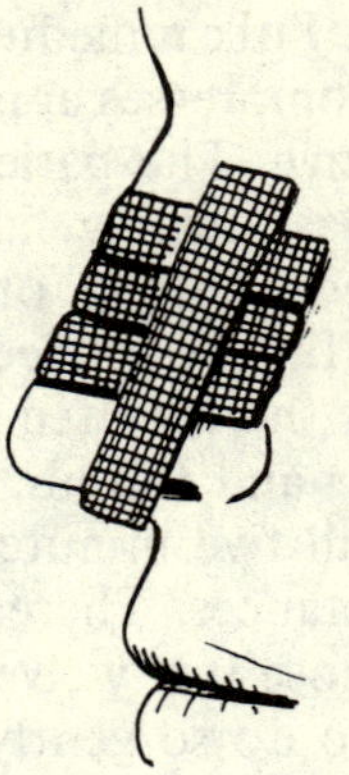

Figure 1

It is necessary to wait for some ten to fifteen minutes to be sure that the bleeding has stopped and, before leaving, the patient's pharynx should be inspected to be sure that no blood is trickling down the back of the throat. The situation should be reviewed in a few hours, and if the bleeding has not recurred the pack should be left *in situ* and the patient advised to rest in bed for forty-eight hours, avoiding smoking or alcohol. The prescription of a mild sedative such as diazepam, 2 mg or 5 mg three times a day, may be helpful at this stage. After forty-eight hours half the pack should be removed, and the remaining half should be extracted the following day.

If the bleeding has recurred, or if the initial packing has not been successful (sometimes, especially in elderly patients the bleeding may have originated from an inaccessible site such as the ethmoids), referral to an Ear Nose and Throat or Accident and Emergency Department is necessary, with a possible view to posterior packing, which should be performed under a general anaesthetic.

Patients with recurrent nose bleeds associated with respiratory infections and crusting are sometimes helped by the topical application of white or yellow soft paraffin BP two or three times a day to soften the discharge. If there is evidence of impetigo a local antibiotic ointment such as neomycin and bacitracin should be used.

If recurrences are frequent the general practitioner may cauterize the bleeding point, after anaesthetizing the mucous membrane with a solution of 5 per cent cocaine and 1:1,000 adrenaline, by using a silver nitrate stick or a very fine wisp of cotton-wool dipped in trichloracetic acid. Alternatively the patient may be referred to an Ear Nose and Throat Department for electrocautery.

Finally it is helpful to reassure anxious patients and their relatives that the amount of blood on handkerchiefs, clothing and pillow-cases often gives a falsely inflated impression of the total blood loss. Nose bleeds are often alarming but rarely dangerous.

References

[1] Morrell, D.C., Gage, H.G. and Robinson, N.A. (1971): Symptoms in General Practice. *Journal of the Royal College of General Practitioners, 21,* 32

[2] Hodgkin, K. (1973): *Towards Earlier Diagnosis, A Guide to General Practice, 3rd ed.* Edinburgh: Churchill Livingstone

[3] Royal College of General Practitioners, Office of Population Censuses and Surveys, Department of Health and Social Security (1986): *Morbidity Statistics from General Practice 1981–82*. HMSO Series MB5 No. 1

I am indebted to Dr. A.G.D. Maran, Ear, Nose and Throat Surgeon, Edinburgh Royal Infirmary, for helpful criticism and advice in the preparation of this chapter.

3.25 The patient complaining of sore throat

J.J.C. Cormack

Sore throat is one of the commonest presenting symptoms in general practice. Dunnell and Cartwright[1] found 12 per cent of the adults (and 8 per cent of the children) reported a sore throat in the two-week period studied. In the National Morbidity Survey[2] 57 consultations per annum were for acute pharyngitis, tonsillitis, laryngitis or tracheitis for every 1,000 patients. A practitioner with a list of 2,000 patients may expect some 120 consultations each year on account of sore throat. It is clear that sore throats are an important cause of morbidity accounting for about 2 per cent of consultations in general practice per annum.

Although throat infections are common from infancy onwards children under 4 years of age are rarely brought with a complaint of sore throat. The symptom is predominantly one presented by children, adolescents and young adults; it is comparatively rare after the age of 45.

Presentation

Sore throat may be a concomitant of other upper respiratory infections, especially the common cold and influenza. Most often, however, it is presented to the practitioner as a complaint on its own, usually of gradual onset and fairly short duration (1 to 5 days), with pain present continuously, but made worse by swallowing. In very young children the presenting symptom of acute pharyngitis or tonsillitis may be complaints of vomiting, fever and abdominal pain, sore throat or difficulty in swallowing either being denied or only admitted on direct questioning.

Causes

Streptococci. – By far the most common bacterial pathogen causing sore throats is the B-haemolytic streptococcus. Epidemiologists have reported isolation rates in various studies of between 25 and

60 per cent of sore throats presenting in general practice. Staphylococci and *Haemophilus influenzae* may also be isolated from the pharynx but their role is probably more commonly commensal than pathogenic. The importance of the streptococcus lies in the possibility of the development of post-streptococcal sequelae: rheumatic fever and acute glomerulonephritis. The prevalence of these post-streptococcal complications has dropped quite dramatically in recent years. It has been suggested that this phenomenon was directly related to the widespread use of penicillin in the treatment of sore throats, but in fact the decline in prevalence started before the introduction of antibiotics. Some studies suggest a decline in the virulence of the organisms from natural causes, but there may also be an increase in host resistance due to better nutrition and housing.

Viruses.– A number of viruses have been implicated in the pathogenesis of non-streptococcal sore throat. These include herpesviruses, influenza viruses, enteroviruses, rhinoviruses and adenoviruses. In one study the isolation of all these viruses with the exception of enteroviruses was significantly higher in the winter than in the summer months, in contrast to streptococcal isolations which showed no seasonal distribution.

Irritants.– Sore throats may from time to time be caused by physical irritation, especially from tobacco smoke and also from the overuse of antiseptic lozenges.

Infectious mononucleosis (glandular fever).– This is probably the commonest cause of a sore throat which fails to resolve in four or five days, especially in adolescents and young adults. Occasionally, and unfortunately, the diagnosis may be made if the practitioner has prescribed ampicillin for the sore throat and a widespread and vivid rash appears. Involvement of other nodes should be looked for, and a full blood count and positive 'monospot' or Paul Bunnell reaction should establish the diagnosis.

Thrush.– This is usually confined to infants or very young children, although the possibility should be borne in mind in adults in association with oro-genital sexual practices or the use of steroid inhalers for asthma. The white curdy appearance of candida infection usually provides the clue and a throat swab should be taken.

Vincent's angina.– Here the infection is often unilateral, though it may spread to the margins of the gums. A throat swab should reveal the fusiform and spirochete organisms.

Diphtheria.– Now extremely rare in this country (although one may need to have a high index of suspicion with recent immigrants), this is obviously a diagnosis of major importance. A greyish adherent membrane and the characteristic smell (probably only now recognized by the most senior of practitioners), combined with severe systemic upset, should call for an immediate throat swab and urgent communication with the bacteriologist for rapid confirmation of the result.

Blood dyscrasias.– Leukaemia and agranulocytosis can present as sore throat, usually with necrotic mouth ulcers, systemic upset, fever and sometimes epistaxes or bleeding gums. The history of drug ingestion is important and a blood count essential as soon as the diagnosis of a blood dyscrasia is suspected.

Quinsy.– One fairly uncommon but severe form of sore throat is caused by quinsy or peritonsillar abscess. This can usually be diagnosed by appearance alone – a unilateral inflamed swelling of the fauces – but there may be some doubt, as many such abscesses subside without incision following antibiotic therapy.

History and examination

The history to be taken when a patient complains of sore throat should include enquiries about:

1. Duration
2. Pain on swallowing
3. Fever
4. Associated respiratory symptoms
5. Other systemic upset
6. Smoking habits
7. Self medication.

The examination will usually consist of:

1. Inspection of the pharynx
2. Temperature
3. Palpation for enlarged or tender tonsillar nodes (felt just below the angle of the mandible).

The only other physical examination which is likely to be useful is a search for other enlarged nodes, and liver and/or splenic enlargement when infectious mononucleosis is suspected.

The question of whether or not to take a throat swab is a vexed one and depends upon local laboratory resources, availability of time and the practitioner's own overall assessment of the situation. Ross[3] maintains that throat swabs should be taken from at least all children presenting with sore throats. On the other hand, Everett[4] presents a less purist view, and bases his treatment on more empirical grounds. It is certainly well established that the state of the pharynx and/or tonsils generally gives no evidence as to the etiology of the sore throat: a normal throat may look red and infected, and a heavy growth of streptococci may be obtained from swabbing quite innocent looking throats. Thus, if the practitioner elects to pursue a policy of selective swabbing only, he must at the same time be quite clear that his subsequent management is based on pragmatic and not precise clinical indications.

There would be general agreement that throat swabbing is indicated in closed communities (such as a nurses' hostel or a boarding school) to establish a base for planning isolation or the treatment of subsequent cases. A swab would also be indicated to establish or refute a diagnosis when relatively rare causes of sore throat, such as thrush, Vincent's angina or diphtheria, were suspected. If throat swabbing is undertaken to isolate streptococci, the whole throat including both fauces and the uvula should be swabbed and a specimen of saliva also obtained and transported in the same container as the swab.

The only other investigation which may be indicated is the taking of blood for a full blood count and 'monospot' or Paul Bunnell test in cases of suspected infectious mononucleosis, and blood for a full count and film if there is any reason to suspect one of the blood dyscrasias.

Management

By far and away the two commonest causes of sore throats presenting to the general practitioner are streptococcal and viral infections. Equally, it is established that the two cannot be distinguished in any way on clinical grounds. The purist will take a throat swab and treat symptomatically until the result is available. The realities of life in general practice are discouraging to the purist, and the pragmatist with reasonable justification will make his decision on the basis of the severity of the symptoms and the tolerance of the patient (or his parents), and indeed of the doctor himself, for apparent therapeutic inactivity.

It has been shown that the exhibition of penicillin may reduce the persistence of the symptoms of sore throats caused by streptococci by only some twenty-four hours, as compared with the natural resolution of symptoms caused by the mobilization of the body's defences. It is not clear that the prescription of the antibiotic (at least at the stage when the patient presents) will necessarily prevent the development of post-streptococcal sequelae; in other words the damage may already have been done, if it is going to be done at all, by the time medical aid is sought.

The natural history of sore throat, whether caused by virus or bacterium, is that of a self-limiting condition resolving in a matter of days. A throat infection, however, may be a relatively severe illness, especially if associated with systemic manifestations such as significant pyrexia, vomiting or further spread characterized by enlarged and tender tonsillar nodes, and in such cases the prescription of penicillin is justifiable, if only to reduce marginally the length of the illness.

Penicillin (by injection if the symptoms are especially severe, but in the vast majority of cases oral therapy is quite sufficient) is the antibiotic of choice: haemolytic streptococci have remained penicillin sensitive, whereas resistance to tetracycline is common. Having embarked on antibiotic therapy it should be continued for seven to ten days, in order to eradicate the organisms completely. There is at least the theoretical objection to shorter courses that infection may flare up again and possibly that antibiotic resistance might be encouraged by insufficiently thorough treatment. For adults the dosage is phenoxymethylpenicillin, 250 mg four times daily (the antibiotic is best absorbed on an empty stomach and patients should be instructed to take their tablets half an hour before meals). In children the dosage is 125 mg four times daily: that is 5 ml of paediatric penicillin syrup – and two 100 ml bottles provide a ten-day course.

When penicillin is contraindicated because of a history of hypersensitivity, erythromycin is the appropriate substitute. There is no point in selecting an antibiotic with a broader spectrum: if the throat is bacterially infected the offending organism is almost certain to be the streptococcus. There is a real fear that if ampicillin is prescribed in an indiscriminate fashion coliform organisms in the gut (which can cause urinary infections) may develop resistance which could be transferred by means of R-factors to enteric organisms, and thus give rise to a situation where typhoid could become untreatable.

Those who agree with Everett will prescribe penicillin in all cases; those who agree with Ross will await the result of a throat swab and treat appropriately on the receipt of the result. Others may agree that a sore throat alone, in the absence of any supporting symptoms or signs, can be safely and adequately managed by advice to refrain from smoking or other irritants and the use of soluble aspirin (one 300-mg aspirin soluble tablet B.P. dissolved in a cup of warm water and used as a gargle and then swallowed, every four to six hours).

For infectious mononucleosis treatment is symptomatic and the course of the illness may be lengthy. Rarely steroids may be indicated.

Thrush will usually respond to nystatin or to amphotericin

lozenges, and in resistant cases the old-fashioned, if messy, 1 per cent aqueous solution of gentian violet is almost invariably effective.

The organisms of Vincent's angina will respond to penicillin, but more definitive treatment is metronidazole, 200 mg thrice daily for a week.

The confirmation of diphtheria should lead urgently to consultation with or referral to a specialist in infectious diseases.

The suspicion of a blood dyscrasia should likewise indicate urgent specialist help.

Quinsy may require surgical intervention if the abscess fails to show some signs of resolution within 24 hours of the start of penicillin therapy.

The question of the indications for referring patients for tonsillectomy is a controversial one.[5,6] The criteria suggested by Wood and colleagues[7] provide a reasonable guideline: that is, children suffering five or more sore throats causing more than three weeks off school in one year. Rarer indications are recurrent quinsy and tonsillar hypertrophy causing gross obstruction.

Many children between the ages of 5 and 8 suffer from recurrent sore throats as part of the 'catarrhal child' syndrome. Pressure may be put on the general practitioner by anxious parents to refer such children for tonsillectomy. Individual factors, such as claims of the near-magical effects of such a procedure on an older sibling, will, of course, influence the doctor, but the natural history of the catarrhal child syndrome is that the incidence of symptoms diminishes markedly after the age of about 8 years. Hence, it is normally more helpful to treat acute infections as they arise and indicate that such episodes, while inconvenient, may help the child in his development of improved resistance to respiratory infections ('it's a little like learning arithmetic – tough at the time but useful later') rather than submit the young child to the trauma of hospital admission and the remote but nonetheless existent dangers of an operative procedure.

Conclusion

In Howie's study of respiratory illness in general practice,[8] a consensus emerges to indicate that 'severe throat infection' merits treatment with penicillin. It may be impractical in general practice conditions to await bacteriological confirmation before beginning treatment in the majority of cases of sore throat and therefore the doctor must rely on his clinical judgement and tolerate its inaccuracy and inherent uncertainty.

By prescribing penicillin the practitioner may shorten (marginally) the course of a self-limiting but unpleasant symptom. He may also possibly prevent the development of post-streptococcal sequelae. On the other hand, the ingestion of penicillin may theoretically encourage the emergence of drug-resistant organisms (though fortunately there is as yet no evidence of this happening in relation to penicillin and the streptococcus). The prescription of penicillin may contribute to the population's belief that biologically active and potentially hazardous remedies have to be sought for what can be relatively minor and self-limiting conditions.

The dilemma is inescapable – its resolution may perhaps best be determined pragmatically by the presence or absence of associated symptoms or signs, therapy being based on what is thought to be clinically desirable, with or without bacteriological proof.

References

[1] Dunnell, K. and Cartwright, A. (1972): *Medicine Takers, Prescribers and Hoarders.* London: Routledge and Kegan Paul

[2] Royal College of General Practitioners, Office of Population Censuses and Surveys, Department of Health and Social Security (1986): *Morbidity Statistics from General Practice 1981–82*. HMSO Series MB5 No. 1

[3] Ross, P.W. (1971): Accuracy of clinical assessment of the microbial etiology. *The Practitioner, 207,* 659

[4] Everett, M.T. (1975): Antibiotics in the treatment of tonsillitis. *Journal of the Royal College of General Practitioners, 25,* 317

[5] Hickish, G. (1975): The case for the removal of tonsils and adenoids. *Update, 11,* 73

[6] Carne, J. (1975): The case against unnecessary removal of tonsils and adenoids. *Update, 11,* 82

[7] Wood, B. and Theodoridis, C.G., (1972): Paediatricians look at children awaiting adenotonsillectomy. *Lancet, ii,* 645

[8] Howie, J.G.R. (1973): A new look at respiratory illness in general practice. *Journal of the Royal College of General Practitioners, 23,* 895

3.26 Lumps in the neck

Michael Tellis

Lumps in the neck can be caused by a wide variety of conditions but they are a relatively uncommon cause of a 'first patient-initiated consultation'. Morrell and his colleagues with a practice of about 4,500 patients saw only 32 patients presenting with this condition in a year. The patient presenting with a lump in the neck is usually able to demonstrate it to the doctor, as opposed to the patient complaining of a lump in the throat, who cannot. The latter is often a subjective symptom but the former is objective.

Causes

The cervical lymph nodes are normally palpable in children up to the age of 14 years. They respond as do the tonsils and adenoids to the challenge of repeated upper respiratory tract infections by increasing in size. They are very variable in position, but tend to be symmetrical and occur most commonly in the anterior triangle and deep to the angle of the jaw (the tonsillar nodes). They are soft and sometimes slightly tender. Tender, enlarged tonsillar nodes in a pyrexial child may be caused by acute tonsillitis and the pharynx should be examined. Acute tenderness and pain over an enlarged node may result from staphylococcal invasion of the node which may proceed to abscess formation. This occurs most commonly in young children.

The lymph nodes are not normally palpable in adults and an enlarged lymph node in an adult requires careful investigation and an adequate explanation. If this cannot be found malignancy will have to be excluded, by biopsy. Malignant lymph nodes are often not tender and are more usually hard or rubbery. They usually grow slowly. There may be lymphadenopathy in other areas along with splenomegaly and hepatomegaly in the reticuloses, or evidence of a primary in the lung, breast or stomach. The primary site, however, is often not obvious and indeed may never be found, the diagnosis of the primary lesion being inferred from the histology of the gland.

Other causes of lymph-node enlargement in the neck are secondary infection from a soft tissue infection of the head or face: the primary infection may not be volunteered by the patient and a careful search of the scalp may be necessary to find it. Infestation with lice is still a not uncommon cause of lymph-node enlargement in the posterior triangle. Tonsillitis usually presents as a sore throat in adults, but in children there may be marked lymphadenopathy with no complaint of sore throat. Symmetrical enlargement of the occipital nodes is a common feature in rubella, and may be the presenting symptom. Particularly in young adults enlarged cervical lymph nodes often accompanied by sore throat, malaise, tiredness and muscular pains may indicate infectious mononucleosis. This can usually be established by the typical changes in white cell morphology and the monospot test.

Thyroid swellings can usually be distinguished from other lumps in the neck by their position and their movement in swallowing. The swelling may be a diffuse enlargement of the whole gland or a localized enlargement. The gland is soft and diffusely enlarged when it is due to thyrotoxicosis or a 'simple goitre'. The latter tends to occur at puberty and in pregnancy, and the thyroid status of the patient is normal. Thyrotoxicosis can be distinguished by the other stigmata of the disease and appropriate blood tests. Occasionally the enlargement may cause obstructive symptoms in the neck. Hashimoto's thyroiditis causes a firm enlargement of the gland, tends to occur in middle-aged women and is associated with the presence of thyroid antibodies in the serum.

Localized thyroid enlargement poses a considerable diagnostic problem. The vast majority of cases are due to a simple thyroid adenoma but, unfortunately, it is not possible to differentiate clinically in a reliable way between these and carcinoma of the thyroid.

A dental abscess may present as a soft, painful swelling beneath, but attached to, the jaw. Such abscesses may be surprisingly large, up to 5 cm in diameter, and can puzzle the new entrant to general medical practice. The diagnosis is usually confirmed by finding the associated carious tooth which will be excruciatingly sensitive to touch.

A stone in the duct of the submandibular gland may cause an intermittent swelling of the gland beneath the jaw. The swelling is largest just before and during meals and subsides afterwards. Sometimes, the stone may be palpable in the duct.

Mumps may occasionally present as a swelling of the submandibular gland but more often as enlargement of the parotid glands.

There are other rare causes of lumps in the neck, e.g. thyroglossal cyst, branchial cyst, tuberculous glands, but these will probably not be seen more than once in a lifetime in general practice and are not described here.

History and examination

When the patient has completed his description of the lump the doctor will usually ask a few preliminary questions about how long it has been present and whether there is tenderness or pain before proceeding to examination of the site. The best method of examining the neck is to seat the patient and to palpate the area from a standing position behind the patient's chair. If it is suspected that the lump arises from the thyroid gland the patient may be asked to drink a glass of water as a lump within the thyroid capsule will move up and down on swallowing.

This initial examination of the lump will often be followed by further examination and questioning directed by the preliminary findings. Enlarged tender tonsillar lymph nodes in a child will prompt an examination of the pharynx and tonsils, and information will be sought about the child's temperature, liveliness and degree of unhealth. A soft diffuse enlargement of the thyroid indicates that the patient's thyroid status should be further examined. Is there any evidence of myxoedema or thyrotoxicosis? When no abnormal lump is obvious the patient should be asked to indicate its precise position and to demonstrate it. If no lump can be found, and the patient is not thought to have an intermittent lump, e.g. a salivary gland blocked by a stone, it may be postulated that the patient is feeling a normal part of the neck and interpreting it as abnormal. In this case the remainder of the consultation may explore the possible reasons for this. Is the patient hypochondriacal and over anxious? If so, why?

Management

Moderately enlarged, soft, slightly tender cervical nodes occurring in an otherwise healthy child are a normal reaction to repeated upper respiratory-tract infections and require no active treatment. Parents sometimes fear that the child has leukaemia. If there is no other reason to suspect this, the cause of the lymphadenopathy should be clearly explained to the parent. If the enlarged nodes are due to leukaemia, it is unlikely that the child would seem otherwise healthy. To embark on a series of investigations or consultant referral would cause unnecessary worry and suffering to the child and the parents. If, after adequate explanations, the parents still seem doubtful, then a further appointment may be made in the near future. When the child is seen again it is probable that the nodes will have become smaller. By making another appointment the doctor will have demonstrated his interest in the problem. Exploration of the cause for inappropriate parental anxiety may occasionally be necessary.

The acutely tender node which is thought to be progressing towards abscess formation should be treated with an antibiotic to which it is expected the organism will be sensitive. The likely sensitivity of the organism, usually *Staphylococcus aureus*, may be known from the pattern of sensitivity of other staphylococcal infections in the area. Flucloxacillin is the likely antibiotic of choice. Unfortunately, some of these infections will progress to abscess formation in spite of antibiotics, and will require incision under general anaesthesia. Early referral, as soon as pus is suspected, is important.

The cause of enlarged cervical lymph nodes in an adult should be pursued vigorously. If an adequate explanation cannot be found, the patient should be referred to a surgeon. Because of the difficulty of distinguishing clinically between an adenoma and carcinoma of the thyroid, lumps in the thyroid should also be referred for a surgical opinion.

Patients suffering from a dental abscess should be referred to their dental practitioner. If there is a delay before they are able to see him, an analgesic should be prescribed with phenoxymethylpenicillin in appropriate doses. The syrup preparation may be preferred even in adults because of associated pain and difficulty in swallowing.

Diffuse swellings of the thyroid gland sometimes require surgical intervention, but it is often more appropriate to share the decision about surgical referral with a physician than to refer the patient directly to a surgeon. Many treatment options in addition to surgery are open in these cases, including treatment with thyroxine for patients with simple unloculated goitres and Hashimoto's thyroiditis, and radioactive iodine and anti-thyroid drugs for thyrotoxicosis. Practitioners with experience and an interest in the thyroid may treat some of these patients without referral.

The usual initial regime for treating thyrotoxicosis is carbimazole 10 mg given eight hourly for a period of six to eight weeks. After this the dosage can be gradually reduced to the minimum required to keep the patient euthyroid as judged by clinical response and thyroid function tests. After the initial six weeks the drug can be taken in a single daily dose and treatment should be continued for eighteen months to two years.

The most serious side-effect of carbimazole is agranulocytosis and patients on the drug should be warned that they should stop taking it and report to the doctor if they develop sore throats.

The relapse rate after treatment with antithyroid drugs is high (30–50 per cent) and failure of a course of treatment should be an indication for specialist referral for consideration of more definitive treatment, either by surgery or radio-iodine. In the initial stages of treatment the use of propranolol 20–40 mg every eight hours can be a helpful addition to suppress sympathetic overactivity and provide some symptomatic relief.

Lumps in the neck, because of the wide variety of possible causes, may tax the skill of the most competent practitioner. The response to them may vary from simple reassurance in a child with cervical lymphadenopathy due to repeated upper respiratory-tract infections to urgent referral to a surgeon of a hard, possibly malignant lump in an adult.

3.27 The patient with difficulty in swallowing

M.E. Preston-Whyte

The complaint of difficulty in swallowing, or dysphagia, is uncommon in general practice. Morrell[1] records it as the presenting symptom in only four patients among 5,361 new patient-initiated consultations, but it may also occur as pain in the throat, a common symptom in general practice. It is, however, a precise symptom which warrants further investigation.

The normal swallowing mechanism involves the transfer of food and liquid from the mouth to the stomach by a sequence of reflexes. The first stage, in which the bolus is forced into the pharynx from the mouth, is under cortical control and can be voluntarily inhibited. This explains the child's inability to swallow tablets, and the old, or depressed or anorexic patient's ability to swallow saliva but not food. The second stage of swallowing is controlled by the autonomic nervous system: a peristaltic contraction moves the bolus down the oesophagus to the cardiac sphincter which relaxes to allow the bolus through into the stomach. When intragastic pressure rises the circular fibres of the sphincter contract to prevent gastro-oesophageal reflux.

Dysphagia may arise for a number of reasons, pain due to sore throat being the most common cause, or as a result of interruption of the nervous control of the swallowing mechanism. It may arise from disease of the muscular wall of the oesophagus, or obstruction arising within the lumen or within the wall or outside the wall of the oesophagus.

Presentation

Patients may present with difficulty in swallowing alone, or the complaint may be part of a symptom complex: e.g., in bulbar palsy, for instance, dysarthria and dysphagia occur together. Patients' ideas of what happens to food and drink when swallowed vary widely and the various sensations of food 'sticking', 'burning' or 'coming back into the mouth' may all be interpreted as 'difficulty with swallowing'. It is essential therefore for the doctor to discover what exactly is the difficulty the patient experiences on swallowing. It may simply be pain.

True dysphagia is the sensation of an obstruction occurring during or within 15 seconds of the pharyngeal phase of swallowing. Pseudo-dysphagia is a sensation of a lump in the throat which does not interfere with swallowing and disappears while swallowing, or a sensation that food has stuck or is sitting in the neck and chest which comes on after a meal. Globus hystericus is a group name for the complaint of 'a lump in the throat' manifested by anxious patients as a symptom of emotional stress with no organic basis. In a series of 25 cases[2] of so-called globus hystericus, however, 22 were found to be associated with reflux oesophagitis and the symptoms improved or were eradicated following an antacid regime.

If the main problem is of food sticking, the position that the patient indicates as the site of the obstruction is unlikely to represent the actual site of the lesion. For instance, a lesion in the lower third of the oesophagus may produce symptoms at the top of the sternum. The type of food which sticks is more helpful in deciding what the lesion is likely to be: solids, particularly meat, are likely to cause difficulty first in an obstructing lesion. If swallowing is painful, hot liquid, alcohol or acid fruit juice may be precipitating factors.

Causes

Commonest causes of dysphagia

1. Sore throat
2. Globus hystericus
3. Carcinoma of oesophagus
   Carcinoma of cardia
4. Reflux oesophagitis with stricture formation
5. Achalasia of the cardia.

Other causes

A.	Lesion in the lumen	Foreign body
B.	Lesion in the wall	Strictures following trauma or corrosives Post-cricoid web (Paterson-Kelly syndrome), sideropenic dysphagia (Plummer-Vinson syndrome) Benign tumours Muscular disorders: scleroderma, dermatomyositis, dystrophia

		myotonica, myasthenia gravis Neurological disorders: cerebral arterial disease, preganglionic (diabetic autonomic neuropathy), postganglionic (diffuse oesophageal hypertrophy, diffuse spasm, Chaga's disease)
C.	Lesion outside the wall	Pharyngeal pouch Retrosternal thyroid Mediastinal lymph nodes and tumours Aortic aneurysm Para-oesophageal hiatus hernia Peri-oesophagitis after vagotomy Tight oesophageal hiatus repair

The common causes

Sore throat.– This is usually self evident.

Globus hystericus.– This is a diagnosis of exclusion. The possibility of a more serious cause should be excluded by a careful history and examination of the neck and throat even though the presentation of symptoms combined with an evaluation of the patient's personality immediately suggests the diagnosis. In view of the study[2] which suggests that globus symptoms may be associated with a reflux oesophagitis, an antacid regime might be tried before resorting to sympathetic counselling and mild tranquillizers.

Cancer of the oesophagus is either a squamous cell carcinoma or an adenocarcinoma ascending from the stomach. The incidence is one-fifth that of gastric carcinoma. It is uncommon under the age of 45 years; the incidence from then on increases with age, men and women being equally affected. Symptoms have usually lasted for less than a year, patients complaining of sudden onset of block to solids and subsequent rapid worsening of symptoms, with progressive dysphagia for liquids. Pain is not a feature except in the early stage, as the tumour destroys nerve endings as it grows. Loss of weight is common. When a patient eventually seeks medical advice, about 40 per cent will have evidence of distant tumour spread and 60 per cent will appear to have operable growths. The operative mortality lies between 10 and 20 per cent. Of those who survive, 20 per cent will die in the first year, while 10 per cent will survive for five years.

Treatment aims at increasing survival time and relieving distressing symptoms. Radiotherapy is palliative with or without the insertion of tubes to enable saliva and fluid nutrition to be swallowed.

Stage of Tumour	*Five-year Survival Rates*
If tumour resectable	10%
If tumour less than 4 cm long	20%
If no spread to local lymph nodes	40%

Table I. – Survival rates in carcinoma of the oesophagus

As the table[3] shows, earlier diagnosis is of the utmost importance so that when an unexplained dysphagia occurs as a symptom in general practice it should be investigated radiologically with as much urgency as bleeding from any orifice.

Reflux oesophagitis with stricture formation. — Oesophagitis is recorded as occurring at all ages with an overall consulting-rate of 1.3/1,000 for men and 1.7/1,000 for women. The maximum rate is highest (3.7/1,000) in the age group 65–75.

There is commonly an associated hiatus hernia, but in a study[4] of 95 hospital patients with no appreciable gastro-intestinal symptoms, small sliding hiatus hernias were found in 33 per cent. This high incidence was not related to age, sex or weight. Thus the finding of a hiatus hernia radiologically may not of itself explain the symptoms, particularly if the symptoms are inappropriate. Symptoms have usually been present for longer than a year.[5] Patients say that food or hot liquid seems to move over a 'raw patch' or 'stick' for a few seconds in the chest. Constant pain suggests an ulcer from which bleeding can occur. This is usually occult and can cause an iron-deficiency anaemia. The regurgitation of acid or 'vomit tasting' liquid into the mouth ('heartburn') on stooping, bending or lying down is pathognomonic of oesophageal reflux.

Strictures commonly develop with few preceding symptoms of reflux and develop particularly quickly in people over the age of 60. Alkalis usually help to relieve the symptoms of oesophagitis.

Achalasia of the cardia (synonyms: cardiospasm, megaoesophagus). — The incidence of achalasia is about half that of peptic stricture and squamous carcinoma of the oesophagus. It occurs at all ages and is due to a variable proportion of the ganglion cells of Auerbach's plexus disappearing with inability of the sphincter to relax completely in swallowing. This causes an obstruction to the outflow of food and liquid which is partially overcome by increasing intra-oesophageal pressure. Normal quantities can be eaten and drunk provided this is done very slowly (post-vagotomy and post-hiatus-hernia repair patients have similar symptoms). The oesophagus becomes distended and regurgitation is variable in volume and time after swallowing. Pain unrelated to swallowing (spontaneous pain) is typical and is relieved by drinking cold water.

Some uncommon causes

Post-cricoid web is mainly a disease of women in which a sheet or web of normal looking oesophageal mucosa partially occludes the upper end of the oesophagus. It is associated with a microcytic anaemia and koilonychia. *Pharyngeal pouch* arises as a result of incoordination of pharyngeal swallowing with premature closure of the cricopharyngeus. A pouch of mucous membrane is formed into which food enters compressing the oesophagus. Turning the neck or external pressure over the pouch will cause food to return to the mouth. The characteristic story is that the patient notices that it is food eaten hours or sometimes days earlier.

History

History-taking should aim at differentiating the benign from the malignant and the organic from the functional and, if possible, to determine the possible site of the lesion. A flow chart arranges the questions to be asked in an orderly sequence so that only those are asked which are relevant to the solution of the remaining part of the problem. The diagnostic trees (Flow Charts 1 and 2) are a simplified version of an algorithm[5] which in use proved more accurate than a combination of random history taking, radiology and oesophagoscopy. The importance of making a presumptive diagnosis is that the appropriate action will be taken.

Examination

Physical examination of the neck and chest, including an inspection of the pharynx and a search for supraclavicular or cervical lymphadenophathy, often reveals nothing abnormal if the disease is primarily in the oesophagus. Spread of malignant disease, however, may produce secondary liver involvement with ascites and jaundice.

When dysphagia occurs as part of a generalized disease, other signs may be apparent: e.g., anaemia in the Paterson-Kelly and

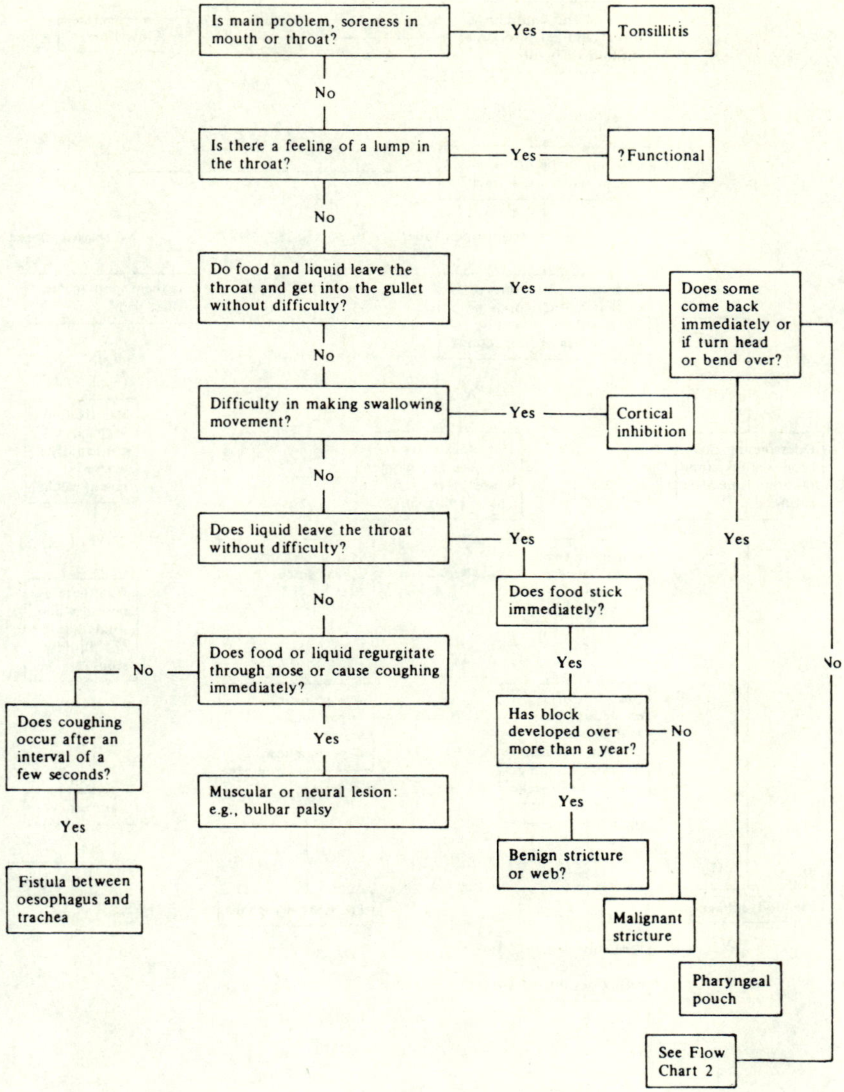

Flow Chart 1.– The diagnosis of pharyngeal causes of dysphagia

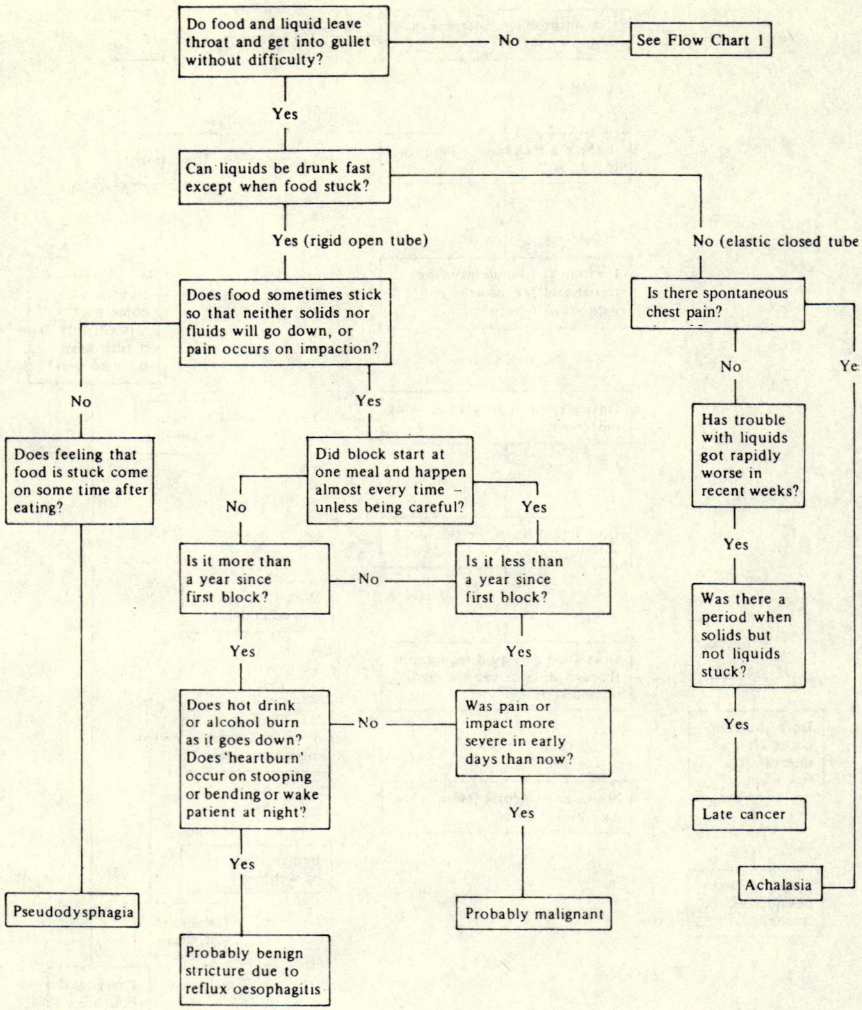

Flow Chart 2.– The diagnosis of oesophageal causes of dysphagia

Plummer-Vinson syndromes, or as a result of occult blood loss in reflux oesophagitis, or contractures and deformity of joints as in scleroderma.

Management

Confirmation of the clinical diagnosis will require referral for special investigation and unless the general practitioner has open access to contrast-media X-ray facilities this will mean referral for consultant opinion. If the general practitioner suspects a benign lesion and can arrange for a barium swallow to be done, the value of a presumptive diagnosis, made after a careful history has been taken, will be that the radiologist will be given a clear indication of where and what the suspected lesion is so that a specific search can be made. The main cause of error in the diagnosis of pharyngeal and oesophageal lesions is failure to give the radiologist the relevant details. Ring and fibro-muscular strictures and achalasia are often missed if a radiologist examines the patient in the erect position only: an anti-gravity swallow in 10° head-down position is essential.

If the results of contrast-media X-ray examination are inconclusive or further confirmation of the diagnosis is necessary, the consultant may attempt to visualize the lesion using a fibre-optic oesophagoscope. The findings vary, however: in achalasia nothing abnormal may be seen and ring strictures and fundal carcinoma may be missed completely.

As a general principle, patients with obstructive symptoms (food sticking) should be referred for urgent specialist investigation to exclude carcinoma or a remediable condition. Patients with symptoms of oesophagitis, i.e. pain on swallowing and heartburn, without the complaint of food sticking may be treated symptomatically with alkalis. The following *British National Formulary* preparations are cheap and effective: magnesium trisilicate compound tablets, or magnesium trisilicate compound powder — half a 5-ml teaspoon in water hourly may be prescribed if renal function is normal. If it is impaired, 30-ml of aluminium hydroxide suspension can be prescribed each hour. The frequent medication is necessary to maintain the antacid effect on the gastric contents so that if reflux occurs less damage will be caused to the oesophageal mucosa. Anticholinergic drugs are ineffective and serve only to decrease the volume of alkaline saliva. There is no evidence that metoclopramide increases the tone of the gastro-oesophageal sphincter but it may help to diminish symptoms in a small number of cases. Gaviscon, which is alginic acid plus sodium alginate compounded with alkalis, is a preparation which must be chewed, to produce a foam. This foam may float up into a herniated loculus when the patient is erect but it seems to follow the air bubble to the pyloric antrum when the patient lies down. The patient should be instructed to sleep propped up and to have a biscuit and a glass of milk or alkali at hand on the bedside table.

Achalasia is best followed up by the surgeon so that increasing dilatation of the oesophagus can be watched for, as the danger of regurgitation at night with aspiration pneumonia becomes more likely as the condition progresses. Inhalation of amyl nitrite taken half-way through a meal will cause relaxation of the sphincter and is useful in the elderly and those unfit for operation.

Dysphagia appearing as part of generalized disease should be managed by treating the cause, if possible. Protection of the larynx against spillage is the most important consideration. When this cannot be prevented the patient may need to be admitted to hospital in order to be treated by naso-gastric intubation and drip-feeding.

References

[1] Morrell, D., Gage, H.G. and Robinson, N.A. (1971): Symptoms in general practice. *Journal of the Royal College of General Practitioners*, *21*, 32

[2] Ardren, G.M. and Delahunty, J.E. (1970): Globus hystericus — A manifestation of reflux oesophagitis? *Journal of Laryngology*, *84*, 1049

[3] Leading Article (1976): Cancer of Oesophagus. *British Medical Journal*, *2*, 135

[4] Dyer, N.H. and Pridie, R.B. (1968): Incidence of hiatus hernia in asymptomatic subjects. *Gut*, *9*, 696

[5] Edwards, D.A.W. (1970): Flow charts, diagnostic keys and algorithms in the diagnosis of dysphagia. *Scottish Medical Journal*, *15*, 378

3.28 The patient complaining of cough

J.G.R. Howie

Although cough is the commonest single symptom presented to the general practitioner as well as a common symptom in respiratory or cardiovascular disease syndromes, it causes only occasional difficulties to the experienced general practitioner. This, however, does not imply that the conduct of the consultation for cough is uniform in terms of history taking or physical examination or that management is agreed by all doctors. In truth it is in some of the dissimilarities between doctors in their handling of the patient with cough that much of the legitimate criticism of the clinical respectability of general practice and general practitioners arises.

Precise estimates of the incidence and prevalence of cough are difficult to make because of the epidemic nature of acute respiratory infections in the community, patients' differing perceptions of the symptom and the varying geographical incidence of chronic respiratory illness. The best available estimates suggest that the average patient experiences four respiratory illnesses a year and consults his doctor for only one in every ten of these. Cough is probably the commonest symptom of these illnesses among both the consulting and non-consulting populations with the result that cough is present in one in eight episodes of general practice illness.

Unpublished data from a large multi-doctor survey of new episodes of respiratory illness showed that cough was present in over two-thirds of 7,500 such illnesses and, if not the presenting symptom, coexisted with the presenting symptom in the majority of all diagnoses recorded except allergic rhinitis, tonsillitis and otitis media. Even in these three categories 40 per cent of consulting patients included cough as a symptom offered to, or elicited by, the doctor.

Presentation

In the surgery.– When the patient is an adult or school-age child the probability is that impatience with the persistence of the symptom or interference with sleep (and not necessarily the patient's sleep) has prompted the consultation. In some cases anxiety that the illness is 'going into the chest' is the reason for consultation, and advice or reassurance rather than medicine is being sought. Similar reasons may bring a mother with her baby or small toddler, but in this age-group the cough may be used to introduce a request for information on more general problems such as feeding and sleep difficulties. This more often applies in the case of first children than in second or subsequent children.

At home.– Although it is, of course, naive to assume that all requests for house calls imply more serious illness than is seen in the surgery, the home visit for cough has its own hallmarks. At one end of the scale is the patient whose viral malaise makes him unwilling to go to the surgery and whose real request is for a sickness certificate rather than advice. The potential irritation caused by this – usually the fault of employers rather than patients – must not, however, prevent consideration of the possibility that serious illness may nevertheless be present or developing. At the other end of the scale the respiratory embarrassment experienced in pneumonia, acute asthma, bronchitis or heart failure may be summarized and presented by anxious patients or relatives simply as cough and the seriousness of the illness under-emphasized.

The emergency call.– Many of the points relating to house calls apply also to the discussion of cough as a presenting symptom of the emergency call. With experience the doctor quickly learns to regard descriptive terms like 'dreadful' and 'terrible' with detachment and to accept that the symptoms will invariably be presented as having lasted 'all day' or 'all night' without a break. Careful questioning may help to decide whether the consultation is about anxiety and the need for advice or about illness and the need for professional assessment. Telephone consultation has serious limitations: many doctors will recognize the risk of making decisions this way, and generally visit patients even with this apparently innocent presentation. Falling into a recognizable sub-group in this category is the 'after-closing-time' type of call where a domestic social crisis is converted into a request for a visit to a coughing child – or even adult. The doctor-patient aggression often accompanying such calls – sometimes on both sides – must not deflect the doctor from attempting a careful assessment of the underlying priorities of the request.

Other presentations.– Although this chapter has dealt mainly with the way cough is presented to the general practitioner, brief comment should be made of occasions when cough, although a significant component of illness, is not reported to the doctor.

This apparently illogical reaction is part of the sometimes well-founded anxiety of smokers consulting because of persistent respiratory symptoms or vague malaise with or without loss of weight. In this setting it may require direct questioning to elicit the presence of cough – and even of the spitting of blood.

Causes

Cough is a reflex act occurring in response to irritation of the lining of the respiratory tract. Classification of the numerous causes can be oriented towards the history taking and physical examination or to decisions on management. The traditional approach to classification by pathological process retains merit even outwith the hospital environment.

Infective.– Infection underlies most coughs seen in general practice. The majority of these are viral in origin and the collaborative work of the Medical Research Council and Public Health Laboratory Service has demonstrated the wide variety of respiratory syndromes associated with different infecting agents. Most viruses are associated with short-lived illnesses but a number are associated with risk of bacterial superinfection, especially in patients with asthma or chronic bronchitis, and this must be suspected in prolonged or recurring illness in this category. The respiratory syncytial virus (R.S.V.) is a common cause of more severe respiratory illness in children as is influenza A virus in adults, and persisting cough during epidemics of these infections requires careful re-assessment. Cough may, of course, be due to bacterial infections existing on their own or superimposed on chronic bronchitis or asthma. Occasionally it may also be due to mycoplasma or fungal infection. Knowledge of the natural history of infections caused by the whooping-cough and tuberculosis bacilli and the measles virus is important. Coliform and staphylococcal infections are normally found only in debilitated patients or in patients with bronchiectasis or after recent hospital admission.

Physical and chemical.– The effect of cold and of smoke (especially from tobacco) in aggravating, prolonging or causing cough is well known. The importance of tobacco smoke is so great that it merits a classification to itself and its positioning is second only to infective causes in frequency and importance.

Circulatory.– Particularly in the elderly, a persistent dry cough may be found in the early stages of cardiac decompensation. Although confirmatory physical signs may be absent, the frequency with which a short course of diuretic therapy relieves the symptom suggests the diagnosis to be a real one. Less commonly pulmonary infarction may present as cough.

Allergic.– Cough, in particular night cough, may occur in patients with an allergic diathesis with or without wheeze. The catarrhal child may conveniently be thought of in this category, as may the mild or established asthmatic and some adult patients with allergic alveolitis. It is often the persistence and usually episodic nature of the symptoms that come to suggest the diagnosis, which may again be confirmed by therapeutic trial.

Psychosocial. — Before looking for rare causes in the patient not already covered by one of the categories described, the possibility of coexisting psychological or social problems must be remembered, such as habit cough as a form of nervous tic.

Neoplastic. — Low in the order of frequency but high in the list of fatal causes of cough is bronchial neoplasm. The legitimate view that the usually anaplastic bronchial carcinoma is in some ways better left undiagnosed till symptomatic relief is needed, must be tempered by recognition that some cell types are more amenable to surgery than others, that Hodgkin's disease is now treatable, that an isolated secondary deposit may justify treatment and that occasionally tumours are not malignant.

Other causes. — The causes of most coughs will be found in those listed. When this is not so other more significant symptoms or signs will probably be present. Inhaled foreign body is possibly the main exception to this statement. The possibility of disease being secondary to cough or superadded to a disease in which cough is a prominent symptom, may occasionally be relevant: pneumothorax and cough fracture of the ribs are examples of this.

History and examination

Discussion of history taking and physical examination in patients with cough requires a cautious compromise between views based on facts recorded at consultations by doctors who knew they were being observed and the tales of instant medicine so well known to the public and profession. There is no point in denying that many patients receive treatment for cough without an adequate history having been taken or any examination performed. Complete out-of-hand criticism of this procedure is probably both inappropriate and illogical as many doctors are now attempting to encourage normally fit patients to self-medicate for the uncomplicated cough, realizing that decisions to consult often indicate doctor-dependence rather than degree of illness. In the reported studies of doctor behaviour at the consultation for cough there seems fairly widespread agreement that a brief history is normally sufficient and that physical examination of the chest is required. The taking of an extensive history and the carrying out of a more complete respiratory or other general examination are usually restricted to patients who are very young, are looking ill, or are failing to make the normal progress to recovery which would be expected. Clearly patients with coexisting symptoms suggesting the greater probability of serious disease being present (haemoptysis and weight loss for example) will also be handled in a manner different from the normal, perhaps making use of specialized investigations.

The following paragraphs attempt to steer a middle course between brevity and over-simplification on the one hand, and detail of the kind to be found in a specialist textbook. The first priority is to determine the seriousness and time scale of the illness. The possibility that the presentation of the symptom is an excuse to discuss a psychosocial issue exists but will not be developed in detail here.

Acute serious disease.– Acute serious illness is normally suggested by breathlessness, sometimes by chest pain, and often by facial appearance: the presence of cyanosis or of ashen pallor is more worrying than the flushed skin of high fever. Coexisting wheeze may alert the doctor to an illness in this group but the serious implication of airways obstruction that has passed from the wheezy to the non-wheezy stage cannot be over-stressed. Illnesses in this group are often associated with restlessness and distress – physical and emotional – and signs of fatigue. Recognition of this important group of coughing patients initially depends more on general assessment than on history taking or physical examination. Specific questioning and examination are then readily directed to the differential diagnosis between asthma, croup, acute bacterial infection, non-asthmatic obstructive airways disease (including inhaled foreign body), pulmonary collapse and pneumothorax.

Non-acute serious disease.– Non-acute serious illness is suggested by the continuation of cough beyond the normal natural history of acute treated bacterial or viral illness in the absence of a history suggesting obstructive or allergic respiratory disease. The patient in this category is frequently middle-aged or elderly, more often a man than a woman and commonly a heavy cigarette smoker. Haemoptysis and loss of weight aid categorization of patients to this group but more often vague malaise with possibly loss of appetite is the only feature. Physical examination is often completely negative. The possible presence of tuberculosis or malignant disease is usually regarded as an invariable indicator that x-ray examination at least is required.

Acute self-limiting disease.– Acute self-limiting illness is characterized by a history compatible with an acute infective process (coryza, influenza) and the absence of the general signs of serious illness already described. The patient may have the headache, myalgia and malaise of the acute underlying process or may have passed from that early stage to one in which cough is the only significant complaint. Here the history taking normally aims to identify any tendency to chest trouble (asthma and chronic bronchitis in particular) and the nature and colour of any sputum being produced. Chest examination will allow exclusion of signs of localized infection but the management decision is usually established on the basis of the history alone. Mothers expect their children's chests to be examined and, if for no other reason, this is a wise policy. The elderly – often barricaded in by layers of clothing – may seem happier not to be examined but the frequency with which basal crepitations are recognized justifies overruling this wish. The routine chest examination of adults with a short history of cough will continue to be advocated because no-one is courageous enough to proclaim its irrelevance in print.

Persisting or relapsing illness.– Outwith these categories lie the coughs of a persisting or relapsing nature. Among these, particular mention should be made of three common 'coughing syndromes': namely night cough in children, often associated with the catarrhal child syndrome; 'whooping-cough', again usually a childhood complaint; the 'smoker's cough' with its inescapable and often unnoticed progress to chronic bronchitis.

The child with persistent or recurrent episodes of cough, worst at night, is a common cause of anxiety, especially to young parents. The child is often at the stage of attending school or play-group for the first time and may have a past history of croup or eczema. A family history of allergic respiratory illness may coexist. The common pattern is one of recurrent bouts of acute wheezy respiratory infections interspersed by periods of comparative health often, however, including nights interrupted by persisting dry cough. The tendency for the child to be well and free of abnormal signs when seen by the doctor may create the unfair impression of fussing parents. Careful history taking will identify the syndrome, and the possible additional precipitating causes of animal or plant allergy may be identified on specific questioning or a home visit.

A second common problem is the whooping-cough outbreak which will be found most years during the winter months.

Characterized by persisting spasms of severe cough often without physical signs or other symptoms (except perhaps loss of appetite and sickness during bouts), the syndrome is a common cause of parental anxiety. The child has usually been fully immunized and often been treated earlier in the illness with antibiotics. The relevant information required for handling this problem is the level of the parents' tolerance of expectant management.

The third category is the smoker's cough syndrome. In this situation the patient, perhaps in his middle thirties, complains of little more than fatigue or breathlessness on exertion and does not mention cough because he has come to regard this as a normal occurrence each morning. Recurrent production of sputum and even of purulent sputum may also not be mentioned because of their regular presence. Examination is again usually negative and the only significant symptoms may be of decreasing exercise tolerance. Peak-flow readings provide objective evidence of diminishing lung function. This syndrome merges inexorably with the typical picture of chronic bronchitis which is all too familiar to general practitioners.

Treatment and management

Reassurance, advice, prescription, observation, investigation and referral cover in appropriate priority the options on management of patients with cough.

Reassurance. — Commonly visits concerning cough represent patient or parental concern that a cold is 'settling in the chest'. If appropriate, the positive use of reassurance is indicated, prescribing being at best a secondary course of action. Reassurance and patient education are closely linked and the more medicine and less reassurance offered, the greater is the likelihood of future dependence on prescribed medicine. Reassurance may also have an important therapeutic role in persistent cough, particularly after measles or during a 'whooping-cough' outbreak. In the adult with cough who consults because of persisting symptoms, fear concerning malignancy may be a significant feature. For such patients the level of action necessary for reassurance will vary from auscultation of the chest to referral for X-ray, according to the patient's insight. It may be, however, that for a heavy smoker a little therapeutic anxiety is indicated and the interval waiting for an X-ray to be reported clear may be filled by appropriate attempts at health education. The parent of the young child with a catarrhal tendency requires, and should be given, reassurance that the frequent recurrences of cough around the time of starting school are common and represent a short although anxious time in the lives of many families.

Advice. — The random way in which patients decide between self-treatment and consultation emphasizes the significant need for advice in treating coughing patients. Genuinely troublesome interference with sleep and ability to work can be alleviated by adequate fluid intake, proprietary preparations containing lemon or blackcurrant, honey, and even — at night — small quantities of alcohol. Inhalation of steam is often rapidly helpful. Sleeping on an extra pillow may help adults with a nocturnal cough; paradoxically, young children who cough at night due to catarrh irritating the back of the throat should sleep without a pillow. The moderate use of cough mixtures may have a useful sedative effect. Patients already on regular medication should perhaps be encouraged to avoid self-medication, although most risks of drug-interaction are theoretical rather than real. Advice on smoking habits is most likely to be effective during an illness when the patient has actually requested care, or when advice is sought about a child with a persistent cough where one or both parents smoke.

Prescription. — If cough is present in a patient with a history of chronic bronchitis, asthma or recurrent chest infection, antibiotics may be prescribed prophylactically on this ground alone. When the lungs are chronically diseased tetracycline, co-trimoxazole, and ampicillin appear of equal merit; when this is not the case simple penicillin is preferable — except of course in the presence of allergy to the drug. Tetracycline is specifically indicated for mycoplasma pneumonia.

If cough coexists with otitis media or tonsillitis these conditions require to be treated as a priority and abnormal chest signs or a purulent sputum are widely regarded as further indications for antibiotics. There is evidence that cough and purulent sputum, in the absence of chest signs, do not require antibiotic treatment and the controversy extends to whether such purulent sputum originates in the upper or lower respiratory tract. Outwith these groups, too many patients with cough receive antibiotics in the mistaken belief that this saves time at a later stage in the illness. Recurrent consultations are equally likely in the treated and untreated, and the side-effects of antibiotics are a real hazard. Dependency on antibiotics is responsible for many minor illnesses being brought unnecessarily to medical care.

Much of what has been said about antibiotic dependency applies to cough mixtures. The sedative effect of the antihistamines they contain probably offers symptomatic relief but few of the other claims made for them appear substantiated. Troublesome night cough, especially in children, may be relieved by a sedative linctus (my own prejudice), or an antispasmodic (salbutamol), this indicating the possible allergic aetiology of this symptom. Mucolytics may help a smaller number of patients with chronic cough as may bronchodilators; drugs for management of cardiac decompensation are appropriate when indicated.

The management of whooping cough makes demands on the parents and the medical attendants. There is little evidence that antibiotics influence the natural history of the illness unless there is secondary infection. A course of erythromycin (100 mg six hourly for ten days) will, however, make the patient non-infective and thus protect other members of the family. Some authorities recommend a prophylactic course of erythromycin for vulnerable contacts in the household — that is infants under the age of six months and unimmunized toddlers. In the very young with repeated vomiting there may be problems in maintaining fluid and electrolyte balance which will require hospital admission. Relief of the paroxysms and whoop is difficult. Some paediatricians favour phenobarbitone, which will reduce anxiety and possibly the frequency of paroxysms. There is no evidence that atropine or its derivatives are of value although frequently used. In severe cases, high humidity and oxygen may be necessary.

When cough is due to malignant disease diamorphine is the drug of choice, and may be given in the form of one of the elixirs described in the *British National Formulary*.

Cough is one of the commonest reasons for prescribing without seeing the patient. Each doctor will take his own position on this, influenced by features such as knowledge of the physical and personal characteristics of individual patients, his own level of tolerance of anxiety or uncertainty, the accessibility of patients to the practice or pharmacists and so on. Certainly on occasions a cough can be reasonably handled in this way but the doctor must couple the prescription with advice to the patient on the circumstances under which he wishes to be notified of progress or its lack.

Observation. — Such is the short or intermittent natural history of cough that its persistence is a strong indication of the need for further investigation. Middle-aged patients seen because of cough should either be seen again or requested to return if symptoms persist. Similarly observation has a diagnostic role in the recognition of allergic cough and an important supportive, educational and therapeutic role in handling anxious patients or anxious parents.

Investigation. — Radiological examination of the chest may be arranged to exclude pneumothorax in an emergency or malignant disease or tuberculosis when the symptom persists or standard indications are present. In malignant disease a clear X-ray may give misleading reassurance. Sputum culture has little part to play in the management of general practice illness.

Referral. — Uncomplicated cough rarely requires acute referral to hospital. Referral may be useful for diagnostic purposes when malignancy or tuberculosis is suspected in cases of persistent or recurrent symptoms, for obtaining confirmation of the nature of obstructive lung disease, or for reassurance of anxious patients or parents.

No mention of management would be complete without reference to the need for awareness of possible coexisting or dominating psychosocial factors, and to the desirability of a new emphasis in the preventive field leading to less need for patients to seek professional help for this complaint.

Conclusions

Cough is one of the commonest symptoms presented in general practice. The cause is usually not serious and this influences the general approach to history taking, examination and management. On the other hand, the occasional presence of treatable life-threatening illness requires the doctor to develop his routine consultation in a way which offers the maximum sensitivity to these critical occasions. As in all aspects of general practice, the doctor must be aware that problems of the patient's reaction to illness or the presence of concurrent psychosocial problems may exist and these must be recognized and treated as effectively as the apparently dominant physical complaint.

Reference

Leading Article (1974): Antibiotics and Respiratory Illness. *British Medical Journal*, *3*, 1

3.29 The patient with dyspnoea

Ian Gregg

The term dyspnoea strictly means abnormal breathing but, by convention, it is used to denote only those situations in which this is perceived in consciousness as an unpleasant sensation, ranging from mere discomfort to intense distress. Since in normal persons strenuous exercise gives rise to an awareness of the need to increase the depth and rate of respiration, dyspnoea is of pathological significance only when the amount of exertion which induces it would not have done so in a healthy person of corresponding age and physique.

Dyspnoea is one of the commonest symptoms encountered by the general practitioner: its subjective nature makes it also one of the most difficult to evaluate.

The significance of dyspnoea

The appreciation in consciousness of proprioceptive impulses which monitor respiration is central to an understanding of the genesis of dyspnoea. Normally, these impulses are not perceived and they become so only when their intensity exceeds a certain threshold, consequent upon an increase in the work of breathing. In patients with impaired pulmonary or cardiac function, the amount of exertion which requires a compensatory increase in the work of breathing is much less than in normal subjects. Other causes of dyspnoea, due to increased work of breathing, are obesity and severe anaemia.

Dyspnoea may also occur as a result of psychic influences which lower the threshold at which proprioceptive impulses enter consciousness. These may be of a non-specific kind, such as depression or anxiety-tension, but a more important cause is the fear of having life-threatening disease of the lungs or heart. In this situation, proprioceptive impulses acquire a special significance and, by seeming to substantiate the fear, their perception serves to perpetuate the liability to dyspnoea. In patients with established disease of the lungs or heart, the fear of their possible consequences, including death, may be responsible for their dyspnoea being quite disproportionate to the severity of their underlying condition. A similar explanation applies to patients who complain of dyspnoea but in whom no organic disease can be identified.

In patients with organic disease, dyspnoea generally indicates that the latter is of severe degree. However, the converse does not necessarily hold true. Thus, dyspnoea may be absent even when respiratory or cardiac function is considerably impaired, especially in patients with sedentary occupations, the reserve capacities of the lungs and heart being sufficient to compensate for their impairment during light or moderate exertion.

In patients with chronic bronchitis or emphysema their respiratory reserves have usually been eroded to a substantial extent by the time they first become aware of dyspnoea. Moreover, in patients with advanced chronic bronchitis which has led to respiratory failure, the absence of dyspnoea is responsible for a dangerous situation in which they make no attempt to rectify hypoxaemia and carbon dioxide retention.

Presentation

Dyspnoea may be the only symptom of which a patient complains or it may be one of several. Its onset may be very abrupt or it may have been slowly progressive over many years. The patient may have noticed it only during unwonted physical activity or it may have occurred very acutely, awakening him or her from sleep.

When dyspnoea is very severe it is only too evident to bystanders. The patient appears distressed and apprehensive. Respiratory effort and rate are greatly increased, making it impossible to speak more than a few words at a time.

It is essential to ascertain the circumstances in which dyspnoea occurs and the amount of exertion necessary to provoke it. Its severity can be assessed by whether it is associated only with running (for instance, to catch a bus), or walking up inclines, or has become a virtually permanent feature of the patient's life, occurring with light housework, dressing or washing, or even at rest.

Clinical assessment

The differential diagnosis of dyspnoea is very large. It may not be due to a single cause but to a combination of respiratory, cardiac or other diseases, especially in elderly patients. Nevertheless, it is essential to identify the predominant cause, since this will determine the patient's management both in the short and long term.

A carefully taken history is often a more reliable guide to diagnosis than physical examination, whose principal purpose should be to confirm or refute the possibilities suggested by the history and to assess the severity of the underlying disorder.

History

The greater a doctor's ability to interpret a patient's description of dyspnoea and to ascertain the circumstances in which it occurs, the more valuable will the history prove to be in elucidating its cause. As the patient recounts the history, it is necessary to intervene with questions designed to confirm or exclude the various possibilities which it suggests.

Sometimes the history immediately suggests the diagnosis. For example, it is highly probable that a patient who has been awakened with a feeling of suffocation and has to sit upright has acute pulmonary oedema. Patients with asthma typically describe a sensation of 'tightness' of breathing, accompanied by wheeze, which is usually most pronounced in the early hours of the morning. When dyspnoea is associated with pain on one side of the chest, likely causes are pneumonia and pleurisy or a spontaneous pneumothorax. Dyspnoea arising from fear of lung or heart disease is characteristically described as a sensation of being unable to take a satisfyingly adequate breath, occurring at rest but not during exertion, and enquiry often discloses that the patient sighs frequently: this form of dyspnoea may be accompanied by discomfort in the left sub-mammary region.

Consideration of whether or not dyspnoea has occurred previously and whether its onset has been acute or insidious will often provide valuable pointers to its underlying cause.

Examination

Four considerations must be borne in mind during physical examination and in the evaluation of any abnormalities which are detected.

1. Dyspnoea may be caused by obstruction to airflow in the upper or middle respiratory tract (i.e. from the naso-pharynx to the larynx), by disorders within the thorax, or by other conditions such as obesity or anaemia.
2. When dyspnoea is due to intrathoracic disease, an attempt must be made to differentiate between respiratory and cardiac causes, though both may be contributory, especially in elderly patients.
3. In the identification of respiratory causes of dyspnoea, a distinction must be made between conditions which are generalized and those which are localized, by comparing expansion,

percussion note and breath sounds in the two sides of the chest.

4. In some patients with chronic pulmonary or cardiac disease, abnormal signs may be a permanent feature and are not necessarily relevant to the dyspnoea which is currently being experienced.

The physical signs associated with abnormalities of the respiratory and cardiac systems are so well known as to require no description of them here. It is desirable, however, to consider various principles which should be adhered to when carrying out an examination and also to review recent advances in the understanding of how certain abnormal signs are generated and, hence, their interpretation.

Inspection. — The value of inspection is often overlooked, especially if patients are examined without having undressed adequately. Unequal expansion of the chest, the use of accessory muscles of respiration, and indrawing of the suprasternal and intercostal spaces, may contribute information about the severity and nature of the underlying cause. Cyanosis is difficult to detect in artificial light, especially if this comes from fluorescent illumination: when present, it is an indication of severe hypoxaemia.

Percussion. — Except when performed by clinicians with great experience, percussion is only likely to yield reliable information if the degree of dullness or hyper-resonance is very marked.

Auscultation. — It is essential to enlist the co-operation of the patient, who should be told to open the mouth and take deep breaths. In patients with airflow obstruction, due to asthma, chronic obstructive bronchitis or emphysema, a forced expiration may reveal wheeze which was not present during tidal breathing: the time required to complete a forced expiration is an indication of the severity of airflow obstruction.

Certain adventitious sounds are highly suggestive of the type of pathological disorder present.

Rhonchi are snoring or whistling sounds which are generated by airflow through narrowed bronchi. A localized rhonchus is suggestive of stenosis of a large airway — for instance, by a carcinoma.

Wheeze is a high-pitched sound which is generally more pronounced in the expiratory phase of respiration. Recent studies have disproved the widely held belief that high-pitched, sibilant rhonchi originate in small airways and low-pitched, sonorous rhonchi in large airways. It has been shown that wheeze occurs only when the calibre of an airway is reduced almost to the point of closure.

The presence of wheeze indicates that there is obstruction to airflow in the bronchi. This may be *variable* (reversible), due to muscle constriction and/or mucosal oedema, as in asthma, or *irreversible*, due to structural damage of the bronchi or lung parenchyma, as in advanced chronic bronchitis or emphysema.
No reliance can be placed upon the loudness or pitch of wheeze as a guide to the severity of airflow obstruction: indeed, if obstruction is very severe, airflow may be reduced so greatly that it generates no sound. The 'silent chest' in severe asthma is a sign of grave danger.
The attempt to identify or assess airflow obstruction by auscultation is analogous to estimation of blood pressure by palpating the radial pulse. Therefore, every general practitioner should possess the means for measuring airflow obstruction and assessing its reversibility. The most convenient test for this purpose is peak expiratory flow (PEF), whose applications are described in the appendix to this chapter.

Crepitations are short, repetitive sounds. It used to be thought that they were caused by fluid or mucus in the alveoli or airways and they are still often referred to as 'moist sounds'. Coarse crepitations (or rales) can certainly be caused by excess mucus in the large airways, as occurs in bronchiectasis and in stuporose or dying patients who cannot clear their airways by expectoration. However, it is now known that fine crepitations (or 'crackles') are miniature explosions caused by a sudden equalization of gas pressure, when small airways open up in regions of the lungs which have become deflated. This occurs in several different types of pathology involving the lung parenchyma, crackles being a characteristic sign of pneumonia, atelectasis and alveolitis. In left ventricular failure, crepitations are probably caused in a similar manner, due to the elastic properties of the lungs being altered by interstitial oedema.

Absence of abnormal findings in a dyspnoeic patient

The failure to detect any abnormalities on physical examination must not be interpreted as signifying that dyspnoea is of psychogenic origin. Recurrent small pulmonary emboli give rise to no abnormal signs and the diagnosis can be made with certainty only by special investigations. Patients with this condition are frequently regarded as neurotic, sometimes with disastrous consequences. To avoid this error, the diagnosis of psychogenic dyspnoea should be made only when there is positive evidence of its existence and not simply on the basis of negative evidence of an organic cause.

Differential diagnosis

This is conveniently considered by categorizing the various causes of dyspnoea according to their mode of onset and history of previous episodes.

Sudden onset in a patient who has never previously experienced dyspnoea

Acute, severe dyspnoea is a medical emergency. Although treatment directed to its relief must be given with the least possible delay, it is all-important to attempt to reach a diagnosis of its cause, since this may indicate the need for entirely different forms of treatment.

Asphyxia. — The most common cause is obstruction of a large airway by an inhaled foreign body.

Croup. — Acute laryngotracheitis, usually due to infection by parainfluenza viruses, can cause obstruction in infants and young children. Stridor is the characteristic sign of obstruction in the upper airways.

Bronchiolitis. — This occurs in young children, generally due to infection by respiratory syncytial virus. It is characterized by rapid respiration, little or no pyrexia, hyperinflation, and crepitations. In infants it may cause severe respiratory distress.

A large spontaneous or tension pneumothorax. — A pneumothorax large enough to cause acute dyspnoea should be readily diagnosed by finding inequality of the percussion note and breath sounds between the two sides of the chest. However, in a patient with pre-existent chronic respiratory disease (e.g. asthma, emphysema or cystic fibrosis — in all of which pneumothorax is a well-recognized complication) even a small pneumothorax, which cannot be detected clinically, may cause severe dyspnoea.

Acute pulmonary embolus. — Acute, severe dyspnoea, usually accompanied by chest pain and shock, are the typical symptoms of a large pulmonary embolus. There are no pathognomonic signs, but it should be suspected in a patient who is shocked and in whom there are no signs of any other cause of sudden dyspnoea.

Acute pulmonary oedema. — This is a common cause of sudden dyspnoea in middle-aged and elderly patients, due to left atrial or ventricular failure. Patients will have tachycardia, a raised jugular venous pressure and bilateral crepitations, sometimes accompanied by wheeze ('cardiac asthma'). The commonest cardiac diseases causing pulmonary oedema are hypertension, ischaemic heart disease and rheumatic valvular disease.

Sudden onset in a patient who has previously had similar attacks of acute dyspnoea

The only two conditions which commonly give rise to recurrent attacks of sudden dyspnoea are left ventricular failure and asthma.

Recurrent acute pulmonary oedema. — This occurs in patients whose heart failure is inadequately controlled by diuretics or digoxin.

Asthma. — There is likely to be a history of similar episodes in the past. The distinctive signs are hyperinflation, rapid respiration and widespread wheeze which is more pronounced during expiration.

Insidious onset during the previous few days or weeks

A large number of conditions have to be considered in the differential diagnosis. Sometimes a definite diagnosis cannot be made until the results of investigations have been received. The history may permit a distinction to be made between dyspnoea which has been steadily progressive (as in pleural effusion, sarcoidosis or cryptogenic fibrosing alveolitis) and dyspnoea whose development has been punctuated by episodes of increased severity (as in chronic left ventricular failure, asthma and extrinsic allergic alveolitis).

Pleural effusion. — When large enough to cause dyspnoea, a pleural effusion should be readily diagnosed by the findings on physical examination.

Sarcoidosis. — This generally occurs in young adults, sometimes being preceded by erythema nodosum. Fine crepitations are the characteristic finding.

Chronic left ventricular failure. — A history of dyspnoea occurring on effort and associated with angina will suggest that the cause is cardiac. A raised jugular venous pressure or peripheral oedema confirm the diagnosis.

Cryptogenic fibrosing alveolitis. — Usually there is marked clubbing of the fingernails. The characteristic finding on auscultation is the presence of crackles which have a peculiar 'leathery' quality. These also occur in patients who have developed pulmonary complications of *rheumatoid disease*.

Asthma. — In many patients with asthma, especially those in whom it first begins in later life, dyspnoea tends to be continuous rather than episodic. In such patients, nevertheless, there is some degree of variability of airflow obstruction causing dyspnoea and wheeze, these symptoms being worst during the night or in the early morning.

All too often, asthma in middle-aged or elderly patients is not recognized, the symptoms being attributed to chronic bronchitis. This error in diagnosis, which is more liable to occur in men if they are smokers, has the important consequence of depriving them of anti-asthma treatment which could have conferred great benefit. Features suggestive of late-onset asthma, as opposed to chronic bronchitis, are a relatively short history of cough and dyspnoea, no history of having been a heavy smoker, and a familial history of asthma. Differentiation on clinical grounds may prove very difficult and the only certain means of confirming asthma is by a trial of corticosteroid.

Extrinsic allergic alveolitis. — Acquired hypersensitivity to certain proteins causes an inflammatory reaction in the alveoli rather than in the bronchi. Repeated exposure may cause fibrosis and permanent lung damage. Extrinsic alveolitis can be distinguished from the cryptogenic form by the absence of clubbing and a history of exposure, often in the course of the patient's occupation. 'Farmer's lung' occurs after repetitive exposure to mouldy hay. 'Bird-fancier's lung' is caused by hypersensitivity to the excreta of budgerigars or pigeons: exposure at the time of cleaning the cage or pigeon-loft may induce acute dyspnoea, sometimes accompanied by fever.

Tumours of the lung. — Dyspnoea is sometimes the presenting symptom of a tumour which obstructs a large bronchus and causes distal collapse, but far more commonly it occurs in the terminal stages of malignant tumours, due to lymphangeitis or pleural effusion.

Recurrent small pulmonary emboli. — The absence of physical signs and the tendency for dyspnoea to be attributed to neurosis has already been discussed. The possibility of pulmonary emboli must, therefore, be considered in any patient in whom no abnormalities are found on examination, but in whom the features of dyspnoea do not conform to those typically present in psychoneurosis. The absence of deep vein thrombosis or other source of emboli in no way excludes the diagnosis.

Psychoneurosis. — Psychogenic dyspnoea is generally described as a sensation of being unable to fill the lungs adequately. It may progress to overt hyperventilation, when it is accompanied by paraesthesiae or tetany, due to alkalosis resulting from excessive elimination of carbon dioxide. If directly questioned, patients often admit that they sigh frequently and that dyspnoea occurs when their minds are unoccupied, but not when they physically exert themselves. There may be clear evidence of anxiety or depression, often arising from some inescapable situation, such as impending final examinations in students. Many patients will admit to fear of lung or heart disease, the onset of dyspnoea coinciding with a close relative or acquaintance having been found to have a life-threatening condition of the lungs or heart.

Anaemia. — Dyspnoea may be a symptom of severe chronic iron-deficiency anaemia, due to menorrhagia or gastro-intestinal bleeding, or of pernicious anaemia.

Progressive development over many months or years

Chronic obstructive bronchitis. — This is the most common cause of slowly progressive dyspnoea. Its principal feature is habitual expectoration and the majority of patients are current or former cigarette smokers or have occupations in which they are exposed to dust, fumes or other irritants. Hypersecretion of mucus is accompanied by structural damage of the bronchi and, in patients who also have emphysema, of the lung parenchyma. Dyspnoea is due to irreversible airflow obstruction and by the time that it occurs on only moderate exertion a patient's peak expiratory flow (PEF) is usually less than 200 l/min.

It is important to bear in mind the possibility that patients with the symptoms of chronic bronchitis may, in reality, have late-onset asthma, in which case some part of their airflow obstruction will be reversible, though it may not respond to a bronchodilator but only to a course of corticosteroid. The steps which should be taken to distinguish between reversible and irreversible airflow obstruction are described in the appendix to this chapter.

Emphysema. — When this occurs without co-existent chronic bronchitis, airflow obstruction is caused by the bronchi lacking the elastic support normally provided by the surrounding lung parenchyma. The breath sounds are poorly heard and expiration is greatly prolonged. Very low or even unrecordable values of PEF will be found. Dyspnoea is very severe but patients remain oxygenated and accordingly are often described as 'pink puffers'.

Fibrosis. — This is still common in older patients who have had pulmonary tuberculosis which has healed by contraction and is sometimes associated with bronchiectasis. Generalized fibrosis occurs in some patients with sarcoidosis and in both the extrinsic and cryptogenic forms of alveolitis. It is also the predominant abnormality in pneumoconiosis.

Clinical investigations

If clinical assessment suggests that dyspnoea is due to airflow obstruction, estimation of PEF and its response to a bronchodilator should be regarded as an integral part of the clinical examination. Other investigations which the general practitioner can undertake are a chest radiograph, blood count and ESR.

Chest radiography. — Interpretation of abnormalities in a chest radiograph depends upon consideration of the possibilities consistent with the clinical evidence. Therefore, the general practitioner should provide the radiologist with information about the clinical findings and any previous history of lung or heart disease. Mention should be made of radiographic abnormalities which have been reported previously to enable the radiologist to distinguish between abnormalities which are longstanding and those which are of recent origin.

While some abnormal appearances are virtually diagnostic — for instance, pneumothorax or pleural effusion, others may be compatible with more than one pathological process. It should be remembered that 'X-rays do not show diseases — they only throw shadows'.

Peak expiratory flow. — Airflow obstruction is probably the commonest cause of dyspnoea encountered in general practice. It is the cardinal abnormality of function in asthma, in which, by definition, it is reversible, and in chronic obstructive bronchitis and emphysema, in which it is irreversible.

When dyspnoea is caused by airflow obstruction, identification of the mechanisms responsible is a pre-requisite of rational treatment. These can be inferred from measurements of PEF and the response to a bronchodilator or a course of corticosteroid. A detailed description of the peak flow meter and the applications of PEF measurements will be found in the appendix to this chapter.

Special investigations

Sometimes diagnosis of the condition which has given rise to dyspnoea cannot be made without special investigations. These may also be necessary for assessing the severity of dyspnoea. Though special investigations are arranged by the specialist after patients have been referred to the out-patient department or have been admitted, the general practitioner should have an understanding of the purpose and interpretation of the various tests available.

Pulmonary function tests. — Estimation of lung volumes, alveolo-capillary gas transfer, and perfusion of the lungs will distinguish between dyspnoea caused by a reduction of *ventilation* (the transport of air to and from the alveoli), impaired diffusion of oxygen from air to blood, and inadequate *perfusion* of alveoli by the pulmonary circulation. By performing an exercise tolerance test the amount of physical work required to induce dyspnoea in a given patient can be determined.

Radiology. — Tomography and, to an increasing extent, various forms of scans can be used to define the location, size and other features of conditions which have given rise to dyspnoea, including both circumscribed lesions and diffuse damage of the lungs, such as emphysema. Lung scans are invaluable for revealing parts of the lungs which are not perfused, especially in patients who are suspected of having had pulmonary emboli.
Bronchography is now rarely performed but is of value for demonstrating localized abnormalities of the larger bronchi, such as bronchiectasis or stenosis, and diffuse changes involving small bronchi, as in chronic obstructive bronchitis.

Other special investigations. — Bronchoscopy, biopsy of the bronchi, regional lymph nodes or lung parenchyma (the latter necessitating an open thoracotomy) are commonly performed in the diagnosis of bronchial tumours, sarcoidosis and alveolitis.
A wide variety of investigations may be necessary in patients whose dyspnoea is caused by cardiac disease.

Treatment

The treatment of dyspnoea depends upon its underlying cause and severity. Rather than attempting a comprehensive review of the treatment of every condition capable of causing dyspnoea, consideration will be given to the management of only two situations: acute dyspnoea presenting as an emergency and dyspnoea due to anxiety.

Dyspnoea presenting as an emergency

Acute dyspnoea may endanger life unless appropriate treatment is given without delay. Accordingly, the severity of the situation must be assessed as rapidly and accurately as possible. This should indicate how much time can be safely spent in taking a history and examining the patient in order to identify the underlying cause.

Acute obstruction of the large airways is usually self-evident. Choking occurs when a foreign body, such as a sweet in children, or a large lump of food in adults, has been inhaled and impacts at the level of the larynx. The patient should be turned head downwards and vigorously thumped. If this is unsuccessful, the only life-saving measure is laryngotomy.

Stridor in a young child is usually due to croup but it also occurs in the much rarer condition of acute epiglottitis. Recognition of the latter is all-important, since complete obstruction can be provoked by an attempt to inspect the pharynx. Acute epiglottitis can be distinguished from croup by the presence of a high fever and the toxic appearance of the child. Immediate admission is essential. This is also necessary in a young child with croup if the time-honoured treatment with inhaled steam has failed to give relief.

Acute obstruction may follow the sting of a wasp which has entered the mouth, particularly when fruit is being eaten. Adrenaline and an antihistamine must be given by intra-muscular injection as soon as possible, failing which laryngotomy may be required.

Hospital admission must be arranged in any patient with acute dyspnoea who appears to be in danger. The ambulance service must be notified that oxygen will need to be brought into the house. While awaiting the ambulance, the general practitioner must give whatever treatment he can. If he carries a portable oxygen cylinder, he should give the patient oxygen. There are no dangers from its administration in any patient with acute dyspnoea.

If time permits, a more detailed examination should be carried out to identify the underlying cause in order that this can be treated appropriately. Two conditions which frequently cause acute, severe dyspnoea and which may be difficult to distinguish are pulmonary oedema and asthma. The importance of the differential diagnosis lies in the contrasting treatment which each requires. In acute pulmonary oedema respiratory depressants, such as morphine or heroin, may be indicated, whereas in asthma all depressants, especially opiates, carry grave dangers. On the other hand, bronchodilators, even those which are selective for beta-2 receptors, are contraindicated in pulmonary oedema because they may increase heart rate or induce dysrhythmia. In some patients with pulmonary oedema, wheeze may be a prominent feature ('cardiac asthma'), and if the general practitioner cannot decide whether the patient has pulmonary oedema or severe asthma, the safest treatment is an intravenous injection of aminophylline and an intramuscular injection of a diuretic.

Anaphylactic shock, while not presenting as acute dyspnoea, is usually accompanied by intense bronchoconstriction. It is liable to occur after the injection of penicillin, contrast media used in radiology, or allergen solutions used in desensitization. Adrenaline must be injected immediately, followed by an antihistamine.

In acute asthma the principal cause of dyspnoea is muscle constriction and this usually responds to a bronchodilator administered either by inhalation or by injection. The agents most commonly used are selective beta-2 agonists, such as salbutamol and terbutaline. Adrenaline by subcutaneous injection has been almost entirely replaced by these newer drugs but some clinicians nevertheless consider that it still has great value, provided that it is given subcutaneously, slowly and with repeated monitoring of the pulse rate. Adrenaline appears to be superior to beta-2 agonists in its ability to counteract mucosal oedema.

If severe asthma has been present for more than a few hours and has been preceded by progressive deterioration over the previous 24 hours, it must be assumed that mucosal oedema and, probably, intraluminal plugging are the main causes of airflow obstruction. Though subjective benefit usually follows the nebulization of salbutamol or terbutaline, it will often be found that PEF measured on completion of the procedure falls far short of the patient's highest value attained when in remission. This deficit represents airflow obstruction which, though potentially reversible, can be abolished only by a corticosteroid. An intravenous or intramuscular injection of hydrocortisone (200 mgm) must be given, together with a large initial dose of oral prednisolone (60 mg in an adult and not less than 20 mg in a child).

Since the initial dose of corticosteroid will have no effect upon reducing airflow obstruction for several hours, a decision must be made whether or not to admit the patient for further treatment and observation. If there is any doubt or if the doctor is unable to see the patient for review within a few hours, admission is advisable.

Anxiety-induced dyspnoea

Mere reassurance that the doctor can find no evidence of organic disease is seldom effective in abolishing the patient's symptoms. It may give rise to the conviction that the doctor was wrong or that the symptoms are caused by a disease which can only be detected by referral to a specialist. The patient may even misconstrue the well-intentioned reassurance as implying that the doctor considers the symptoms to be imaginary.

It is essential, therefore, to give a careful and sympathetic explanation of how awareness of the act of breathing can occur in the absence of disease. Enquiry should always be made whether the patient has already begun to fear that the symptoms may signify heart or lung disease and very often this proves to be the case. If the patient has noticed a tendency to sigh frequently, this will make it easier to explain how a vicious cycle can become established. A chest radiograph and ECG are valuable investigations provided that it is made clear to the patient that their purpose is to confirm the absence of organic disease.

Further reading

Howell, J.B.L. and Campbell, E.J.M. (1966): *Breathlessness*. Oxford: Blackwell Scientific Publications

Gregg, I. and Clark, T.J.H. (1978): Respiratory system. In *Scientific Foundations of Family Medicine*, ed. Fry, J., Gambrill, E. and Smith, R. London: Heinemann pp 441–61

Forgacs, P. (1978): *Lung Sounds*. London: Baillière Tindall

Clark, T.J.H. (1981): *Clinical Investigation of Respiratory Disease*. London: Chapman and Hall

Appendix
Assessment of airflow obstruction by measurement of peak expiratory flow

Estimation of the severity and reversibility of airflow obstruction is essential for rational and effective treatment of asthma, chronic bronchitis and emphysema. No reliance can be placed upon auscultatory signs, such as rhonchi or wheeze, which may sometimes even be dangerously misleading. The presence of airflow obstruction can be identified, and its severity assessed with accuracy, only by means of tests which provide an objective measurement of airflow.

Of the various tests available, peak expiratory flow (PEF) best meets the needs of the general practitioner. Yet it is only within the last few years that the use of peak flow meters, which were first introduced more than 30 years ago, has become commonplace in general practice. The majority of general practitioners now possess peak flow meters, though there is evidence that some make little or no use of them[1], and undoubtedly many are unaware of the applications of PEF measurements, even though these were fully described as long ago as 1964[2].

Peak expiratory flow

Peak expiratory flow denotes the maximum velocity of airflow at the very beginning of a forced expiration, and is expressed in litres per minute (l/min). Although it might seem more logical to express PEF in millilitres per second, since the peak rate of flow is sustained for only a fraction of a second, the notional expression of PEF in litres per minute has become established by convention and has the advantage that values can be expressed as whole numbers. Essentially, PEF is an index of the patency and structural integrity of the bronchi but, in common with all other tests employing forced expiration, it is also determined by the dimensions of the thorax and the muscles which act on it. Hence, levels of normal PEF are lower in children than in adults and are higher in men than in women of the same age and height (the latter being the most convenient index of the size of the thorax).

Performance of the test

The level of PEF which a subject can achieve is highly dependent upon the effort made in performing the test. It is all-important, therefore, that the subject is exhorted to take a maximum inspiration and then to expire as hard and as fast as possible into the meter without any escape of air between the mouth and the mouthpiece. If a subject has never previously carried out the test, the correct manner of performing it must be demonstrated. This is especially important in children: with encouragement, children as young as five years are capable of performing the test. When it is clear that the subject has mastered the technique of the test, the highest of three measurements should be recorded as his or her PEF.

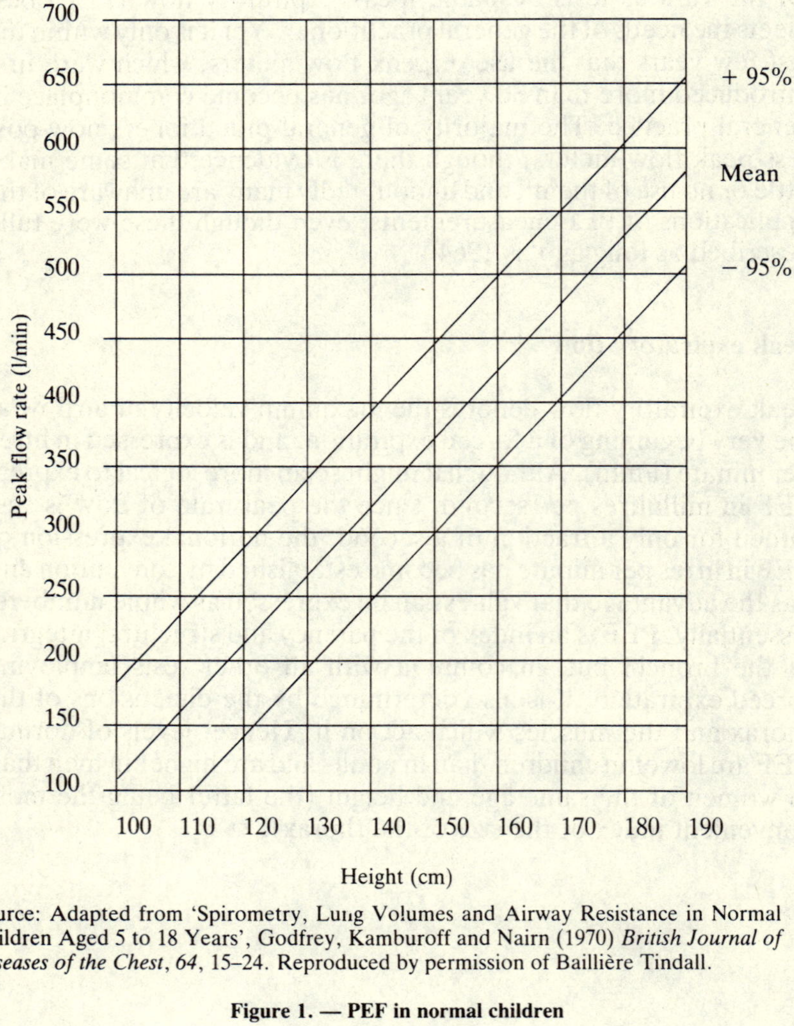

Source: Adapted from 'Spirometry, Lung Volumes and Airway Resistance in Normal Children Aged 5 to 18 Years', Godfrey, Kamburoff and Nairn (1970) *British Journal of Diseases of the Chest*, *64*, 15–24. Reproduced by permission of Baillière Tindall.

Figure 1. — PEF in normal children

Evaluation of PEF

The influence of bodysize and, in adults, of age and sex must be taken into account when assessing the normality or otherwise of a subject's PEF. This is done by comparing the observed value with that which a normal child of the same height or a normal adult of the same sex, age and height can be expected to achieve.
Predicted values of PEF can be found either in tables or from nomograms. The latter show the mean regressions of PEF in normal subjects. In children, the relationship between PEF and height is linear and is independent of age or sex[3]. The nomogram shown in Figure 1 shows normal values of PEF in children between the ages of 5 and 15 years. During adolescence, however, there is a steep rise in PEF which is greater in males than in females. This sex difference is maintained throughout adult life. The relationship between PEF and age in men and women is curvilinear, rising to a maximum level between the ages of 25 and 35 years and thereafter declining gradually with advancing age. The nomogram in Figure 2 is based on unpublished data in 211 men and 219 women between the ages of 15 and 85 years who had never smoked and who satisfied other strict criteria of normality.
The nomogram for adults which is currently issued by the distributors of the Wright peak flow meter and the Mini-Wright meter was based upon an earlier study[4], in which there were few subjects over the age of 60 years. Therefore, when using that nomogram for predicting normal values above this age, it had to be assumed that the gradient of decline of PEF was the same as that in younger subjects. The later study has confirmed that assumption and, in due course, the new nomogram (Figure 2) will replace the one which has been in use up to the present.
In the long term management of asthma, the highest PEF which a patient has previously attained is an invaluable index against which subsequent measurements can be compared. In children account must be taken of growth and only if the previous 'personal best' PEF was recorded within the last six months should it be used for comparison.

Types of peak flow meter

The first instrument suitable for measuring PEF in clinical practice, the Hildebrandt pneumometer, was introduced in Germany in 1955. At about the same time in Britain, Wright designed a peak flow meter for the Medical Research Council which became commercially available in 1959[5]. In 1973 a cheaper instrument, the peak flow gauge, was introduced. It began to enjoy wider use in

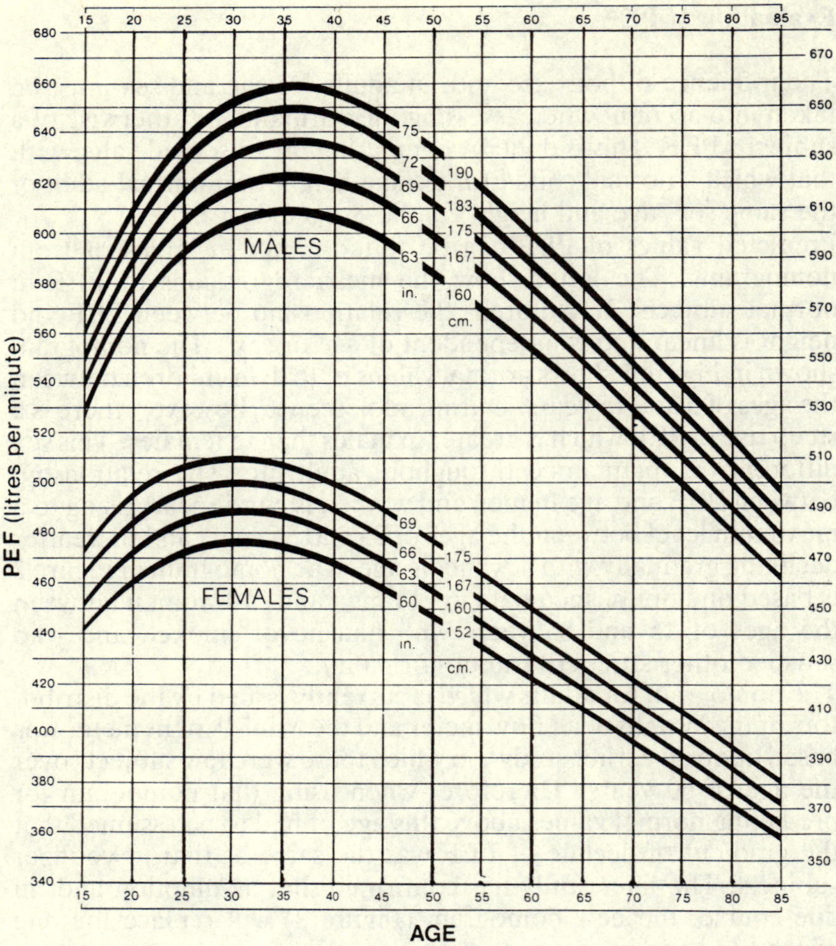

Figure 2. — Peak expiratory flow in normal adults

general practice but proved to be inaccurate and was rendered obsolete when Wright designed his Mini-meter in 1978[6].

The Wright meter is a robust, precision-made instrument. Each is individually checked for its calibration and should maintain its accuracy for many years despite intensive use. The Mini-Wright meter, on the other hand, was originally conceived as a much cheaper instrument which could either be loaned to or bought by patients so as to measure and record PEF themselves. It soon began to be distributed widely to general practitioners by pharmaceutical companies, with the result that the Mini-meter, and not the Wright meter, has become standard equipment in most general practices.

It is important to appreciate that it was never intended that Mini-meters, which are mass-produced, should possess the same accuracy as Wright meters. Only a small sample from each batch produced is checked for calibration: consequently, individual instruments do not give identical values. This is of little consequence when Mini-meters are used by patients to record their PEF, but it assumes greater importance when they are used for diagnosis and assessment. Although one Mini-meter when new should not differ from another or from a Wright meter by more than ± 5%, in the course of time it may lose its accuracy, and, unless the doctor possesses a Wright meter against which its calibration can be checked, there will be no means of knowing this.

Applications of PEF measurements

Airflow obstruction is the commonest cause of dyspnoea encountered in general practice. Measurement of PEF is not only essential for assessing its severity but it also enables the general practitioner to identify the mechanisms which have given rise to it and, hence, to treat patients with airflow obstruction on a rational and effective basis.

While airflow obstruction is the fundamental disorder common to asthma, chronic bronchitis and emphysema, an important distinction must be made between what can be reversed by treatment, as in asthma, and what is irreversible, being caused by structural damage of the bronchi as in chronic bronchitis, or of the lung parenchyma as in emphysema.

Variable (reversible) airflow obstruction

Intermittent or persistent airflow obstruction, which can be reversed by appropriate treatment, is the cardinal abnormality of asthma. The term 'bronchospasm', which is still frequently used, should be discarded since it implies that airflow obstruction is caused by muscle constriction and it ignores the contribution of other mechanisms. These comprise oedema and exudation of the bronchial mucosa and excess secretion of mucus, but, unlike muscle constriction, they respond poorly, if at all, to bronchodilators, and can be reversed only by a corticosteroid. Many of the problems in the management of asthma are due to this inflammatory component of airflow obstruction: surprisingly, it has only recently come to be widely recognized, though studies carried out more than 20 years ago in general practice clearly demonstrated its importance[7].

Irreversible airflow obstruction

In chronic bronchitis, airflow obstruction is due to insidious but progressive structural damage of the bronchi, caused by a prolonged irritation (notably by smoking and dusty occupations) or recurrent infection. A progressively larger number of the smallest, distal airways become obliterated and airflow obstruction is enhanced by excessive secretion of mucus. In emphysema, which may sometimes occur on its own but much more commonly co-exists with chronic bronchitis, airflow obstruction is due to the lack of elastic support in the smallest airways, which is normally provided by the surrounding lung parenchyma.

Irreversible airflow obstruction may be present in some patients with asthma, due either to co-existent chronic bronchitis or to structural changes arising from prolonged, unrelieved mucosal inflammation and plugging. Such patients exhibit variability of airflow obstruction but the highest value of PEF which they can attain never approximates to their predicted values.

Assessment of reversibility

If PEF is measured before and five minutes after inhalation of an aerosol of a rapidly acting bronchodilator, such as isoprenaline or rimiterol, the amount by which it has risen is an indication of how much airflow obstruction is due to muscle constriction. If the post-bronchodilator PEF is much lower than predicted, the deficit must be due either to mucosal inflammation or plugging (both being potentially reversible), to irreversible obstruction, or to a combination of these components. If a patient's maximum PEF has previously been ascertained, any difference between it and the post-bronchodilator value must be due to inflammation. Similar considerations apply in assessing the response to a nebulized bronchodilator in an acute asthmatic attack.

It has already been emphasized that a corticosteroid is the only treatment which can suppress mucosal inflammation or eliminate mucus plugs. Therefore, the ultimate distinction between reversible airflow obstruction which has not responded to a bronchodilator and irreversible obstruction is by a trial of corticosteroid. It is now recognized that many patients who are regarded as having chronic bronchitis may, in reality, have asthma, especially of the late-onset 'intrinsic' type, though in many there will be a large irreversible component in addition to that which is reversible. The steps which should be taken to distinguish between reversible and irreversible airflow obstruction can be represented in the form of a decision tree (Figure 3).

Frequency of measurements in long-term follow-up

PEF should be measured when any patient with asthma, chronic bronchitis or emphysema is seen for the first time and, thereafter, whenever there has been a change of circumstances or if it appears that symptoms are not adequately controlled by current treatment. PEF needs to be measured more frequently in the follow-up of patients with asthma than in those with chronic bronchitis and emphysema because of the much greater variability of their airflow obstruction.

Regular, sequential measurements are far more informative than occasional measurements, especially when they are used to assess the effects of treatment. A characteristic feature of asthma is worsening of symptoms during the night. However, a patient may have had severe breathlessness at night or on waking, yet a few hours later can achieve a level of PEF close to his or her personal best.

The only way to ascertain the variability of airflow obstruction between consultations is to teach patients to measure and record PEF themselves. This also helps patients to gain a better understanding of asthma and the purpose and correct use of their treatment. Impending deterioration can sometimes be detected by a gradual fall in PEF before a patient becomes aware of any worsening of symptoms.

Assessment of nebulized bronchodilators in acute asthma

The considerable subjective relief which is often conferred by a nebulized bronchodilator may not be matched by a commensurate reduction in airflow obstruction[8]. This situation, if not recognized, carries potential dangers. Therefore, on completion of the procedure, measurement of PEF is essential. If it is found that there is

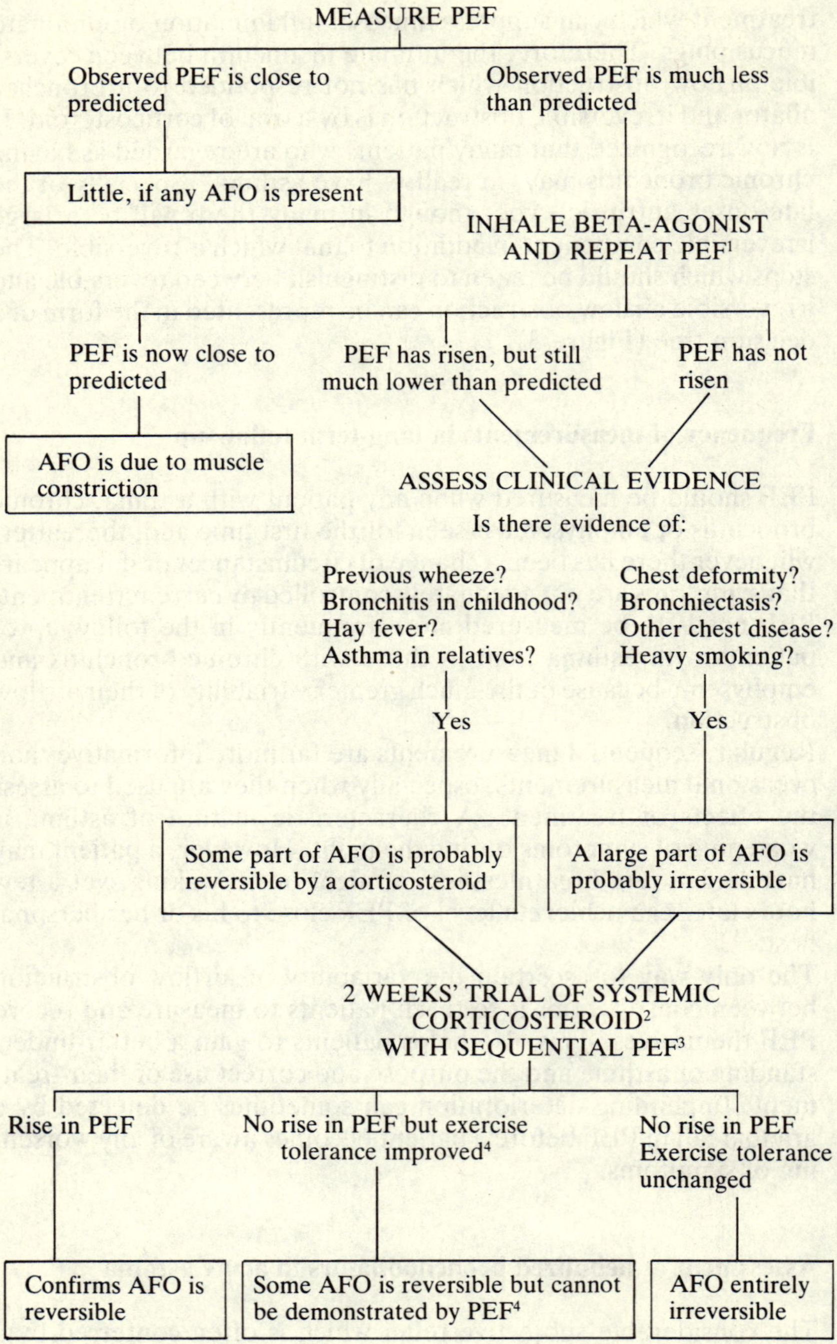

Figure 3. — Schematic representation of the steps that must be taken to identify the mechanisms causing airflow obstruction (AFO)

Steps to be taken — capital letters; Inferences — in boxes

Notes to Figure 3

1. If a rapidly acting beta-agonist aerosol is used, e.g. isoprenaline or rimiterol, any rise of PEF should be complete within five minutes. If salbutamol or terbutaline are used, maximum PEF is not attained until about 10 minutes after inhalation.
2. Prednisolone in a dose of at least 40 mg per day (20 mg per day in a child less than 10 years).
3. Ideally, the patient should record his/her PEF at least twice daily in order to show whether an overall rise in PEF occurs, and a reduction of nocturnal or early morning asthma.
4. Since measurement of PEF entails forced expiration, a reduction of AFO may not be demonstrable by this means if there is a severe degree of structural damage. In this situation the most reliable index of response to a trial of corticosteroid is exercise tolerance.

a large difference between post-nebulization PEF and the patient's predicted or previously highest recorded PEF, it can be inferred that mucosal inflammation or plugging are present and must be treated by a corticosteroid.

Summary

The measurement of PEF to assess the degree and reversibility of airflow obstruction should be an integral part of the clinical diagnosis and management of asthma, chronic bronchitis, and emphysema. Patients with these diseases can only be managed effectively if the mechanisms causing their airflow obstruction have been identified. This is possible by means of inferences based upon observation of the response of PEF to a bronchodilator or corticosteroid.

References

[1] Carne, S. (1985): What do others do? *Modern Medicine*, *46*

[2] Gregg, I. (1964): The measurement of peak expiratory flow rate and its applications in general practice. *Journal of the Royal College of General Practitioners*, *7*, 199–214

[3] Godfrey, S., Kamburoff, P.L. and Nairn, J.R. (1970): Spirometry, lung volumes and airway resistance in normal children aged 5 to 18 years. *British Journal of Diseases of the Chest, 64*, 15

[4] Gregg, I. and Nunn, A.J. (1973): Peak expiratory flow in normal subjects. *British Medical Journal*, *3*, 282–4

[5] Wright, B.M. and McKerrow, C.B. (1959): Maximum forced expiratory flow rate as a measure of ventilatory capacity. *British Medical Journal*, *2*, 1041

[6] Wright, B.M. (1978): A miniature Wright peak-flow meter. *British Medical Journal*, *2*, 1627–8

[7] Gregg, I. (1965): Towards a better understanding of chronic bronchitis and asthma. Proceedings of the Royal Society of Medicine, *58*, 232–4

[8] Gregg, I. (1982): Misplaced confidence in nebulised bronchodilators in severe asthmatic attacks. *British Medical Journal*, *284*, 46–7

3.30
The patient complaining of spitting blood

J.G.R. Howie

Spitting of blood is not a common complaint, being described by Hodgkin[1] as present ('without obvious cause') in only 1.4 patients per 1,000 per year although also part of a number of other named major and minor respiratory illnesses. In the study of Wadsworth, Butterfield and Blaney[2] only 2 of 2,000 adult patients reported coughing up blood in a two-week period, and in the Third National Morbidity Study[3] 'haemoptysis' is recorded as the cause of 1.3 per 1,000 episodes of general practice illness and 0.9 per 1,000 consultations. Hodgkin estimates that the ratio of serious : non-serious causes of the complaint is 1 : 7. In an unpublished series of 7,500 new consultations for respiratory illness, haemoptysis was recorded on 22 occasions. In these patients the provisional diagnosis made at the initial consultation was coryza (four times), bronchitis (three times), cough, sinusitis, influenza, chronic bronchitis and pneumonia (twice each) and tracheitis, pharyngitis and laryngitis (once each).

Presentation

Patients with this symptom present in many ways ranging from the expected to the surprising. The first of these is the expected one where a clearly frightened and anxious patient calls at the surgery or makes an out-of-hours phone call to report the occurrence as soon as it has happened. This event may be part of a previously unreported acute illness or may be a new development in an illness already under the doctor's care. When the symptom occurs while the patient is in apparently good health it is usually a particularly potent cause of alarm.

A second common but perhaps surprising presenting situation is when a patient who has coughed up blood on one or perhaps several occasions consults the doctor about apparently less important related or unrelated symptoms without mentioning the occurrence of this event. It is extraordinary how even apparently comprehensive history taking may fail to elicit this truth and the doctor must ask directly whether blood has been seen in the spit if he wishes to ensure finding this out. Patients who wish to suppress this information may be brought to the surgery by relatives or the doctor may receive tip-offs from the family in advance of an arranged consultation.

A third presentation is that of a patient who consults about a respiratory (or cardiovascular) illness in which spitting of blood has been a minor feature which the patient has not thought of particular significance in the setting of an acute illness. An acute or severe cough, chest pain or sore throat, the copious production of phlegm or previous episodes of production of blood-stained spit may be found to be present and usually dominating the illness. Even if it is less obvious, a degree of anxiety and wish for reassurance are often present, though sometimes only after the doctor's interest in the symptom has become evident.

Causes

Acute respiratory infection. – A variety of acute infective illnesses classified at first consultation as anything from coryza and sinusitis through pharyngitis and acute bronchitis to pneumonia may include spitting of blood in their symptomatology. In some cases the symptom may reflect no more than the trauma of coughing, in others a component of an acute inflammatory exudate and in others part of the process of resolving inflammation.

Other respiratory illnesses. – This group contains illnesses sharing different etiologies. The first etiological division is *infection*, with tuberculosis probably still the single most important diagnosis for consideration. Bronchiectasis also comes within the category of infection and is one of the few causes of recurring small haemoptyses. The second category is *neoplasm*. Either simple bronchial adenoma or bronchial carcinoma may bleed quite profusely and this symptom is a common mode of presentation of these tumours. Finally chronic bronchitis may be associated with either staining of the sputum or frank haemoptysis.

Cardiovascular illness. – Illnesses in this group can again be conveniently thought of under sub-headings.

Cardiac causes. – Till recently mitral stenosis was probably the illness most commonly associated in student teaching with coughing up blood. This condition is uncommon nowadays but spitting blood remains a common accompaniment of left-sided cardiac failure.

Vascular causes. – The most important disorder under this heading is the pulmonary embolism usually occurring in association with deep venous thrombosis following surgery or trauma or after myocardial infarction.

Others. – For completeness spitting of blood following gastro-intestinal and nasal bleeding require to be mentioned. These causes, along with disorders of the mouth, are easily diagnosed provided they are thought of. Blood dyscrasias may occasionally present in this way.

History and examination

History taking and examination in this group of patients follows a more traditional pattern than in many general-practice situations, this reflecting the comparatively major significance of the symptom.

Symptoms. – The first essential is to identify whether the blood is from the gastro-intestinal or respiratory tracts or from the mouth or nasal passages. Leaving aside the obvious larger intestinal bleeds, small quantities of intestinal bleeding will probably be of dark altered blood and normally associated with nausea. Respiratory bleeding will more often be fresh and not infrequently described as pink or frothy in nature. The severity of any related coughing and a description of the contents of any associated sputum should be recorded. The presence of previous episodes should be noted as well as any history of weight loss, the smoking habits of the patient and any previous inoculation against tuberculosis. Additional enquiry relating to symptoms of cardiovascular disease may need to be made along usual lines. Ankle swelling, bilateral or unilateral, breathlessness and chest pain may be important symptoms, a past history of rheumatic fever may still be relevant and any recent serious illness or surgical procedure may be associated with deep venous thrombosis.

Examination. – Careful examination is required. Weight loss, heavy nicotine staining of skin, or finger clubbing hint at a serious condition. A cotton-wool probe passed into the nostrils or auriscope examination of the nasal passages may identify a local source of bleeding and a look at the mouth and throat will identify lesions at this level. Careful ausculation of the chest must include the apical as well as basal areas and separate ausculation for cardiac abnormality – particularly mitral stenosis – is essential. More general examination of the cardiovascular system may also be appropriate. Unilateral ankle oedema is, of course, particularly significant and evidence of acute illness (breathlessness and pyrexia) will obviously be relevant.

Investigation. – Information from investigation will not normally be available at a new consultation for this complaint.

Management

Priorities of management become more physically and less psychologically slanted when serious illness is a significant possibility. In patients spitting blood, referral and observation take priority over prescription of medicine, and consideration of concurrent or coincidental psychosocial problems become very much secondary considerations. Reassurance and support, of course, remain important supplements to any management decision and may require to be offered to relatives as much as to patients. Having already grouped the causes of spitting blood in a framework relevant to general practice, it seems appropriate to make general comments on management under the same headings.

Acute respiratory infection. – When an acute and normally self-limiting respiratory infection is identified the initial management should be that of the acute episode. Follow-up should be arranged, at which time appropriate clinical judgment will help to determine whether further investigation is required. The younger the patient, the more acute the original infection, the less suspicious the details of the original symptom and the fewer the features suggesting risk of serious disease – then the greater probability of justifying a decision to take no action. When doubt exists, a normal chest x-ray, erythrocyte sedimentation rate (ESR), and estimation of haemoglobin will often provide doctor and patient with the necessary reassurance. The limitations of these procedures are important and are discussed below.

Other respiratory illnesses. – Spitting of blood not thought to be covered by causes described in the previous section, and not apparently due to cardiovascular illness or oral disease, will normally warrant investigation. Although some doctors will feel reassured by a normal chest x-ray, perhaps backed by a normal ESR value, more are impressed by the frequency with which such reassurances are followed within months by development of the typical picture of malignant disease. Patients in whom malignant disease or tuberculosis cannot be excluded with some confidence should probably be referred directly to a chest specialist. In an established case of chronic bronchitis or bronchiectasis the doctor must decide whether spitting of blood represents the established disease or may be due to new disease. Once again this involves the use of judgment in assessing probability. New cases of chronic bronchitis or bronchiectasis may be diagnosed during investigation of otherwise unexplained spitting of blood.

Explanation of diagnosis and of the significance of treatment to patients spitting blood is a difficult but important part of management. Few doctors claim to be at ease with this and careful preliminary explorations of the patient's insight, fears and desire to hear bad as well as good news will often make the doctor's decision on what to tell an easier one. The techniques of counselling are often helpful in this process.

Cardiovascular and other illnesses. – Nose bleeding is discussed in Chapter 3.24. The management of spitting of blood due to heart disease (whether due to failure or to valvular disease), gastrointestinal bleeding and oral disease is that of the underlying disorder. The outstanding dilemma in this group is in the patient with possible pulmonary embolism, and at the present time the balance of opinion appears to be in favour of short-term anticoagulants being used on an inpatient basis.

Conclusions

Spitting of blood is a relatively uncommon symptom in general practice. Although more often due to simple than serious disorders, it is a frequent presenting symptom of major illness of respiratory or cardiovascular etiology. Knowledge of the probability of serious illness being present in different groups of patients considerably simplifies the making of a decision to refer or not refer for investigation.

References

1 Hodgkin, K. (1973): *Towards Earlier Diagnosis: A Guide to General Practice. 3rd ed.* Edinburgh: Churchill Livingstone

2 Wadsworth, M.E.J., Butterfield, W.J.H. and Blaney, R. (1971): *Health and Sickness: the Choice of Treatment.* London: Tavistock Publications

3 Royal College of General Practitioners, Office of Population Censuses and Surveys, Department of Health and Social Security (1986): *Morbidity Statistics from General Practice 1981–82*. HMSO Series MB5 No. 1

3.31 The patient complaining of chest pain

Aubrey Colling

The physician who has suffered the unpleasant experience of a patient dropping dead soon after being reassured about the harmless nature of his chest pain is the oft-quoted example of how a skilled doctor, even after taking a careful history and making full investigations, is sometimes unable to make an accurate diagnosis. Nevertheless, the general practitioner cannot avoid making decisions and he must give practical advice consistent with the most likely cause of his patient's chest pain, while at the same time avoiding unnecessary alarm. Many times he will relieve his patient's anxiety but add to his own.

Despite this association with serious disease, chest pain is a common experience to everyone. Dunnell and Cartwright[1] interviewed 1,410 people chosen at random and found that 5 per cent had suffered chest pain in the previous two weeks. There was no difference in incidence between men and women, and it was equally common at all ages in adults. Chest pain is an unusual complaint in children, in distinct contrast to abdominal pain (Figure 1).[2]

An analysis of presenting symptoms in a rural practice in Warwickshire[3] showed that 2 per cent of new consultations were for pain in the chest, and were commoner in the lower social classes. A similar survey in London[2] found that 3 per cent of patients had chest pain as the predominant symptom and in less than half of these patients was the doctor able to make an accurate diagnosis. Such lack of precision is common to other painful conditions such as backache, headache and abdominal pain. In the same survey the reported incidence of new complaints of chest pain was 37.3 per 1,000 practice population each year. A similar figure (33.4) was found by Frank in a five-year study of anterior chest pain in general practice.[4] It follows that a general practitioner will be faced by a patient whose main complaint is chest pain about twice a week, only a fraction of those experiencing chest pain at that time in the community.

Clearly then, most people suffering chest pain either receive no treatment or treat themselves. Analgesics and antacids are among the commonest of home remedies and it is unusual for patients not to have tried one or other before seeking medical care. The use of analgesics can sometimes cause gastric irritation and lead to symptoms which add to the diagnostic confusion.

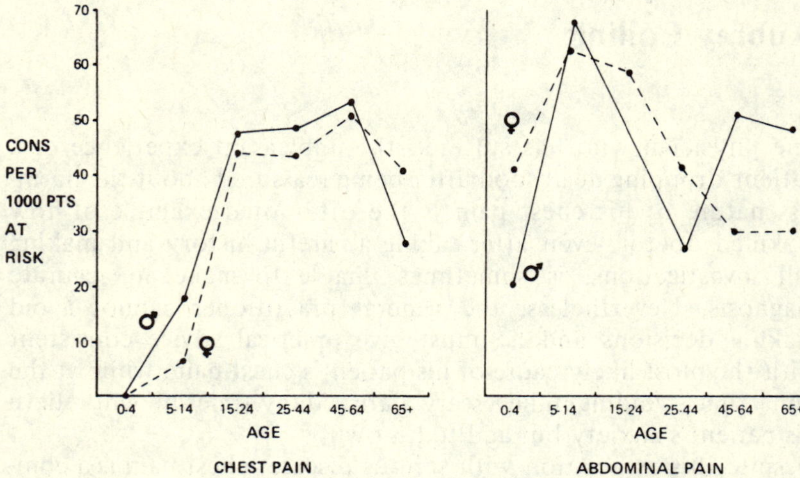

Figure 1. – Age incidence of chest and abdominal pain in patients in general practice

Presentation

When the cause of chest pain is in doubt, examination is rarely of help. It is therefore important to spend time eliciting a precise history to determine what the patient is trying to say and to resist early resort to the stethoscope and sphygmomanometer. Many patients have difficulty describing what they feel; a doctor must give patients time to muster words, sighs and grunts, and he will save his own time if he puts down his pen, sits back in his chair, and listens carefully and watches intently for a minute or two.

It is a combination of verbal expression and non-verbal gestures that gives the doctor his clues; a single hand placed flat across the front of the chest in ischaemic heart disease, sometimes a stationary clenched fist; the slightly flexed fingers pointing to the lower sternum or moving up and down the sternum in oesophageal and gastric disease. A full hand placed over the left or right costal margins is unlikely to be related to the heart. The hands may indicate some radiation of pain, even though the patient does not verbalize, a fleeting movement which may be missed if the doctor is writing at the time. In most cases the diagnosis will not be in doubt but there remains a sufficiently large group in which the diagnosis may be extremely difficult and which poses special problems for the general practitioner in deciding whether to allow his patient to continue to work.

It is most important to assess each patient's response to pain. The general practitioner is in a fortunate position as he may be able to recall a patient's behaviour in a previous illness. It is now considered that a person's pain threshold, that is, the point at which a sensation is perceived as pain, varies only within narrow limits from person to person, yet pain tolerance and the reaction to pain vary considerably.

The World Health Organization[5] has described the pain of cardiac ischaemia as a pain occurring in the front of the chest at the mid or upper sternal level which may radiate to the left arm or both arms, round the chest or into the jaw. It is described by the patient as being tight, heavy, constricting, crushing or even numbing or burning. It can sometimes begin above the left nipple or at any of the sites of radiation. Ischaemic pain is not lancinating or throbbing. It usually lasts a few minutes unless effort is continued. It rarely lasts only a few seconds, or more than half-an-hour unless a myocardial infarction has occurred. It is unusual for it to be relieved by continuation of effort. Tenderness over the site of pain or aggravation by arm movements is against an ischaemic cause. Failure to recognize that ischaemic pain can begin to the left of the sternum in many patients can lead to serious errors of judgment.

It is important to establish the relationship of chest pain to exertion; if it is ischaemic in origin there is little difficulty in diagnosis in most cases, though the mildness of effort angina can sometimes be misleading. It can be masked by epigastric pain or a feeling of indigestion with belching. Sometimes it can be precipitated by emotion, such as watching a wrestling contest or an athletic programme on television, and is commonly aggravated by cold weather and by heavy meals. Some patients, however, may be able to walk or garden without difficulty yet experience typical angina at rest in relation to emotion or even without obvious cause. Episodic angina of this kind is often severe and lasts longer than angina of effort. When patients have previously had a myocardial infarction they often fear a recurrence when they first experience such attacks at rest and may call their doctor. If the doctor arrives very quickly he may wrongly attribute the pain to a further infarction. In these patients the electrocardiogram will show ischaemic changes but they will resolve over 15 minutes or more after an injection of heroin, morphine or pethidine. Other patients suffer angina when lying down. There remains the perplexing problem of angina pectoris in a patient either with known gall-bladder or gastro-intestinal disease, or with symptoms suggesting such conditions. Confusion can also arise with pain from cervical spondylosis. It has been said that when serious consideration has to be given to such differential diagnosis there is a strong possibility that both conditions exist.[6]

The presentation of pain arising from chest muscles or the cervical spine is usually clear, though occasionally pain from the lowest cervical roots can cause pain much lower in the chest than expected, either anteriorly or posteriorly, without any associated pain in the neck. It can usually be reproduced by movement of the cervical spine.

The pain of pericarditis can be overlooked by too hasty an assessment. It has no certain distinguishing features. It is often made worse by deep breathing and may be relieved by sitting forward but can be precordial and constant, uninfluenced by respiration and made worse by movement. Pain from respiratory infection can be very severe, the central pain of laryngotracheitis and the pleuritic pain of lung infections are usually clear but pulmonary emboli and pneumothorax are often forgotten unless dyspnoea is a prominent feature. Sometimes severe reflex spasm of the chest muscles occurs in pleurisy which may distract attention from the underlying cause.

A deep retrosternal pain, often associated with anxiety and a sense of impending death, can be caused by pulmonary hypertension and may be seen in severe asthma, acute or chronic chest infections, and high altitude dyspnoea. Similar distension of the pulmonary arteries occurs in pulmonary embolism. Pulmonary hypertension is caused by constriction of small pulmonary arteries and consequent dilatation of the pulmonary arteries due to low PO_2.

Differentiating between cardiac and alimentary pain may be difficult since oesophageal pain can resemble myocardial ischaemia in both severity and location.

A prospective survey of hospital patients whose primary presenting symptom was chest pain was made by Bennett and Atkinson in Worcester[6] (figure 2). Although most patients were found to have heart disease, nearly one-quarter of these cases of chest pain had an alimentary cause and 1 in 7 had both. General practitioners were correct in 67 per cent of their diagnoses. These authors stress that the clinical features of oesophageal pain may resemble closely those of cardiac pain with identical radiation and precipitation by exercise or emotion. The most diagnostically useful features were dyspnoea associated with cardiac pain and acid reflux into the mouth with oesophageal pain, but these two symptoms, together with faintness, heartburn, vomiting, dysphagia and sweating, all occurred in some patients of both groups.

Spontaneous rupture of the oesophagus due to violent vomiting will cause severe pain in the epigastrium or lower retrosternal area, as severe as a dissecting aneurysm.

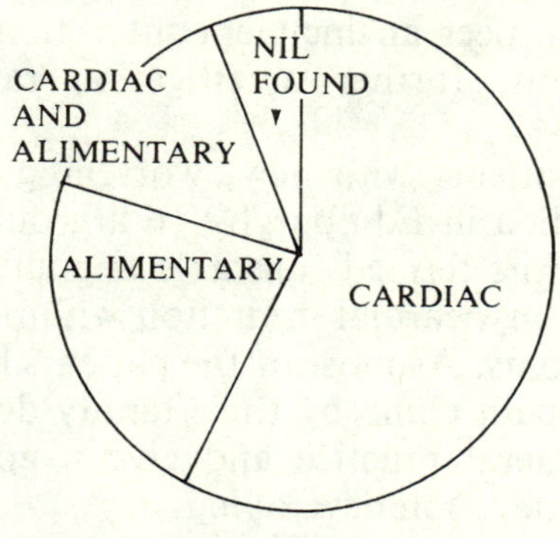

Figure 2. – Causes of chest pain in hospital patients (Bennett and Atkinson[6])

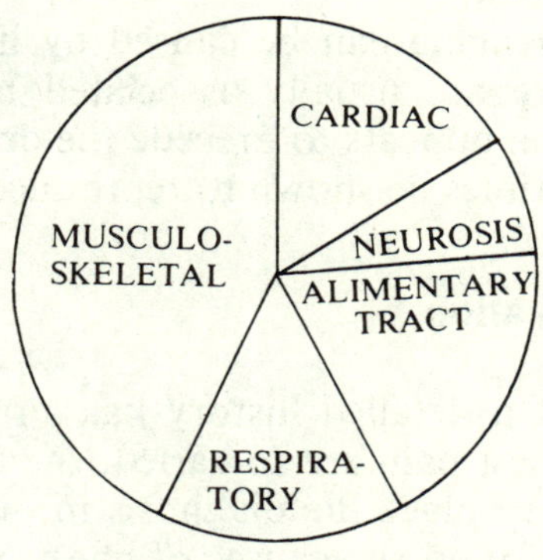

Figure 3. – Causes of chest pain in patients in general practice (Frank[4])

Ischaemic pain can occur centrally in the back at the level of the scapulae. Its relation to exertion may not be suspected by the doctor, or recognized by the patient unless especially perspicacious or intelligent.

One of the most worrying presentations in general practice is angina of recent onset, or worsening angina in a patient who already suffers from angina. Both are known to presage an infarction in a certain number of patients. In a study of nearly 2,000 patients with myocardial infarction on Teesside[7], 20 per cent of those who survived to give evidence complained of new or worsening angina in the days or weeks beforehand. Many had other symptoms such as unusual tiredness, unusual breathlessness, indigestion or vague chest pains. Such premonitory symptoms are now well recognized as part of the 'pre-infarction syndrome' and were shown to be several times commoner in patients than in a control group of people matched for age and sex who had not complained to their doctor. Unfortunately, even though a general practitioner may suspect an incipient infarction from such pre-infarction symptoms, further investigation rarely reveals any abnormality.

The outcome of patients with new, worsening or exacerbations of angina was studied in Edinburgh.[8] In a group of 167 patients with what the authors termed 'unstable angina' they found that 1 in 6 developed a myocardial infarction within three months of the onset of symptoms. As most of the patients had been referred to a special chest pain clinic by their family doctor, the figures are relevant to general practice and give a good guide to the probability of an infarction developing.

Printzmetal angina is an unusual form which occurs at rest, is not precipitated by exertion and is associated with elevation rather than depression of S-T segment on ECG. It is probably caused by coronary artery spasm.

A form of pseudoangina can be caused by hyperventilation. In these patients there are usually associated nervous symptoms, and hyperventilation appears to precede the development of chest pain and can sometimes be shown to reproduce it.

History and examination

The importance of a detailed history has already been stressed. As the causes of chest pain are so varied, the general practitioner must first attempt to place the diagnosis in one of several broad categories. Frank[4] found the causes of chest pain to fall into the groups shown in figure 3. Such preliminary sorting is extremely important in the day-to-day management of patients in a doctor's surgery. Almost half of such patients suffer from musculoskeletal pain. Anxiety about its possible relation to heart disease is usually the reason for the consultation, and reassurance rather than treatment with drugs is all that is necessary. Chest pain due to respiratory disease is usually fairly obvious. The main difficulty is to differentiate between pain of cardiac origin and that arising elsewhere, and in particular to decide whether the patient can safely be allowed to continue work.

Although examination is often unrewarding it must never be omitted. The doctor is sometimes relieved to discover a simple explanation of chest pain, such as the rash of herpes zoster, tenderness of the chest muscles, or chest pain reproduced by movement of the arms or cervical spine. The patient may be febrile in respiratory infections or pericarditis.

The manner of presentation is significant: patients with a variety of symptoms, together with anxiety and agitation, are unlikely to have serious organic disease, in contrast to the quiet distress and concern caused by the pain of myocardial ischaemia. Pain associated with acute respiratory infections rarely presents difficulties in diagnosis but enterovirus infections such as Coxsackie virus and echovirus may be forgotten. Pain over the ribs or at the insertion of the pectoral muscles is common in muscular sprains. Although tenderness of the sternum occurs in reticuloses such as Hodgkin's disease and leukaemia, it is more often present without any serious cause. A small pulmonary embolus may be suspected when there is chest pain and dyspnoea, even though such dyspnoea is slight. Examination and x-rays will not usually give any help but evidence of deep-vein thrombosis should be sought. A major pulmonary embolus will cause severe chest discomfort and may be confused with a myocardial infarction.

Further clues should be sought to try to elucidate the cause of chest pain. Altered breath sounds, crepitations, dullness or hyperresonance on percussion may indicate lung disease. If the pain is of cardiac origin the following might be found, especially if pain is present: abnormal parasternal heave caused by areas of left ventricular dyskinesia, paradoxical splitting of the second heart sound, abnormal murmurs, quiet first heart sound, third and fourth heart sounds. A raised jugulovenous pulse suggests heart failure, pericardial effusion or pulmonary embolus. Abnormalities of the pulse may occur in dissecting aneurysm and should be sought in the carotid, radial and femoral arteries. Measurement of blood pressure and peak flow may also be helpful.

Angina pectoris may be associated with potentially reversible conditions such as anaemia, bradycardia, atrial fibrillation, hypertension and thyroid disorders, which are easily overlooked. A careful examination must be made to detect conditions which may be amenable to surgical treatment, e.g. mitral valve prolapse, aortic and mitral stenosis, aortic regurgitation.

A direct relation to smoking is seen occasionally and paroxysmal dysrhythmias may be suspected from the history. Most underlying causes can be detected on physical examination and confirmed by a full blood count, thyroid function tests and electrocardiography. An x-ray of the chest may reveal a normal heart shadow but it is an essential investigation, if only as a baseline measure. Fasting lipoproteins should also be determined.

The patient presenting with angina of recent onset must have an electrocardiograph which should if possible be taken by the general practitioner or a member of his team. Referral to hospital for an electrocardiogram inevitably means delay, causes difficulties in management of the immediate problem in deciding whether a man can continue to work and may alarm him unnecessarily. In addition, it is known that when patients with chest pain are referred to hospital for electrocardiography, some are found to have had a recent infarction and it is not good sense for them to be driving cars or travelling to hospital on buses.

An electrocardiograph exercise test should not be performed on patients with recent onset or worsening angina even though the resting electrocardiogram seems normal. The Master 2-step is often used in patients with more long-standing angina when the diagnosis is in doubt. There is a small risk of such patients developing cardiac arrest while doing the exercise but this is minimal if care is taken to exclude those with unstable angina. It is always wise, however, to ensure that a doctor is present. A review of stress tests, including the Master 2-step test, by Redwood and Epstein,[9] however, casts serious doubts on its diagnostic value. They say it is insensitive, many patients with angina caused by coronary artery disease having negative tests. There are also many false positive results which indicate a lack of specificity. Indeed, the authors conclude that a careful history is superior, in both sensitivity and specificity, to stress tests in the diagnosis of coronary artery disease.

Management

From the figures already quoted it would seem that the general practitioner has no difficulty in diagnosing musculoskeletal pain and respiratory causes of chest pain, since he does not send such patients to hospital in error. He will usually achieve this by clinical examination but he may need to confirm his impression with x-rays of the cervical/thoracic spine and chest if the symptoms are prolonged or if he suspects serious underlying disease.

Analgesia

The relief of pain caused by acute myocardial infarction requires special mention. Some doctors are in the habit of prescribing fixed amounts of analgesic, sometimes with an anti-emetic, and they may even give them orally. This approach must be condemned as many patients will be left in pain and there is evidence that they will be more liable to disturbances of rhythm. Enough analgesic must be given to relieve pain and even with intravenous injections there may be a delay of ten minutes in achieving complete control. Heroin is the drug of choice but morphine and pethidine are also used. Other widely advertised drugs are not considered to be so effective. Heroin, 5 mg (1/12 grain), should be given intravenously to begin with, followed by a further 5 mg given in ten minutes if there is no relief, either intravenously or intramuscularly depending on the severity of the residual pain. Occasionally, even more may be necessary. The heroin powder may be dissolved in Cyclizine (valoid) 50 mg instead of water; if intravenous injection is impracticable, the upper deltoid should be the site for intramuscular injection. If the pain has been relatively mild, then further control can be obtained with opiate tablets, such as dipipadone or methadone. If the pain is severe, the patient will need to be revisited in a few hours. The doctor should not restrict the use of opiates. His patient will be grateful for adequate relief of pain but will be only too pleased to stop drugs as soon as he can, usually after 24 to 48 hours, to avoid the mental confusion they cause. Some doctors now carry Entonox, a mixture of oxygen and nitrous oxide, which can help to relieve pain in the early stages after a myocardial infarction. Complete relief of pain is essential whether the patient is treated at home or admitted to hospital.

Home care or hospitalization?

There has been debate about the relative benefits of home and hospital care after myocardial infarction and the position is now becoming clearer.[10] Account must be taken of a patient's social state, his medical condition and the distance he is away from a coronary care unit. After the first few hours and with suitable analgesics, most patients are free of pain, have a stable rhythm and can be safely kept at home. Those who have had an arrest and been resuscitated, those who remain in pain or have heart block or other unstable rhythm should be treated in hospital.

For those patients who are seen in the first two or three hours after an infarction, treatment is less well defined. Relief of pain is paramount, and as a general guide a patient should have a stable rhythm and be free of pain before being moved. However, it is not yet known whether home or hospital care is better for these patients, nor are the hazards of moving them fully understood.

If home care of myocardial infarction is undertaken then an electrocardiogram is recorded as soon as possible, though not necessarily at the first visit, and blood is taken for serum enzymes. Further electrocardiograms may be necessary if the diagnosis is unconfirmed, and a second enzyme estimation should be taken the following day, as changes in level are more revealing than a single reading. When similar pain is alimentary in origin, the diagnosis may be in doubt for several days until cardiac investigations are complete. It often happens that the history of prolonged chest pain is suggestive of a myocardial infarction though the electrocardiogram shows slight, fleeting or no changes, and the transaminase levels are normal or borderline. Although the doctor may be justified in reassuring his patient, he may nevertheless conclude that there has been a small infarction or the threat of one and proceed with caution for two or three weeks. It would be inappropriate, however, to confine such a patient to bed once the results have been seen.

Dysrhythmias

When there is bradycardia in the early hours after an infarction then treatment is required if the patient is hypotensive, shocked or in persistent pain. It is not usually given unless the heart rate is less than 55 to 60 per minute. There is less need to treat bradycardia which is observed some hours after the attack. Atropine should be given intravenously in aliquots of 0.3 to 0.6 mg, the dosage being related to the response in heart rate. Occasionally an undesirable tachycardia follows which is believed to be caused by the release of sympathetic overactivity and may require treatment with beta-blockers. Atropine will also be appropriate if there is heart block.

Tachycardia occurring soon after a myocardial infarction may be associated with transient hypertension. A modest tachycardia of 100 to 110 may be watched carefully but higher rates will increasingly require treatment. An intravenous beta-blocker, such as sotalol in 5 mg aliquots, should be used.

Ectopic beats, especially when coupled, multifocal or showing an R-on-T phenomenon may be given lignocaine in a dosage of 75 mg intravenously, administered slowly. If the patient is being transferred to hospital then a 300 mg intramuscular bolus could be given at the same time.

Adequate relief of pain alone is believed to prevent or alleviate dysrhythmias in many cases.

Angina

The management of unstable angina is extremely difficult. When a patient presents with angina for the first time or with an exacerbation of existing angina, full physical examination and investigations, including resting electrocardiograms, will not usually reveal any underlying cause. Some of these patients will develop a myocardial infarction soon afterwards and, although the risk is not great, it can never be ignored. With tact and reassurance it is wise to persuade such patients to stay at home for a week or two while investigations are completed. How seriously the doctor takes the symptoms will depend on how severe the pain has been and how long it lasted, whether it occurred at rest or only on exertion, and the time-scale of its development.

Associated factors, such as hypertension, anaemia, diabetes mellitus and dysrhythmias, will require special care but it is the larger group of patients, in whom no cause can be found, that is of concern. The doctor clutches at therapeutic straws for comfort. Anticoagulant therapy is sometimes given but it is clumsy for the general practitioner to use because of the difficulties of control, and its value is not proven. Beta-blocking drugs may be used to reduce angina and may control dysrhythmias should an infarction occur. A small dose of aspirin each day to limit platelet stickiness may prove to be of some value. Patients should be advised to avoid heavy physical work and to stop smoking. They should continue light activities. The borderline between a complete and a partial occlusion of a coronary artery is a fine one and it would seem reasonable in someone with new angina or an exacerbation of existing angina to use the same degree of caution in resuming full activity and exercise as if an infarction had occurred.

The recognition of vague chest pains when associated with other symptoms of the pre-infarction syndrome is of little help to the general practitioner. With our present knowledge he appears to be in more danger of causing crippling iatrogenic disorder than of preventing myocardial infarction.

The treatment of established angina is well understood by doctors though the investigation of underlying causes is often neglected. In particular, the general practitioner is well placed to see that weight reduction is pursued and maintained in the obese. What is more important is that angina may reflect abnormal patterns of behaviour in the family. Risk factors of ischaemic heart disease are common to all members but manifestations may appear first in the male. When the situation is presented to the family in this way they may be prepared to increase their activity and to reduce their food intake and cigarette smoking. Exercise should be encouraged as there is evidence that patients who exercise can decrease the severity of their angina by a considerable increase in maximum oxygen uptake and a decrease in myocardial oxygen consumption on exertion.

It is better to encourage an optimistic approach to fitness and activity than to become preoccupied with drugs, which should be seen as an adjuvant to treatment. In many cases no drug therapy is required as the symptoms are mild or occur on strenuous exertion only. Glyceryl trinitrate has stood the test of time but many patients still do not take full advantage of its benefits and only use it at the onset of pain rather than prior to exertion. Beta-blocking drugs taken regularly help many patients and a doctor should become familiar with a few of those now available. Unfortunately they are contraindicated in patients with bronchospasm, heart block and bradycardia. Obstructive airways disease and heart failure are not absolute contraindications to beta-blocking drugs but they must be used with circumspection in such patients.

If the angina cannot be satisfactorily controlled with glyceryl trinitrate plus a beta blocker, a second line drug should be added. The choice lies between long-acting nitrates and calcium channel blockers. The long-acting nitrates (isosorbide dinitrate or isosorbide mononitrate) are given in divided doses two or three times a day, the dosage being tailored to the symptomatic response. Between the two most commonly used calcium channel blockers, nifedipine (Adalat) and verapamil the choice depends on whether or not a beta blocker is used as a first line drug: verapamil should not be added to a beta blocker as the cumulative effect on slowing the heart rate and decreasing atrio-ventricular node conduction could induce heart block. The action of nifedipine is more predominantly arteriolar dilating, and it can therefore be combined safely with beta blockers.

The place of percutaneous glyceryl trinitrate in the form of patches or ointment has not yet been fully assessed.

Patients with unstable angina (angina occurring at rest) should be admitted to hospital as an emergency. Patients with stable angina (i.e. infrequent angina or angina only occurring on exertion) should be referred for specialist assessment if they are aged less than 45 years, if they have frequent severe angina or if they are not responding adequately to double medical therapy (beta blockers plus long acting nitrates, beta blockers plus nifedipine or long-acting nitrates plus verapamil). Such assessment is likely to include exercise electrocardiography and coronary arteriography, with a view to possible coronary artery bypass surgery, or transluminal angioplasty.

The management of severe chest pain when there is difficulty in differentiating between cardiac, gall-bladder and alimentary-tract disease, can sometimes be vexing. Minor electrocardiographic changes have been reported in gall-bladder and oesophageal disease and the transaminases can be raised in both if there is liver involvement. Gall-bladder disease usually becomes obvious with the passage of time as the symptoms and signs become abdominal. When oesophageal disease is suspected as an alternative to a myocardial infarction, the doctor should keep the patient at rest for a few days until tests are complete. Usually the electrocardiogram and transaminases will be found to be normal. Meanwhile it is important to nurse such patients sitting up, either in bed or in a chair. Since such symptoms often recur it is helpful to arrange a barium meal. Gastric reflux or hiatus hernia may be demonstrated

but their absence does not preclude such a presumptive diagnosis. Endoscopy may be necessary in some cases.
Anginal chest pain is sometimes associated with belching and heartburn. The association with cardiac disease may be clear when symptoms occur in relation to exertion. Often, however, the symptoms are not so obvious and they may occur at rest. When there is considerable doubt it is possible that both angina and oesophageal disease co-exist. It may take some weeks to make a firm diagnosis, which is aided by the patient making more accurate observations of aggravating factors, and the different response to glyceryl trinitrate and drugs for the relief of oesophageal inflammation. Sometimes the exacerbation of oesophageal symptoms may be wrongly attributed to a worsening of existing angina and a doctor may unnecessarily alarm or restrict his patient if he suspects an incipient myocardial infarction.

Conclusion

A doctor will inevitably make occasional mistakes in the care of patients with chest pain but they will be fewer if he 'listens' carefully to what his patient is communicating, both in words and in non-verbal signals.

References

[1] Dunnell, K. and Cartwright, A. (1972): *Medicine Takers, Prescribers and Hoarders*. London: Routledge and Kegan Paul
[2] Morrell, D.C., Gage, H.G. and Robinson, N.A. (1971): Symptoms in General Practice. *Journal of the Royal College of General Practitioners, 21*, 32
[3] Hull, F.M. (1969): Social Class Consultation Patterns in Rural General Practice. *Journal of the Royal College of General Practitioners, 18*, 65
[4] Frank, P.I. (1970): *Anterior Chest Pain in Family Practice*. M.D. Thesis, University of Liverpool
[5] World Health Organization. *Hypertension and Coronary Heart Disease: Classification and Criteria for Epidemiological Studies*. Technical Report Series No. 168. HMSO
[6] Bennett, J.R. and Atkinson, M. (1966): The Differentiation Between Oesophageal and Cardiac Pain. *Lancet*, *ii*, 1123
[7] Colling, A., Dellipiani, A.W., Donaldson, R.J. and MacCormack, P. (1976): Teesside Coronary Survey: An Epidemiological Study of Acute Attacks of Myocardial Infarction. *British Medical Journal*, *2*, 1169
[8] Fulton, M., Lutz, W., Donald, K.W. *et al* (1972): Natural History of Unstable Angina. *Lancet*, *i*, 860
[9] Redwood, D.R. and Epstein, S.E. (1972): Uses and Limitations of Stress Testing in Evaluation of Ischaemic Heart Disease. *Circulation*, *46*, 1115
[10] *Coronary Care in the Community*, ed. Colling, A. (1977). London

3.32 The patient complaining of palpitations

David Illingworth

This complaint ranks with indigestion in its lack of precise meaning. Being a symptom and not a sign, the term should be avoided by doctors except in attempts to discover what the patient is trying to convey. The National Morbidity Survey[1] reports 'palpitations' presented by 1.5 per 1,000 patients per year.

Morrell and his colleagues[2] noted that 'disturbance of a heart rhythm' was, in one year, reported by 12 patients: seven men and five women, in a practice population of 4,455. Dunnell and Cartwright[3] invited 1,410 patients to recall symptoms over a two-week period. Six per cent, all of whom were adults, reported 'palpitations or thumping heart' and most of these were in the age-group 45 to 75 years. Women outnumbered men in the proportion of two to one. It is therefore likely that, while the symptom is sometimes offered by the patient, it may need to be elicited by enquiry. Furthermore, it is remarkable how often one encounters patients with disordered heart rhythm who remain unaware of the fact. Modern textbooks of medicine and cardiology, with two exceptions,[4,5] devote little or no space to discussion of the significance of palpitations.

Presentation

The complaint may be volunteered or evoked by the doctor's questioning. Although the doctor may define palpitations as an uncomfortable awareness by the patient of his heart's action, a statement that palpitations exist is meaningless without a precise account of the experience.

After such a description it should then be possible to decide whether the problem is a *true palpitation* in the medical sense of disordered rhythm, or a *spurious palpitation* which covers a profusion of symptomatology — often unrelated to the heart.

True palpitation is surprisingly rare. It is likely that the disturbance of heart rhythm reaches a level of perception more easily in older people, in higher social classes and, in particular, in those who are anxious.

Spurious palpitation is a complaint related, at least in part, to geographical area and dialect. Patients have presented with 'palpitations' and then described their experience as sinking feelings in the stomach, hiccough, flatulence, giddiness, shortness of breath, or angina pectoris.

Palpitation may also be observed by the patient who has other manifestations of heart disease. The symptom may then be only a minor incidental complaint dwarfed by overt heart disease.

Causes

It is astonishing how seldom true palpitation is experienced by those with fixed arrhythmia or organic heart disease. The corollary is that it is almost always possible to reassure those who *do* experience the true forms of palpitation, that it is a common symptom in people with normal hearts. When lying in bed at night, especially on the left side, many people are aware of cardiac action. Some even report the matter to the doctor and rarely, if ever, is any cardiovascular defect discovered.

The commonest cause of palpitation is sinus tachycardia. When under mental or physical stress many of us are aware of rapid heart action. It is worth remembering, however, that the powerful apical thrust of hyperthyroidism or aortic incompetence may also produce an uncomfortable awareness of the heart's presence. Extrasystoles are also frequent explanations of the patient's symptom of palpitation. Increasing the heart rate by gentle exercise in the consulting-room may be expected to eliminate these.

Undoubtedly it is the intermittent, episodic arrhythmias which most impress patient and doctor — in contrast to the unconscious acceptance of the fixed arrhythmias. Paroxysmal atrial tachycardia is the classical and most dramatic cause of the complaint of palpitations. The onset of this regular heart rhythm is usually given a precise moment by the patient. Chest discomfort of ischaemic origin may coexist if the episode continues for a time. Some patients are aware of procedures which abort their attacks. Vagal stimulation may be self-employed through eyeball pressure, the Valsalva manoeuvre, epigastric pressure or inducing vomiting. The tachycardia may cease equally suddenly but this is not a significant feature.

The examiner will note the rapid regular cardiac action at 160 to 180 beats per minute and may well have the supreme satisfaction of confirming his clinical diagnosis by employing carotid sinus pressure, on one or other side, to stop the attack.

While fixed atrial fibrillation hardly ever produces palpitations the intermittent variety is usually observed by the patient. It may presage the fixed variety in heart disease or may occur intermittently for years in perfectly normal hearts. The ventricular response to atrial fibrillation is totally irregular at about 130 to 150 beats per minute. The paroxysmal variety may be associated with ischaemic chest pain. The duration of the episode has little effect in pain production in contradistinction to the discomfort of paroxysmal atrial tachycardia.

There are a few rare causes of true palpitation such as atrial flutter and the Wolff-Parkinson-White syndrome but they are not within the scope of this book.

The patient who has true palpitation is usually an educated, sensitive introvert — often under nervous strain. Furthermore, the word 'palpitation' may have a significance varying with the locality. Women complainers far outnumber men, while the long-established etiological platitudes relating to the consumption of tea, coffee and spiced food have little relevance in modern practice, although occasionally provocative factors such as smoking or alcohol or some drugs may be identified and eliminated.

History and examination

The patient's account is all important and enables the practitioner to make immediate distinction of true from spurious palpitation. Disturbance of rhythm may best be elicited by having the patient reproduce his disturbed heart beat by tapping the doctor's desk with his finger. When is the sensation experienced? Is the onset sudden or gradual? How long do the episodes last? Are there precipitating factors such as nervous tension or lying on the left side? Do the episodes cease slowly or abruptly? What can the patient do to help himself? (Keeping a diary of events and diet may be helpful in identifying possible precipitating factors.) Palpitation may not be the primary or only complaint. Enquiry must be made about other cardiac symptoms, such as chest pain or breathlessness. Occasionally the patient will enhance the value of the interview by revealing that the symptom is present. The doctor and the patient can then share the experience and the benefit of an immediate probable diagnosis.

The previous history may be of the greatest importance. One may elicit an account of rheumatic fever, joint pain or streptococcal infections. Hypertension and all forms of coronary artery disease may be found, on enquiry, to pre-exist. The family history of the patient with palpitations should be considered. Not only is the familial factor important in ischaemic heart disease but the individual neurotic inheritance can also be significant.

During the history taking the doctor will be observing the patient. Is this a nervous person? Is there anaemia, tremor, a goitre or other signs of hyperthyroidism? Do the facies suggest heart failure or possible hypertension?

The physical examination of the patient will include comprehensive coverage of the cardiovascular system. Even though it is clear that the 'palpitation' is not of cardiac origin it is impossible to give proper reassurance without examining the cardiovascular system. When feeling the pulse the fingers are easily examined for tremor, nicotine staining and koilonychia. Touching the palms may tell one much about vasomotor control and emotional state. Palpation of the thyroid gland should not be forgotten, along with measurement of the blood pressure and auscultation of the heart.

Not only is it important to assess heart size and heart sounds, but particular attention should be paid to the cardiac rhythm while listening at the apex of the heart. It may be helpful to ask the patient to indicate, during the auscultation, if he feels his palpitations. Not infrequently, extrasystoles will be noted by both parties at the same moment. Diagnosis is thus greatly facilitated. In general, if valvular disease coexists with palpitation it is of mitral origin. It is therefore often helpful to listen to apical heart sounds with the patient lying on his left side.

The type of palpitation will usually be obvious from the history and examination. Although an electrocardiogram may not add more information it can help to confirm the diagnosis and often has a certain therapeutic value as well.

Management

The patient must understand at once that the complaint, though uncomfortable, is a symptom and not a disease. It should be made clear that most palpitations occur in perfectly normal hearts. The patient's account will separate spurious from true palpitation and the former will not be considered further.

All types of palpitation will benefit from the doctor's reassurance. Attempts at adjustment in life style, when indicated, are worth while to reduce stress and pressure in the individual's environment. Unphysiological habits, such as smoking, physical lethargy and obesity are worthy of attention: the degree of success is in proportion to the practitioner's enthusiasm and optimism.

Organic causes for palpitation such as hyperthyroidism and fixed atrial fibrillation with heart failure require the treatment indicated for the underlying lesion.

The common innocent intermittent arrhythmias, such as extrasystoles, paroxysmal atrial tachycardia and paroxysmal atrial fibrillation may need only explanation, simple advice and self-help. Extrasystoles which are particularly troublesome may merit mild sedation with benzodiazepines and, on rare occasions, beta-blocking drugs.

Paroxysmal atrial tachycardia may be easily dealt with by the patient's own manipulations though a few may require carotid pressure from the doctor. Short, frequent bouts of paroxysmal atrial tachycardia are particularly troublesome for some patients and in these cases drug therapy is reasonable. Beta-blockers may be useful to prolong atrioventricular nodal conduction. Digoxin in maintenance doses remains the most useful drug for a small number of patients. Those with paroxysmal atrial fibrillation tend to do well on either beta-blockade or digoxin.

The calcium channel blocker verapamil is a useful drug increasingly used in the treatment of supraventricular tachycardias. It should, however, not be administered parenterally in patients already receiving beta blockers as further prolongation of the atrioventricular nodal conduction time could cause hypotension and asystole. Amiodarone (Cordarone X) should probably be reserved for use under specialist supervision: side-effects include photosensitivity and disturbance of thyroid function.

Quinidine may itself precipitate arrythmias and, according to many cardiologists, should seldom be used. It is of interest and significance, however, that its popularity is slow to wane.

There is usually no therapeutic haste in treating the patient with palpitations and referral for specialist opinion is seldom necessary, before at least a trial of the simpler forms of management outlined above.

References

[1] Royal College of General Practitioners, Office of Population Censuses and Surveys, Department of Health and Social Security (1986): *Morbidity Statistics from General Practice 1981–82*. HMSO Series MB5 No. 1

[2] Morrell, D.C., Gage, H.G. and Robinson, N.A. (1971): Symptoms in General Practice. *Journal of Royal College of General Practitioners, 21,* 32

[3] Dunnell, K. and Cartwright, A. (1972): *Medicine Takers, Prescribers and Hoarders*. London: Routledge and Kegan Paul

[4] Julian, D.G. (1973): *Cardiology*. London: Baillière Tindall

[5] Owen, S.G., Stretton, T.B. and Vallance-Owen, J. (1968): *Essentials of Cardiology*. London: Lloyd-Luke

3.33
The patient who looks blue

Ian Gregg

Cyanosis is the term used to describe the blue or dusky complexion of the skin which, except under very rare circumstances such as methaemoglobinaemia, is due to the superficial capillaries containing blood with a high level of reduced haemoglobin.

Classification

Peripheral cyanosis. – If the rate of flow of blood through the superficial capillaries is reduced, there is greater time for the tissues to extract oxygen and therefore the amount of reduced haemoglobin in the blood is increased. This form of cyanosis is termed *peripheral.*

Central cyanosis, on the other hand, is a manifestation of generalized hypoxaemia due to inadequate uptake of oxygen by the blood as it passes through the lungs.

It is important to appreciate that not uncommonly cyanosis may have both a peripheral and a central component.

Causes

The patient must be examined in a good light. Cyanosis may be impossible to detect in the light given off by fluorescent tubes. Cyanosis only becomes detectable if the blood in the superficial capillaries contains at least 20 per cent of reduced haemoglobin. Clinicians differ greatly in their ability to detect cyanosis.

Peripheral cyanosis is most liable to occur in exposed areas, such as the face and hands, and is enhanced by cold. The presence of central cyanosis should be sought in those parts of the body which are naturally warm, such as the tongue and buccal mucosa.

The significance of central cyanosis. – Because of the shape of the oxygen dissociation curve, the saturation of haemoglobin is maintained even when the partial pressure of oxygen (pO_2) in the arterial blood is moderately reduced. Two corollaries follow from this. If cyanosis is entirely central in origin, indicating that the blood is at least 20 per cent unsaturated, the pO_2 in the arterial blood must have fallen from its normal level of about 100 mm Hg to about 45 mm Hg. This can only have arisen as the result of a serious reduction in the uptake of oxygen in the lungs: due to disease either of the lungs themselves or of the cardiovascular system. On the other hand, because hypoxaemia of only moderate degree does not give rise to central cyanosis, absence of the latter does not preclude the existence of respiratory or cardiovascular disease.

Inadequate oxygenation of venous blood in the lungs can result from a disorder of any of the three components of respiratory function. Interference with the conduction of atmospheric air to the alveoli (*ventilation*) occurs in asphyxia due, for instance, to an inhaled foreign body or severe obstruction of the airways as in status asthmaticus. *Diffusion* of oxygen across the alveolar-capillary membrane is impaired if the latter is thickened (as in fibrosing alveolitis) or if the alveoli are filled with exudate (as in pneumonia and pulmonary oedema). If part of the pulmonary circulation passes through capillaries which are not in contact with atmospheric air, blood cannot be fully oxygenated: such a defect of *perfusion* occurs in those forms of congenital heart disease in which there is a right to left shunt: e.g., septal defects accompanied by transposition of the great vessels.

Common disorders giving rise to cyanosis

Peripheral cyanosis.– This occurs when there is a localized obstruction to, or stasis of, blood supply in the superficial tissues. It is enhanced by cold and therefore is best seen in the extremities. Peripheral cyanosis occurs in the fingers and toes with Raynaud's disease and in the lower limbs in obliterative arterial disease. Peripheral cyanosis and oedema of the neck and face occur in superior vena caval obstruction. The malar flush of patients with mitral stenosis is due to peripheral cyanosis associated with a low cardiac output. General causes of peripheral cyanosis include shock, heart failure with a low cardiac output, primary polycythaemia and secondary polycythaemia (the latter occurring as a compensatory mechanism in hypoxaemia).

Central cyanosis.– An acute onset of central cyanosis in a previously healthy person may occur with asphyxia (due to obstruction of the larger air passages by a foreign body, croup or diphtheria), pneumonia or acute pulmonary oedema. The commonest cause of central cyanosis which has not arisen suddenly is severe, chronic disease of the lungs. In chronic obstructive bronchitis it is caused by an imbalance of ventilation and perfusion and gives rise to the 'blue bloater' appearance. Central cyanosis also occurs in the advanced stages of pneumonoconiosis and other forms of pulmonary fibrosis. In an infant cyanosis is strongly suggestive of congenital heart disease with a right-to-left shunt.

If emphysema is not complicated by chronic obstructive bronchitis, patients maintain a normal level of pO_2 by hyperventilation and therefore central cyanosis does not occur until the terminal stages of the disease. The characteristic appearance of such patients being described as 'pink and puffing'.

Clinical elucidation of the causes of cyanosis

Having decided whether cyanosis is peripheral or predominantly central, history taking and physical examination should be directed towards finding the cause of hypoxaemia. The history will immediately distinguish between an acute onset (as in arterial obstruction to a leg, pneumonia or pulmonary oedema) and its pre-existence in chronic lung or heart disease or in Raynaud's disease. During physical examination the following signs should be especially looked for: clubbing, the jugular venous pressure, adventitious sounds in the lungs and the presence of murmurs during ausculation of the heart. A plethoric appearance suggests polycythaemia and splenic enlargement may be found in primary polycythaemia. Where this diagnosis is suspected, a full blood count and venous haematocrit should be carried out.

Treatment

Clearly treatment must be directed to the underlying cause of hypoxaemia, but an attempt to restore oxygenation of the blood by the giving of oxygen must be made if cyanosis has occurred acutely as in pneumonia or pulmonary oedema, since other measures of treatment will take some time before they are effective.

Long-term oxygen therapy may be indicated for patients with chronic hypoxaemia but in those with chronic obstructive bronchitis it must be given under careful control because of the insensitivity of the respiratory centre to high levels of pCO_2.

If the hypoxaemia is relieved in these circumstances the patient's respiratory drive may be lost and dangerous CO_2 retention occurs. In any patient therefore with acute respiratory failure due to an exacerbation of chronic obstructive bronchitis provoked by a respiratory infection, oxygen should not be given unless the levels of arterial pO_2 and pCO_2 are monitored, and this can only be carried out in hospital.

If primary polycythaemia is diagnosed, the patient should be referred to hospital for advice. The high blood viscosity associated with this condition carries with it a serious risk of cerebrovascular and cardiovascular complications which can be reduced by regular venesection and, in some cases, the use of radioactive phosphorus.

In secondary polycythaemia, the reduction of a very high haematocrit by venesection may also produce symptomatic improvement in some cases and specialist advice should be considered.

3.34
The patient who looks pale

David Morrell

In community surveys of anaemia it has been repeatedly shown that women have lower mean haemoglobin values than men. In one study[1] the mean haemoglobin in men aged 15 to 24 years was 14.07 g/100 ml (standard deviation (SD) 0.81), falling to 13.15 g/100 ml (SD 1.07) in men aged 65 to 74 years. In the same survey the mean haemoglobin of women aged 15 to 24 years was 11.87 g/100 ml (SD 0.96) and at the age 65 to 74 was 13.01 g/100 ml (SD 1.10). In men therefore the haemoglobin tends to fall with increasing age, while in women it tends to rise. The higher standard deviation in women indicates the greater variation of haemoglobin levels detected in the survey. Any definition of anaemia must be arbitrary, and in this study the value of 12.5 g/100 ml was accepted as the lower limit of normal for men and 12 g/100 ml for women. With this definition the prevalence of anaemia in men was found to be 2 to 3 per cent between the ages of 15 and 44 years, rising to 8 per cent in the age-group 45 to 64, and 20 per cent over the age of 65 years. In women the prevalence of anaemia was over 25 per cent in the child-bearing years, falling to 12 per cent in the age-group 45 to 64, and rising to 21 per cent over the age of 65 years. Almost all the cases of anaemia detected in this survey were of iron-deficiency type.

Presentation

The complaint of looking pale is relatively uncommon in general practice. When it occurs, it is most commonly presented by women or by parents concerned about their children. It is commonly assumed by the general public, and by some doctors, that pallor is associated with anaemia. It is true that severely anaemic patients may be pale, but pallor of the mucous membranes is a notoriously inaccurate indication of the haemoglobin level in the blood, and its assessment in general practice leads to both false positive and false negative results.[2]

Pallor, as a presenting feature of anaemia, is most common in those experiencing a sudden blood loss, or those with a haemoglobin below 8.5 per cent, when the patient or his relatives may notice a change in appearance. Pallor may also be presented in other conditions. In myxoedema changes in the skin and a general slowing of the circulation may cause pallor, and in depression tiredness and pallor may draw attention to the illness.

In population surveys[3] it has been shown that there is little correlation between the commonly accepted symptoms of anaemia, such as tiredness, shortness of breath, palpitations and haemoglobin levels, until these fall below 9.5 g/100 ml. On the other hand it is important to recognize that there is a difference between population surveys which reveal chronic anaemia, to which the patient has adapted, and new symptoms which may have been produced by a sudden fall in haemoglobin levels. It is, however, pertinent to point out that in randomized controlled trials, in which iron was administered to patients detected in the survey to have low haemoglobin levels, there was no difference in the rate of remission of symptoms between those receiving iron and controls, despite a rise in haemoglobin. It is equally important to remember that in a screening survey the symptomatic patients may have selected themselves out by consulting their doctors and receiving treatment.

These studies reveal the complexity of the problem of anaemia in general practice. While it is easy to attribute vague symptoms of tiredness and depression to a low level of circulating haemoglobin, there is ample evidence that merely raising the haemoglobin level does not inevitably cure the symptoms. The finding of a low haemoglobin, however, should provoke the doctor to look for a cause for both the anaemia and the associated symptoms, rather than lead to immediate therapy without first elucidating the cause of the anaemia.

Causes of anaemia

Hypochromic anaemia.—The most common cause of iron-deficiency anaemia in general practice is excessive menstrual blood loss which is not compensated for by an adequate diet. Use of the intra-uterine device as a contraceptive measure may contribute to this in some cases. Bleeding from the bowel is the second most important cause. This may result from the use of analgesics or anti-inflammatory agents, or from chronic peptic ulceration, hiatus hernia, oesophageal varices, malignant disease, particularly of the colon, or haemorrhoids. Rarely an inadequate diet may cause the hypochromic anaemia; this is most commonly seen in the aged and in some immigrants, particularly those who are vegetarians.

Macrocytic anaemia.—Pernicious anaemia is by far the most common cause of a macrocytic anaemia seen in general practice.

Rarely, drugs, myxoedema, or the malabsorption syndrome causing folate deficiency will be encountered.

Normocytic and normochromic anaemias.—With the exception of acute blood loss these are relatively uncommon in general practice. The average general practitioner is unlikely to have more than one patient in his practice with a congenital or acquired haemolytic anaemia. In practices with large immigrant populations, however, sickle cell anaemia and thalassaemia may be more important. The anaemias associated with chronic disease, e.g. Crohn's disease, chronic renal disease, the collagen disorders and carcinoma should always be considered as they may present in general practice with vague symptoms of pallor or tiredness. Aplastic anaemia which is usually idiopathic but may be due to toxic chemicals or drugs presents as a normocytic anaemia, but there is also a pancytopenia and thrombocytopenia.

History and examination

When a patient complains of pallor or the doctor by his clinical observation or history-taking suspects that the patient is suffering from anaemia, there is little to be gained by an extensive history or examination until it is established whether or not the patient is anaemic. This is one of the rare occasions in medical practice when it is sensible to carry out a laboratory test before indulging in an exhaustive history or examination. If the initial clinical impression is confirmed, and the patient is indeed anaemic, then time may be set aside for a full exploration of the cause of the anaemia. If, on the other hand, the blood test is normal, the time may be equally well occupied in attempting to identify the cause of symptoms of tiredness and general malaise in the presence of a normal haemoglobin and a normal erythrocyte sedimentation rate. In the absence of these laboratory results, time may be completely wasted pursuing totally irrelevant channels of enquiry. Before dismissing completely the value of an immediate history and examination, however, it is important to stress that there will be some patients who present with symptoms of syncope or the passage of black stools. These are relatively rare, but clearly need immediate investigation and often require admission to hospital.

Patients presenting with symptoms suggestive of anaemia, and in whom this is confirmed by blood examination, may be divided into those who, on the basis of the haematological investigation, show signs of iron-deficiency anaemia, those who are reported to have a macrocytic anaemia, and those who have a normocytic anaemia. The first group is by far the most common. History-taking in these patients will be directed to determining the cause of the iron deficiency. Specific enquiry should be designed to identify any cause of abnormal blood loss. In women there should be questions about the amount and duration of menstrual bleeding. If this exceeds six days in duration or requires the use of more than 18 to 20 sanitary towels, it may be regarded as excessive. In both sexes a history of epigastric pain, passage of dark stools, ingestion of aspirin or similar anti-inflammatory agents, or bleeding piles should be sought. A knowledge of the patient's past medical history may be helpful in identifying the cause, such as a history of partial gastrectomy, thyroidectomy or chronic diarrhoea. In all patients there should be some enquiry about the appetite, diet and change in bowel habit. Unexplained anaemia in a man or post-menopausal woman should always suggest a silent neoplasm of the colon. Thalassaemia, a haemolytic anaemia seen in patients of Mediterranean origin, usually presents as a mild hypochromic anaemia with characteristically microcytic cells.

In patients with megaloblastic anaemia specific enquiry about drug treatment is important. A number of drugs, of which the anticonvulsants are the most important, have been implicated. Changes in appetite or loss of weight may be suggestive of a neoplasm of the stomach, while loss of appetite accompanied by weight gain may suggest myxoedema. A past history of thyroidectomy, treatment with I^{131}, a general slowing of the reactions, loss of concentration and bradycardia would confirm this suspicion. Specific questions should be asked about the possible neurological complications of pernicious anaemia such as changes in power or sensation in the lower limbs, or unsteadiness of gait. The family history of the patient and his occupation may give a clue to the cause of the anaemia.

Normocytic anaemias may be caused by sudden blood loss, and the history should indicate this by the mode of onset of symptoms. It may also occur in haemolytic disease. This may be hereditary, in which case a family history may give a clue to the cause of the disorder. It may also be caused by the ingestion of drugs or toxic chemicals, and specific enquiry about this should be made.

Sickle cell anaemia is seen mostly in West Indian or West African immigrants. Clinically, there is a chronic haemolytic anaemia, a susceptibility to infection, gall stones and infarctive damage to a variety of organs, particularly the spleen. The history is of a life punctuated by crises. The most common are infarctions usually brought on by infection, hypoxia or exposure to cold. They present with pain in the hands or feet in children or in the limbs, back or thorax in adults. Hypoplastic crises may also occur in response to infection leading to severe anaemia. In children splenic sequestration crises lead to rapid enlargement of the spleen and a rapid fall in haemoglobin.

Patients who complain of pallor and other symptoms suggestive of anaemia, but who have a normal haemoglobin may rarely be suffering from myxoedema or some other organic disease. Most commonly, however, they are suffering from depression or general anxiety about their health. In these cases a careful history should be taken, focusing on such factors as sleep disturbance, loss of concentration, suicidal thoughts and frank feelings of depression with weeping. A careful social history should also be obtained.

The examination of the patient will be influenced by the results of the haematological investigations. In the presence of a low haemoglobin it should be systematic and designed to look for specific abnormalities. Examination of the tongue may reveal glossitis. The skin may show petechial haemorrhages, suggestive of a serious haematological disorder. The nails may be spoon shaped in iron-deficiency anaemia. In severe anaemia the pulse rate may be raised with a wide pulse pressure, and in advanced cases, there may be signs of congestive heart failure. Examination of the reticulo-endothelial system may reveal widespread lymphadenopathy, suggestive of leukaemia or Hodgkin's disease. The spleen may be enlarged in haemolytic anaemias, Hodgkin's disease, leukaemia or in cirrhosis of the liver, where bleeding oesophageal varices may be the cause of the anaemia. The sudden onset of symptoms, particularly if accompanied by faintness should prompt a rectal examination when frank or occult bleeding may be revealed. In cases of abnormal menstrual loss a vaginal examination is indicated.

In patients with a megaloblastic anaemia a full neurological examination of the lower limbs should be carried out. The signs of subacute combined degeneration of the cord may occasionally be detected, with loss of vibration and deep sensation accompanied by an extensor plantar response.

Investigation

A full blood count, followed by a careful history and examination, will elucidate the cause of most cases of anaemia presenting in general practice. In some caes, however, confirmatory evidence will be desirable before treatment is instituted. Appropriate ways to proceed in respect of the different types of anaemia are indicated in Figures 1 to 4.

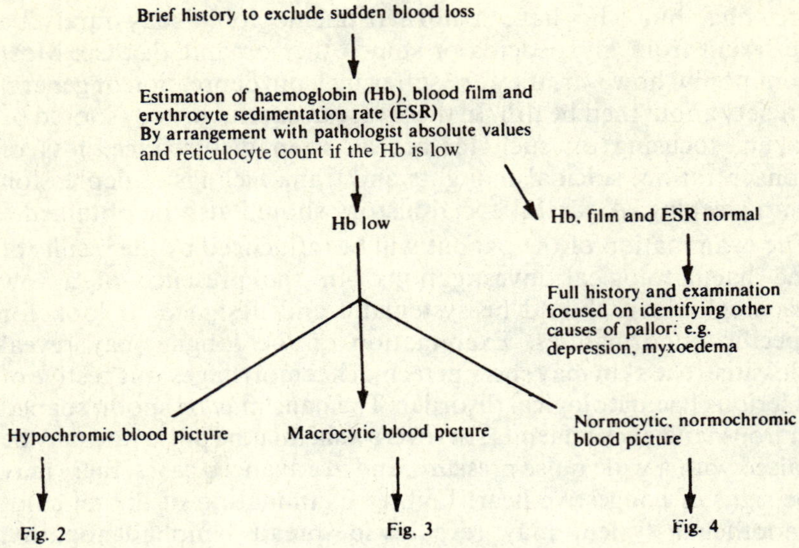

Figure 1.—Schematic outline of method of procedure in patients presenting with pallor or symptoms suggestive of anaemia

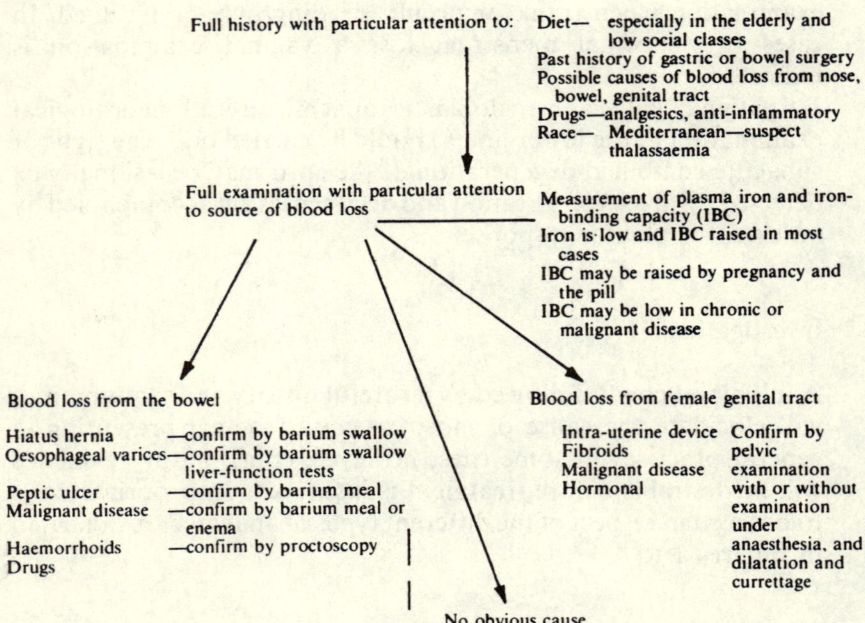

Figure 2.—Schematic outline of method of procedure in patients with a hypochromic blood picture

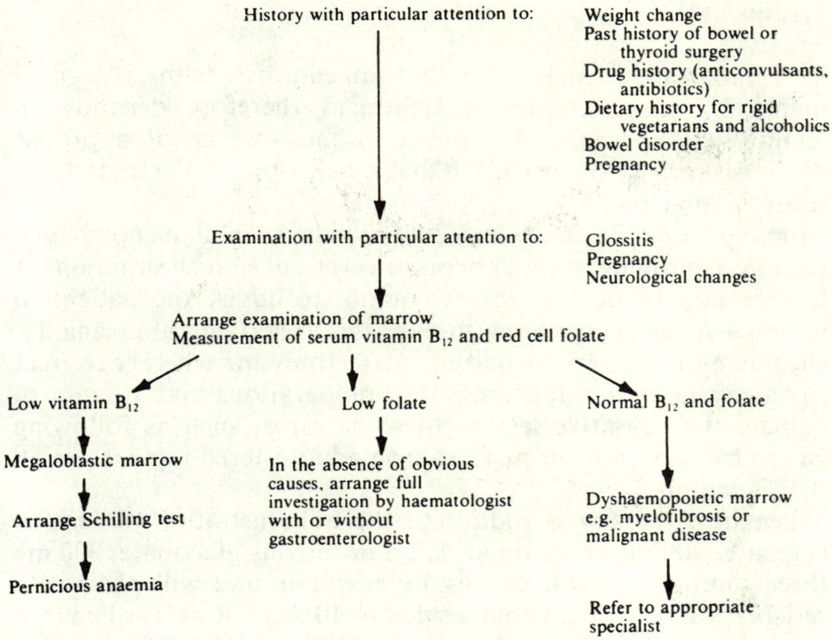

Figure 3.—Schematic outline of method of procedure in patients with macrocytic anaemia

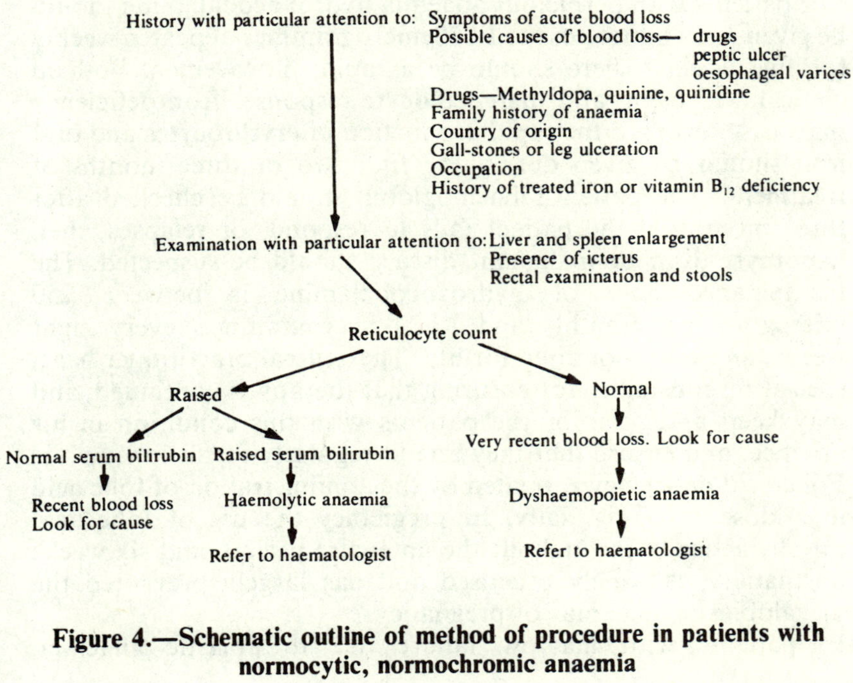

Figure 4.—Schematic outline of method of procedure in patients with normocytic, normochromic anaemia

Treatment

It is important to remember that anaemia is a clinical sign of underlying disease. Correct treatment therefore depends on identifying the cause. Treatment in the absence of a precise diagnosis may be dangerous in that it may obscure the underlying cause of anaemia.

In many cases the cause may be obvious, such as menorrhagia, chronic aspirin ingestion or peptic ulceration. In such situations, it is necessary to decide whether or not to advise the patient to undergo medical measures to cure the underlying abnormality, such as hysterectomy or partial gastrectomy, or whether to treat the anaemia by administering iron preparations and attempt to palliate the causative lesion. In some cases, such as following gastrectomy, treatment by extra iron administered regularly is all that is required.

When iron therapy is indicated, the administration of ferrous sulphate, 200 mg three times daily, or ferrous gluconate, 300 mg three times daily, will usually be adequate and will produce a reticulocyte response within a week to 10 days. Rarely, when iron must be administered urgently, as in the last trimester of pregnancy, or when the patient cannot tolerate oral preparations, injections of iron dextran (Imferon), 50 to 250 mg daily, may be given intramuscularly, or the patient may be admitted to hospital for an intravenous infusion.

For patients with pernicious anaemia hydroxocobalamine should be given in an initial dose of 1,000 microgrammes, repeated weekly for five weeks. There should be a rapid improvement both in clinical well-being and in reticulocyte response. Iron deficiency may arise owing to the rapid production of erythrocytes and oral iron should be given during the first two or three months of treatment. The patient's haemoglobin should be checked after three months; if the patient fails to respond, or relapses, then hypothyroidism or malignant disease should be suspected. The maintenance dose of hydroxocobalamine is between 250 microgrammes monthly and 1,000 microgrammes every eight weeks, and must continue for life. The general practitioner has a special responsibility for ensuring that therapy is continued, and may keep a register of the patients with this condition in his practice, and ensure that they attend regularly for follow-up.

Folic-acid deficiency is treated by the administration of folic acid in a dose of 5 mg daily. In pregnancy the use of folic acid prophylactically throughout the antenatal period, and six weeks postnatally, is widely practised and has largely prevented the megaloblastic anaemias of pregnancy.

In patients with marrow failure due to aplastic anaemia,

leukaemia, myelofibrosis or malignant infiltration, the management will usually be passed into the hands of the specialist. It may include repeated blood transfusions, chemotherapy, splenectomy or even bone-marrow transplant.

The treatment of crises in sickle cell anaemia needs hospital admission. Early treatment of even minor infection may sometimes prevent a crisis. Special care is needed if these patients require surgery or go into labour, and their records should be suitably marked.

Patients with sickle cell 'trait' have about 50 per cent of their haemoglobin as 'Hb S' and are normally healthy. If, however, two patients with the trait marry, 50 per cent of their offspring are likely to suffer from sickle cell anaemia. This may present the general practitioner with a difficult pre-marriage counselling role.

The general practitioner has an important role to play in the prevention of anaemia in women with heavy menstrual periods, in pregnancy, and in the elderly. This prevention is concerned with both dietary advice and the administration of iron when required. He has an equally important part to play in recognizing anaemia as a clinical sign of underlying disease and identifying the cause of the disease, and in ensuring continuity of care for those suffering from pernicious anaemia or folate deficiency, as well as in monitoring patients who have had gastric, thyroid, or bowel surgery. In addition there are many rare and obscure anaemias which he may encounter once in a year or once in a professional lifetime; these he must recognize and then seek help from his specialist colleagues.

References

[1] Kilpatrick, F.S. (1961): Prevalence of anaemia in the general population. *British Medical Journal*, *2*, 1736

[2] Hodgkin, K. (1973): *Towards Earlier Diagnosis*. 3rd ed., p. 182. Edinburgh: Churchill Livingstone

[3] Elwood, P.L. (1970): Some epidemiological aspects of iron-deficiency relevant to its evaluation. *Proceedings of the Royal Society of Medicine*, *63*, 1230

It is a pleasure to acknowledge the help I have received in preparing this chapter from the late Professor G. Wetherley-Mein of St Thomas's Hospital Medical School.

3.35
The patient with swollen legs

A. G. Donald

In approaching the problem of swelling in the legs, it is essential to have an understanding of the fundamental aspects of the pathophysiological process that may produce this symptom which is presented in almost 1 per cent of patient-initiated consultations[1] and which is recorded as present (in the form of oedema) in 4.7 consultations per 1,000 patients at risk per annum. The symptom predominates in women.

Swollen legs are almost always due to an excessive accumulation in the tissues of extracellular fluid. Extracellular fluid occupies an intermediary position between the intracellular fluid and the blood, with both of which it is in constant exchange. The volume of extracellular fluid is influenced by the arterial pressure within the capillaries pushing fluid out through the semi-permeable membrane of the capillary wall, assisted by the attraction through osmotic pressure of the existing extracellular fluid. The force responsible for the reduction of extracellular fluid is, most importantly, osmotic attraction of the blood (due mainly to plasma protein) assisted by the relative firmness, or elasticity, of the tissues. The drainage of the area is through the venous and lymphatic systems. The venous flow in the capillaries normally operates at about one-third of the hydrostatic pressure of the arterial end thus facilitating the return of fluid into the blood.

Total body sodium also influences the extracellular volume through the osmoregulatory system controlled by renal and adrenal hormones responding to renal perfusion. Reduction in total body sodium results in a reduction in extracellular fluid.

All these factors work together in a quite remarkable way to produce a dynamic equilibrium which ensures a constant circulation of extracellular fluid without any excessive accumulation in the healthy individual. Swelling, in the form of oedema, results when one or more of these factors is disturbed.

The composition of extracellular fluid in oedema varies with its cause. The oedema of inflammation cannot, for example, be moved about through the tissues as in other forms of oedema and is less influenced by gravity because inflammatory fluid is rich in protein and probably contains a network of fibrin. In lymphatic obstruction, the 'lymphoedema' is also rich in protein and becomes organized by fibroblasts so that it tends to be irreversible and leads eventually to a characteristic brawny thickening of the skin. The fluid of congestive oedema, on the other hand, is loose in the tissues and readily changes its position under the action of gravity so that it first appears in the dependent part showing the characteristic of 'pitting on pressure'. The oedema of renal disease resembles that of congestive oedema but is less influenced by gravity, the protein content and specific gravity being lower than in cardiac oedema.

Presentation

Although swollen legs are often themselves the overt presenting symptom in a consultation, especially when the oedema is secondary to venous obstruction, when the cause is a general one (most commonly heart failure) the leg swelling may only be presented as a secondary feature, the main complaints being breathlessness or tiredness, or only elicited in the course of systematic enquiry or on examination. The patient with swollen legs is most often seen first in the course of a surgery consultation as the swelling from almost all causes (with the possible exception of phlebothrombosis) is of gradual onset and is rarely, if ever, classed by the patient or doctor as an emergency.

Causes

General causes. — The most important general cause is congestive heart failure, in which a variety of factors, including salt retention, hypoproteinaemia, increased hydrostatic pressure and increased capillary permeability, play a part in inducing oedema.
In renal oedema the principal factors are a decrease in plasma protein and increased salt retention due to faulty renal function. Diabetes mellitus may be responsible for renal damage and may therefore precipitate renal oedema. The other general causes include hepatic oedema due to a lower production of plasma proteins causing reduction in osmotic pressure in the blood aggravated by increased congestion from obstruction to the venous return. Reduced plasma protein will also occur when there is a protein-losing enteropathy and may therefore be associated with swelling in the leg. Hypothyroidism can be associated with swelling, the so-called 'myxoedema' due to mucin deposition in the subcutaneous tissues.

Local causes. — Swelling in the legs may be due simply to a postural obstruction to venous return and this is often seen in the elderly who sit for long periods in a chair, so that a dependent oedema is produced from pressure on the veins behind the knee and by the immobility which removes the muscle-pumping action encouraging venous return. In a similar way, swelling of the legs is caused by prolonged sitting during journeys by air or car, particularly in warm weather. Patients with varicose veins will also experience swelling in the legs due to venous congestion of the superficial veins, especially if a constricting garter is worn. Varicose veins are more common in women and the swelling will be most prominent towards the end of the day, especially when there is prolonged standing which increases the hydrostatic pressure in veins for long periods. The swelling will be aggravated if the patient is overweight.

Perhaps the most important local cause of swelling is phlebothrombosis (deep-vein thrombosis) although it should be noted that this condition must be extensively established before it causes swelling since oedema in this case occurs due to inflammatory involvement of the lymphatic system causing obstruction to return flow. The deep-vein thrombosis may occur at any point in the deep venous system but the calf, pelvis and feet are the most common sites, and swelling will occur peripheral to the obstruction and may therefore involve the whole leg. In women taking oral contraceptives, the risk of developing deep-vein thrombosis is 6 times that of a non-user.[3]

Less common causes. — Obstruction due to effusion into the knee joint or into the semimembranosus bursa will cause swelling below the knee especially when a crêpe support has been applied. Local inflammatory causes of swelling due to toxic damage to capillary walls include cellulitis and gout. The hereditary condition of obstruction to lymphatic return (Milroy's disease) is rare but there is a tendency, predominantly in otherwise healthy women, to develop thickening of the legs due to an increase of subcutaneous tissue, from chronic lymphoedema due to lymphatic inadequacy. This type of chronic lymphoedema renders the patient especially prone to cellulitis and, whilst it usually involves both legs, this is not exclusively the case. The lymphatic return can also be obstructed when the patient has had radiotherapy or there are metastases in the inguinal glands. Obstruction to the venous return can also occur from intra-abdominal tumours and, rarely, from a gravid uterus.

In angioneurotic oedema, there may be a local or general production of swelling due to a hypersensitivity reaction to an antigen causing severe local oedema by increasing capillary permeability. The drug carbenoxolone, used in the treatment of gastric ulcers, causes salt retention and potassium loss and may be responsible for causing oedema. Other rarer causes include enlargement of the leg due to arterio-venous fistulae which may be either congenital or acquired as the result of a penetrating wound.

History

The practitioner must bear in mind the mechanisms producing swollen legs so that questioning may be pertinent, particularly if swelling is absent at the time of examination. He will appreciate that swollen legs may be a manifestation of a general systemic illness, of which the two most important are heart failure and renal disease, or alternatively may be due to some local cause. It is therefore important to establish for how long the swelling has occurred, whether or not swelling affects both legs equally, whether the swelling is influenced by duration of posture and the time of day, the level in the legs to which swelling extends and whether the swelling has been accompanied by pain.

Accurate medical records will indicate relevant previous medical history. In women, it is important to remember that retention of fluid can occur premenstrually and may aggravate other causes of swelling. Because of the association with thrombo-embolism, history-taking should note if the woman is on the 'Pill'.

Examination

The examination of the patient will begin with the legs to confirm the presence or absence of swelling. This may be obvious on inspection and particular note should be made around the margin of shoes where pitting may be present or at the site of any garter or similar constriction in the legs. Firm pressure (which may be quite unpleasant, and therefore the patient should be duly warned) over the dorsum of the foot, or over the lower anterior tibia, may be necessary to produce even minimal pitting. Where the swelling is more obvious, its character should be noted with particular reference to looseness in the tissues. Where a unilateral swelling is suspected but is not obvious, it may be necessary to measure the girth of the legs at selected points, such as at mid-calf, while inspection of the superficial veins for varicosities or any increased venous flow will be an essential part of preliminary examination. Any local tenderness should be noted but, if a deep-vein thrombosis is suspected, forcible dorsi-flexion of the foot should be avoided because of the danger of dislodging a thrombus.

Examination of the joints for any intra-articular effusion is important, particularly at knee level where the presence of an enlarged semimembranosus bursa can be responsible for obstruction to the venous return.

When examination of the legs is complete, the examiner should ensure that there is no lesion within the pelvis that may be causing obstruction. A general examination may then be required with particular reference to the cardiac and renal systems and to the other general causes of swelling in the legs already listed. It will be important to note the patient's weight since an accumulation of water cannot be detected clinically, from a general cause, until five or six litres have collected.

Laboratory investigations will be dictated by the suspected cause of the swelling but may include examination of the urine for protein and sugar and of the blood for haemoglobin, sedimentation rate, urea, electrolytes and plasma proteins.

Treatment

The treatment of patients with oedema is related to the underlying cause and in particular whether that cause is a general or a local one. In patients in whom the cause is a general systemic condition, restriction of salt intake is indicated. This can be assisted by avoiding the addition of salt at the table, the restriction in the consumption of food with a high salt content, such as ham, bacon, sausages and kippers, and, if necessary, by avoiding salt in cooking. If this regime is inadequate, then a diuretic may be used as part of the regimen for the treatment of the general condition.

The treatment of local causes will be dictated by the nature of the underlying condition but it is worth remembering that when oedema is due to an obstruction in the venous or lymphatic return existing in the lower limbs only, the use of a diuretic must be approached with caution since this will act centrally to disturb the normally functioning kidneys.

When there is a chronic impairment of the lymphatic return, or when the swelling is the result of impaired functioning of the venous return, the swelling can be reduced by the use of elastic stockings. When swelling extends above the knee, a two-way stretch stocking should be prescribed but where the swelling is confined below the knee, it may be appropriate, especially in men, to prescribe a one-way stretch stocking since this is more self-supporting. The use of Tubigrip should be avoided since this is not shaped to the leg and therefore causes differential pressure which can aggravate obstruction like an over-tight garter. In patients with severe arterial disease, an elastic support may rarely embarrass arterial flow but otherwise wearing elastic support stockings, properly measured, can make an important contribution to the control of swollen legs.

General measures to avoid excessive standing, or restriction of the venous return for those who are confined to chairs, may produce a substantial improvement while the factor of obesity is as relevant to swelling in the legs as it is to almost every other medical complaint.

References

[1] Morrell, D.C., Gage, H.G. and Robinson, N.A. (1971): Symptoms in General Practice. *Journal of the Royal College of General Practitioners*, *21*, 32.

[2] Royal College of General Practitioners, Office of Population Censuses and Surveys, Department of Health and Social Security (1986): *Morbidity Statistics from General Practice 1981–82*. HMSO Series MB5 No. 1

[3] The Royal College of General Practitioners (1974): *Oral Contraceptives and Health.* London: Pitman Medical.

3.36 Itch

David Morrell

The simple complaint of itching is rare in general practice with two exceptions. These are itching of the anal and vulval areas. In most other conditions itching is complained of in association with a skin rash, although there are rare systemic disorders in which generalized itching may be prominent. The detailed description of rashes which may be irritant is considered in chapter 3.37. This chapter will review briefly the sort of conditions which may underlie the complaint of itching.

Causes

Skin infestations.– Scabies is probably the most common infestation which presents in general practice as itching. This is particularly troublesome at night. Its presentation and management are described in Chapter 3.37

Infestation with body lice is now uncommon, but head lice and occasionally pubic lice are still encountered, particularly in inner city practices. The cause of the itching in these cases will usually be seen crawling among the hairs, or the 'nits' will be seen attached near the base of the hairs. A pointer to infestation with head lice is often provided by extensive excoriation of the skin of the neck caused by the vigorous scratching.

A variety of insects such as fleas, mosquitoes and bed bugs may cause irritation of the skin. Flea bites tend to be aggregated together, not uncommonly along a line where further exploration of the skin is limited by a tight garment, such as the upper or lower limit of a brassiere or the waistband of pants. They appear as small 1 to 2 mm red spots. Mosquito bites may also be limited by clothing but are seen most commonly on the exposed parts of the body and present as urticarial papules. Bed bugs and house-dust mites cause papules and urticaria.

Skin diseases.– The most irritant skin diseases are atopic and primary irritant eczema. Their characteristics and management are described in Chapter 3.37. Other characteristically itchy skin diseases also described in that chapter are lichen planus, dermatitis herpetiformis and fungal infections of the skin.

Systemic disorders.– The most important systemic disorders causing generalized pruritus are Hodgkin's disease and other reticuloses, obstructive jaundice and cirrhosis of the liver, diabetes mellitus, and pregnancy. Angioneurotic oedema and urticaria, which result most commonly from the ingestion of substances to which the individual is allergic, are probably the most common systemic causes of itch in general practice.

Pruritus ani.– The most common cause of anal itching is probably threadworm infestation in children. The ingestion of broad-spectrum antibiotics almost certainly comes next. This may result in diarrhoea followed by irritation, or it may lead to secondary monilial infection of the natal cleft. By the time the problem is presented to the general practitioner there will usually be excoriation of the anus and possibly secondary infection. Continued scratching tends to perpetuate the lesions, and once established the condition is often difficult to eradicate. Frequently, patients attempt to treat the problem themselves. This treatment almost always includes frequent washing with soap and water, which may simply make matters worse if the soap is not completely removed from the natal cleft. In some cases the patient obtains medicated creams from the pharmacy and not uncommonly obtains from a doctor cream or ointment containing antihistamines, local anaesthetics or antibiotics. All of these may complicate the problem by producing a primary irritant eczema, and unravelling the primary cause from the secondary effects of treatment may be complex. Rarely seborrhoeic eczema or psoriasis may cause irritation of the natal cleft.

Pruritus vulvae.– The most common cause in general practice is vaginal moniliasis, which is predisposed to by the use of systemic broad-spectrum antibiotics. It is also common in patients taking oral contraceptives. It produces a vaginal discharge and the diagnosis may be confirmed from direct smears of the discharge or from vaginal swabs transported to the laboratory in Stuart's medium. Direct observation of the white patches of 'thrush' on the vaginal walls, however, is diagnostic in most cases without recourse to the laboratory. By causing a persistent discharge and excoriation of the vulva, other vaginal infections may also produce pruritus, and the patient's response to this symptom, which often includes repeated washing with soap and water, may complicate the picture by producing a primary irritant eczema. Another common cause of pruritus vulvae is irritation from cosmetics. These may be 'bubble baths', or similar scented bath additives, or the direct application of deodorants to the vulva in the form of aerosols or lotion. Occasionally rubber or chemical contraceptives may be implicated. The initial irritation caused by such irritants leads to scratching and a vicious circle of scratching and itching leads to lichenification of the skin and persistent irritation.

Specific infections of the skin may cause pruritus vulvae. Tinea cruris develops in the fold of the groin and spreads outwards over the thigh and inwards over the labia majora with healing at the centre and extension of the rash at the periphery. Seborrhoeic eczema may develop in the groin and spread to the vulva and natal cleft with excoriation and weeping. Monilial infection may complicate this. Less commonly psoriasis may affect the vulva and cause itching.

Contamination of the vulva by urine is an important cause of pruritus. In all cases the urine should be tested for sugar. In infancy contamination may lead to a napkin dermatitis. At the other end of life stress incontinence may lead to pruritus vulvae, a cause that may be overlooked as many elderly women do not complain of stress incontinence, accepting it as a normal process of ageing.

In post-menopausal women atrophy of the vagina and vulva may lead to itching and scratching. This in turn causes lichenification, and a vicious circle of itch and scratch is established.

Pruritus vulvae may occasionally be the presenting symptom of a psychosexual disorder. In these patients itching tends to be associated with soreness of the vulva which often precludes sexual intercourse. Rarely, this symptom may be presented by a patient indulging in lesbian or solitary sexual practices. The patient may be anxious about the acceptability or possible complications of such practices but may find it impossible to present this problem directly to the doctor. When such a possibility is considered it is appropriate in identifying the cause of the pruritus to inquire delicately into the patient's sexual life; this may open up a new diagnostic problem (Chapter 3.61).

Lichen simplex.– A variety of lesions of the skin from minor trauma through ichthyosis to stasis eczema may cause itching. The individual responds by scratching. As a result areas of skin become lichenified and continue to itch. This results in the development of patches of lichen simplex. These are localized areas of abnormally thickened skin in which the condition is perpetuated by scratching. The importance of psychiatric disturbance in precipitating this cycle of events is not clear but in some cases stress may increase the sensitivity to itching and may predispose the individual to scratching.

History and examination

It is important to ask the patient complaining of itching whether this is generalized or localized, and to establish the time of onset in relation to other events. Generalized itching, particularly in the absence of cutaneous abnormalities, is suggestive of some systemic disturbance. This may include the accumulation of normal metabolites which provoke itching, such as occurs in jaundice or pregnancy, or it may be due to the abnormal release of proteinases or circulating antigens due to an allergic phenomenon such as drug hypersensitivity. The history in such cases should be designed to identify any relationship between the presenting symptom and possible causes. These are numerous and questions should be asked about injections, drug therapy, including the taking of proprietary drugs purchased at the chemist, and the ingestion of unfamiliar foods. Rarely the cause may be immediately evident in that the patient is known to be suffering from some predisposing condition or receiving drug therapy. More often it remains obscure. Occasionally, generalized itching may be caused by exposure of the whole body surface to some primary irritant such as 'bubble bath', or by general infestation of the skin, such as scabies. A history of itching in other members of the family should be inquired for, and is strongly suggestive of an infestation.

Localized itching may be associated with an obvious skin rash which will lead to an appropriate history concerning the time and site of onset of the rash, and the mode of spread. In some cases, however, there may be only excoriation due to the scratching, and no history of a preceding skin lesion. In these cases a careful history should be taken concerning the use of possible primary irritants or allergens, such as soaps, detergents, cosmetics, deodorants or even medically prescribed preparations containing potential irritants or allergens such as local anaesthetics or antibiotics. The time relationship between exposure and onset is all-important in these cases. Sometimes the systemic administration of antibiotics may lead to localized itching due to an overgrowth in the skin of monilia; this is a common cause of pruritus ani and vulvae. The history should therefore include enquiry about such treatment. Rarely drug ingestion may lead to hypersensitivity of the skin to sunlight, resulting in itching followed by solar dermatitis. The phenothiazines, thiazides and sulphonamides are particularly likely to be responsible. Itching of the eyes is a common feature of hay fever, and a history of seasonal attacks may be obtained in such patients.

The extent of the examination will depend very much on the findings in the history. In some cases it will be necessary to seek for evidence of skin diseases, such as atopic eczema and in particular for evidence of infestation such as scabies, lice or simple fleas or mosquito bites. In some cases of pruritus due to ingestion of food or drugs to which the individual is hypersensitive, the skin may be very sensitive to minor trauma and a mild scratch will lead to weal formation. It is uncommon for itching to be the first symptom of liver disease or reticulosis but, if such conditions are suspected by other symptoms suggestive of general ill health, clearly further examination and investigations will be undertaken. Where a monilial infection or tinea is suspected the diagnosis may be confirmed by taking swabs or skin scrapings for examination.

Management

The treatment of itching can be dramatically successful in some but in others may cause almost insuperable problems. In cases due to such conditions as scabies, tinea, threadworm infestations or monilial vaginitis a precise diagnosis of the cause will lead to appropriate therapy and complete cure. The treatment of scabies, tinea and insect bites is described in Chapter 3.37; the treatment of vaginitis in Chapter 3.59. Threadworms respond to treatment with piperazine compounds for a period of one week in a dose determined by the age of the patient. Thus for piperazine phosphate the dosage is: adults, 2 grams daily; children of 5 to 12 years 1.5 grams daily; those aged 2 to 4 years 750 mg daily.

Atopic and primary irritant eczema respond to local steroids such as 1 per cent hydrocortisone cream, and seborrhoeic eczema to a combination of steroids and nystatin e.g. Nystaform-HC. The detailed treatment of these conditions will be found in Chapter 3.37, as also will the treatment of papular urticaria.

Acute and recurrent urticaria.– This may be extremely difficult to manage. It may present as an acute response to the ingestion of a food or drug to which the individual is allergic. The itching may be almost intolerable. Initial treatment should be by the use of systemic antihistamines such as promethazine, 25 mg three times daily, or trimeprazine tartrate (Vallergan), 10 mg three times daily. The latter is also available as an injection, 25 mg in 2 ml, for use in acute allergic reactions. Patients being prescribed antihistamines should be warned that sedative side-effects occur and that the drugs may interact with alcohol. Cooling lotions such as calamine lotion or calamine lotion containing 1 per cent phenol may be of value. In severe cases, however, steroids should be used, starting with a large dose such as prednisone, 10 mg six hourly, and rapidly tailing this off as the patient responds to treatment.

Some patients develop recurrent attacks of urticaria in the absence of any obvious precipitating cause. Such patients, if the condition is severe, should be treated with high doses of steroids for short periods of time, and these should always be withdrawn gradually. An appropriate dosage regime is 40 mg of prednisone for two days, followed by 30 mg, 20 mg, 10 mg, and then 5 mg, for two days respectively. A sedative antihistamine such as promethazine may be used concurrently.

Pruritus ani. – A precise diagnosis of the cause of this complaint is important. Careful examination of the natal cleft and surrounding skin may indicate, for instance, a fungal infection (tinea cruris) with lesions spreading out onto the inner thighs and scrotum. This will be treated appropriately (Chapter 3.37). A soggy pale appearance of the natal cleft may suggest a monilial infection; a history of antibiotic therapy would support this diagnosis and treatment with nystatin cream combined with hydrocortisone would be appropriate. An angry red, inflammatory reaction which is both tender and extremely itchy suggests a primary irritant eczema. One per cent hydrocortisone cream is the treatment of choice.

In all cases it is important to stop all the treatment which the patient is carrying out at the time of presentation, as this condition is so often iatrogenic. The patient should be instructed to have a daily bath, but otherwise indulge in no other washing or cleaning procedures. The appropriate therapy which should be simple and where possible specific should be applied at eight-hourly intervals. As the condition resolves the treatment should be gradually withdrawn. Creams containing antibiotics, anti-histamines, or local anaesthetics should never be used in treating this condition. Occasionally, local conditions such as haemorrhoids or an anal fissure may be precipitating the symptoms. These will be diagnosed by rectal examination or proctoscopy and should be treated appropriately (Chapter 3.48).

Pruritus vulvae. – As in the case of pruritis ani, a precise diagnosis of the cause may lead to a rapid and complete cure. Monilial vaginitis can be treated with nystatin or clotrimazole pessaries and cream and other vaginal infections as indicated by the causative organisms (Chapter 3.59). The management of tinea cruris, pediculosis pubis, psoriasis and seborrhoeic eczema is described in Chapter 3.37. Primary irritant eczema caused by cosmetics responds to hydrocortisone cream. As with pruritus ani it is important to stop all previous medication and to limit washing to a daily or, if necessary, twice daily bath. Washing with soap and water must be banned as it is almost impossible to remove all the soap from the creases of the vulva unless the patient is immersed in a bath. Many general practitioners have suspected that the wearing of nylon pants covered by nylon tights and held in place by a further pair of nylon pants (a degree of security initially demanded by the mini skirt) predisposes to vulval irritation and infection. There is no hard evidence that this is so but it seems reasonable to recommend that a single pair of cotton pants might be the appropriate covering for an inflamed and itching vulva.

In post-menopausal women atrophy and a change in pH of the vagina and vulva may predispose to infection and itching. The administration of oestrogens such as ethinyloestradiol, 0.01 mg daily, or topical dienoestrol cream may produce dramatic improvement. If stress incontinence is present this should be treated surgically.

Generalized pruritus. – Itching may present as a serious problem in the management of obstructive jaundice or reticulosis. Unfortunately there is no really effective systemic anti-pruritic. In such cases sedative antihistamines such as promethazine or simple sedatives such as diazepam or phenobarbitone may be useful. In liver disease the phenothiazines are contraindicated but they may be valuable in treating itching due to the reticuloses. Patients not suffering from organic systemic disorders may complain of generalized itching. This is most common in the elderly and in some of these cases is due to ichthyosis. These patients may be helped by the use of emulsifying ointment or oilatum emollient added to the bath instead of soap and aqueous cream applied to the dry areas of the skin. If the patient is elderly and is advised to use emulsifying ointment he should be warned that this may make the bath very slippery and exceptional care must be exercised in getting in and out.

A number of patients with psychoneurotic disorders may occasionally complain of generalized itching. In such cases the phenothiazine drugs may be of value, such as chlorpromazine, 25 to 50 mg three times daily. It should always be remembered that very minor skin lesions may lead to itching. In the predisposed personality the vicious circle of itching and scratching is set up and an incurable patch of neurodermatitis may develop. Early intervention by the general practitioner is important in preventing this almost incurable disability.

3.37
The patient complaining of a rash

David Morrell

Estimating the prevalence of skin diseases in the community is fraught with difficulties. In particular the imprecise nature of the diagnostic labels applied to skin diseases and the difficulty of satisfactorily grouping the conditions found in order to report results complicate the task. In a community survey of skin diseases in Lambeth, London[1] the prevalence of skin lesions requiring medical care was estimated to be 22 per cent of the population sampled. The 92 conditions found in this survey were classified into 13 groups. The most important groups were eczema with a prevalence of 6 per cent and acne with a prevalence of 3·5 per cent. The prevalence of psoriasis was 0·6 per cent.

Similar problems of labelling are encountered in general practice studies reporting consultation rates for skin disorders. In the Third National Morbidity Study[2] an over-all consultation rate of 13.4 per 100 was recorded for diseases of the skin and subcutaneous tissues, with females consulting more often than males, and, with the exception of the age-groups 15 to 24 years, a gradual decline in consultations with increasing age. All skin disorders do not present to the general practitioner as a rash. Many present as individual spots, sores or ulcers, and these will be considered in a subsequent chapter. Patients, however, often do complain of a rash as a presenting symptom, and in a study designed to measure the frequency of symptoms[3] a rash accounted for 5 per cent of all new symptoms presented in general practice, and was exceeded in frequency only by the symptoms of cough and sore throat. Rashes were most commonly presented in children under the age of 5 years and declined in frequency with advancing years.

In studying the way in which rashes are presented to the general practitioner, it is possible to discern two broad groups of diagnostic problems. There is a large group of patients, most commonly children, who present with a rash of recent onset which is usually symmetrical in distribution and becomes generalized within a period of twenty-four to forty-eight hours. This group poses a different problem from a second group who present with a localized rash, or a more widespread rash which has developed over weeks or months. Inevitably, there will be exceptions to this rather arbitrary division of the way in which rashes present, but identifying this difference may be helpful in unravelling the diagnosis of rashes in general practice and it will be used in this chapter.

Before considering these separate modes of presentation, it is important to define certain terms which will be used in this chapter:

Macule	– A flat spot which differs in colour from the surrounding skin
Papule	– A raised spot on the surface of the skin
Nodule	– A lump deeply set in the skin
Scale	– A flake of horny cells loosened from the skin surface
Crust	– Dried serum adherent to the skin
Vesicle	– A skin bleb filled with clear fluid
Bulla	– A blister filled with clear or blood-stained fluid
Pustule	– A skin bleb filled with pus
Urticaria	– An irregular white or pink pruritic weal.

PART I. – THE PATIENT COMPLAINING OF A GENERALIZED RASH

Part I will be concerned with rashes which develop symmetrically over a period of less than forty-eight hours and ultimately cover at least one-half of the surface of the body.

Mode of presentation

Patients presenting with generalized skin rashes are most commonly either children or young adults. They can be divided into three broad groups:

1. Those presenting with a generalized skin rash which is accompanied by constitutional upset such as fever, malaise and upper respiratory catarrh
2. Those presenting with a generalized itching rash with little or no constitutional disturbance
3. Those presenting with a symmetrical rash but with minimal pruritus or constitutional upset.

Causes

Generalized rashes accompanied by malaise and fever

These are nearly always due to specific infectious diseases.

Measles. – The onset is with a catarrhal illness with a particularly irritable cough and conjunctivitis. The child is usually miserable and pyrexial. At this stage the characteristic Koplik spots resembling grains of salt may be seen on the mucous membranes of the cheek, opposite the molar teeth. After three or four days the rash appears at first behind the ears and at the hairline, and rapidly (over twenty-four hours) spreading to the trunk and limbs. It consists of dusky red macules with some slightly raised maculo-papules which coalesce to form irregular blotches. After two to three days the rash fades leaving behind brownish staining. The fever subsides in the absence of complications, but the child usually remains catarrhal for a further week or two.

Rubella. – The onset is one of mild malaise accompanied by slight conjunctivitis. About 24 hours after the onset of the illness the rash first appears behind the ears and on the face and consists of pale pink macules. It spreads rapidly over the trunk and limbs. On the trunk it may become confluent to produce a pink flush. It usually remains discrete on the limbs and never produces the ugly dusky red irregular blotches of measles, or the punctate erythema of scarlet fever.

Scarlet fever. – The onset is abrupt with fever and tonsillitis, and in children may be accompanied with vomiting. Headache is sometimes a prominent symptom. The rash follows within forty-eight hours. It appears as a red flush on the face, in contrast with pallor which surrounds the mouth. It spreads down over the trunk and limbs as a background erythema with red punctate lesions superimposed upon it. The rash persists for two to three days and then fades, and is followed by desquamation. At onset the tongue is characteristically furred with enlarged papillae projecting through the fur (the white strawberry tongue). Later the fur peels off to leave a red glazed punctate surface (the red strawberry tongue).

Chickenpox. – Chickenpox may be presented to the doctor as one or two isolated spots, but it usually comes to his attention when there is a fairly widespread rash which is most commonly the first sign of the illness. In adults there may occasionally be a mild prodromal period with malaise, fever and headache. The rash develops as macules which rapidly progress to umbilicated papules and vesicles. The lesions appear first on the trunk and later on the face and limbs. Successive crops of lesions appear so that at any one time all stages of the rash may be seen. The distribution is essentially centripetal. One or two lesions are almost invariably present in the mouth. Differentiation from smallpox is rarely demanded of the general practitioner in this country. Smallpox is accompanied by far greater constitutional disturbance, by a centrifugal distribution of the rash, and the absence of cropping: i.e. all the lesions are at the same stage of development.

Non-specific viral infections. – A large number of virus infections produce catarrhal illnesses accompanied by erythematous or macular rashes. Clinically they are often indistinguishable from mild rubella, but lymphadenopathy is a more prominent feature of this latter illness. Most of them fade within twenty-four to forty-eight hours and produce no serious complications.

Glandular fever. – In infectious mononucleosis a raised erythematous eruption occurs on the trunk, buttocks and extensor surfaces of the limbs in about 10 per cent of cases. If ampicillin is given to a patient with glandular fever a widespread, maculo-papular, erythematous eruption occurs in most cases. The other features of the illness, including a severe membranous tonsillitis, lymphadenopathy and often splenomegaly, suggest the diagnosis.

Secondary syphilis. – In general practice, this is a rare cause of a symmetrical rapidly evolving rash which occurs six weeks to one year after a primary infection. It consists of a reddish papular eruption of the trunk and limbs. It is often accompanied by some malaise and lymphadenopathy. The palms and the soles often have papulo-squamous lesions. There are often lesions on the mucous membranes described as snail track ulcers, and condylomata should be looked for around the anus or genitals. Serological tests for syphilis are always positive at this stage.

Generalized rashes in which acute pruritus is the predominant feature

Drug eruptions. – Almost any drug may produce a drug eruption in a sensitive individual. The eruption may appear on the first occasion that the person is exposed to the drug, or it may appear in a person who has been taking the drug without any trouble over a period of time. Because the eruption is in response to a drug circulating in the body, it is usually of abrupt onset and widespread. It commonly appears as an acute erythematous response, and is sometimes accompanied by urticaria, severe pruritus and angioneurotic oedema. There may be some malaise, fever or fleeting joint pains.

Morbilliform eruptions. – These are maculo-papular eruptions resembling measles but often with an urticarial element. They are most commonly caused by ampicillin. Other drugs producing this type of eruption are phenylbutazone, barbiturates and phenothiazines.

Erythema multiforme. – This type may be caused by sulphonamides and penicillin.

Purpuric eruptions. – Drug-induced purpura is most commonly seen on the legs and may be caused by non-steroidal, anti-inflammatory agents, quinidine, barbiturates and thiazide diuretics.

Photosensitivity. – Some drugs sensitize the skin to sunlight, and in these cases an erythematous lesion often leading to blistering may occur. The extent of the lesion depends on the part of the body exposed to sunlight. The most common causes are phenothiazines, tetracyclines, nalidixic acid and sulphonamides.

Urticaria and angioneurotic oedema. – This is widespread and usually highly irritant. The urticaria is often most prominent on the pressure points. Dermographism may be present. It is most commonly caused by the penicillins, and injections of serum and salicylates may cause exacerbations. Less common causes are anti-thyroid drugs and monoamine oxidase inhibitors. In severe cases, often referred to as serum sickness, there may be considerable constitutional upset and arthralgia.

Non-specific urticarial eruptions. – These consist of irregular white or pink transient pruritic weals. They may be produced by ingestion of food or drugs, but in some cases they are recurrent, and no cause can be found. Occasionally, they are related to exercise or emotion, and in these cases may appear and disappear within a period of a few hours.

Generalized eruptions in which there is minimal constitutional upset or pruritus

Erythema multiforme. – This tends to occur in young adults. The lesions consist of slightly raised macules up to one centimetre in diameter. They may coalesce, and typically show concentric rings (iris or target lesions) of different shades of red and purple. There may be a small vesicle in the centre of each lesion. The lesions occur most profusely on the extremities and involve the palms of the hand and the soles of the feet. Lesions may also occur on the buccal mucous membranes and the genitalia. A severe form of the disease with extensive skin, conjunctival, and mucous-membrane lesions (Stevens-Johnson syndrome) is occasionally seen in children. Milder forms of the disease resolve spontaneously in three or four weeks. Erythema multiforme may be idiopathic, provoked by drugs or, less commonly, be a sequel to recurrent herpes simplex infections.

Pityriasis rosea. – In general practice this is a relatively common condition, seen in young adults. A widespread symmetrical eruption occurs on the trunk and later spreads to the upper arms and thighs. It rarely spreads to the lower part of the limbs or the face. The typical lesion is oval in shape, the long axis lying in the natural line of cleavage of the skin. The edge of the lesion is slightly scaly. Not uncommonly the generalized rash is preceded by a single large scaly patch (the herald patch) by several days. There is little constitutional upset, minimal pruritus and the rash clears in six to eight weeks. Once a patient has had pityriasis rosea, the illness does not recur.

History and examination

It is important to record the mode of onset of the rash. Rarely, a long-standing localized rash may rapidly spread to involve the whole body. More often the rash spreads gradually over a period of hours from its site of onset to involve in symmetrical fashion the surface of the skin. The exact site of onset and mode of progression should, if possible, be determined. A history of any constitutional disturbance should be sought. The presence of upper respiratory catarrh, conjunctivitis, cough or sore throat may suggest the cause of the lesion. The patient should be asked specifically about drugs ingested in the preceding two weeks or immunization procedures undertaken. Enquiries should also be made about diet, particularly the ingestion of any unaccustomed food such as shell fish. Exposure to external irritants is a less common cause of generalized rashes, but this possibility should be explored and the patient's occupation ascertained. The patient should be asked about contact with infectious disease and about the presence of illness in other members of the family.

Examination of the skin should include the mucous membranes and conjunctivae. The nature of the rash, erythematous, macular, papular, vesicular, urticarial or a combination of these features, should be ascertained. The distribution and mode of spread are often all-important in reaching a diagnosis. The examination should be extended to look for signs of throat, ear or chest infection and enlarged lymph nodes and spleen.

Investigations are rarely helpful in reaching a diagnosis, although in a few specific conditions such as glandular fever a blood count or specific test may be necessary to confirm the diagnosis.

Diagnosis

The possible diagnostic pathways which may be followed in attempting to identify the cause of a generalized rash presenting in general practice are illustrated in figure 1. This is based entirely on the accompanying symptoms and physical signs which may be present in patients complaining of a generalized skin rash. If the knowledge of the individual lesions observed in the rash is added to this diagnostic scheme it is likely that most generalized rashes seen in general practice can be diagnosed.

Management

The sudden appearance of a widespread rash almost always causes considerably anxiety in patients. It is important for the doctor to explain to the patient the probable cause and natural history of the disease. In most cases the patient will be anxious to know whether the rash is infectious, and the doctor should be able to give appropriate advice in those conditions where the patient may be infectious to those around him.

Measles. – The rash in this condition is incidental to the catarrhal reaction in the respiratory tract and requires no specific treatment. In most cases symptomatic treatment will suffice for the respiratory symptoms, but careful watch must be kept for complications and the child's parents can be informed that these are usually indicated by a recrudescence of fever as the rash fades. This usually indicates bacterial infection of the middle ear or chest, and demands appropriate treatment with antibiotics. Prophylactic administration of penicillin is advocated by some for children with a history of recurrent otitis media or bronchitis.

Rubella. – This condition requires no treatment. The relationship between rubella and congenital malformations does, however, demand close enquiry about possible contacts between the patient and women in early pregnancy. Should these be established then serological confirmation of the disease is desirable and serological investigation of the pregnant patient should be undertaken to establish whether or not she has pre-existing antibodies.

Scarlet fever. – Treatment is simple and requires the administration of phenoxymethylpenicillin by mouth which should be given in a dose of 125 to 250 mg depending on age, four times daily before meals. Treatment should be continued for a period of ten days. Review eight weeks after the illness is

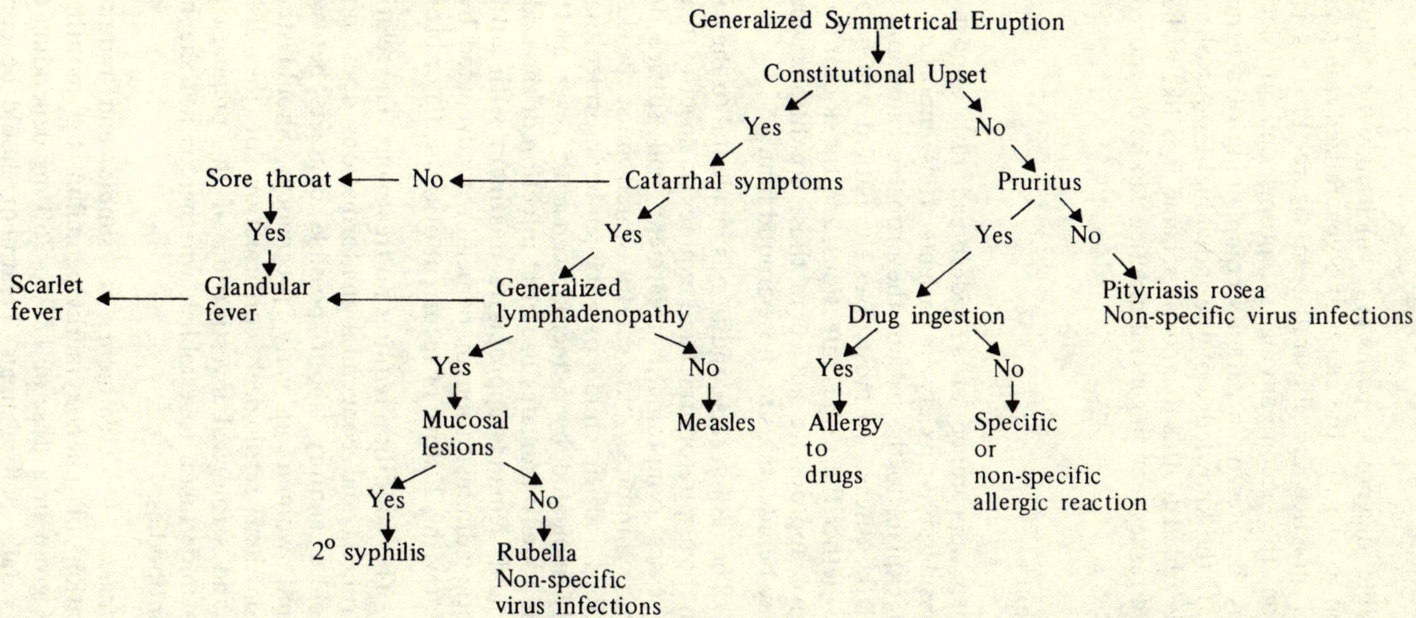

Figure I. – A diagnostic tree for the common generalized symmetrical rashes of rapid onset

desirable, and should include a urine test for albumen and examination of the cardiovascular system.

Non-specific virus infections. – A variety of virus infections, particularly in childhood, present non-specific skin eruptions. Some may be given names such as erythema subitum, or sixth disease. Many others are not associated with specific infections, but may accompany infections with a variety of viruses. Treatment should be symptomatic.

Secondary syphilis. – When this condition is suspected clinically the correct management is referral to a specialist in venereal disease. This alone will ensure adequate contact tracing and treatment.

Drug eruptions. – In mild cases treatment with antihistamines and local cooling lotions such as calamine lotion will suffice. In severe cases of angioneurotic oedema, or in the presence of severe pruritus, a short course of steroids given in high doses initially, but rapidly tailed off is indicated, such as prednisone, 40 mg on the first day, and reduced by 5 mg daily for a period of eight days. As many of these acute allergic reactions are produced by antibiotics, the introduction of steroid therapy in such cases should be accompanied by administration of an alternative antibiotic if the infection which provoked the initial antibiotic therapy has not resolved.

Non-specific urticarial reactions. – These are notoriously difficult to control. Antihistamines may be helpful. In most cases they are subject to acute exacerbations and prolonged remissions, and the intermittent use of steroids may control the major exacerbations.

Erythema multiforme. – Treatment must be related to the cause of the condition. If it is drug induced the drug must be withdrawn. In some cases the haemolytic streptococcus is implicated and here penicillin therapy is indicated. The condition is usually self limiting and local symptomatic measures such as the application of calamine lotion will be adequate. In severe cases such as the Stevens-Johnson syndrome, the condition may be life-threatening, or potentially damaging to eyesight, and requires admission to hospital and treatment with steroids, together with antibiotic therapy to counter secondary infection.

Pityriasis rosea. – This condition is self limiting. There is no specific therapy. If pruritus is troublesome, local treatment with calamine lotion will produce symptomatic relief.

PART II. – THE PATIENT PRESENTING WITH A LOCALIZED RASH

This part is concerned with rashes presented to the general practitioner which are usually of gradual onset and affect initially a localized part of the skin surface. They may or may not be symmetrical.

Causes

A consideration of the causes of localized rashes entails a review of the whole of dermatology. This section will concentrate on the differential diagnosis of those conditions commonly seen in general practice, and the characteristics and distribution of the rashes which they produce. The general practitioner is presented with a rash on the hand, the elbow or the flexures, and it is from this point that he must make a provisional diagnosis and seek confirmatory evidence. Before considering the differential diagnosis of rashes at particular sites, it is necessary to consider the main characteristics of the most common skin diseases seen in general practice.

Eczema

This denotes a sequence of inflammatory changes in the skin, in which redness and swelling are followed by blistering, scaling and ultimately thickening of the skin. The particular lesion seen depends on the site, the cause and the chronicity. In acute cases the skin is red and swollen with white papules, vesicles, exudation and crusting. In more chronic conditions the skin is thickened, red, scaly and dry, sometimes demonstrating considerable fissuring. In almost all cases pruritus is a troublesome feature. Eczema is a non-specific response of the skin to a variety of challenges. It is helpful to identify certain classes of eczema based on cause and clinical features, but it is important to realize that cases fall outside any classification, and cases seen early may be quite impossible to classify.

Primary irritant eczema. – Powerful irritants will produce an eczematous reaction in almost any skin. Some skins are more sensitive, and react when others would not. The rash may be caused by short exposure to a very powerful irritant, e.g. alkalis or solvents, or repeated insults by less powerful agents, e.g. detergents and soaps. The distribution of the rash and the occupation of the patient will usually lead to a correct diagnosis. Housewife's dermatitis affecting the hands and wrists is due to repeated contact with detergents, and is by far the most common example in general practice.

Allergic eczema. – This occurs when the skin is in contact with a substance to which the patient is allergic. The most common causes are:

Rubber and elasticized garments	E.g. rubber gloves, brassières and roll-ons which cause lesions on those parts of the skin covered by these garments.
Metals	Nickel is the commonest cause of contact eczema and may be found in jewellery clips, brassière clips and suspenders.
Dyes	These most commonly cause trouble from clothing, including shoes. Dye in clothes is particularly liable to cause eczema in the flexures due to perspiration at this site. Hair dyes are a common cause of eczema and may be seen in men as well as women.
Cosmetics	These include lipsticks, eye shadows, nail varnishes (the rash caused by nail varnishes may appear on the side of the face or neck) and deodorants.
Leather	This most commonly affects the feet due to contact with the shoes, but is also seen in hat bands and watch straps.
Therapeutic agents	Topical antibiotics, antihistamines and local anaesthetics are common causes of contact eczema.

Gravitational or stasis eczema. – This may be due to incompetent perforating varicose veins. It is seen in the lower limbs and may proceed to ulceration. It will be considered in detail in Chapter 3.39.

Industrial eczemas. – Many of the eczemas seen in general practice in the working population are caused by contact with irritant substances in the course of their work. They are most likely to occur on the hands or face. Most of these are primary irritant eczemas. The most common irritants are acids and alkalis, chemical solvents and various oils and greases. There may be a history of inadequate provision of or careless use of protective clothing. Some industrial eczemas are allergic in origin due to a wide variety of substances.

The complexity of modern industrial processes makes it impossible for the general practitioner to know about all the possible hazards, but he should try to be acquainted with the industrial processes taking place in his own practice area. Many large industrial plants have medical officers available for consultation. When an industrial eczema is suspected the industrial medical specialist may be able not only to identify the precise cause but also give advice on prevention and future employment prospects.

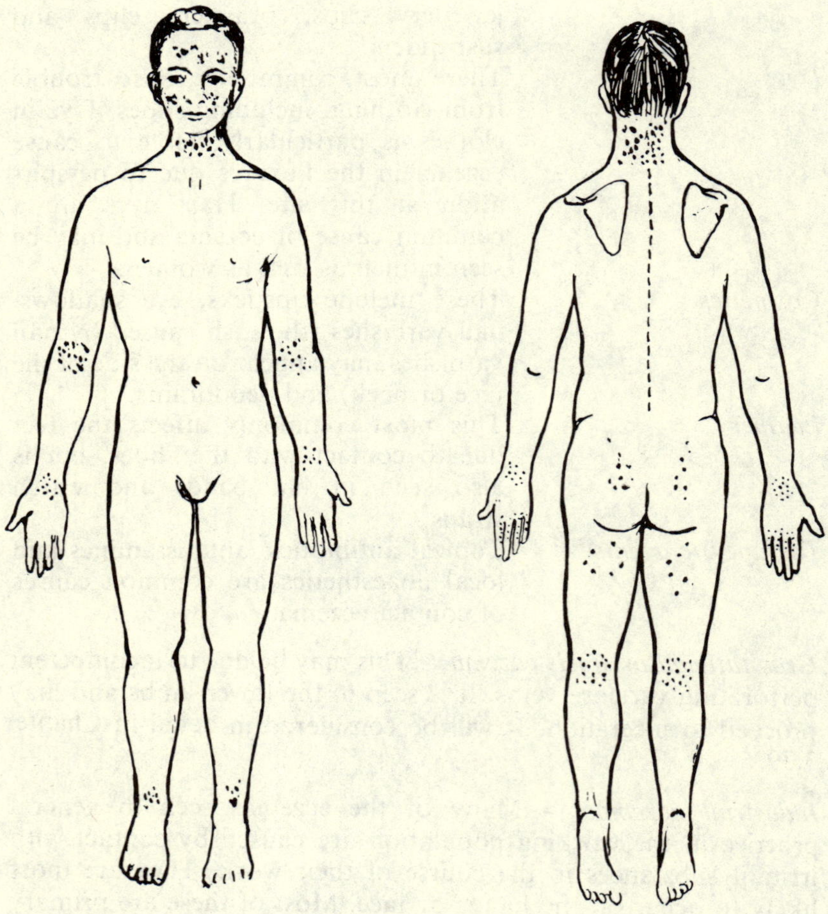

Figure 2. – Distribution of atopic eczema

Atopic eczema – This is part of the eczema-asthma-hay-fever syndrome. Onset is most commonly in the second year of life. The lesions tend to appear in the flexures of the elbows and knees. It often affects also the neck, face, wrists and buttocks. In infantile eczema it may become generalized, but most commonly persists in childhood as a recurrent flexural eczema.

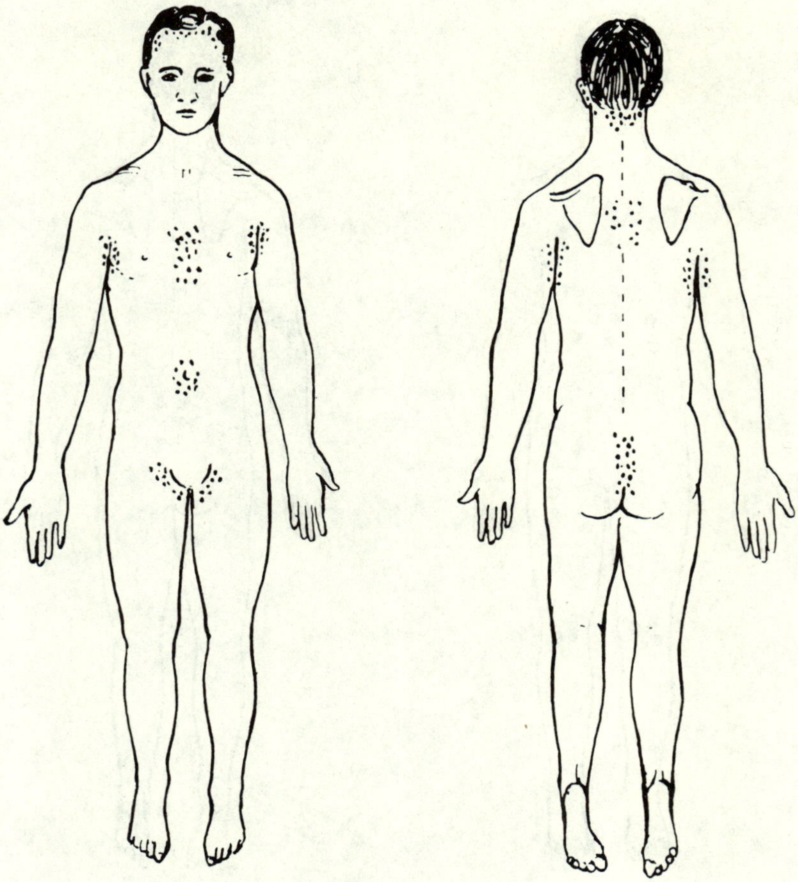

Figure 3. – Distribution of seborrhoeic eczema

Seborrhoeic eczema. – This is most commonly manifest as pityriasis capitis (dandruff) and an exudative eczema affecting characteristically the hair margins, ears, nasolabial folds and presternal and interscapular areas. It is sometimes also seen in the axillae and groins. In the obese it commonly occurs in the submammary region and in the umbilical region. Here it is often referred to as intertrigo, and may be complicated by bacterial or monilial infections.

Nummular eczema. – This tends to occur in adults. It is usually symmetrically distributed and the lesions assume a coin-like appearance. It occurs on the trunk and the extensor aspects of the limbs.

Pompholyx eczema. – This occurs on the hands and feet. It appears as small blisters between the fingers or in the instep.

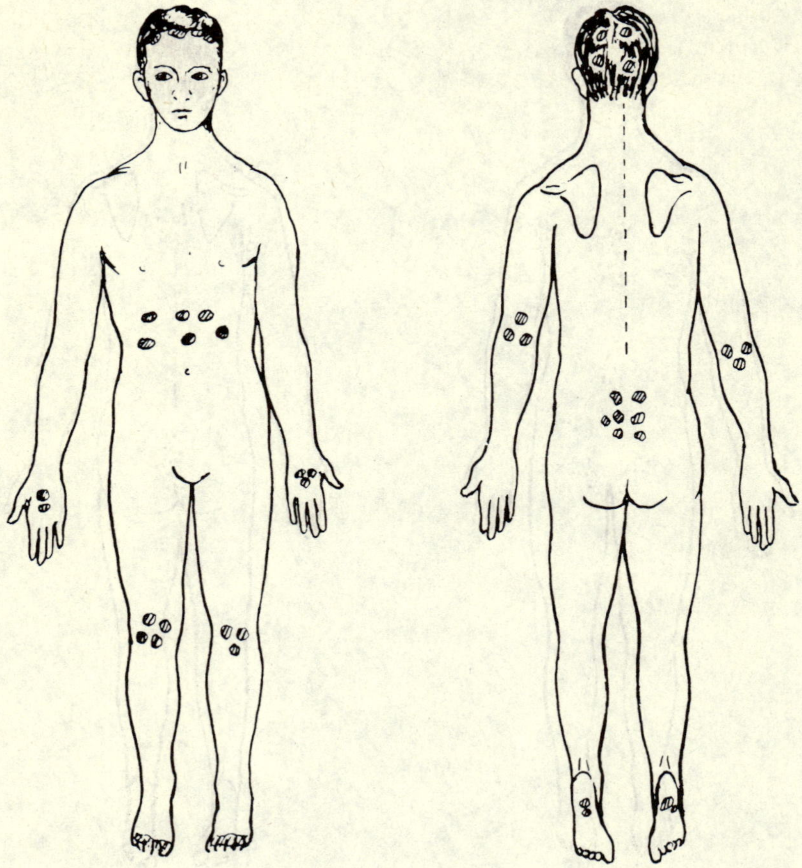

Figure 4. – Distribution of psoriasis

This characteristic is related to the character of the skin on these parts of the body. It is usually worse in hot weather. The blisters may rupture and produce a weeping area affecting a large proportion of the hands and feet.

Psoriasis

Psoriasis most commonly presents in early adult life. The characteristic lesion is a raised red scaly plaque with a sharp margin. The scaling tends to be silvery. Lesions occur most commonly on the knees, elbows, sacrum and scalp. If the easily detached scales are gently scraped off the lesion capillary bleeding points will be revealed. Less commonly psoriasis presents as a rash on the thorax with small lesions 0·5 to 1 centimetre in diameter scattered over the skin surface (guttate psoriasis), usually precipitated by streptococcal infections. It may also occur on the palms and soles as thick scaly lesions. When psoriasis affects the nails it produces a characteristic pitting. Rarely, psoriasis becomes confluent over the trunk (erythrodermic psoriasis) or pustular. Psoriatic arthritis is seen in about 10 per cent of cases.

Fungal infections

A number of fungus infections affect the skin and are referred to as tineas. They tend to develop as a small inflammatory lesion which spreads outwards to form an annular lesion with healing in the centre. The most common sites of infections are the feet (tinea pedis, one form of athlete's foot), the groins (tinea cruris), the trunk or limbs (tinea corporis) and the scalp (tinea capitis).

Tinea pedis. – This presents as maceration or scaling of the skin between the toes which may spread on to the plantar surface of the foot. Occasionally a scaling dermatitis of the instep area of the foot may occur.

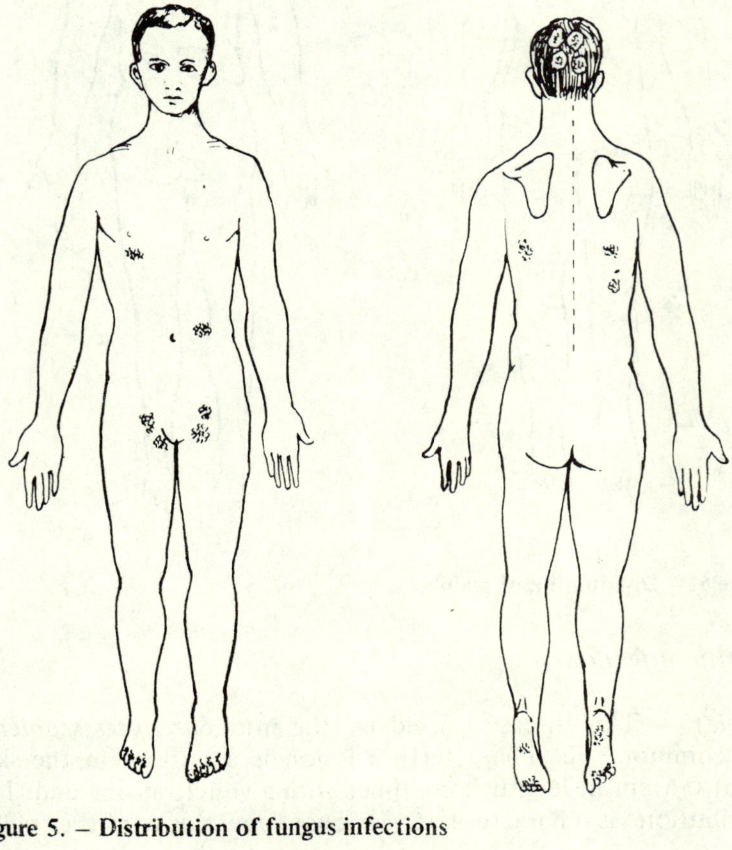

Figure 5. – Distribution of fungus infections

Tinea cruris. – This begins in the crural fold as an erythema and spreads out with a raised annular scaly margin.

Tinea corporis. – The lesion begins as a red papule and advances as a small ring (ringworm). It occasionally develops as a granulomatous ulcerating lesion.

Tinea capitis. – This presents as a discoid patch on the scalp, usually in children, with loss of hair due to the hair breaking off just above the surface of the skin. The skin is usually scaly but may rarely become pustular.

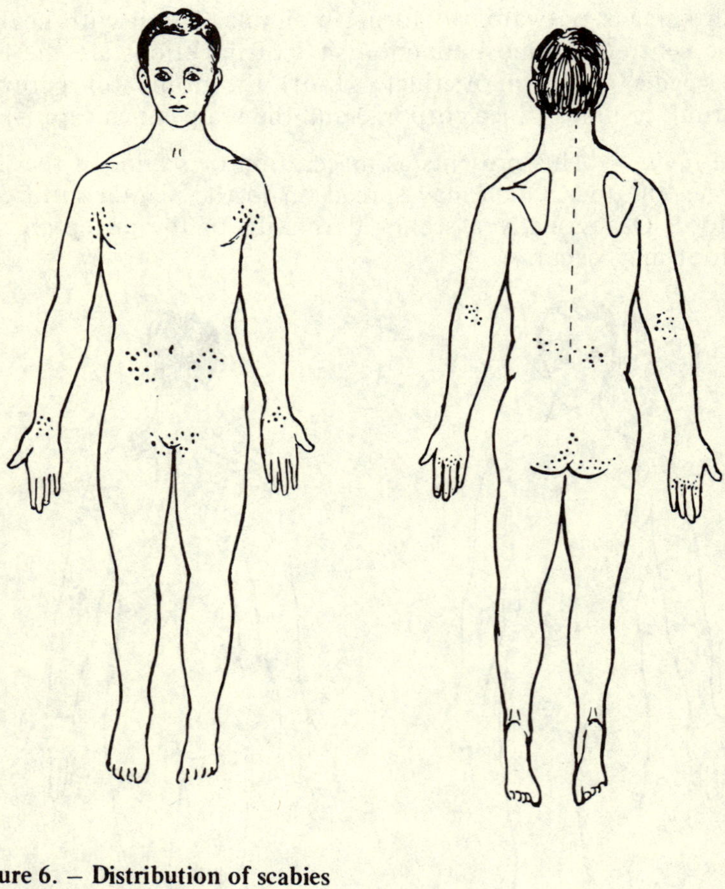

Figure 6. – Distribution of scabies

Parisitic infections

Scabies. – This disease caused by the mite *Sarcoptes scabiei* is still common. The characteristic lesion is a burrow in the skin about 0·5 cm in length, sometimes with a vesicle at one end. The distribution is characteristic, lesions appearing on the palm, between the fingers, the front of the wrists, the elbows, the anterior axillary fold, the breast, the buttocks and the external genitalia. The lesions are extremely irritant, particularly at night, and when presented to the doctor may be complicated by excoriation, eczematization, and impetigenization.

Papular urticaria. — This represents an urticarial and vesicular response to a variety of insect bites. The lesions are most commonly seen in children on exposed areas of the limb. They may be caused by fleas or bedbugs, but have in some cases been attributed to the housedust mite.

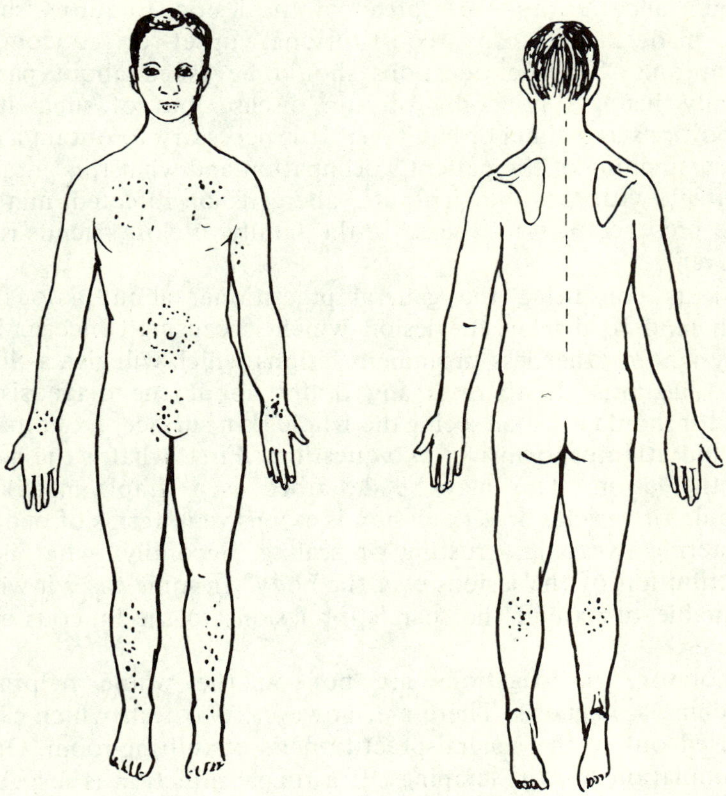

Figure 7. – Distribution of lichen planus

Lichen planus

This is a papulo-squamous eruption affecting most commonly young adults. The typical lesion is a flat-topped papule, polygonal in outline, about 5 mm in diameter, violaceous in colour and crossed by white streaks. The most common site is the wrists, but the lesions may be widespread and occasionally may coalesce to form plaques. There are characteristic lesions on the mucous membrane of the mouth and genitalia in many cases.

History and examination

In general practice the patient may present a skin lesion at a stage in its natural history before it has exhibited any diagnostic characteristics. As the condition develops, it may reveal its etiology by its appearance or distribution. In taking a history it is important to establish, if possible, the exact site and time of origin, and the mode of spread of the lesion. Enquiries should be made about any constitutional upset or concomitant symptoms. Specific questions should be asked about past or family history, not only of skin disease, but of such atopic conditions as asthma or hay fever. It is necessary to obtain a clear understanding of the patient's occupation and what this entails in contact with possible irritants, allergens or infected material. The presence of skin disease in the family or close friends is also relevant.

Patients consulting the general practitioner about a localized rash tend to display the lesion which is causing concern. They may ignore other less prominent lesions which will give a clue to the diagnosis. If there is any doubt about the diagnosis the doctor should insist on seeing the whole skin surface. Examination should attempt to answer two questions. First, what is the nature of the lesion? This may be described as a simple macule, or papule or vesicle, or if the lesion is extensive in terms of oedema, blistering, weeping, crusting or scaling. Secondly, what is the distribution of the lesions over the body? In some cases it will be desirable to extend the search for lesions to the mucous membranes.

Laboratory investigations are not on the whole helpful in reaching a diagnosis. There are, however, two tests which can be carried out in the general practitioner's consulting-room. One is examination of skin scrapings. If a fungal infection is suspected, scrapings from the skin may be placed on a microscope slide, and a few drops of 5 per cent potassium hydroxide are added. This dissolves the keratin and, after warming the slide for a few minutes, examination under the microscope may then reveal the hyphae or spores of the fungus or yeast. If scabies is suspected, scraping the burrow with a blunt scalpel and examination of the scrapings under a microscope may reveal the acarus itself or its eggs.

Distribution of rashes

Rashes affecting the hands. – The most common cause of rashes affecting the hands in general practice is primary irritant eczema, resulting from the use of soaps, detergents and other cleaning materials. The lesions in this case tend to affect the total skin surface of the hands and often spread on to the wrist and forearms. Less commonly, a rubber dermatitis, due to the use of rubber gloves, may produce a similar lesion.

Cheiropompholyx tends to affect predominantly the sides of the fingers with vesicular lesions, worse in hot weather.

Scabies characteristically affects the webs of the fingers and the fronts of the wrists. It may become eczematized or impetigenized by scratching.

Psoriasis is an uncommon cause of a rash affecting mainly the palm of the hand, while lichen planus may affect the flexor aspect of the wrist.

Rashes affecting the flexor aspects of the arms and legs. – Atopic eczema is by far the most common cause of a rash in the flexures of the elbow and knee. It is characteristically seen in young children, but may persist into adult life.

Rashes affecting the feet. – Tinea pedis is probably the most common cause of rashes on the feet. It tends to affect the skin between the toes and the plantar surface of the feet. Contact eczema due to leather or dye from shoes may affect the feet, when the lesions tend to be more prominent on the dorsum of the foot. Psoriasis may rarely affect the soles of the feet. Podopompholyx causes a vesicular eruption of the plantar surface of the foot, mainly in the instep area.

Rashes affecting the extensor surface of the limbs. – Psoriasis characteristically occurs on the elbows and knees. Erythema multiforme affects the extensor aspects of the hands, forearms and feet, and dermatitis herpetiformis is commonly seen as vesicular lesions on the knees, elbows and buttocks.

Rashes affecting the groin area. – These are most commonly due to tinea cruris. Seborrhoeic eczema of the groin area is another fairly common cause and is usually accompanied by seborrhoeic eczema elsewhere on the body.

Rashes affecting the axilla. – Contact eczema from deodorants or depilating agents is probably the commonest cause of rashes in this area. Less common causes are seborrhoeic eczema, folliculitis and tinea.

Rashes affecting the scalp. – Seborrhoeic dermatitis accompanied by pityriasis capitis is the most common cause of scalp lesions in general practice. Psoriasis may also affect the scalp and there may be evidence of psoriasis elsewhere. Tinea capitis is recognized by the essentially circumscribed lesions which it causes, as also is impetigo of the scalp which may complicate pediculosis capitis (lice).

Rashes affecting the trunk. – Seborrhoeic dermatitis develops in the presternal and interscapular areas of the trunk. Guttate psoriasis produces widespread 'rain-drop-like' lesions over the trunk. Nummular eczema tends to produce symmetrical discoid lesions on the trunk. In widespread lesions on the trunk pityriasis rosea and secondary syphilis must also be considered.

Rashes affecting the buttocks. – These are most commonly caused by scabies, psoriasis, dermatitis herpetiformis and atopy.

Lesions of the mucous membranes. – Some skin lesions are accompanied by lesions of the mucous membranes, and these lesions may be helpful in reaching a diagnosis. The skin rashes most commonly associated with mucosal lesions are:

Monilia	This produces the white patches (thrush) which may occur in the mouth or vagina.
Syphilis	This characteristically produces 'snail track' ulcers in the mouth.
Lichen planus	This may produce whitish papules on the inside of the cheek or on genital mucous membrane.
Erythema multiforme	This may produce a vesicular lesion in the mouth or genitals.

Management

Certain general principles govern the management of all rashes. These will be modified where specific remedies are appropriate, but they may be summarized in terms of the vehicle in which the medicament is delivered.

1. Moist or weeping rashes should be treated by lotions.
2. Oedematous but not exudative lesions should be treated with creams.
3. Dry lichenified fissured lesions should be treated with ointments.

Eczema. – Very acute exudative rashes should be treated with wet dressings, which are kept constantly moist with normal saline. This type of lesion is rarely encountered in general practice. Less acutely inflamed lesions may be treated with hydrocortisone lotion, proceeding to hydrocortisone cream as the rash resolves. Patients with eczema should avoid using normal soap preparations; these may be replaced by emulsifying ointment. The baby with infantile eczema should be bathed daily in a bath in which one tablespoonful of oilatum emollient is added to the bath water.

Steroids are invaluable in the management of eczema. In most cases 1 per cent hydrocortisone lotion or hydrocortisone cream will be adequate to control the eruption. Rarely it may be necessary to use the stronger preparations containing triamcinalone or betamethasone, but it should always be remembered that these are absorbed and should be used with care in patients with extensive moist lesions and in infants. If the rash becomes infected then an antibiotic, e.g. gentamicin, gramicidin, or bacitracin, should be added to the steroid preparation.

In prescribing steroid preparations it is important for the doctor to instruct the patient carefully on their use, and as with the use of steroids in other conditions it is usually helpful to apply the preparation fairly often during the early part of treatment when the lesion is acutely inflamed, and gradually withdraw treatment. To stop treating a lesion abruptly with a steroid will almost always lead to rapid exacerbation. This is the cause of a great deal of dissatisfaction among patients who use these preparations and of most cases of failure to produce a cure.

Seborrhoeic eczema presents special problems. Pityriasis capitis, which is often present, should be treated by the use of regular shampoos, such as 5 per cent cetrimide and the application of scalp lotions containing coal tar (liquid Polytar). Hydrocortisone lotion or cream may be applied to the axilla and groins. Scaly lesions of the presternal and interscapular region may be treated with 2 per cent sulphur in aqueous cream, B.P. If there are many adherent scales on the lesions of the scalp or trunk a preparation containing 2 per cent salicylic acid and 2 per cent sulphur in aqueous cream, B.P. should be used. Seborrhoeic eczema in the axilla, groin and sub-mammary region is not uncommonly complicated by bacterial and monilial infection. In such cases a steroid cream incorporating nystatin and clioquinol (Nystaform-H.C.) may be useful.

Psoriasis. – Many of the cases of psoriasis seen in general practice run a chronic course and affect only limited areas of the skin. Acute new lesions and psoriasis in intertriginous areas are best treated with steroid creams. The chronic scaly lesions may be treated with 5 per cent coal tar in Lassar's paste. Clearing of the most chronic lesions may be promoted by the use of 0·1 per cent dithranol in Lassar's paste. This should be applied overnight and covered with stockinette. The dithranol content of the paste may be increased to 0·2 per cent. It may, however, cause an acute reaction and will usually be employed under specialist supervision.

Acute and extensive psoriasis is relatively uncommon in general practice. It presents serious problems in management and usually demands specialist advice. Special textbooks should be consulted about the treatment of this distressing condition. Not uncommonly, psoriasis of the scalp presents a problem in general practice. Regular shampooing with 5 per cent cetrimide is helpful. A number of proprietary preparations containing coal tar (e.g. liquid Polytar) designed specifically for use on the scalp are now available. In very chronic cases a preparation containing 10 per cent coal tar and 5 per cent salicylic acid in emulsifying ointment, B.P. may be used but it is very messy. It should be used twice weekly at night and the hair shampooed in the morning.

Fungal infections. – Superficial fungal infections of the body or feet may be treated successfully with an ointment containing benzoic acid (Whitfield's ointment). In addition there are many proprietary preparations on the market containing miconazole nitrate (Dermonistat, Daktarin) which are effective, and most general practitioners have selected one which they find satisfactory. Acute lesions of the feet are often best treated with soaks of potassium permanganate. Patients should be advised to add sufficient permanganate crystals to turn the water in the basin pink. The feet should then be soaked for five minutes, dried and powdered with one of the proprietary powders available.

Fungal infections of the finger nails should be treated with oral griseofulvin, 125 mg four times daily for six months. Infections of the nails are very resistant to treatment and may require more than a year to obtain a lasting response. Fungal infections of the scalp and chronic fungal infections of the skin may be treated with griseofulvin four times daily for a month.

Parasitic infections. – Scabies can be eradicated by appropriate treatment. The patient should have a bath, following which all underclothing should be properly laundered. The whole skin surface below the neck should be painted with 25 per cent benzyl benzoate solution. Twenty-four hours later the patient should have a second bath and once more change the clothing. As a more cosmetically acceptable alternative, 1 per cent lindane may be used and applied as a cream, or a lotion (Esoderm, Quellada).

Papular urticaria must be treated by eliminating the insects causing the hypersensitivity response in the patient. The first step in the treatment is convincing the patient or parent that this is a reaction to insect bites. Treatment is directed to eliminating the insects. A thorough hoovering of the house and bedding should be accompanied by the treatment of any pets with dicophane powder (DDT). The powder may also be applied to the child night and morning. It is possible to obtain veterinary analysis of the brushings of pets to identify the cause.

Lichen planus. – This will usually respond to local steroids. In some severe cases in which pruritus is a serious problem systemic steroids may be used but this will usually be on the advice of a specialist.

Conclusion

This chapter has been concerned with the diagnosis and management of common rashes in general practice. The rashes discussed probably account for 90 per cent of the dermatological consultations in general practice. Now and again there will be rashes which the general practitioner cannot recognize. Such conditions as dermatitis herpetiformis, pemphigus and leprosy will be seen perhaps once in twenty years in general practice. Sometimes the general practitioner will see rashes at a stage in their natural history, or presenting in an atypical way, which again will make it impossible for him to reach a diagnosis although the condition concerned may be relatively common. In these cases he requires the advice of a dermatologist. Management has also concentrated on the common conditions and the commonly successful remedies. Inevitably, there will be patients who fail to respond to these remedies or whose lesions are so extensive that more complex treatment is required. Once again the general practitioner will turn to his specialist colleagues for advice.

The diagnosis of certain diseases depends largely on the visual recognition of the lesions displayed. In association with this Handbook some of the excellent illustrated guides of dermatology will be found valuable.[3,4]

References

[1] Rea, J.N., Newhouse, M.L. and Halil, T. (1976); Skin Disease in Lambeth. *British Journal of Preventative and Social Medicine, 30*, 107

[2] Royal College of General Practitioners, Office of Population Censuses and Surveys, Department of Health and Social Security (1986): *Morbidity Statistics from General Practice 1981–82*. HMSO Series MB5 No. 1

[3] Fry, L. (1973) ***Dermatology– an illustrated guide***, London: Update Publications

[4] Levene, G.M. and Calnan, C.D. (1974): ***A Colour Atlas of Dermatology***. London: Wolfe Medical Books

It is a pleasure to acknowledge the helpful criticism of Dr Martin Black, Consultant Dermatologist to St Thomas's Hospital, in the preparation of this chapter.

3.38 The patient complaining of spots

David Morrell

The complaint of a spot or spots usually means that the patient has noticed one or more isolated skin lesions. The separation of this complaint from the complaint of a skin rash is to some extent artificial, but there are several well-defined conditions which lead a patient to complain of spots rather than a rash.

Presentation

In childhood the most common are impetigo, warts, insect bites and the early lesions of chickenpox. Between puberty and middle age this symptom is complained of more commonly by women than by men,[1] although the incidence of the underlying conditions such as boils, carbuncles and acne are probably the same in the two sexes and the complaint reflects the greater sensitivity of women to skin lesions. In the elderly the complaint is uncommon.

Causes

Virus infections

Herpes simplex. – The virus produces small groups of blisters on an erythematous base. The appearance of the eruption may be preceded by a burning or a tingling sensation at the site. The most common site is the lips, but the virus may produce the characteristic grouped lesions at other sites, in particular other parts of the face, the genitals and the fingers. Eruptions due to herpes simplex are often recurrent, usually at the same site, and frequently brought on by a feverish illness or exposure to wind or strong sunlight.

Herpes zoster. – Most commonly this presents with pain, and three to four days later characteristic groups of blisters rather larger than those of herpes simplex appear along the distribution of a sensory nerve, most often on the trunk. The lesions are always unilateral and very tender. The blisters dry into crusts over a period of about a week and these gradually fall off leaving scarring with pain which may persist for weeks, months or rarely years. Zoster affecting the ophthalmic division of the fifth nerve may involve the cornea.

Chickenpox.– In its early stages this may be presented to the doctor as individual spots or blisters. There may be a history of contact with an infected subject. The passage of time with the development of new lesions will usually clinch the diagnosis.

Warts.– These are usually presented by the patient with the correct diagnosis. Plantar warts may present as a single painful spot on the sole of the foot but they are often multiple.

Molluscum contagiosum.– This presents as a characteristic umbilicated small papule. It is pearl white in colour and firm to touch. Auto-inoculation from the original lesion often occurs, giving rise to satellite lesions usually limited to one area of the body. It is most commonly seen in children and may become extensive in patients with widespread atopic eczema.

Bacterial infections

Folliculitis.– One of the most common causes of spots is infection of the hair follicles. If the infection is limited to the follicle it is referred to as folliculitis. Infection of multiple follicles in the beard area is called sycosis barbae. Frequently infection of a follicle spreads into the surrounding dermis leading to a tender nodule. In two to three days the infection becomes walled off, the centre becomes necrotic and discharges. This is the common boil or furuncle. Less commonly a number of furuncles aggregate to form a carbuncle giving rise to a very painful lesion which progresses to a purulent ulcer which ultimately discharges. It is often associated with malaise and fever. The causative organism in most follicular infections is *Staphylococcus aureus.* In addition to the skin lesion there may be spread of infection to the regional lymph nodes. Some patients suffer from recurrent boils due to carriage of the organisms, most commonly in the nose, axilla or perineum.

Impetigo.– This is caused by an infection of the epidermis by *Staphylococcus aureus.* The early lesions are vesico-pustules which are soon covered by a loosely adherent crust. Satellite lesions appear fairly rapidly and lesions may also develop on more distant parts of the body by the transfer of infection. This is still a common cause of consultation for children. Lesions occur most often on the face and hands or at the site of minor skin trauma or other skin diseases such as eczema.

Diseases of the sweat and sebaceous glands

Acne vulgaris. – The spotty adolescent is a common sight, and his spots are most commonly due to acne. The basic lesion is in the pilo-sebaceous gland, the mouth of which becomes blocked by keratin and sebum. The 'blackhead' (comedone) is the cardinal sign of acne vulgaris but infected sebum may burst into the surrounding dermis and form an inflammatory cystic lesion, or the sebum may break through to the surface where it is seen as a pustule. Lesions tend to develop on those areas where there are large numbers of pilo-sebaceous glands and are characteristically seen on the forehead, perinasal area and chin; they are common also on the chest and back. The condition rarely occurs before puberty, lasts a variable period, often clearing in two to three years, but sometimes persisting much longer. The severity of the lesions also varies greatly and in some cases extensive inflammatory reactions and cyst formation may lead to persistent scarring.

Naevi and skin tumours

Pigmented naevi.– These may be presented to the general practitioner because they are unsightly, or because the patient is worried that they may become malignant. They vary enormously in appearance from small flat pigmented spots, 1 to 2 mm in size, through slightly raised lesions, often with coarse hairs growing from them, to raised verrucose lesions and to extensive areas of pigmentation several centimetres across.

Seborrhoeic warts.– These are common: raised, slightly pigmented, greasy looking lesions, which develop in middle and old age. They are seen most often on the face or trunk, and may be very numerous. They are benign, but do not regress like viral warts. Skin tags, which may be quite numerous, are also common in the elderly; they are seen most often on the neck and around the axilla.

Haemangiomas.– Four common types are encountered. The mature haemangioma (port wine stain) is present at birth, appears as a macular lesion varying in size from a few millimetres to several centimetres, and does not regress. The immature haemangioma (strawberry naevus) appears in the first week of life, grows rapidly, is raised and bright red. It reaches its maximum size by about 18 months and disappears by the age of 5 to 6 years.

De Morgan spots (cherry angiomas).– These are small raised bright red angiomas which appear on the trunk in the middle-aged and elderly. They have no clinical significance.

Spider naevi.– These have a small central 'feeding' vessel from which superficial dilated capillaries radiate outwards. Pressure on the centre of the lesion causes these capillaries to blanch. They are sometimes associated with liver disease. They are common in pregnancy and often cause some anxiety to the patient but usually disappear after confinement. Remaining spider naevi can be easily treated by applying cold point cautery to the central 'feeding' vessel.

Other causes of spots

Insect bites and fungal infections of the skin are not uncommonly presented to the doctor as a single spot. These have been described in Chapter 3.37.

History and examination

The patient will on most occasions present the lesion for inspection to the doctor and in many cases simple inspection will be sufficient to reach a diagnosis and prescribe treatment. In others, however, a careful history and examination will be required. It is always important to determine where the first lesion appeared and how and over what period of time it developed. If subsequently other lesions develop it is important to discover their relationship to the first in time and distribution. Septic lesions of the skin are commonly tender or even painful and may be accompanied by general malaise and fever. In conditions such as chickenpox, fever and malaise may precede the appearance of the first spots. Some spots are itchy and this is particularly so of insect bites and primary contact eczema which may present as a single spot or patch at the site of contact. Enquiry should be made about the patient's occupation and, if septic lesions are presented, about the presence of similar lesions in other members of the family or close associates. Patients presenting with recurrent septic lesions should be asked about symptoms suggestive of diabetes mellitus and the urine should be examined for sugar.
The extent of the examination carried out depends almost entirely on the nature of the spot presented. In septic spots, surrounding skin should be inspected for cellulitis or spreading lymphangitis and the regional lymph nodes examined for enlargement or tenderness. A single verruca or wart should lead to a search for other lesions on the usual sites on which these occur and which the patient may not have noticed. Where the

diagnosis is not clear from the spot presented a full examination of the whole body surface may bring to light other lesions, the distribution and characteristics of which may be diagnostic, such as chickenpox and insect bites.

Many of the spots presented in general practice reflect only minor illness and the doctor will adapt his history and examination to suit each individual case. As with other minor illnesses in general practice it is always worth considering whether the patient's behaviour is out of character with the doctor's previous experience of that patient, which may indicate that the patient is using his spots to obtain access to discuss some more serious anxiety. The repeated presentation of minor skin lesions in a child may be an indication of undue maternal anxiety or depression or marital or social disharmony.

Management

Many of the spots seen in general practice represent mild benign conditions in which reassurance to the patient that the condition will clear up spontaneously is more important than actual treatment. There are, however, specific treatments for some of the conditions mentioned in this chapter.

Herpes zoster. — There is evidence that early treatment of herpes zoster by painting with idoxuridine will shorten the natural history of the disease and reduce the duration of post-herpetic neuralgia. To be effective, however, treatment must be started within twenty-four hours of onset of the rash. It should be applied as a 5 per cent solution in dimethyl sulphoxide (Herpid) four hourly for five days. In the management of herpes zoster of the ophthalmic branch of the fifth cranial nerve idoxuridine eye ointment may be used. For the same purpose the new antiviral agent acyclovir (Zovirax) is also prepared as an eye ointment. Cases seen later in the disease are unlikely to benefit and should be treated with a drying lotion such as calamine lotion. The condition is painful and the patient should be warned that pain may continue after the rash has disappeared and adequate non-addictive analgesics should be provided. Especially in the elderly, post-herpetic pain may last months or years. In these cases nerve block may be of value. This is most successful if administered early and referral to a pain clinic should be made if symptoms are not beginning to diminish in four to six weeks.

Herpes simplex. — As with zoster, early application of idoxuridine continued for four days may reduce the severity of the eruption. An important advance in treatment is the development of acyclovir which inhibits the replication of some herpes viruses. If applied early as a cream it reduces the severity of the eruption and is probably superior to idoxuridine but much more expensive. In recurrent herpes simplex it does not unfortunately eradicate the virus from the skin. If secondary infection occurs in herpetic lesions, a topical antibiotic may be necessary, or antiseptic such as povidone-iodine (Betadine). Prevention of herpes simplex in those in whom it is brought on by exposure to sunlight or wind is an important part of management and the use of a barrier cream such as mexenone cream may be helpful.

Warts. — A great deal of general practitioners' time and that of their nurses is spent in treating warts. The wide variety of treatments available suggests that none is entirely effective. A quick, painless and effective method is the cryocautery which uses nitrous oxide gas under pressure to freeze the lesion. It may require two to three treatments at weekly intervals. The initial expense of equipment (about £350) may well be a worthwhile investment for the larger group practice. Less sophisticated methods which work over a period of time are the application of 10 per cent salicylic acid in collodion which is applied nightly, or podophyllin ointment 20 per cent applied under an occlusive (zinc oxide) strapping and changed weekly. Small plane warts are better left untreated.

A simple treatment for plantar warts is to soak the wart for fifteen minutes daily in a saucer containing 5 per cent formalin solution for about three weeks. Tender parts of the skin such as the webs of the toes must be protected from this solution. The dry skin should be pared away twice weekly.

Warts on the face should not be treated with strong acid or astringent; the most satisfactory treatment is electric- or cryo-cautery.

Peri-anal or genital warts, which are often numerous, may be treated by painting with 25 per cent podophyllin in spirit. The surrounding skin should be protected with white soft paraffin and the podophyllin should be washed off about twelve hours after use. Three or four applications at weekly intervals will usually produce a cure.

Molluscum contagiosum. — This does not regress spontaneously. The lesions can be cured by piercing each one with a needle or sharpened orange stick dipped in 1 per cent phenol.

Folliculitis, boils and carbuncles. — Most of the boils seen in general practice require only hot fomentations such as kaolin poultice, followed by drainage when they point, and most patients should be encouraged to cope with this themselves. Boils causing extensive cellulitis, boils on the face and carbuncles may be treated with systemic antibiotics, in addition to local treatment. The antibiotics to which the staphylococcus is most likely to be sensitive in general practice are flucloxacillin or erythromycin. If pus is accessible from which to take a swab before treatment, the information obtained may be valuable later if the patient does not respond to the antibiotic prescribed. Carbuncles may require surgical drainage under general anaesthetic. Folliculitis of the beard area may be difficult to clear if the patient continues to shave. Swabs should be taken from the nose and from pus from the follicles and local antibiotic treatment as indicated by sensitivity tests to both these sites after shaving may be helpful.

Recurrent furunculosis can be very troublesome. Management should include taking swabs from the boils and testing for antibiotic sensitivity. A course of treatment by the appropriate antibiotic administered systemically and the appropriate local antibiotic administered to the anterior nares, accompanied by the use of hexachlorophane soap in a daily bath may break the vicious circle of infection and re-infection. The urine should always be tested for sugar in these cases.

Impetigo should be treated with local antibiotics which are not used systemically, such as gentamicin, or a mixture of polymyxin B and bacitracin (Polyfax) applied twice daily after careful removal of all crusts. The cream should also be applied to the anterior nares where the organisms may be carried. The child should be isolated until the infection is cleared up.

Acne. — The successful treatment of acne requires careful attention to detail by the patient and regular supervision by the doctor. Treatment is aimed at keeping the skin clean and free from grease by regular use of soap and water, and producing a mild erythema or peeling by use of keratolytic agents. The most useful of these is benzoyl peroxide which also has a mild antibacterial action, and tretinoin solution. Benzoyl peroxide is marketed as 'benoxyl' and is available as a lotion and a cream. Preparations containing 5 or 10 per cent of benzoyl peroxide are prescribable and may also be combined with sulphur. Tretinoin, which possesses vitamin A activity, is marketed as 'retin-A lotion'. The principles of treatment are the same using either preparation. In initiating treatment, the lotion should be applied, and kept on for about two hours only, on consecutive days. Mild burning, redness or discomfort may occur. Gradually the duration of treatment can be prolonged until the lotion is applied nightly. The objective is to produce mild peeling; if the skin reacts too violently treatment may be stopped for one or two nights. The strong preparations should only be used if the patient is resistant to milder ones and should be introduced with the same care. Tretinoin may be more successful where comedones pre-

dominate, and benzoyl peroxide where papules and pustules are the main features.
Ultra-violet light acts in the same way by producing mild desquamation and should likewise be introduced slowly. A few minutes' exposure twice weekly may gradually be extended to longer periods.
In cystic or pustular acne tetracyclines can be effective. It is usual to start with oxytetracycline 500 mg twice daily for two months. If the patient responds to this, the dose may be halved for a further two months and then gradually tailed off. In some cases erythromycin is successful when tetracycline has failed to produce improvement. In treating acne it is important to explain to patients that the tendency to develop acne may persist for a few years and that intermittent attention to the skin may be needed throughout this time if it is to be kept clear. Patients often enquire about the value of special diets and they can be reassured that there is no sound evidence that diet influences the activity of the disease.
Circulating androgen is important in sebum production and oestrogens lower sebum production by reducing the release of gonadotrophins. Some high dose combined contraceptives containing 50 mcg ethinyloestradial e.g. Minovlar may reduce sebum production by reducing the release of gonadotrophins and improve acne. Anti-androgens e.g. cyproterone acetate also reduce sebum production. A combination of cyproterone 2 mg and ethinyloestradial 50 mcg (Diane) is marketed specifically for the treatment of acne in females. It is administered cyclically and also acts as a contraceptive. It should be given initially for three months and stopped when the acne has resolved. In the present state of knowledge long term administration is not recommended. If amenorrhoea occurs a pregnancy test should be carried out before resuming treatment as feminization of a male foetus is a theoretical risk. In severe cases of acne not responding to the regimes described the possible use of oral treatment with isotretinoin should be considered. This is still at an experimental stage and should only be given with advice from a dermatologist. It appears to be very effective but causes many side-effects and may be teratogenic.

Naevi and haemangiomas. — The management of these conditions is usually concerned with the explanation of the natural history of the condition and appropriate cosmetic therapy. The removal of pigmented naevi, even for cosmetic reasons, should always be surgical and with adequate removal of the surrounding normal skin. Melanomas should always be referred to a dermatologist if there is any suspicion of malignancy. This may be indicated by (1) sudden enlargement of the melanoma, (2) alteration in the pigmentation of the melanoma or the appearance of a halo of pigmentation around the lesion, (3) bleeding or ulceration of the lesion, (4) a lesion exposed to recurrent trauma.

References

[1] Morrell, D.C., Gage, H.G. and Robinson, N.R. (1972): Interpretation of Symptoms in General Practice. *Journal of the Royal College of General Practitioners*, *22*, 297.

It is a pleasure to acknowledge the advice I have received from Dr Martin Black, Dermatologist to St Thomas's Hospital, in preparing this chapter.

3.39
The patient complaining of skin ulcers

David Morrell

The term 'skin ulcer' covers a wide spectrum of disorders. In the National Morbidity Survey,[1] 1.7 per 1,000 patients per annum consulted their general practitioner with chronic ulcers of the skin. Hodgkin[2] reports a similar incidence of 3 per 1,000 population. In a recent population survey of leg ulcers[3], a point prevalence of active ulcers under treatment was 1.5 per 1,000 with a female to male ratio of 2.8:1.

This chapter deals mainly with leg ulcers, because these provide the main problems of skin ulceration in general practice. In the survey referred to above, 87 per cent of the population receiving treatment were being managed in the community. Brief reference will be made to less common ulcers occurring in other parts of the body.

Causes

Of the more common types of skin ulcer, venous ulceration is best understood. It results from damage to the calf muscle pump mechanism. This may be due to incompetence of the saphenous or perforating veins as part of the varicose process. It may be the result of past deep venous thrombosis with damage to the valves. High pressures developing within the calf muscle pump during exercise are transmitted to the overlying capillary circulation via the calf perforating veins whose valves have been rendered incompetent. This high pressure causes capillary distension and leakage of fibrinogen with the development of a lipodermatosclerosis seen in the skin of the calf as induration and pigmentation. In due course the nutrition of the skin suffers from the deposition of fibrinogen and anoxia results in ulceration[4]. Initial healing of venous ulceration produces fibrous tissue and scarring which almost inevitably breaks down with the passage of time to form even more indolent forms of ulcer in the fibrous tissue. Stiffness of the ankle as a result of scarring and pain then leads to atrophy of the calf muscle and therefore a reduction in the effectiveness of the muscle pump. As a final addition there may be tertiary changes due to interference by the patient or her doctor through the use of preparations which produce a contact dermatitis. The treatment of this by topical steroids can for instance cause skin atrophy.

Although venous ulcers are the most common variety of leg ulcer, there are several other conditions which should be considered in the differential diagnosis of leg ulceration. Peripheral vascular disease and diabetes mellitus, by their impairment of the arterial and arteriolar circulation, produce ulceration of the lower limb. These ulcers are usually found on the foot, and the precise location may be determined by local trauma due to unsuitable footwear. Rheumatoid arthritis, the rarer connective tissue disorders, allergic vasculitis and sickle cell anaemia, can all cause damage to the arterioles which feed the skin. The ulcer thus produced is an infarct of the skin supplied by the affected arteriole and is visible as a deep ulcer which is well demarcated from the surrounding normal skin. The skin in these cases shows no evidence of lipodermatosclerosis. Tuberculosis is now a rare cause of leg ulceration. A painful penetrating ulcer of the calf occurring in young women (Bazin's disease) is an occasional manifestation. The way in which local pressure produces sores is easy to understand. Compression of the blood vessels causes tissue anoxia and ultimately necrosis. Surface conditions of the skin also play a part in the development of a pressure sore. A skin which is wet with urine and abraded by starched sheets will, with additional trauma, be at risk to pressure ulceration.

Trauma to skin already compromised by circulatory problems often produces ulceration in the legs. Occasionally trauma to the legs with a normal vasculature will produce ulceration. This is particularly likely to occur in 'horse-shoe flap' lacerations over the tibia when the base of the flap is peripheral.

Occasionally in general practice cases are encountered where ulceration is self-induced 'dermatitis artefacta'. In these cases ulcers are most likely to be presented on the upper limbs, the face and the trunk and the ulcers typically have a square rather than a rounded outline.

Rodent ulcers are basal cell carcinomas. They are most commonly seen on the face, but can occur anywhere on the skin and may be misdiagnosed unless they are considered in the differential diagnosis. Squamous cell carcinoma of the skin may occur on the face or any areas exposed to sunlight and tends to be associated with prolonged solar irradiation, although other forms of chronic irritation may also produce this lesion.

In considering the more unusual types of skin ulceration, the appearance, site and distribution of the lesions will all help in making a diagnosis. In dermatitis artefacta the appearance of the individual ulcers can be very bizarre and will vary according to the trauma used.

Some generalized skin eruptions ulcerate. If transient these are usually regarded as vesicular or bullous lesions. If the lesions become chronic, then they become ulcers. Pyoderma gangrenosum is such a condition in which the raised nodule forms a pustule which ulcerates to form a chronic ulcer. About half the patients with this condition have underlying ulcerative colitis. Other skin conditions like pemphigoid and 'summer ulceration' must be considered, but may require biopsy for diagnosis.

History

Leg ulcers may be present for many years before the patient consults the doctor and in many patients leg ulcers are recurrent and the patient may give a history of previous episodes of ulceration. A history of deep vein thrombosis in the past is highly suggestive of venous ulceration as also is a history of varicose eczema. Ulcers due to arterial insufficiency may be accompanied by intermittent claudication or rest pain, but these symptoms may only be brought out by careful enquiry and are not always presented. Patients should always be asked about their smoking habits which may also suggest an ischaemic cause of their symptoms. A common pitfall in general practice is to miss an unusual cause for a common condition. Important but less common causes of leg ulcers include diabetes, rheumatoid arthritis and blood dyscrasias, and these must be included in the history.

Pressure sores are an important part of skin ulceration in general practice. The history usually reveals that the patient has been rendered immobile as a result of a variety of disabilities, such as stroke, paraplegia, acute trauma or indeed just old age and general infirmity. Occasionally pressure sores may develop for reasons which are not immediately obvious, such as unconsciousness, due to drugs or alcohol.

Basal cell carcinomas (rodent ulcers) are a less common cause of ulceration in general practice. Because of the insidious onset and slow rate of growth the significance of these is often underestimated by the patient. Malignant melanoma and squamous cell carcinoma can also be insidious in onset but the history of a sudden change in appearance may be important in bringing them to the attention of the patient and the physician.

Examination

In addition to their appearance, the site and distribution of ulcers is important in making a diagnosis. Venous ulcers of the leg occur predominantly in the gaiter region above the ankle, particularly in the skin above the medial malleolus. The ulcer usually develops in a patch of indurated thickened pigmented skin (lipodermatosclerosis). The ulcers vary in size and shape and occasionally encircle the leg. The base of the ulcer can appear infected with an adherent grey slough of necrotic tissue which may progress to frank suppuration. Healing is accompanied by improvement in the basal granulation, presenting a clean red velvety appearance. Although venous ulcers are usually superficial, infection can lead to damage of underlying structures and spreading cellulitis.

Pressure sores occur most frequently in the skin of the heels, buttocks and sacrum. The first sign is induration of the skin and subcutaneous tissue. This is followed by reddening of the surface of the skin which then progresses to a necrotic lesion, which breaks down to form an ulcer. The sores can be small and superficial or involve the full thickness of soft tissue. In these deeper pressure sores, the size of the mouth of the ulcer often reflects poorly the extent of the tissue damage.

Rodent ulcers occur most commonly on the upper two-thirds of the face. Initially they resemble a seed or pearl lying on the surface of the skin. The lesions gradually enlarge and ulcerate in the centre to produce an ulcer with a raised rolling edge. The ulcer enlarges slowly but without treatment will erode and destroy adjacent structures.

Management

It is most important to separate venous from arterial ulcers.

Venous ulcers

The treatment of venous ulcers follows logically from an understanding of the aetiology. Ideally they should be prevented. The two main strategies are the prevention of deep vein thrombosis by early mobilization after surgery, and the referral of patients with severe varicose veins for surgical treatment, including ligation of the perforating veins. In people with a history of deep venous thrombosis, preventive measures include protection of the skin and reduction of the capillary pressure with the use of suitable elastic stockings.

The ideal treatment of venous ulcers is to elevate the legs in order to eliminate the effect of the excessive hydrostatic venous pressure and reduce local venostasis. This should of course be accompanied by regular exercises of the calf muscles. For many patients, this is impossible or inconvenient and they must be treated while remaining ambulant. Treatment consists of debridement of the ulcer combined with compression bandaging using 'viscopaste' or 'calaband' bandages. These should be covered with elastocrepe or tubigrip bandages which allow the exudate from the ulcer to be absorbed while maintaining adequate compression. Local antibiotic preparations should not be used because they are ineffective and may produce sensitization or allergic reactions. The dressings should be changed weekly at first, but this period may be extended as healing occurs and the exudation decreases.

Some patients cannot tolerate this treatment or do not respond. They may be treated by daily wet dressings applied by the district nurse using hydrogen peroxide 3 per cent solution or chlorhexidine 0.05 per cent solution and compression bandages. The eczema surrounding an ulcer may be treated with 1 per cent hydrocortisone cream or 0.025 per cent beclamethasone cream.

Failure of conservative management requires admission to hospital. An initial period of bed rest by leg elevation and cleaning of the ulcer may, if unsuccessful in producing healing, be followed by excision and skin grafting.

Once the ulcer has healed, continuing support and protection of the leg is necessary. Supportive bandages are unsatisfactory because they tend to slip and do not provide adequate compression. The ideal support is provided by Sigvaris or Venosan stockings. Unfortunately neither of these are available on NHS prescriptions in general practice. They may be obtained from hospital or on private prescription. Alternatively elastic yarn two way stretch below knee stockings are prescribable by the general practitioner. Once healing has occurred, it may be useful to obtain an opinion from a surgeon who is interested in venous ulceration to establish whether or not any surgically remedial lesion exists in the leg veins.

Arterial ulceration

The importance of differentiating venous from arterial ulceration has been stressed. The reason for this is that compression bandaging of an ischaemic ulcer will be disastrous resulting in further skin breakdown. Ischaemic ulcers need urgent referral to a surgeon who may be able to carry out reconstructive arterial surgery to improve the blood supply to the leg.

The punched out deep ulcers associated with rheumatoid arthritis and allergic vasculitis may be very resistant to conservative treatment; in some cases they may be treated by skin grafting.

Pressure sores

These should be prevented. Patients who are confined to bed and immobile for whatever reason should be considered at risk of developing pressure sores. Turning such patients every two hours changes the areas of skin pressure sufficiently often to avoid the development of sores. The areas of skin affected by pressure can be changed in an automatic fashion by air-filled mattresses. The control of urinary incontinence is an important element in the prevention of pressure sores. If a pressure sore develops, the patient should be nursed in such a way as to avoid any weight bearing by the affected area of skin. As with varicose ulcers, removal of the causative condition is the most important aspect of treatment. Local applications should be simple and safe. Ulcers with a grey slough of necrotic tissue in their base can be cleansed by eusol. Swabs should be sent at regular intervals for identification of the bacterial flora, but treatment with antibiotics is only indicated if there are signs of surrounding cellulitis. Non-adherent dressings such as paraffin-impregnated gauze are useful in keeping the ulcer clean and in making the task of changing dressings much easier.

In some of the larger and deeper pressure sores affecting the sacrum and buttocks there is a tendency for the mouth of the ulcer to close before there is healing of the deeper structures. Referral to the plastic surgeon is worthwhile in this situation, since exposure of the ulcer base will allow for full drainage of the ulcer. Progressive ordered healing can then occur from the ulcer base. Some patients with varicose ulcers and pressure sores may have had a deficient diet. In these patients the rate of healing may be improved by Vitamin C.

Rodent ulcers

The histological confirmation of rodent ulcers requires an excision biopsy of the lesion. This in itself is often curative. Such patients may, in addition, require radiotherapy, which in this condition is very effective.

Conclusion

This chapter has concentrated on common leg ulcers seen in general practice. The more unusual ulcers are often the manifestation of systemic disorders and in these cases a full physical examination will be even more important than usual, and treatment is then largely that of the underlying problem; for example, Bazin's disease where the ulcer of the calf is associated with tuberculosis.

Emphasis has been laid upon the treatment of venous ulcers, as energetic treatment is most rewarding and can transform a miserable, housebound, old lady into an active member of the community. The all too frequent sad story of chronic venous ulceration with secondary infection and eczematous change is entirely avoidable and a major proportion of medical care should be directed towards patient education. It is a condition in which the doctor, health visitor, district nurse and the patient all play their part. The plan of management as outlined should be understood by the whole team, including the patient, so that confusion does not occur.

References

[1] Royal College of General Practitioners, Office of Population Censuses and Surveys, Department of Health and Social Security (1986): *Morbidity Statistics from General Practice 1981–82*. HMSO Series MB5 No. 1

[2] Hodgkin, K. (1973): *Towards Earlier Diagnosis*. 3rd ed. Edinburgh: Churchill Livingstone.

[3] Callam, M.J., Ruckley, C.V. et al. (1985): Chronic ulceration of the leg: extent of the problem and provision of care. *BMJ*, *290*, 1855–1856.

[4] Browse, N.L. and Burnand, K.G. (1982): The cause of venous ulceration. *Lancet*, 243–245.

We are grateful to Mr K.G. Burnand of St Thomas's Hospital Medical School for his advice and help in the writing of this chapter.

3.40 The patient complaining of varicose veins

Allan Forsyth

The condition is so common in Western civilization that it is important to place in perspective the whole range of patients with varicose veins, from those who require surgical treatment to those who will never seek advice on the subject. There is great disparity between the incidence in the community and the consultation rate at the surgery. The incidence may be as high as 50 per cent in an adult European population[1] although in the UK National Morbidity Survey consultation rates on varicose veins were 8·8 per 1,000 patients per annum with a female to male ratio of more than 2 to 1.

Presentation

The most common presentation of varicose veins in general practice is as a minor complication of pregnancy. Between pregnancies or after the child-bearing years the consequences of varicose veins may bring the patient to the doctor with symptoms ranging from aching legs, skin irritation and varicose eczema to phlebitis or varicose ulcer. Sometimes the patient may complain only for cosmetic reasons but in most cases the patient's diagnosis of varicose veins is correct. In a minority of cases what are claimed to be varicose veins are, in fact, superficial angiectases for which little can be done.

Trauma to the skin that overlies varices and results in a complicated wound is a common starting point to the treatment of the pre-existing condition. Many people with gross manifestations procrastinate when it comes to seeking advice but are compelled to have treatment for the inevitable complications. Alternatively, the condition is one that can be kept in reserve as a respectable symptom that would merit a consultation. Thus it can become psychosomatic, and the unrelated condition of anxiety, stress or family problem may be the underlying reason for presenting at that particular time.

Two other conditions which may be described by the patient as varicose veins are thrombophlebitis migrans and erythema nodosum.

Causes

There is insufficient evidence to define a common cause for varicose veins and there is great dispute over many conflicting theories. Sufficient to say that there are many factors that are associated with an increased prevalence of varicose veins. Heredity, standing occupations, multiparity and obesity can be listed. The condition is scarcely to be found in rural African and Asian populations and dietary fibre as well as ethnic factors may have a bearing on this condition as it does on haemorrhoids.
Trauma which damages a valve leads to incompetence in a perforating vein which allows the pressure from the deep vein to be transmitted to superficial veins. Local filling is followed by retrograde flow, and dilatation of veins proximally in the superficial system in turn spreads the cusps so that they cannot close. Thus secondary valvular incompetence progresses proximally. This theory certainly accounts for the remarkable return to normal flow that occurs when treatment is carried out at a fair distance from some of the varicose lengths of vein. These secondarily incompetent valves have the potential to function well again when treatment causes a sequential reduction in flow-volume, pressure and dilatation.[2]

History

Questions relating to the length of time the varicose veins have existed and whether the onset was related to pregnancy, trauma or other event should be asked. In particular, definite information should be sought as to the occurrence of a deep venous thrombosis in the past: e.g. the use of anticoagulants and prolonged postpartum bed-rest. The general medical history may be relevant and diabetes mellitus and peripheral vascular disease should be noted. The ability of the patient to walk briskly and exercise for an hour without limitation from arthritis, dyspnoea, or pain in the affected leg will have a bearing on the choice of treatment. In a high proportion of cases in this country the problem is one of recurrence, and dates and details of previous treatments should be gathered.
The patient's occupation, the family history of varicose veins and the patient's own reasons for initiating the consultation may all be of value.

Examination

The presence of obesity which would make compression

bandaging difficult is noted along with the general configuration and equality of the two legs. The condition of the skin, the presence of oedema or the presence of old scars can be seen and the flexibility of skin over the deep fascia can be felt. Anything more than slight oedema should raise the suspicion of deep venous obstruction. A quickly drawn anatomical map of the veins of both legs that are prominent can give more useful information than laborious writing. When the veins are palpated, areas will be identified where dilatation, pressure, heat and pain are greatest and here a deficiency in the deep fascia may be felt as a punched-out hiatus. This is a probable site of an incompetent valve in a perforating vein which has permitted reverse flow from deep to superficial veins.

The practitioner who proposes to carry out sclerotherapy himself will need to extend the examination. If the cough impulse is transmitted at the sites of incompetent valves (which should be marked) it may be concluded that there is no deep venous occlusion. The same manoeuvre of palpating the cough impulse should be used to test the competence of the valve at the termination of the long saphenous vein in the fossa ovalis in the groin and the short saphenous vein in the popliteal fossa. Palpable incompetence here has a decisive influence on treatment.

The *Trendelenberg test* will confirm these findings. The patient lies down and the leg is elevated to empty the superficial veins (another test of pelvic vein patency). With digital pressure applied at the sapheno-femoral junction the patient stands and the leg is observed to see the level at which veins first fill. If there is no filling until the pressure in the groin is released there may be simple sapheno-femoral incompetence. More commonly, filling occurs from incompetent perforators in the calf and there may be an increase when pressure from above is released. Localization can be done quite simply by excluding proximal superficial filling with a light tourniquet and applying digital pressure to marked distal sites in turn with the patient off and on the couch to empty the veins between each test.

After all this has been done it may well be shown that the filling of a whole complex of varices may occur through incompetence at only one or two sites, but it is important to know whether these are above or below the knee and whether there is incompetence at the terminations of the saphenous veins.

Management and treatment

In the past twenty-five years the treatment of choice has swung from the terminal ligation and full-length stripping of the long and/or short saphenous veins or the subfascial ligation of veins in the calf, to the ambulant outpatient technique of compression sclerotherapy,[2] when sodium tetradecyl is injected at selected sites where perforators are primarily incompetent and the patient plays a part in the treatment on rising from the couch and walking with compressed veins for one hour that day and every day thereafter for six weeks. The results of the latter technique compared so favourably with surgery after three years that this method of Fegan gained wide acceptance. At six-year follow-up, however, there was a recurrence rate of 65 per cent, particularly when there had been sapheno-femoral incompetence in the groin.[3] When this is found it is usually now an indication for flush tie as the odds are too long against the vein regaining competence as it should theoretically do after perforators have been dealt with distally. Varicose veins above the knee may likewise require surgical ligation as compression is admittedly difficult in an adipose thigh.

A well-defined range of cases emerges who are fortunately suitable for compression sclerotherapy. This technique is sometimes used in general practice, but the adherence to the details in Fegan's technique is as vital for success as the enthusiasm that is transmitted from doctor to patient. The reader should therefore refer to the original source.[2]

The object of treatment is to relieve the patient of:

(a) the pain from aching and swollen legs

(b) the dangers of poor circulation in the skin.

Patients seeking cosmetic results may also need treatment under one or both of these categories but those who do not should be discouraged for the following reasons. Injection often results in some pigmentation of the skin and ligation scars may be discoloured and tender.

For those with genuine need who refuse operative treatment or where there will be a long delay, all is not lost. Considerable relief and clinical improvement can be achieved by wearing elastic stockings with or without foam rubber compression at the sites of a 'blow-out'. It should be pointed out to them that this will never effect a cure but relief of symptoms will last for as long as they wear the proper stockings. These should be the full-length 'standard yarn-circular' type which come in three sizes and leave the toes free. If it is explained that these should be worn as a foundation garment under ordinary tights or stockings, the patient's initial resistance will be overcome. With the two-way stretch of the circular weave they extend a more uniform pressure than the older 'flat-bed' variety. Men prefer the below-knee length but these will only be satisfactory if the varicosity is restricted to the lower leg. For other men and pregnant women who cannot wear a girdle, a button should be sewn on to the tops of the stockings and an extra long elastic over the shoulder can be worn. Patients who spend long hours standing should be instructed to walk or constantly exercise their foot or calf muscles. This will only be effective if stockings are effectively compressing the calf and the thigh.

Finally, the practitioner should take every opportunity to educate a patient with varicose veins to the dangers of bleeding and the simple method of treating this emergency by applying pressure and lying the patient down with the leg elevated.

If the patient does not have a competent valve between his right atrium and his ankle, he must have this knowledge.

References

1 Leading Article (1975): The Treatment of Varicose Veins, *Lancet, ii,* 311

2 Fegan, G. (1964): *Varicose Veins. Compression Sclerotherapy*. London: Heinemann

3 Leading article (1975): Tailored Treatment for Varicose Veins. *British Medical Journal, 1,* 593

3.41 The patient who is too fat

Denis Craddock

Obesity is usually regarded as being present if an individual is 10 per cent or more above the optimum weight for his or her height and build as recorded in the New York Metropolitan Life Assurance Society tables. This definition accords with clinical experience and most patients who complain that they are too fat are obese by this criterion.

There is no accurate information about the prevalence of overweight in adults in the United Kingdom, but recent surveys indicate that for both men and women this rises from about 20 per cent of the population in the third decade to 50 or 60 per cent of the population in the fifties and sixties. There are regional variations in the prevalence of obesity but from these figures it is possible to estimate that there are at least 300 obese adults in the average general practice looking after 2,000 individuals.

Presentation

The problem of obesity may be presented to the general practitioner in a variety of ways. Some patients complain of being too fat and, having made ineffective attempts at weight loss themselves, seek help from the doctor. Some present symptoms often attributable to other diseases but made worse by obesity. Shortness of breath may be caused by gross obesity alone but is more often associated with cardiovascular disease and exacerbated by the obesity. Pain in weight-bearing joints is a frequent common presenting feature in patients with arthritis who are also obese and treatment of the obesity may relieve the symptoms. Gastro-oesophageal reflux is not uncommonly associated with obesity and may be relieved by weight loss.

An increasing number of patients present with conditions unrelated to obesity, but the doctor noticing that they are overweight recommends weight reduction. This is particularly likely to occur in childhood and pregnancy, at the time of an insurance examination or when hypertension is diagnosed. If such obesity can be corrected this will increase life expectation and reduce morbidity.

Causes

Genetic factors.– It is well known that some people can eat what they like without putting on weight, while others eat little, become fat and remain so. The tendency to put weight on easily is inherited and is associated to a major extent with body build. As long ago as 1954 Sheldon, the American anthropologist, showed that the typical slim-built ectomorph was able to remain thin throughout life without any effort while the shorter, broadly built and round-headed endomorph usually put on weight steadily during his early adult life, often despite trying desperately to avoid this weight gain. While one-half of men are on the endomorphic side of the spectrum, Sheldon showed that about three-quarters of all women have a tendency to endomorphy. This is one of the reasons why women tend to put on weight more readily than men. Studies with identical twins also show that the tendency to put on weight easily is mainly inherited, as does the fact that adopted children take after their natural parents rather than their adoptive ones.

Alterations in energy balance.– Most individuals in the countries of western civilization do not take enough exercise and those with a genetic tendency to put on weight can, in some cases, use up only half as many calories as slim individuals of the same weight, even while they are sitting and standing. Excluding grossly obese patients, many surveys have shown that the average obese individual does not in fact eat more than his lean counterpart. Many individuals put on weight when a change in their way of life reduces their energy output while their energy food intake remains the same due to habit.

Social factors.– Most individuals in western civilization can afford to eat more than they need, and do so. They have usually been conditioned from childhood to eat sweets or sweet-tasting foods for comfort and conversely are deprived of them for punishment. As foods containing sugar or refined carbohydrates, such as white processed cereals and white flour, are part of most children's normal diet they tend to create an artificial appetite. After a satisfying savoury meal or between meals, food of this nature is eaten for pleasure rather than to satisfy hunger. Cleave[1] and Burkitt[2] have both produced epidemological evidence to show that when a community has been affluent for about a generation these refined foodstuffs associated with an absence of natural fibre in the diet are at least partially responsible for an increase in many disease processes. These include diabetes mellitus, coronary artery disease, constipation, diverticular disease, haemorrhoids, varicose veins and possibly carcinoma of the colon and peptic ulcers.

Psychological factors.– Those with a genetic tendency to overweight have usually a good appetite and as they have been conditioned to eat sweets, chocolates, biscuits and the like for comfort when they are young, it is natural that these foods should be taken to comfort themselves when they are tense, bored, unhappy or even merely vaguely worried. These people eat for comfort instead of smoking, drinking or biting their nails. In some individuals a vicious circle ensues. They hate the look of themselves when they are overweight. This makes them more unhappy and they tend to eat all the more for comfort while at the same time cursing themselves for so doing. In a few individuals in addition to a psychological addiction to carbohydrate, there is a true physiological addiction as the increased insulin needed to cope with their carbohydrate intake can give them a reactionary hypoglycaemia and a physiological craving for carbohydrate.

History and examination

Body weight is a physiological variable and obesity is not a disease, although the metabolic abnormalities associated with long-standing obesity will in many cases lead eventually to disease unless they are reversed by weight loss. In taking the history it is important to try to determine when, how and, if possible, why excessive weight gain occurs. There may be a family history of obesity. The patient may have been fat as a baby or child, or excessive weight gain may have occurred at puberty and persisted into adult life. In women administration of an oral contraceptive or a pregnancy may have been associated with excessive weight gain. Sudden increase in weight in adult life should lead the doctor to suspect a major change in life pattern or the occurrence of some stressful event and he should specifically enquire about these, if he is not already aware of them.

The patient should be asked about his present eating habits. Does he feel that he has an excessive appetite? Does he eat between meals? When does he have his main meal? He should be asked to give examples of a typical day's menu. In women who are at home all day particular care should be taken to estimate the quantity of tea and coffee consumed. Some patients eat when they are bored, lonely or depressed and they should be asked about this.

It is important at the outset to find out if the patient sees his problem as one of excessive food intake or denies that his eating habits are unusual. It is also important to determine why the patient wishes to lose weight and his expectations of the

doctor.
Physical examination usually adds little to the information obtained from the history. In children and young adults it is rarely necessary to do more than to measure the body weight and height. In older patients obesity may be associated with diabetes mellitus, hypertension and hyperlipidaemia. For this reason the urine should be tested for sugar, the blood pressure recorded and in all men and post-menopausal women a specimen of blood should be sent for measurement of serum cholesterol and triglycerides.
Endocrine causes of obesity are rare in general practice. If the possibility of Cushing's disease, acromegaly and myxoedema are borne in mind the appearance of the patient is likely to prompt further examinations where these are appropriate.

Management

Those patients who can lose weight easily, constituting approximately half the obese or potentially obese population, do not come to their doctor, so that those who do come have usually a strong genetic tendency to put on weight easily, or a strong emotional need to eat for comfort, or both. It is essential therefore to elucidate the etiological factors as outlined and to estimate the patient's degree of motivation to lose weight.

Diet.– This is the cornerstone of treatment. A variety of diets advised by a variety of enthusiastic doctors and nutritionists have been successful, at least in the short-term. In the long-term, however, the diet must involve the patient in a radical change in eating habits. It is important to stress this to the patient at the first interview. Nearly all obese patients have either a sweet tooth, a liking for bread and butter or cakes, or drink alcohol to excess. All these are taken for pleasure rather than to satisfy hunger, and the patient must be convinced that there is no easy way to lose weight and, with rare exceptions, sacrifices must be made.
A start is usually made with one of the so-called 'free diets'. These allow the patient to eat as much as he wishes of certain natural foodstuffs to satisfy his hunger. He is rationed on only a few items. The patient should be given a copy of one of these diets together with notes as to how it can be carried out.[3] My modification of Marriotts' diet is included as an appendix to this chapter. This will cause weight loss initially in almost all patients who stick to the diet properly. Successful adherence to a

diet demands interest and sympathy and supervision by the physician. In many patients the determination to continue the diet seems to wear off after about two weeks and this is the time when they should be seen again by the doctor and encouraged to continue.

An alternative to the 'free diet' is the calorie-controlled diet. This is useful for short-term weight reduction, but must be well balanced. It should contain a minimum of 800 Calories (3,360 kJ) a day for an adult and 1,500 Calories (16,300 kJ) for a growing teenager. Below this level protein may be burned instead of fat and this may lead to weakness and malaise.

On an 800-Calorie diet most people will lose at least 3 to 4 pounds (1,360 to 1,820 grams) a week initially and can maintain a loss of 2 to 3 pounds (900 to 1,360 grams) a week as long as they keep to the diet. After the initial effort the diet may be relaxed to 1,000 Calories (4,200 kJ) and it has been shown that all adults will continue to lose weight if they adhere strictly to this. Clearly the calorie content of the diet must be related to the patient's occupation and activities and these generalizations apply to those in sedentary occupations. Calorie-controlled diets are usually employed for short-term treatment but some individuals with a strong genetic tendency to obesity, and others who are immobilized by physical disability, may need to continue on a diet below 1,500 Calories a day to control their weight.

Drugs.– Anorexiant drugs are, as their name implies, thought to act solely by diminishing appetite. As the obese patient reverts to a normal weight the metabolic changes observed in the obese also revert to normal.

Problems of addiction associated with the use of amphetamines in treating obesity make most general practitioners cautious in the use of potentially addictive drugs in treating a condition which can only be cured by a major change in habits. There has, however, probably been an over-reaction to the dangers of drug therapy in a condition which is itself associated with a high morbidity but in using these drugs certain precautions should be taken:

1. They should never be used as the first treatment. Their particular value is in helping those patients who by diet alone have lost a significant amount of weight but have reached a plateau below which they cannot obtain any further weight loss.
2. They should not be used for long periods of time and should not be continued if weight loss is not occurring.
3. The patient should be seen every two weeks.
4. They should not be used in patients who are depressed or have a past history of depressive illness.

The drug of choice for those with a good appetite is the non-amphetamine, diethylpropion. It is cheap, side-effects are uncommon and it is effective in a dose of one sustained action tablet (75 mg) in the morning increased cautiously to one-and-a-half or two if necessary. The very mild stimulant effect which occurs occasionally will not lead to addiction if prescriptions are given at fortnightly intervals and are renewed only if weight loss continues. The one exception to this rule is in some women in whom premenstrual fluid retention temporarily masks a loss of fat. Some individuals continue to lose weight for many months on this drug.

If patients are tense, fenfluramine is suitable. Drowsiness is the commonest side-effect. It can cause depression, and sudden cessation of the drug can also lead to depression within a few days in normal individuals. Apart from drowsiness, side-effects, including abdominal pain, nausea, diarrhoea and general malaise, are sufficiently common to cause between 10 and 20 per cent of patients to stop using the drug. It is usual to prescribe one or two tablets (20 mg) in the morning and at tea time, advising patients that if they are not drowsy on one tablet they can immediately double the dose.

Mazindol (2 mg) is given as one tablet before midday. It produces more side-effects than diethylpropion but is justifiable as a second-line treatment. Phentermine, given as one 15- or 30-mg capsule in the morning, suits a few patients although there is a one in five chance of insomnia being produced.

Behaviour therapy.– As has been noted, patients with a difficult weight problem can be helped by investigating their eating patterns. They are asked to write down in detail everything they eat and drink over a period of a week or more and to record the way in which they eat and their emotions at the time. They are also asked to try to eat more slowly and to reduce the amount of fattening foods kept in the house. They should be promised rewards for weight loss by their family or friends.

Group therapy.– Those doctors who feel they cannot afford the time to see patients at fortnightly intervals might well consider setting up a weekly group in their own practice.[4] This should be led by a health visitor or a member of the practice staff who has successfully coped with a personal weight problem. Alternatively, a successful dieter should be enrolled as an assistant. Group therapy by commercial groups has brought fresh hope to hundreds of thousands of overweight individuals but success to only a few. Silhouette and Slimming Magazine Groups are cheaper than the authoritarian American-orientated Weight Watchers and all of them have similar results on follow-up.

Difficult cases.– Fasting in hospital and the currently popular dental splintage both give disappointing results on long-term follow-up. For those individuals who are desperate and have tried everything else, intestinal bypass, which is reversible, is the procedure of choice. It should only be considered for patients who are approaching at least twice their normal weight and are willing to put up with one or two years of hectic offensive diarrhoea before their weight approaches normal.

The future

Education in sensible eating habits, particularly during the antenatal period, is the only way of reducing to any extent the number of overweight individuals in the community. Of 167 children between 3 and 17, whose mothers have been under my care during the antenatal period, only three have been even moderately obese, while of a similar number born outside the practice, 14 have been obese, many of them considerably so.

References

[1] Cleave, T.L. (1974): *The Saccharine Disease.* Bristol: John Wright

[2] Burkitt, D. (1973): Some Diseases Characteristic of Modern Western Civilization. *British Medical Journal, 1*, 247

[3] Craddock, D. (1976): *Obesity and its Management.* 3rd ed. Edinburgh: Churchill Livingstone

[4] Craddock, D. (1974): Special Clinics: Obesity. *Update*, 7, 1309

Appendix

High fibre reducing diet

This diet contains no sugar, is low in fat and moderate in protein. It is high in high fibre carbohydrate foods. Because it allows such a wide choice of foods without counting calories it is sometimes referred to as a 'Free Diet'.

1. Satisfy your hunger by eating as much as you like of the following:
   Lean meat, including poultry, offal, rabbit, lean ham, grilled bacon or sausages.
   Fish, boiled or steamed.
   Eggs.
   Nuts.
   Cottage cheese, medium fat cheeses, e.g. Camembert, Edam, processed cheeses.

Vegetables, including potatoes boiled or baked in their jackets.
Fresh fruit or fruit bottled without sugar, sweetened with saccharine.
Salads.
Thin soups, sour pickles, condiments, Worcestershire sauce.
Tea, coffee, Oxo, Bovril, low-calorie squashes and other low-calorie drinks.
Starting a meal with soup and drinking water or low calorie drinks with meals may help to fill you up and make you less hungry.
Medium fat cheeses, dried fruit and nuts should only be eaten as part of a main dish.

2. Daily allowances:
   (a) Up to half-a-pint of skimmed milk *OR* five ounces of fresh milk *OR* two ounces of ice-cream.
   (b) Half an ounce of butter or margarine *OR* one ounce of St. Ivel Gold or Outline *OR* one ounce of double cream *OR* two ounces of single cream.
   (c) Three ounces of wholemeal bread *OR* six ounces of starch-reduced bread *OR* six pieces of crispbread.
   (d) One helping of a whole grain cereal product.

   Wholemeal bread and brown cereals are better than the white refined alternatives and they are also more satisfying.

3. You may have NOTHING ELSE WHATEVER. Note especially that this means:
   NO bread or cereals, except as above.
   NO biscuits, cakes or pastry.
   NO thick sauces or thick soups.
   NO puddings.
   No sugar, syrup, chocolate, sweets, honey, jam. (Many packaged foods contain sugar.)
   Weigh yourself before you begin and once a week afterwards on the same scale in the same clothes at the same time of day.
   You may eat up to three or four meals a day. Do not eat between meals. You should lose between five to fifteen pounds per month.
   If your weight loss slows down it will help to omit the following items:
   Avocado pears, medium fat cheeses, dried fruit, fruit juices, ham, bacon, goose, duck, fish canned in oil, fatty fish such as eels, herrings, kippers, mackerel.
   NOTE:
   (1) The weight can vary by up to two or three pounds in the course of a day, usually being higher in the evening.
   (2) A glass of beer or a short drink is equivalent in food value to one ounce of bread, and may be substituted for it.

(3) For those who cannot resist sweet things, one ounce of a favourite item may be taken instead of one ounce of bread.

THE IMPORTANCE OF EXERCISE IN WEIGHT REDUCTION

More weight is lost by exercise if it is taken one or two hours after food as some of the food is turned into heat instead of fat. Vigorous exercise has an added bonus in that the bodily processes are speeded up for many hours after the exercise is finished with a consequent loss of calories in the form of heat.

3.42 The patient who is too thin

Denis Craddock

Few patients present to the general practitioner complaining that they are too thin. Rather more present with complaints of weight loss. The former group tend to be physically fit thin people who are dissatisfied with their slender physique or lack of secondary sexual characteristics. The latter group include individuals suffering from serious organic disease leading to weight loss. This may be caused by inadequate intake or absorption of food, by increased or abnormal metabolic processes or by excessive loss in the stools. Conditions which come into consideration include low-grade fevers, thyrotoxicosis, diabetes mellitus and wasting diseases such as tuberculosis and carcinoma.

Causes

1. *The patient is thin due to weight loss*
   - (a) *Weight loss is due to recent stress*. The largest group
   - (b) *Weight loss is due to disease*. A small but important group
     Diabetes mellitus
     Thyrotoxicosis
     Carcinoma
     Tuberculosis
   - (c) *Anorexia nervosa*. This is a small but important group almost entirely confined to girls between the ages of 12 and 20. There is a large preponderance of patients in social class I.
2. *The patient is thin but the weight is stable*. The patient has no complaint apart from being thin.

History and examination

A patient complaining of loss of weight often mentions the amount he claims to have lost in a certain length of time. He usually overstates his case, possibly to emphasize his concern and to make certain that the doctor takes it seriously. When a

patient's case records show that he has been weighed previously, the loss of weight is rarely as great as has been suggested.
History taking must be directed towards the various serious possibilities outlined above. The state of the appetite and bowels are always important considerations. Special attention should be paid to the possibility that recent stress may have caused the loss of weight, as this is by far the most common cause. Physical examination can be therapeutic as well as diagnostic if loss of weight is due to psychological causes. The state of the heart, lungs, blood pressure and urine is assessed. Abdominal, rectal or vaginal examinations are undertaken if necessary. If no obvious cause for weight loss has been found after history taking and clinical examination, a full blood count, including the erythrocyte sedimentation rate (E.S.R.) and a radiograph of the chest should be carried out, together with thyroid function tests when this is indicated by the clinical picture.
If a physical cause for weight loss has not been found in a teenage girl, anorexia nervosa should be considered, especially if there is a history of previous dieting for overweight, if the girl has a poor relationship with one or both parents, has an obsessional personality or appears somewhat immature. Although questioning may reveal an adequate food intake, the girl may have secretly made herself vomit or purged herself, or both, so that she may enjoy her food without developing the rounded contours and sexual attractiveness of the normal girl at puberty. She is not yet emotionally ready to encourage young males to regard her as sexually desirable. When the weight drops below the critical level of 47 kg plus or minus 2 (103 pounds, plus or minus 5) secondary amenorrhoea may supervene and this is an important diagnostic point.
If there is no history of recent weight loss without obvious dieting, an attempt should be made to find out why the patient is determined to remain thin. The common cause usually lies in her emotional attitude to the other sex.

Management

As in all syndromes with a complex mixture of causes this depends entirely on the accuracy and completeness of the diagnosis. Organic disease if found will be treated. If it has been excluded to the satisfaction of the patient and doctor, those individuals who have lost weight due to recent stress will be relieved of their fear of disease and this itself will be therapeutic. If the stress situation which provoked the weight loss is in process of resolution, the patient should be told to report back in a month if weight is not being gained. If there is a depressive element in the illness, amitriptyline or a similar tricyclic antidepressant may be helpful, the patient being closely followed up for a period of weeks or months. Among the major tranquillizers, chlorpromazine may be helpful.

Anorexia nervosa.– This represents a difficult problem of management, but if the practitioner is on the look out for the condition he may be in a position to prevent the established syndrome from developing. It is essential to establish a good rapport with the girl. If rapport is hard to establish, it is best to refer to a psychiatrist with an interest in the condition. Success is likely if the patient can be made to feel that the doctor is treating her as an equal, that he understands her difficulties and is not on the side of the establishment as represented by her parents. Her attitudes to her own maturing body and mind should be explored at regular consultations. She should be seen alone and, if considered necessary, with her consent the parents should also be seen separately at intervals. There is often a depressive element and amitriptyline may be needed and helpful. If the girl is afraid of developing the secondary sexual characteristics which will lead to involvement with boys and young men, she has to be helped to a more mature attitude to her body. Some girls are helped by being given an inducement to gain weight, such as a particular treat when she reaches a certain mark, or a promise by her parents of a certain sum of money for each pound gained. If support, encouragement and simple psychotherapy do not soon bring about a weight increase, psychiatric help should be obtained as the girl may need to be removed from the stress of her environment before she can come to terms with her problems.

The thin fit patient is usually a slim built (ectomorphic) individual with poor musculature as a result of genetic endowment. A man needs reassurance that his body build is compatible with physical fitness, a long life and virility. Although he can build up muscle groups to some extent by static exercises, weight lifting or sport, he will have to come to terms with the fact that he can never look a typical 'he-man' type. He will usually be pleased to learn that he is less likely to develop coronary artery disease, diabetes mellitus or gout. A woman must understand that she can only become less thin by increasing muscle bulk or laying down fat. Increased muscularity is most unlikely to assist her feminine image and fat will be laid down in a genetically predetermined order which could easily make her look less attractive. She should settle for a long life and a slim one, realizing that many of her fat friends will envy her.

3.43 Heartburn, waterbrash and wind

John Fry

These are three symptoms that may mean different things and have different implications for patients and doctors. It is not possible to measure gases or record and visualize heartburn, waterbrash and wind. This being so a practical clinical approach is required so that we may be able to assess, diagnose and help our patients with these symptoms.

The first decision to be made is whether they are 'functional', or whether there is any 'organic' disorder causing them. Yet another assessment is required when an apparent 'organic' cause is found, such as a hiatus hernia or gall-stones. It may be that the organic condition detected is not the true cause of the symptoms. It is well known from experience that treatment, often surgical, of the apparent cause, such as hiatus hernia, gall-stones or peptic ulcer, is unsuccessful in curing the symptoms. The frequency of these three symptoms is uncertain because of the differing recording and diagnostic habits of physicians. Apart from 'wind' in infancy, they are all most prevalent between the ages of 20 and 65.

Presentation

The patients generally complain of indigestion and in the mix that often goes to make up this homely syndrome are the three symptoms of heartburn, waterbrash and wind. It is the practitioner's task to endeavour to unravel the history and to try to extract from it some guidelines to make a holistic diagnosis that must include the patient as an individual, his family and social environment as well as any physical signs. Indigestion with heartburn, waterbrash and wind may be a feature of many conditions ranging from cancer of the stomach or large bowel, peptic ulcers, malabsorption, the irritable bowel syndrome, to anxiety, depression, aerophagy and others.

Heartburn

Causes. — Heartburn is produced by a reflux of gastric acid into the lower oesophagus through the cardia. Conditions that interfere with the functioning of the cardia or the whole of the gastro-oesophageal mechanism and lead to reflux of gastric contents into the oesophagus may cause heartburn. It is common in the later weeks of pregnancy and usually disappears after delivery. It is also commonly associated with obesity and may be relieved by weight reduction. The relationship between hiatus hernia and reflux is confusing. It has, for instance, bcen shown that in about one-third of volunteers a sliding hiatus hernia can be demonstrated despite the absence of any gastrointestinal symptoms. Conversely, in only about one-third of patients with hiatus hernia is there heartburn or regurgitation.[1] Oesophageal reflux and heartburn may accompany peptic ulceration, when it is presumably related to hyperchlorhydria. The possibility of excessive alcohol intake should also be considered in patients presenting with upper gastrointestinal symptoms which may include heartburn. It may also be caused by anti-inflammatory drugs such as aspirin, indomethacin and a variety of the other agents used in treating rheumatic disorders.

Symptoms. — The characteristic symptoms are retrosternal and upper abdominal discomfort described as a soreness or burning sensation. This symptom is often aggravated by stooping, bending forward, lifting and on lying down flat in bed. The victim may be awakened by the discomfort. There may be a reflux of bitter tasting fluid into the mouth or even of undigested food. The heartburn tends to occur an hour or more after a meal. It is relieved by antacids, milk or a light meal. It tends to be aggravated by a heavy meal with lots of fluid. Gaseous drinks may also bring on the symptoms. The course of the symptom is unpredictable. The heartburn may be shortlived, as during a pregnancy, and not be repeated in future pregnancies. It may be intermittent and occasional, associated with certain food and physical activities and may, for no good reason, cease spontaneously and for ever. On the other hand, it may continue for many years. There is a strong tendency for the symptoms to improve spontaneously.

Examination. — There are no specific abnormal physical signs, although there may be those of associated conditions such as pregnancy, obesity, new growths or peptic ulcer.

Investigations. — The purpose of investigation is to discover a possible underlying cause that may be treatable. No special investigations are indicated during pregnancy. A barium meal examination with head tilting will show up evidence of gastro-oesophageal reflux, hiatus hernia or peptic ulcer. This may be supplemented by gastrointestinal examination with fibre-endoscopy in some units. Fibre-endoscopy should not, however, replace barium studies because it will fail to demonstrate reflux and hiatus hernia in about one-third of the patients examined.[2] Measurement of gastric acidity is rarely necessary.

Treatment. — The symptoms may often be improved by simple dietary advice. Small frequent dry meals are better than large infrequent meals washed down with copious fluids. Gaseous drinks, hot and strong tea and coffee, neat spirits and highly seasoned foods should be avoided. Large meals taken at night tend to exacerbate this symptom, and physical activity, particularly the bending involved in gardening and housework, should be avoided immediately after meals. The association of obesity with heartburn may lead to appropriate advice concerning weight loss. Antacids taken after meals or when the symptom is present are helpful and a tablet of aluminium hydroxide or magnesium trisilicate dissolved slowly in the mouth is the best method of administration. Anticholinergic drugs are contraindicated in oesophageal reflux and indeed cholinergic drugs, e.g. bethanechol chloride (Myotonine) 10 mg thrice daily may be helpful. Increasing the viscosity of the gastric contents by use of a mixture containing alginic acid and sodium bicarbonate (Gaviscon) has been shown to produce symptomatic improvement. By reducing gastric acid output cimetidine (Tagamet) and ranitidine (Zantac) have been shown to reduce symptoms due to oesophagitis. The latter in a dose of 150 mg twice daily is probably the drug of choice in men as it does not have the anti-androgen effects of cimetidine which produces gynaecomastia and it does not interfere with the metabolism of phenytoin, warfarin or theophyllines. Another drug of value in treating oesophagitis is metoclopramide in a dose of 10 mg three times daily. It increases the tone of the oesophageal sphincter and promotes gastric emptying. It should be used with care as it may produce extrapyramidal symptoms as a side-effect. If the symptom is particularly troublesome at night the patient should be well propped up in bed or the head of the bed raised on bricks.

The possibility of surgical intervention for hiatus hernia may rarely be considered if the symptom is intractable. It produces a cure in about 80 per cent of cases with an operative mortality rate of about one per cent. More often, associated symptoms of peptic ulcer or bleeding from oesophagitis may prompt a surgical approach.

Waterbrash

Waterbrash is defined as the sudden appearance of watery fluid in the mouth often in association with a history of indigestion. The fluid is tasteless and clear and must be distinguished from thicker mucus that may occur with some oral lesions and from the reflux of bitter acid with conditions associated with heartburn. It may occur at any time and is sometimes associated with meals. It may be of a sizeable volume causing the subject to spit up a cupful or more of the watery fluid.

The significance of waterbrash is that it may be associated with a duodenal ulcer or oesophageal disorders. The cause of the waterbrash is uncertain.

Management. — The presence of waterbrash is an indication for investigations to discover an associated lesion. Thus contrast-media radiography of the stomach and duodenum is indicated, followed, possibly, by fibre-endoscopy. Once diagnosed the cause demonstrated should be treated on accepted lines. A trial of cimetidine (Tagamet) may be justified if the symptom is persistent; if effective there should be a dramatic response within two days.

Wind

'Wind' is a most unreliable and confusing symptom. In infancy it is the parents' presentation of a disturbed and distressed child who suffers repeated attacks of crying and drawing up of the legs. Whether these symptoms are ever caused by 'wind' is impossible to say and it is therefore a dangerous and incomplete diagnosis for a doctor to make. In adults it may mean abdominal fullness or discomfort; it may signify excessive eructations, burping, and flatulence; it may mean colicky abdominal pains and distension and constipation; or it may mean excessive passage of flatus. The practitioner presented with a 'windy' patient must never accept it as a diagnosis but must proceed to try to arrive at a diagnosis in terms of a physical, emotional or social disturbance.

Causes. — Excess of wind in the gut must be due either to excessive swallowing of air (aerophagy), the formation of gas within the bowel or a failure to pass wind per rectum. Aerophagy is by far the most common cause. This may be a habit, particularly in anxious and tense patients. Such patients not uncommonly have hurried meals and the working lunch is particularly conducive to this habit. In babies, aerophagy may occur during feeding if the teat is too small or the flow of breast milk too slow and is commonly caused by crying. Patients who suffer from other symptoms of indigestion due to peptic ulcer or gall-bladder disease also tend to swallow air and complain of excessive wind. Very rarely, disorders of malabsorption, e.g. coeliac disease or sprue, may be associated with wind in the small bowel, and subacute intestinal obstruction due to Crohn's disease, neoplasms or adhesions may cause accumulation of wind in the bowel. In the irritable bowel syndrome, the large bowel may be distended with wind and passage of excessive flatus may be associated with bowel irregularity and abdominal discomfort. Loss of tone in the musculature of the large bowel, particularly in old age, may lead to constipation and distension from flatus. Rarely, drugs such as methyldopa or the tricyclic antidepressants may contribute to this problem.

Symptoms. — These may differ depending on the sites to which the wind is attributed by the patient. 'Wind' in the upper gastrointestinal tract leads to retrosternal and epigastric discomfort, frequent burping and often associated heartburn. Although rarely mentioned by the patient, a history of constant swallowing of air is generally present. Vomiting is unusual. 'Wind' in the mid gut leads to abdominal distension. There may be colicky abdominal pains if the wind has built up quickly, as in intestinal obstruction, or there may be a more general discomfort with a longer history. 'Wind' in the lower bowel generally means excessive and embarrassing passages of flatus, or gas, through the anus. If associated with the irritable bowel syndrome, there may be intermittent left-sided abdominal pain relieved by the passage of wind and often accompanied by bowel irregularity.

History and examination. — The history is all important and should be concerned with not only the symptoms experienced but also the patient's way of life, eating habits, and the like. It is not uncommon to observe a patient swallowing air as he recounts his symptoms. In the absence of any other symptoms indicating organic disease, e.g. a change in bowel habit, or abdominal pain, it is unlikely that examination or further investigation will be helpful in reaching a diagnosis.

Management. — Aerophagy: This is frequently associated with bad eating habits. The patient should be advised to have regular meals taken at leisure. The working lunch is particularly to be avoided. The eating habits of many of these patients reflect their personalities and they are often tense and driving people. Counselling such patients is the most helpful measure in encouraging them to develop a more relaxed life-style. There is little place for drug treatment. The association of any specific upper gastrointestinal disease, e.g. oesophageal reflux or peptic ulcer, will lead to appropriate treatment of that disorder.
Irritable bowel syndrome: This should also be treated initially by advice concerning eating habits and life-style. If symptoms persist, a high roughage diet should be supplemented with methyl cellulose or ispaghula husk of which there are many different proprietary preparations. They should all be taken with at least half a pint of

water. In some cases, an antispasmodic, e.g. mebeverine hydrochloride (Colofac) or hyoscine butylbromide (Buscopan) may be helpful.

'Three month colic': The relationship between this syndrome, sometimes also called 'paroxysmal fussing', and wind is difficult to determine. There is no doubt that crying in a baby is associated with air swallowing and distension of the stomach with wind. Air swallowing may also occur when a hungry baby sucks on a teat with a small hole or a breast from which milk is flowing too slowly. Crying in turn may be caused by hunger or pain of any description. The syndrome is characterized by continuous crying, usually late in the day. It is most common in first-born children, starts in the first trimester of life, always improves with admission to hospital with or without the mother and is associated in many but not all cases with evident lack of confidence in the mother in handling her baby.

This latter finding suggests that prenatal advice on mothering and support in the early weeks of life, in particular for those mothers who do not have cohesive family support, may be important measures in preventing the disorder. Once established, it is important to seek for a cause for the crying, of which hunger may be important in a breast fed baby whose mother may become fatigued and short of milk late in the day. In this case, supplementary feeds in the afternoon and early evening may solve the problem. The baby should not be left to cry for long periods and the mother should be encouraged to pick him up and comfort him. In some cases, the use of a dummy is helpful. The use of antispasmodics e.g. dicyclomine (Merbentyl) which has been recommended in the past is contraindicated in infants under the age of six months as there is some evidence that it is associated with sudden death in small infants. A small dose of chloral or infant Gaviscon may, however, be useful.

This syndrome can be very confusing and distressing to the parents and may lead to baby battering. The doctor should not hesitate to admit a very distraught mother and baby to hospital, if the situation cannot be safely managed at home.

References

[1] Price, S. and Castell, D.O. (1978): Esophageal mythology. *Journal of the American Medical Association*, *240*, 44.

[2] Gear, M.W.L. and Barnes, R.J. (1980): Endoscopic studies of dyspepsia in general practice. *British Medical Journal*, *280*, 1136.

Appendix
Developing a practice policy in the management of dyspepsia

This appendix describes a practice policy developed by a general practitioner, who was asked by his partners to establish guidelines for the management of dyspepsia. In his literature search, he selected a paper by Saunders et al.[1] as his main guide to management. It was selected for the following reasons:
- The study was based on patients identified by general practitioners.
- The patients selected were clearly defined, dyspepsia being defined as 'epigastric or retrosternal pain or discomfort that was usually related to meals and had been present for at least 2 weeks'.
- The clinical diagnosis was confirmed by endoscopy.
- A well designed randomized control trial of ranitidine was described with endoscopic follow-up. Appropriate statistical tests were carried out.

Results of the study

A total of 604 patients were recruited to the study by 106 general practitioners. Of these patients 559 were endoscoped and 496 finally entered the trial.
The most common endoscopic diagnoses were oesophagitis (29%) followed by duodenitis (21%), duodenal ulcer (17%), gastritis (16%) and hiatus hernia (15%). Gastric carcinoma was found in one patient on endoscopy. No abnormality was found in 31% of the patients. The general practitioners' clinical diagnosis agreed with that of the endoscopies in only 50% of cases, with the highest correlation in the diagnosis of duodenal ulcer.
Overall, symptomatic response to placebo was 55% at 6 weeks, compared with 76% of the patients treated with ranitidine. Of the patients in whom no abnormality was detected on endoscopy, 81% responded to ranitidine and 66% to placebo. There was no significant difference in the side-effects reported by patients receiving ranitidine 150 mg twice daily, or placebo.
Follow-up 12 months after a 6-week course of treatment indicated that about 50% of patients had a recurrence during this period of time.

Practice policy

(1) Patients presenting in the practice with dyspepsia, as defined in the study, and of more than 2 weeks' duration, should initially be treated with a 6 week course of ranitidine 150 mg twice daily, without investigation, with the exception of patients presenting with dyspepsia for the first time over the age of 50 years, or patients complaining in addition of weight loss or anorexia.
(2) All patients treated in this way should be followed up for a period of one year. About 80% will respond to the initial course of treatment. Of these, 50% may relapse during the subsequent year. These patients should be referred for endoscopy in order to establish a firm diagnosis, which may lead to a decision to institute intermittent treatment with H_2 blockers to introduce other drugs such as carbenoxalone or the new anticholinergic pirenzepine, or to recommend for surgical treatment.
(3) Patients who fail to respond to treatment (20%) should be carefully reassessed. They may be suffering from some disease other than acid peptic disease, such as cholecystitis, ischaemic heart disease or a functional disorder associated with stress. A decision must then be made in terms of further physical investigation, such as endoscopy, cholecystogram, ECG, etc., or a more careful assessment of psychological factors in the aetiology of their symptoms.
(4) General practitioners will be reassured that only one patient in this study was found, on endoscopy, to be suffering from gastric carcinoma. The early diagnosis of this condition has little influence on the prognosis, and fear of this diagnosis should not prompt referral of a very large number of patients suffering from 'acid peptic diseases' for expensive investigations.

Effect of practice policy

Many patients will be protected from unpleasant, invasive investigations. Investigations which do not contribute to the management of patients with dyspepsia will be kept to a minimum, thus saving the health service large sums of money, and there is no evidence that patients will suffer as a result.
Ranitidine is preferred to cimetidine in the treatment of dyspepsia because it does not have the same tendency to produce gynaecomastia in males, nor does it interfere with the oxidative drug metabolism in the liver which may slow the metabolism of warfarin, phenytoin and theophylline. The relative costs of 4

weeks' treatment are ranitidine 150 mg twice daily, £27, and cimetidine 400 mg twice daily, £17 (1986 prices).

References

[1] Saunders, J., Oliver, R., and Higson, D.L. (1986): Dyspepsia: incidence of non-ulcer disease in a controlled trial of ranitidine in general practice. *British Medical Journal*, *292*, 665

3.44
The patient complaining of nausea and vomiting

John Fry

Vomiting is a relatively common presenting symptom in general practice and is twice as common in children as in adults. In a random sample of adults questioned about the symptoms they had experienced in the preceding two weeks, 3 per cent admitted to vomiting. It is a non-specific symptom covering a wide range of possible causes which will be identified only by piecing together other clinical features of the illness presented.

Presentation

The mode of presentation is very variable. In babies it may be presented as a non-acute problem of food regurgitation following feeds. Less commonly it presents as the most prominent feature of a pyrexial illness or as projectile vomiting in an otherwise healthy infant. In children vomiting is often a concomitant of fever from a variety of causes, and equally commonly presents as a syndrome of vomiting, colicky abdominal pain followed by diarrhoea. A similar syndrome is seen less often in adults in whom vomiting may be associated with headache as in migraine, travel as in motion sickness, or amenorrhoea as in pregnancy. All these presentations are acute in onset. In middle age vomiting is more often presented as part of a more chronic gastro-intestinal disturbance when abdominal pain may be a more prominent symptom. In any age-group the combined presentation of abdominal pain and vomiting will lead the doctor to exclude acute appendicitis or intestinal obstruction.

Causes

Nausea and vomiting may result from local, central, or general causes. Locally, the most likely cause is 'acute gastritis', a useful label for the syndrome of vomiting, abdominal pain and malaise. Presumably it is caused by an infective agent or some other ingested gastric irritant (in particular excessive alchohol consumption). It is not uncommonly followed by diarrhoea. Central causes include acute vertigo associated with nausea and vomiting (as in Menière's syndrome or acute labyrinthitis), motion sickness, migraine and much rarer conditions such as vestibular neuronitis and tumours. General disorders that may cause vomiting and nausea are reactions to drugs such as digoxin and aspirin, uraemia, diabetes mellitus and rarities such as Addison's disease.

In general practice the physician is faced with the earliest stages of diseases and it is often difficult to arrive at a definitive diagnosis. The patient may present with symptoms such as nausea and occasional vomiting that may require time and observation for the natural history of the disorder to develop and become sufficiently clear to make a diagnosis. For example, the earliest features of infective hepatitis are often severe nausea and anorexia and these may be present for as long as two weeks before jaundice is noted. Sudden and profuse vomiting with abdominal pain may signify a dramatic but benign bout of acute gastritis but they may also be the beginning of acute intestinal obstruction, myocardial infarction, a catastrophic cerebrovascular accident, or an acute vestibular neuronitis. 'Vomiting' may also occur in food rejection with anorexia nervosa or allied psychopathic disorders. 'Vomiting' may be normal in babies who regurgitate small amounts of milk. On the other hand projectile vomiting may raise the question of pyloric stenosis.

Thus, there are many possible causes of nausea and vomiting and it requires time, observation and a degree of clinical experience and awareness to decide on the cause and nature of the problem and on the correct management. It may be easy and straightforward, or it may be a most difficult and worrying situation for the physician. The following are among the more likely or important causes of nausea and vomiting.

Infancy: 0–1 year
Feeding problems
Gastro-enteritis
Pyloric stenosis
Any acute infection including meningitis

Childhood: 1–5 years
Gastro-enteritis
Acute infections:
  tonsillitis
  acute otitis media
  meningitis
  pyelonephritis

5–45 years
Dietary indiscretion
Gastro-enteritis
Pregnancy
Infective hepatitis
Migraine
Motion sickness
Acute labyrinthitis
Acute appendicitis
Drugs and alcohol

45 years and over
Dietary indiscretion
Gastro-enteritis
Drugs and alcohol
Menière's disease
Intestinal obstruction
Carcinoma of stomach, pancreas and large bowel
Cholecystitis
Cerebro-vascular disturbance
Renal failure

History

The history will give guidance to a likely diagnosis. Systematic enquiry should be made on how the symptoms began and how long they have been present. Any nausea and/or vomiting that goes on longer than three to four days, in the absence of pregnancy, must raise possibilities of some significant underlying cause. The timing of the vomiting may be noteworthy. Vomiting of relatively unaltered food soon after a meal suggests an oesophageal obstruction, present some time, to allow the oesophagus to become dilated as an inert receptacle as in achalasia of the cardia, or benign stricture of the oesophagus. Pyloric stenosis is associated with large offensive vomitus but with no evidence of bile. A gastro-colic fistula characteristically produces faeculent vomit. Associated features such as vertigo, loss of weight, changes in bowel habits, micturition and menses, general malaise, drowsiness, abdominal pain and jaundice will help in diagnosis but may take some time to appear.

The possibility of nausea and vomiting being part of a psychiatric disturbance is unlikely. They are not features of an anxiety state, except in acute situations in certain individuals, or of a depression, but they may occur in the much more complex condition of anorexia nervosa and its variants. Although refusal and abstention from eating are the main symptoms there also may be induced vomiting.

Examination

The many possible causes of vomiting make it necessary to carry out a full physical examination of patients presenting with this symptom. Associated symptoms, however, may direct particular attention to certain areas.

The pyrexial infant or child who presents with vomiting will lead the practitioner to look particularly for neck stiffness, signs of inflammation in the ears and throat, and abdominal tenderness. In the presence of respiratory distress or cough he will try to elicit signs of pulmonary infection. In the absence of any abnormalities in these systems he will examine a mid-stream specimen of urine bacteriologically. Very often vomiting in infancy is caused by mild gastroenteritis, when the practitioner's main concern will be with eliciting signs of dehydration, in the absence of which rapid recovery may be expected. A question about the frequency with which the infant is wetting his nappies is a useful guide to impending dehydration. In the apyrexial infant in the first few weeks of life pyloric stenosis may be suspected by the presence of projectile vomiting and the doctor will then examine the infant during a feed in order to identify a pyloric tumour.

The apyrexial adult presenting with vomiting associated with colicky abdominal pain and possibly diarrhoea is almost certainly suffering from an acute dietary indiscretion or gastro-intestinal infection. In these cases it is always wise to examine the abdomen for localized tenderness to exclude appendicitis.

Nausea and vomiting associated with vertigo or headache should lead to a careful neurological examination with particular examination of the optic fundi for signs of raised intracranial pressure, eye movements for nystagmus, and for signs of ataxia in the limbs. The ears should also be examined.

Nausea and vomiting of gradual onset will draw special attention to the gastro-intestinal tract. The practitioner should look for signs of weight loss, abdominal masses, visible peristalsis and abdominal distension and should carry out a rectal examination.

In young adults infective hepatitis often presents with nausea, and jaundice and liver tenderness should be looked for. In young women an unwanted pregnancy not uncommonly presents with nausea and this may be confirmed by a vaginal examination or pregnancy test.

Investigations

These will depend on the results of the history and examination. In the vast majority of patients presenting in general practice with vomiting they will add nothing to the diagnosis. In the second half of life, patients presenting with nausea and vomiting of gradual onset may often require full investigation to exclude organic bowel disease.

Management

In selecting the treatment for patients presenting with nausea and vomiting, the first priority is to make a diagnosis. In infants and children most cases will be due to feeding problems, gastro-intestinal infections or infections of the upper respiratory tract. Feeding problems are most commonly due to faulty technique rather than faults in the content of the feed. They require time for diagnosis and not only must a careful history be taken but the mother must be observed feeding her infant. In many cases the health visitor is the appropriate person to treat these problems and can give the time and attention which a mother needs in this situation.

In treating acute gastro-intestinal infections in children, or adults, the most important step is to stop all solid food and to ensure an adequate intake of simple fluids, of which water is the most appropriate. Under the age of 1 year milk feeds should be stopped and the infant prescribed a balanced electrolyte solution containing sodium and potassium chloride (e.g. Rehydrat). Each sachet is reconstituted with 250 ml of freshly boiled water and the infant should be allowed to take this on demand. Usually, vomiting will cease within 24 hours and the infant can be slowly returned to a normal feeding pattern. In children over the age of 1 year it is usually sufficient to stop all normal feeds and to recommend clear fluids only for 24 hours, e.g. water flavoured with orange or blackcurrant. If the infant or child does not respond to the treatment and signs of dehydration become apparent admission to hospital is indicated. Mothers are often worried about starving children in this way and should be positively reassured that the child will come to no harm as long as adequate fluids are administered.

Acute infections in childhood other than gastro-intestinal should be treated with the appropriate antibiotic. In the vomiting child this should normally be administered by intramuscular injection. Parents in this situation should be particularly warned not to use aspirin which may exacerbate the gastro-intestinal upset.

In adults the most common cause of vomiting is a dietary indiscretion or gastro-intestinal infection. Treatment consists of bed rest, withdrawal of all solid food and adequate simple fluids. Very commonly diarrhoea follows the gastric symptoms and may be relieved by a kaolin mixture or codeine phosphate, 30 mg four hourly.

The specific causes of nausea and vomiting demand appropriate remedies. Vestibular disorders, e.g. motion sickness, acute labyrinthitis and Menière's disease may be relieved by cinnarizine (Stugeron) 15 mg three times daily, or prochlorperazine maleate (Stemetil, Vertigon) 5 mg three times daily. This drug is also available as an injection 12.5 mg or a suppository 25 mg which is useful when vomiting precludes oral therapy. Metoclopramide (Maxolon) which acts both centrally and on the gastro-intestinal tract may be used in a dose of 10 mg three times daily by mouth and is also available as an intramuscular or intravenous injection. It is particularly valuable in the treatment of nausea and vomiting following cytotoxic therapy. All these drugs may produce dystonic reactions if used over a long period e.g. in the treatment of Menière's disease.

Vomiting in pregnancy will usually resolve without specific treatment but with reassurance and advice about taking something by mouth before rising in the morning, and small frequent snacks, rather than large meals, during the day. The more resistant case may be helped by use of meclozine hydrochloride (Ancoloxin) 25 mg, which has stood the test of time and for which there is no evidence of teratogenicity.

Vomiting may be a troublesome symptom in migraine. Metoclopramide 10 mg taken at the earliest warning of an attack and followed by an analgesic appears to offer a real advance in the treatment of the condition. Alternatively, prochlorperazine maleate 5 mg by mouth or 25 mg by suppository may be helpful.

In terminal illness, particularly that due to gastro-intestinal neoplasms or in patients treated with cytotoxic drugs, vomiting may be troublesome. The use of morphia for pain may exacerbate this symptom. In these cases metoclopramide 10 mg three times daily, chlorpromazine 25 mg three times daily or prochlorperazine 5 mg three times daily may provide relief.

3.45
The patient complaining of abdominal pain

John Fry

Abdominal pain is one of the commonest symptoms reported to general practitioners, and of the commonest symptoms it is the one which gives rise to the greatest diagnostic uncertainty. Morrell and his colleagues[1] in their analysis of the frequency with which 98 different symptoms were presented in general practice found that abdominal pain was the fourth most common symptom (after cough, rashes and sore throat) but that the doctor was confident in reaching a presumptive diagnosis, as opposed to a symptomatic or provisional one, only in less than a quarter of cases.

The majority of cases of abdominal pain seen in practice will be due to dietary indiscretion, minor muscular strains or such vague entities as 'indigestion', 'colic', 'dyspepsia' or 'gastritis'. It is neither surprising nor worrying that diagnostic certainty is rarely achieved in such instances. What is important is that the practitioner should be able to identify the potentially life threatening – the 'acute appendix', the perforated ulcer or the ruptured ectopic pregnancy – and for the rest, judge the point at which toleration of uncertainty should give way to more vigorous investigation.

The questions facing the general practitioner presented with a patient with abdominal pain are:

1. Is this an 'acute abdomen' that has to be admitted to hospital at once, or can the patient be managed and observed at home and, if so, how often should he be seen and assessed?
2. Is there an identifiable surgical or medical cause for the pain?
3. If the general practitioner decides to accept the care of the patient, how should he be investigated and managed?

The clinical approach to the management of abdominal pain must be systematic and thorough if mistakes are not to be made and patients' lives put at risk.

There is still no better statement and description of such an approach than the late Sir Zachary Cope's book *The Early Diagnosis of the Acute Abdomen*.[2]

History

In many ways, a good history, with the patient being allowed and encouraged to tell his or her story, is more useful in diagnosis than a physical examination. The general practitioner may be at an advantage in knowing his patient and the patient's family over many years. This may help in providing a personality background, although it may also give rise to a dangerous prejudice or bias. It is well to remember that even the most chronic neurotic, anxious and depressed patients will suffer at times from abdominal diseases.

As a start, some information on the *time relationships* of the pain is necessary. When did it start? Has the pain been constant or intermittent or recurrent? Has anything made it worse or better? What does the patient think may have brought it on?

Determining the *character* of the pain is often helpful. Is it dull and aching, or sore or sharp or stabbing or colicky? Is it a nuisance in interfering with what the person is doing, or is it so agonizing that the victim is completely immobilized, prostrate or collapsed?

What is the *site* of the pain? Does it shift, or has it shifted? Does the pain radiate elsewhere during attacks?

Are there any *associated features*

- Is there *nausea and/or vomiting*?
- Has there been any alteration in the *bowel habits*?
- Is *micturition* normal?
- Are the *menses* normal? When did the last menstrual period start? Is the patient taking an oral contraceptive pill or has she been fitted with an intra-uterine device?

What of the patient's *previous history*? Have there been bouts of abdominal pain or indigestion? What major illnesses have been experienced and, in particular, have there been any previous abdominal operations? The *family history* should also be investigated for gastro-intestinal and other major diseases.

Finally, an enquiry should be made about whether the patient has been abroad recently.

Examination

The patient's *general demeanour and appearance* should be noted. If the patient is known to the practitioner, any loss of weight will be apparent, as will any features of anxiety, tension or depression.

A note should be made of the *temperature* and the *pulse rate*. The *tongue* should be inspected to assess hydration. Once or twice in a professional lifetime inspection of the *skin* may reveal spots or rashes of a general disorder that may be responsible for the abdominal pain, as in herpes zoster or typhoid fever.

The *abdomen* should be inspected before it is palpated. Does it move freely? Is there any swelling, distension or asymmetry? Palpation should be gentle, with a warm hand, and starting away from the site of the pain. Is there any tenderness, guarding or rigidity on superficial or deep pressure? Are there any palpable masses or lumps? Is there any rebound tenderness? If there is any distension or swelling is it dull or resonant to percussion? Auscultation with the stethoscope may reveal a silent or noisy abdomen and either finding may be highly significant. Examination of the groins to check for the possible presence of herniae, and (in the young male) of the testes to exclude torsion, should complete the routine.

If the diagnosis is in doubt, examination may be extended to include the chest, back and central nervous system. A rectal and/ or vaginal examination may be necessary to clarify the diagnosis or exclude disease in the pelvis.

Investigations

In the majority of patients with abdominal pain, who suffer from relatively minor conditions of short duration or from more major or dramatic acute disorders that require urgent admission to hospital, no investigations will be required. Faced, however, with a patient with abdominal pain where the diagnosis is not quite clear or requires confirmation, a series of investigations may be indicated, and these should be ordered selectively.

The *urine* must be examined not only to diagnose a possible urinary-tract infection but also to exclude diabetes mellitus or the rare porphyria.

Examination of the *faeces* may be necessary for occult blood (a test which can be performed simply with the use of 'Hemastix' in the consulting-room), or for ova or cysts – probably best carried out in the laboratory.

The *blood* may need to be tested for: signs of anaemia from blood loss; signs of infection such as a raised white count and erythrocyte sedimentation rate; raised blood sugar, serum amylase and evidence of liver dysfunction; rarely, and more specifically, for malarial parasites.

Indications for *radiography* will depend on the presenting clinical features. A straight radiograph of the abdomen may be helpful to demonstrate distended obstructed loops of bowel and to show fluid levels, but normally such patients will have been admitted to hospital. A barium meal will be indicated when gastric or duodenal conditions are suspected, with a follow-through for possible disorders of the small bowel. In some areas open-access *endoscopy* is now available and may be helpful to supplement contrast media radiography. A barium enema in association with sigmoidoscopy will be helpful to define possible lesions of the large gut. Less commonly, an intravenous pyelogram and a chest X-ray may be indicated for special reasons when chest or urinary-tract disorders are suspected. Ultrasound may be useful in identifying gallstones.

A practical etiological classification

A practical classification of abdominal pain as encountered in general practice is to divide the types simply into those of acute and non-acute onset.

Acute abdominal pain. Acute abdominal pain of recent onset (within a few days) may be major or minor.
Major types of acute abdominal pain occur at an annual rate of 10 per 1,000 or 15 to 20 in a practice of 2,000. The most common is spontaneous abortion, but here it is bleeding rather than pain that is the predominant symptom. The most common major diagnosis where pain predominates is acute appendicitis. This occurs at all ages but is most prevalent in children and young adults.[3] In an average-sized practice of 2,000 patients about four cases of acute appendicitis can be expected each year.
Acute intestinal obstruction, although less common than acute appendicitis, may be expected to affect two or three patients each year in a typical practice. The most likely causes of the obstruction are strangulated hernia, new growth, intussusception and bands or adhesions. Perforations from peptic ulcers, diverticulae and new growths can be responsible for dramatic acute abdominal pain. Other causes of acute abdominal pain include: in women, ruptured ectopic pregnancy or twisted ovarian cysts; in young men, torsion of the testis; and in elderly men, acute urinary retention.
There is also a number of non-surgical disorders that can cause acute abdominal pain and which have to be remembered in the differential diagnosis. Renal and biliary colic, caused by acute infection or calculi in the urinary or biliary tracts, are important medical causes of acute abdominal pain. Much more rarely, acute pancreatitis can present as an acute abdominal emergency. Pneumonia, particularly in one of the lower lobes, can give rise to pain, tenderness and some guarding in the upper abdomen. Bornholm disease, or epidemic myalgia, can arise as sudden severe upper abdominal pain with pain on breathing. In acute myocardial infarction the pain may be referred to the epigastrium and in the early stages of infective hepatitis there are pain

and tenderness in the right upper quadrant of the abdomen. Pain in the pre-rash stage of herpes zoster has confused many a doctor, and when the lower thoracic or upper lumbar nerve roots are affected an acute abdominal emergency may be suspected. Possibly once or twice in a general practitioner's career he will come across a ruptured abdominal aorta, uncontrolled diabetes mellitus, porphyria and possibly typhoid fever or malaria as causes of acute abdominal pain.

Table I shows the expected incidence of various major causes of abdominal pain in one year in a practice of 2,000 patients.

Acute medical		
Cholecystitis or biliary colic		4
Renal or ureteric colic		3
Acute pancreatitis		< 1
Acute surgical		
Spontaneous abortion		8
Appendicitis		4
Acute intestinal obstruction		2
Perforated ulcer		1
Acute urinary retention		1
Torsion of testis	each	< 1
Torsion of ovarian cyst	each	< 1
Ruptured ectopic pregnancy	each	< 1

Table I. – Expected incidence in one year of various major causes of acute abdominal pain in a practice of 2,000 patients

Having listed some major causes of abdominal pain, it is necessary to remember the possibility of the Munchausen syndrome. Rare in general practice, but not uncommon in hospital emergency departments, are patients who present with plausible symptoms and signs of an acute abdominal emergency, who seek and even demand potent analgesics and who tend to disappear if these are not given. Some display multiple scars from previous operations.

Numerically, there are many more *minor* than major causes of acute abdominal pain. Acute gastro-intestinal infections with pain, vomiting and often diarrhoea occur in equal annual prevalence (25 per 1,000) at each decade from five to 80, but are much more common in young children (100 per 1,000 a year). Dietary indiscretion or abuse is a not infrequent cause of abdominal pain, particularly in children. The 'little belly-acher' or the 'periodic syndrome' is a common clinical picture in practice. The child, aged three to seven, is brought by the mother with the

complaint of sudden and recurrent mid-abdominal pain. There is often pallor and occasionally vomiting. There are no abnormal physical signs. The condition ceases spontaneously with time,[4] but a few 'little belly-achers' become 'big belly-achers' as adults.
Most commonly, however, the causes of minor acute abdominal pain remain undiagnosed, and resolve with the passage of time and perhaps simple symptomatic remedies. In many of these instances, strains of the muscles of the anterior abdominal wall may play at least some part.

Non-acute abdominal pain. Causes of non-acute pain in the upper abdomen are gastric and duodenal ulcers, cancer of the stomach and gall-bladder and liver disease. Other causes include a congested liver from heart failure, and cancer of the pancreas. Pain in the mid-abdomen may occur in cancer of the pancreas, which is very rare, or regional ileitis (Crohn's disease), ileocaecal tuberculosis, and sprue and other causes of malabsorption.
Pain in the lower abdomen may be due to cystitis, cancer of the colon or rectum, diverticulitis of the large bowel, ulcerative colitis, spastic colon or the 'irritable bowel syndrome'. In women, lower abdominal pain may be found in a variety of gynaecological conditions, such as dysmenorrhoea, ovulatory (or mid-cycle) pain, salpingitis and tubo-ovarian infections, ovarian cysts, and fibroids or new growths of the uterus. Retroperitoneal tumours of the lymphatic system or other tissues may also cause vague and uncertain pains in the lower abdomen.
Table II shows the expected incidence of some minor acute and more serious non-acute causes of abdominal pain in one year in a practice of 2,000 patients. A further classification of abdominal pain, in relation to site, is shown in figure 1.

Abdominal pain – cause not established (including 'gastritis', 'colic', indigestion, dyspepsia and muscular abdominal pain)	60
Acute gastro-intestinal infections	60
Cystitis	40
Peptic ulcer	20
Dysmenorrhoea	12
'Periodic syndrome'	4
Cancer of gastro-intestinal tract (stomach, colon, rectum)	2
Irritable bowel syndrome/spastic colon	2
Diverticular disease	2

Table II. – Expected incidence in one year of minor acute and more serious non-acute causes of abdominal pain in a practice of 2,500 patients

The long list that can be given of possible organic causes of non-acute abdominal pain is often inadequate to account for the patient's continuing, persisting or recurring symptoms. There are patients who have been investigated in detail and in whom no organic explanation can be discovered. They are often depressed and anxious, with numerous personal and family problems to account for their persistent symptoms.

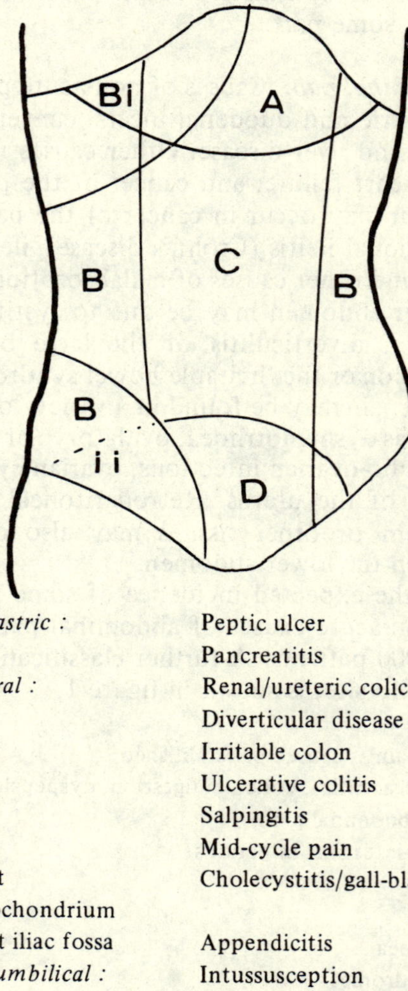

A –	*Epigastric :*	Peptic ulcer
		Pancreatitis
B –	*Lateral :*	Renal/ureteric colic
		Diverticular disease
		Irritable colon
		Ulcerative colitis
		Salpingitis
		Mid-cycle pain
Bi –	Right hypochondrium	Cholecystitis/gall-bladder colic
Bii –	Right iliac fossa	Appendicitis
C –	*Peri-umbilical :*	Intussusception
		'Periodic syndrome'
		Appendicitis (early)
D –	*Hypogastric :*	Cystitis
		Dysmenorrhoea
		Obstruction

Figure 1. – Common sites for various causes of abdominal pain

Clinical types at various ages

The probability of disease varies at different ages and is summarized in table III.

Infancy
Colic
Acute gastroenteritis
Acute respiratory infections
Intussusception

Children
Acute gastroenteritis
Tonsillitis
Otitis media
Urinary infections
'Periodic syndrome'
Appendicitis

Young adults
Acute gastroenteritis
Dysmenorrhoea
Abortion
Ruptured ectopic pregnancy
Appendicitis
Peptic ulcer
Testicular or ovarian torsion
Trauma

Middle age
Appendicitis
Cholecystitis/gall-bladder colic
Renal/ureteric colic
Cystitis
Peptic ulcer
Spastic colon/irritable bowel syndrome
Neoplasms

Old age
Diverticulitis
Peptic ulcer
Cholecystitis
Acute urinary retention
Neoplasms

Table III. - Common causes of abdominal pain classified by age groups

Children. In infants and very young children the most likely causes of abdominal pain are 'evening colic' and acute gastroenteritis. The cause of evening colic is unknown, though many conflicting theories have been advanced, but the condition is a common one and distressing to both infant and parents. The baby, otherwise apparently well and happy during the day, has attacks of inconsolable crying in the evening with drawing up of the legs, and does not settle with lifting or 'winding'. The condition usually settles by the age of about three months.[5]

In acute gastroenteritis the cause is either bacterial (*E.coli*) or viral, and the onset is sudden with pain, vomiting and then diarrhoea. The attack is normally short-lived, over in two to three days, and quite benign. In infancy, however, there is danger of dehydration.

The 'periodic syndrome' is a label given to bouts of recurring abdominal pain in children, usually between three and seven years of age. The pain is always referred to the peri-umbilical region. It is often associated with pallor, malaise and irritability. Vomiting may occur, and so may headache in older children. The attacks may be associated with anxiety, such as on starting school. There is often a family history of similar attacks or of 'biliousness' and migraine in the parents. There are no abnormal physical signs during an attack and the condition appears to settle naturally by the age of 10, sometimes to be followed by migrainous headaches a few years later.

In infants and young children 'pain in the tummy' may be caused by acute otitis media, acute throat infections or pneumonia. The ears, throat and chest must therefore be examined in all children with abdominal pain.

Infections of the urinary tract, sometimes associated with congenital abnormalities, may lead to acute or recurrent attacks of abdominal pain. More frequent in girls than in boys, there is often no complaint of dysuria or frequency by the child or the mother. The presenting features may be fever, malaise, generalized abdominal pain and, in chronic infections, failure to thrive – hence the need to examine the urine for pus cells and organisms in such children.

The more rare, dramatic and potentially dangerous causes of acute abdominal pain are acute appendicitis and intestinal obstruction. Acute appendicitis in young children is particularly dangerous because of the speed with which perforation and peritonitis develop. In children, the condition is one of general illness with fever, vomiting and often diarrhoea and generalized abdominal pain. The lower abdomen is usually tender and distension and absent bowel sounds may be found within a few hours.

Intestinal obstruction in children may occur from intussusception, strangulated or obstructed inguinal herniae or from congenital bands or other intestinal abnormalities. Intussusception presents between six months and two years of age with sudden abdominal pain, occurring in attacks with drawing up of the knees. Vomiting may occur early or later. A sausage-shaped lump may be felt in the abdomen and the passage of 'red currant jelly' per rectum is diagnostic, but this may be noted only on rectal examination.

Young adults. The most common cause of abdominal pain is acute gastroenteritis. It is an annoying but short-lived condition. Much less common is acute appendicitis, characteristically with central abdominal pain shifting to the right iliac fossa, with tenderness and guarding. The pain is continuous and may wake the patient

from sleep. There are often associated symptoms of anorexia, malaise and vomiting and there may be a low-grade fever. The tongue is coated and the breath smells.
In girls, dysmenorrhoea, abortion and other possible complications of early pregnancy, as well as mid-cycle pain occurring with ovulation must be remembered.
Peptic ulcers are unusual at this age, but delayed effects of closed trauma may cause unsuspected rupture of the spleen or liver with sudden collapse and severe abdominal pain.

Middle age. From middle age on, new growths of the stomach, pancreas and large bowel have to be considered as possible causes of persisting abdominal pain, and whilst only two or three new cases will occur each year in an average-sized practice, their early diagnosis is important. There are no specially distinctive clinical features, but any persisting abdominal pain accompanied by malaise, anorexia, vomiting and changes in bowel habit must be considered.
Spastic colon, or the irritable bowel syndrome, is a vague title for a vague or persistent aching pain in the left side of the abdomen, accompanied by loose or, in some patients, 'pellety' stools and tenderness along a palpable tubular descending and pelvic colon. The cause is uncertain, but it does seem to occur in persons who tend to be depressed and anxious.
In this age-group renal/ureteric colic and cholecystitis can present as acute abdominal emergencies. The history of very acute pain, with the patient restless and unable to find a comfortable position, and the localization of the pain to one or other loin with radiation down towards the groin and often associated urinary urgency will usually establish the diagnosis of urinary-tract colic without too much difficulty. In cholecystitis or gall-bladder colic, nausea and or vomiting tend to be associated symptoms, and the pain and tenderness are located in the right hypochondrium. The pain may radiate to the right subscapular region, and Murphy's sign (a sudden accentuation of pain on deep inspiration while the examiner's fingers press on the right hypochondrium) may be elicited.
In peptic ulceration the history is commonly of pain related to meals and often associated with stress. The pain is usually well localized and the 'finger-pointing' sign (the pain located by the use of a single finger pointing to a spot in the epigastrium) can be diagnostic. There is often a family history of peptic ulcer.

Elderly. In addition to new growths, gastric ulcers and gall-bladder disease, diverticulitis of the colon is more common in the elderly than in younger persons. Diverticulae of the descending and

pelvic colon are found in the majority of persons over 65 years of age. Most are symptomless and trouble free, but a few may become obstructed and infected and lead to pericolic infection, obstruction and even generalized peritonitis.
Acute intestinal obstruction gives rise to colicky abdominal pain, vomiting and absolute constipation. There is visible peristalsis and borborygmi are heard on auscultation. Strangulation of a hernia is indicated by a smooth tender swelling in the groin.
In elderly men, acute urinary retention secondary to prostatic enlargement may present as acute abdominal pain.

Management

General. The patient should be seen as soon as possible and a systematic history taken and an examination carried out. Unless this is done mistakes will be made and sooner or later a patient's life will be in jeopardy.
Is it an acute abdomen? This is the first question to be answered. A specific diagnosis is unnecessary in the early stages of dealing with the problem.
Is it an identifiable medical or surgical condition?
Should the patient be admitted to hospital? This must depend on the likely diagnosis. If it is considered to be an acute surgical condition, urgent admission to hospital is imperative. Likewise, if the diagnosis is uncertain and further close observation and investigations are considered necessary, there should be no hesitation in admitting the patient. It is much safer to have the patient admitted and find, in retrospect, admission was unnecessary than to take the risk of leaving the patient at home with an undiagnosed progressive abdominal emergency.
If kept at home, what care? Once it is decided that the patient with, say, renal colic or acute gastroenteritis, can be kept at home, then he should be seen again within twenty-four hours and instructed to call the doctor if there is any deterioration.

Specific treatment. Details of treatment of all the possible causes of abdominal pain cannot be given here but a few general principles can be stated. The simpler the treatment the better for both patient and doctor. Be honest and cynical enough to question periodically the true efficacy of the treatment you have come to prescribe by habit. Reassess the need for long-term medication, because it often does little more than keep the patient as a patient.

Non-acute abdominal pain. Here there is more time to think and act, but a systematic approach is essential in the history, examination and investigation. If the practitioner has access to pathological and radiological facilities, he should be able to assess, investigate and diagnose most of the more serious cases of abdominal pain. It may be that the symptoms and signs are so suggestive of a diagnosis that few confirmatory investigations are necessary. In fact, the case which requires a lot of investigation is often one in which no organic diagnosis can be made. There are relatively few causes of non-acute recurrent or persistent abdominal pain: peptic ulcers, hiatus hernia, gall-bladder disease, the irritable bowel and new growths of the large bowel or stomach account for most of these symptoms.

Acute gastroenteritis. The causes are uncertain. The majority are likely to be virus infections. It is therefore quite useless to use antibiotics or chemotherapy for a short-term, self-limiting illness of a few days. If medication is considered necessary in addition to a fluid diet, kaolin mixture BPC or codeine phosphate is sufficient.

Infantile colic. The most important point in managing infantile evening colic consists of explanation and reassurance to the mother that, although this is distressing, it is a benign condition, which often passes by the time the baby is about three months old. Dicyclomine (Merbentyl) has been recommended in the past but is now contraindicated in infants under the age of six months. Paediatric chloral mixture or Infant Gaviscon may be effective in some cases.

'Periodic syndrome'. The reassurance of a full history and examination, supplemented possibly by simple investigations, such as a barium meal, may be accompanied by simple explanation along the lines of 'while the pain is real and can be distressing, there is no serious disease going on and it may be a bit like the sort of headaches adults sometimes get when they are tired or under stress'. The keeping of a diary card or chart may help to identify possible precipitating factors, and regular, but not too frequent, follow-up visits can serve to show that the condition is being taken seriously. Occasionally, the advice to take some milk, or the prescription of simple antacids to be taken at the onset of pain, may improve the situation, perhaps more by placebo effect than anything else.

When all else fails the prescription of a small dose of diazepam can be very effective.

Gall-bladder colic. The pain of acute gall-bladder inflammation should be treated with morphine sulphate, 15 to 20 mg intravenously or intramuscularly, along with propantheline bromide, 30 mg intramuscularly, to relieve spasm. Alternatively parenteral pethidine 100 mg may be effective. After such initial treatment the patient should be given a supply of a suitable oral analgesic (such as phenazocine hydrobromide (Narphen) 5 mg which appears to have both an analgesic and an antispasmodic effect) to be taken in a dosage of one to two tablets every four hours if required. For at least twenty-four hours the patient should take a fluid diet only, and an anti-emetic (such as prochlorperazine maleate (Stemetil, Vertigon) 5 mg) may also have to be prescribed. The use of antibiotics in acute cholecystitis is a controversial subject, but if the patient is pyrexial, a course of ampicillin should be considered.

After an acute attack has subsided it is usual to refer the patient for cholecystography or ultrasound and, if gall-stones are shown to be present, to consider referral for surgery, which is indicated if attacks are recurring and disabling.

The use of bile acids (chenodeoxycholic and ursodeoxycholic acids) orally to dissolve cholesterol gall-stones has met with some success in hospital practice, and studies are continuing, but it is likely to be some time before such therapy finds a place in general practice. It may, however, be borne in mind that gall-stones are said to be found in 1 in 5 of all adults at necropsy. Few of these have ever caused serious symptoms in life and it is not automatically necessary to refer patients who have been found to have gall-stones, or poor gall-bladder function, for operation. Many will suffer no serious or dangerous troubles.

Renal/ureteric colic. The pain of acute urinary-tract colic is among the most severe which can be experienced, and the initial management is the same as that outlined for the treatment of gall-bladder colic. With a high fluid intake (at least four litres a day), ureteric stones are usually passed spontaneously, but renal stones may require eventual surgical removal.

Peptic ulcers. Peptic ulcers tend to cure themselves in about 80 per cent of instances.[6] Their unpleasant symptoms can generally be controlled by antacids and frequent bland meals. More sophisticated medication and surgery are necessary for the minority. Carbenoxolone (in the form of 'Biogastrone') is often helpful in promoting the healing of gastric ulcers, and more controversially is sometimes used (as 'Duogastrone') in the treatment of duodenal ulcers. A major advance in the treatment of peptic ulcers is the use of H_2 receptor antagonists. Cimetidine (Tagamet) in a dose of 200 mg three times daily and 400 mg at night is frequently successful, producing symptomatic relief within a few days of starting treatment. In males, ranitidine (Zantac) 150 mg twice daily has the advantage that it is not an anti-androgen and thus does not produce gynaecomastia which may occur if cimetidine is used. Ranitidine is also of value in treating patients receiving phenytoin, warfarin or theophylline derivatives. Initially treatment should be continued for at least two months after which the drug should be tailed off. A recurrence of symptoms should lead to a further course of treatment and in some cases long-term treatment, e.g. ranitidine 150 mg at night, should be continued indefinitely.

Spastic colon, *irritable bowel syndrome.* These and other bowel neuroses have to be managed individually, and personal problems defined and helped. Symptoms such as pain and loose stools can be controlled by occasional codeine phosphate (30 mg). Constipation can be relieved best by increasing the bulk of the diet and with extra bran and other roughage; this regime is also helpful in diverticular disease. Some patients find bran unacceptable and in these cases isphagula husk in the form of Fybogel as effervescent granules, one sachet twice daily, or Regulan also prepared as effervescent granules may be preferred. Methylcellulose (Celevac or Isogel) may also be used.

References

[1] Morrell, D.C., Gage, H.G. and Robinson, N.A. (1971): Symptoms in General Practice. *Journal of the Royal College of General Practitioners*, *21*, 32.

[2] Cope, Sir Zachary (1968): *The Early Diagnosis of the Acute Abdomen*. 13th ed. London: Oxford University Press.

[3] Royal College of General Practitioners, Office of Population Censuses and Surveys, Department of Health and Social Security (1986): *Morbidity Statistics from General Practice 1981–82*. HMSO Series MB5 No. 1.

[4] Apley, J. (1974): *Children with Abdominal Pain.* 2nd ed. Bristol: John Wright.

[5] Illingworth, R.S. (1975): *The Normal Child.* 6th ed. Edinburgh: Churchill Livingstone.

[6] Fry, J. (1974): *Common Diseases*. Lancaster: Medical and Technical Publishing Co.

3.46
The patient complaining of diarrhoea

David Morrell

Of a random sample of adults in the United Kingdom who were asked if they had experienced diarrhoea in the preceding two weeks, 2 per cent of men and 4 per cent of women admitted to this symptom[1]. The answers showed no consistent relationship to age. In a similar study[2], limited to a random sample of adults in the London boroughs of Bermondsey and Southwark, 7 per cent admitted to this symptom. Of these individuals, 14 per cent had consulted their doctor on account of the symptom and 26 per cent had taken some form of medication.

In several studies of symptoms presented to the general practitioner, diarrhoea was among the most commonly presented symptoms. It was seen most in children under the age of five years, and the age distribution of patients presenting this symptom resembled that of patients presenting with acute respiratory illness.

Causes

It is convenient to divide patients complaining of diarrhoea into those presenting with new acute episodes and those presenting with long-standing or recurrent diarrhoea.

Acute gastro-intestinal illness

Dietetic indiscretions or a sudden change of diet provoked by a holiday abroad are probably the commonest causes of a sudden change in bowel habit. Usually the patient can relate the illness to his behaviour and does not consult the doctor, but rarely symptoms are sufficiently severe to provoke that level of anxiety which leads to a consultation.

The role of infection as a cause of acute episodes of diarrhoea seen in general practice is still uncertain. In a study in general practice carried out in 1962[3], in which stools were cultured in 84 per cent of episodes, pathogenic bacteria, such as *Shigella sonnei* were rarely isolated in absence of a recognizable epidemic. The introduction of new techniques for isolating such organisms as *Campylobacter jejuni* and *Clostridium difficile* and enteropathic *E. Coli* from stool specimens indicates that these organisms may be an important cause of some cases of diarrhoea seen in the community, but most research has been carried out in hospital series. Advances in virology have also led to the isolation of specific viruses as a cause of diarrhoea and the rotavirus[4] is a particularly important cause in children under the age of five years. In recent years the parasite, *Giardia lambia* has been found particularly in children presenting with diarrhoea.

Diarrhoea due to campylobacter infections is often preceded by one or two days of malaise, fever and aches and pains, before the onset of profuse foul smelling and sometimes blood stained stools.

Diarrhoea due to *Giardia lambia* tends to produce profuse mucoid stools with severe abdominal colic. It most commonly affects children, who despite the diarrhoea remain remarkably well with a good appetite. In babies under six months giardiasis may cause failure to thrive without clear-cut gastro-intestinal symptoms. Most other causes of diarrhoea do not have characteristic clinical features, but the presence of blood and mucus in the stools should lead to a search for enteropathogens.

Another common cause of diarrhoea is drug therapy. Penicillin, ampicillin and tetracycline may all produce loose stools. Rarely severe diarrhoea accompanied by serious systemic disturbance may complicate treatment with antibiotics. This is due to pseudo-membranous colitis caused by the toxin from the organism *Clostridium difficile*. It presents characteristic sigmoidoscopic appearances and is a medical emergency requiring hospital treatment. Many other drugs may cause diarrhoea in some patients, including magnesium trisilicate, anti-inflammatory drugs such as indomethacin, ibuprofen and mefenamic acid derivatives. It also occurs in patients treated with clenodeoxycholic acid for gallstones, in diabetes treated by biguanides and in the treatment of myaesthenia gravis with neostigmine. Occasionally diarrhoea presenting in general practice is due to laxative abuse.

In children acute infections of the urinary tract or ear may present with diarrhoea, and local pelvic inflammatory disease including appendicitis may present in any age group complaining of diarrhoea.

Chronic and recurrent diarrhoea

This refers to illness of more than two weeks' duration. Alternate diarrhoea and constipation is the classical presenting feature of carcinoma of the large bowel. This symptom in the middle-aged or elderly always justifies further investigation. Alternate diarrhoea and constipation in old age is not infrequently associated with constipation and overflow incontinence. This condition can be easily diagnosed by rectal examination and relieved by an enema,

but if this cause is eliminated further investigations must be undertaken.
Conditions such as ulcerative colitis and regional ileitis (Crohn's disease) are relatively uncommon in general practice. The former may be suspected in a young adult presenting with diarrhoea and the passage of blood and mucus per rectum. There is often associated weight loss and malaise. The diagnosis is confirmed by sigmoidoscopy. Regional ileitis is more difficult to diagnose. The main feature is pain due to small-bowel colic, and there may be accompanying diarrhoea or constipation. A raised ESR is common and the diagnosis must be confirmed by a small-bowel barium meal.
Chronic diarrhoea may be presented by patients suffering from metabolic and endocrine disorders. Coeliac disease is a rare cause of diarrhoea in children in general practice, but should always be considered and lactose intolerance may cause attacks of diarrhoea with abdominal pain and distension. It is most common in non-whites and should always be suspected in non-white children presenting with periodic abdominal pain and in non-white adults presenting with the 'irritable bowel' syndrome. Thyrotoxicosis is a not uncommon cause of diarrhoea, and Addison's disease is a rare but important cause.
Iatrogenic diarrhoea may present as an acute episode following the ingestion of an antibiotic or anti-inflammatory drug, but sometimes develops more insidiously and has been present for some weeks before the patient complains. Diarrhoea also presents in more chronic forms following, for instance, gastric surgery, or radiotherapy to the pelvis. Acute or chronic anxiety occasionally presents with diarrhoea, and acute stressful situations, e.g. examinations, are well known to cause this symptom.

History taking

In patients presenting with diarrhoea it is, as with other symptoms, important to understand precisely what the patient is experiencing. Bowel habits vary widely in the population and what is diarrhoea to one patient may be normal to another. It is a change in habit which usually draws the patient's attention to his bowels.
It has been shown that diarrhoea is common and is often treated by patients by self-medication, and it is important to determine why a particular episode of diarrhoea has provoked sufficient anxiety to lead to a consultation. It may be the severity of the symptoms, but it may equally be due to many other factors. These include the patient's or parents' previous experience of this symptom, pressure from relatives or neighbours, the need for a National Health Insurance certificate for sickness absence, or the insecurity of the

patient in the face of illness resulting from factors described in Chapter 1.3. The patient is the best person to provide the answer to this question, and the doctor should not be afraid simply to ask the patient why he has consulted on this occasion. This will often clarify the situation and save a great deal of time.

Focusing on the symptom, it is important to determine its duration and time relationships. Is this an illness of sudden onset and of short duration; or is the patient presenting a chronic and recurrent problem? The vast majority of patients presenting with diarrhoea in general practice are concerned about an illness which has been present for 24 to 48 hours. Rarely, they present a long-standing complaint and in these cases it is important to establish the mode of onset, duration of the symptoms, relationship to meals, stress or any other particular situation to which the patient is exposed, and to identify whether the complaint is of alternating diarrhoea and constipation. Enquiry should always be made about recent travel abroad.

Other symptoms which accompany the diarrhoea must also be established. Does the patient feel ill or feverish? Is there a change in appetite, or vomiting? Is there abdominal pain? It is important to clarify the characteristics of abdominal pain including the site, whether it is colicky in nature or constant, and its relationship to episodes of diarrhoea. In long-standing cases particular attention will be directed to weight loss. Enquiry should be made about the appearance of the stools with a specific question about the presence of blood. The history should also establish the patient's occupation, any current or recent drug therapy, and recent dietary history.

Examination

This will be influenced by the history and the age of the patient. In the new acute case of perhaps 24 to 48 hours' duration, examination in an adult will usually be limited to palpation of the abdomen. In the child under five a similar history will lead to more extensive examination designed to identify pyrexia, the presence or absence of dehydration and the presence or absence of intercurrent infection, particularly of the ears or throat. In long-standing cases, or patients presenting with recurrent diarrhoea, more extensive examination will be carried out and will always include rectal examination. The patient's weight will be recorded as will his general appearance and the pulse rate and blood pressure.

Investigations

On the basis of the history and examination, patients presenting with this symptom will be divided into those with acute episodes of diarrhoea and those in whom the symptom is of long standing. These groups will be investigated quite differently.

Acute episodes of diarrhoea are most often due to dietary indiscretion or viral infections. More rarely they are of bacterial or iatrogenic origin. Virological investigation is currently of intense scientific interest but little practical importance to the general practitioner. Bacteriological investigations, in the absence of an epidemic of diarrhoea are rarely necessary in managing acute episodes of diarrhoea. Exceptions exist where this symptom presents in a patient who is a food handler, or lives in a closed community such as a residential school or a gaol.

If diarrhoea persists for more than a few days, however, bacteriological investigation of the stools is indicated, and if the patient has recently travelled abroad, a fresh specimen should be examined for *Giardia lambia* and, where indicated, for *Amoeba histolytica*.

In patients presenting with diarrhoea of two to three weeks' duration, more extensive investigation is required. This may include sigmoidoscopy and barium enema which will usually be carried out after referral to a specialist. In children, long-standing diarrhoea may suggest the diagnosis of coeliac disease and must exclude the possibility of giardiasis.

Management

Acute episodic diarrhoea

There is no evidence that antibiotics improve the prognosis in acute infective diarrhoea due to *Salmonella*, *Shigella* or viruses and they may also be dangerous by prolonging the carrier state. In certain specific infections, such as typhoid or amoebiasis, specific therapy is indicated. In campylobacter infections erythromycin will eliminate the infecting organism, but does not appear to influence the natural history of the illness. In giardiasis, treatment with metronidazole is curative. Treatment of acute episodes of diarrhoea in general practice should normally focus on three aspects of management.

1. Diet. The patient should be advised to stop eating and to take simple fluids only, such as water, or water flavoured with fruit juices. Hot and iced fluids are particularly liable to provoke attacks of diarrhoea. As the symptoms subside the patient should be advised to take a light diet for a further 48 hours.

In babies it is particularly important to stress the details of feeding. In mild cases it is sufficient to advise mothers to stop all feeds and replace them with three-hourly water (57 to 87 ml or 2 to 3 ounces).

In more severe cases the mother should adhere to the following regime:

The mother should be given a prescription for Dioralyte or some similar preparation of a powder containing dextrose and electrolytes. The sachets of powder should be dissolved in 200 ml (7 ounces) of water. The baby should be encouraged to take as much of this solution as it wishes at three-hourly intervals (200 ml per Kg body weight per day should be aimed at).

If the symptoms subside in 24 hours, then one measure of milk powder should be added to every 200 ml of the electrolyte solution. After a further 24 hours, two measures of milk powder are added to the solution. If the baby tolerates this it is returned to normal feeding.

Almost all children seen in general practice with diarrhoea will respond to this regime. If an advance in the regime leads to a relapse, then the child should be put back a stage in the regime. If signs of dehydration should occur (the absence of a wet nappy every four hours is a useful guide), loss of skin elasticity, or weight loss of 10 per cent of the body weight, then hospital admission is indicated.

In practice the need for hospital admission most commonly results from consideration of the child's social circumstances and the inability of the mother to cope with the problem, rather than objective signs of deterioration in the child. With close adherence to this regime the admission of a child to hospital with diarrhoea would probably not occur more than once in every five years in the life of the average general practitioner, irrespective of the particular cause of the diarrhoea.

2. Drugs. In adults the administration of kaolin and morphine mixture 10 ml three hourly, until symptoms abate is usually adequate combined with dietary restrictions. In severe or obstinate cases codeine phosphate 30 mg or diphenoxylate hydrochloride and atropine (Lomotil) every four hours is helpful. In infants and children, drug therapy plays little part in treatment and may in fact be dangerous.

3. Rest. Most acute infections respond to bed rest. This applies to acute gastro-intestinal illness, as well as to other illnesses, and 24 hours of bed rest combined with dietetic measures and, where necessary, drugs, will settle most acute episodes of diarrhoea seen in general practice.

Chronic and recurrent diarrhoea

Management of this will be directed to the underlying cause and may vary from surgical treatment of an underlying carcinoma to the administration of an enema to an elderly patient with overflow incontinence.

Ulcerative colitis frequently responds to treatment with sulphasalazine (Salazopyrin) 1g four times daily reduced to 0.5g four times daily as control of symptoms is established. Codeine phosphate 30mg three times daily is a useful adjuvant. In patients with proctitis local treatment with enemas of prednisolone may be helpful. When remission occurs maintenance treatment with sulphasalazine should be continued. A small proportion of patients will fail to respond to this treatment and may need systemic steroid therapy or surgical treatment.

Regional ileitis should be treated initially by diet and symptomatic remedies. A bulk-forming agent, e.g. Isogel, may be useful. Pain should be relieved by analgesics and diarrhoea by codeine phosphate. Any intercurrent anaemia should be treated appropriately. In some cases, sulphasalazine may be helpful and corticosteroid treatment may be indicated in severely ill patients. Extensive disease failing to respond to medical treatment and complications of the disease, e.g. intestinal obstruction, will need surgical intervention.

Coeliac disease must be treated with a gluten-free diet. Gluten-free flour, bread and biscuits can be prescribed under the National Health Service for these patients. If lactose intolerance is suspected, a trial of a lactose-free diet should be carried out.

The general practitioner may sometimes be left with the patient in whom all investigations have failed to provide an adequate explanation for diarrhoea. This may be due to a particularly sensitive gastro-colic reflex occurring in an anxious individual, or associated with gastric surgery. These patients may be helped by the use of a parasympathomimetic drug, such as propantheline, bromide (Pro-Banthine) or dicyclomine hydrochloride (Merbentyl), taken half an hour before meals. Other patients with chronic or recurrent diarrhoea may be suffering from the results of totally unsuitable diets and may be helped by appropriate dietetic advice. In some patients chronic or recurrent diarrhoea may be the result of drug therapy for other disorders. In these cases it will be important to try to devise suitable therapy to minimize symptoms. It may rarely be necessary to add specific anti-diarrhoea treatment in order to make a particular form of therapy acceptable. This is most likely to occur in the use of drugs such as guanethidine in the treatment of hypertension, but a change to a beta-blocker is usually preferable, and the wide variety of anti-inflammatory drugs available for treating arthritis make it possible to experiment with different preparations if one causes diarrhoea.

References

[1] Dunnell, K. and Cartwright, A. (1972): *Medicine Takers, Prescribers and Hoarders.* London: Routledge and Kegan Paul

[2] Wadsworth, M.E.J., Butterfield, W.J.H. and Blaney, R. (1971): *Health and Sickness: the Choice of Treatment.* London: Tavistock Publications

[3] Tuckman, E., Chapple, P.A.L., Franklin, L.M., Manser, I.N., Woodall, J.T., Randall, K.J. and McDonald, J.C. (1962): Acute gastro-intestinal illness in general practice. *British Medical Journal*, *1*, 135

[4] Leading article (1975): *Lancet*, *i*, 257

3.47
The patient complaining of constipation

David Morrell

The term constipation may be used to describe infrequent bowel action, hard stools or difficulty in defaecation. In a random sample of patients questioned about this symptom[1] 10 per cent of the adults and 6 per cent of children admitted to constipation in the preceding two weeks. The symptom was found to be more than twice as common in women than men, and to increase in frequency with age.

In a study carried out in an industrial medical centre and in general practice[2] designed to determine the normal frequency of bowel action 99 per cent of 1,455 persons questioned had a frequency of bowel action within the limits of three times weekly and three times daily. From these results it might be suggested that less than three bowel actions a week, or more than three a day may be regarded as abnormal. Studies of this sort are, however, confused by the widespread use of laxatives. About 15 per cent of the patients in this study were taking laxatives and while the frequency of bowel action was not shown to increase with age, the frequency of laxative consumption did. All laxatives, however, are not taken for symptoms of constipation and many are taken for totally unrelated symptoms. Laxative consumption is twice as common in women as in men and 45 per cent of patients keep laxatives in the medicine cabinet in the home.

Presentation of complaint

Constipation is a relatively uncommon presenting symptom in general practice. It is, however, a symptom which is often held responsible for a variety of disorders such as headaches, lack of energy or depression, and treated by patients by self-medication; many patients take regular laxatives assuming that this will improve their general well-being.

Constipation tends to be presented at particular times in life. There is the infant who is presented with infrequent bowel action: a relatively common event. In childhood, parents may attribute behavioural problems to bowel action, and consult the doctor. The pregnant woman not uncommonly presents with constipation and consults fearful of the effect of laxative drugs on her pregnancy. In middle age changes in bowel habit may be often presented with sinister implications. Drug therapy provided by the doctor may cause constipation, and lead to consultation. In the elderly, constipation may for the first time become a serious problem.

As frequency of bowel action varies widely between individuals and it is a change in bowel habit which usually provokes a consultation, it is important for the doctor to determine what the patient is experiencing. Is it infrequent action, hard stools or difficulty in defaecation, or a combination of these? Equally important is it to enquire into any recent changes in dietary habit. A diet designed to reduce weight and particularly in men a change in the consumption of beer may lead to major changes in bowel action. It is also important to inquire into the general well-being of the patient. Has there, for example, been any reduction in energy, drive, concentration? Are there changes in sleep pattern, or overt symptoms of depression? Specific questions about abdominal pain or distension, the presence of blood or mucus in the stools and weight gain or loss should be made. Finally, enquiries should be made about drug taking, in particular drugs taken for depression, hypertension or arthritis. The precise enquiries which the general practitioner undertakes of a patient with constipation will depend on the identification of the problem which the patient is experiencing. In the infant it may simply be lack of knowledge on the part of the mother of the normal bowel function of a baby, or a disparity between the performance of one sibling compared with another. In a young child the problem of constipation may be associated with the problem of negativism.

Constipation is still associated in the minds of many patients with symptoms varying from bad breath to headaches, period pains and recurrent infection. It may be a presenting symptom of a more complex problem. Identification of a patient's problem is crucial to appropriate history taking.

Causes

In childhood. – In spite of the fact that 99 per cent of individuals have a frequency of bowel action between three times daily and three times weekly, there is a widespread belief that a daily bowel action is normal, and that less frequent movement may lead to a variety of symptoms. Those who hold this faith may spend a lifetime regarding themselves as constipated and become regular takers of laxatives. Most habits are developed in childhood. There is some anecdotal evidence that the children of parents with sluggish bowel habits treated by regular laxatives are more often brought to the doctor with complaints of constipation than those children whose parents have a daily bowel opening. This would not be surprising as anxiety in the parent may well be transferred to the child.

In infancy and young childhood constipation is most commonly due to dietetic problems. It may result in infancy from inadequate fluid intake or the ingestion of cow's milk or cow's milk substitutes which contain relatively less digestible protein and inadequate carbohydrate. Rarely, obstinate constipation in childhood accompanied by abdominal distension may be due to Hirschsprung's disease in which ganglia are absent from the rectal wall, or megacolon in which this defect is not present. The former may be suspected in constipation in early childhood accompanied by abdominal distension and an empty rectum with a normal anal sphincter. The latter tends to appear later in childhood with a lax anal sphincter, full rectum and faecal soiling. It may be accompanied by emotional disorders in early childhood.

In young adults.– Constipation as a presenting symptom by young adults in general practice is rare. By far the commonest cause is a change in diet or occupation, and reducing diets are probably the commonest single cause for this symptom. An adequate history will usually establish the diagnosis. Very rarely a change in bowel habits may be associated with systemic upset or weight loss. In these cases, full specialist investigation may reveal regional ileo-colitis or tuberculosis. The latter should be suspected in immigrants, particularly from Pakistan or India. Analgesic ingestion should also be suspected in patients in this age-group, particularly in young women suffering from dysmenorrhoea.

A condition referred to as the irritable-bowel syndrome is not uncommon in this age-group. It is twice as common in women as in men. It is characterized by pain in the descending colon and alternate constipation and diarrhoea. The pain tends to be relieved by defaecation or passage of flatus. The stools are often described as pellet-shaped. Colonic mobility is abnormal in these patients and in some cases this appears to be associated with psychological factors.

In middle age.– Over the age of 40 years a sudden change in bowel habit should always prompt a suspicion of large bowel cancer.

This, however, is by no means the only cause of constipation in this age-group, and probably accounts for less than 10 per cent of all patients presenting with this symptom but, as one of the more treatable forms of cancer, it must be excluded. The other conditions which cause constipation in the middle aged and elderly include myxoedema, depression and diverticulitis. In addition, this age-group is subject to many chronic diseases and exposed to the side-effects of medication for these disorders. Iatrogenic constipation may, indeed, be the most common cause in older patients. Drugs responsible include analgesics, given to relieve the symptoms of chronic arthritis, tricyclic antidepressants, hypotensive agents, drugs for the treatment of peptic ulcer and codeine-containing linctuses used in the treatment of chronic bronchitis.

In the elderly.– Neoplasms of the colon must always be considered in a change in bowel habit in the elderly, but in this age-group major changes in diet and habits are often occurring and there is a steady diminution in activity. Chronic painful diseases are often present and iatrogenic constipation is still probably the most common single cause.

Constipation alone is a relatively uncommon presenting symptom. The doctor's diagnostic decision making is often influenced by

Presenting Complaint		*Differential Diagnosis*
Constipation alone	→	Misunderstanding of normal bowel action. Iatrogenic Dietary change Carcinoma of the colon.
↓		
Constipation + abdominal pain	→	Chronic intestinal obstruction – Carcinoma of colon – Regional ileo-colitis Appendicitis Diverticulitis
↓		
Constipation + abdominal pain + vomiting	→	Acute intestinal obstruction – Intussusception – Carcinoma of colon – Volvulus – Diverticulitis – Strangulated hernia Appendicitis
↓		
Constipation + abdominal pain + rectal bleeding	→	Intussusception Carcinoma of the colon Diverticulitis

Figure 1.– Spectrum of diagnosis in constipation

accompanying symptoms. In figure 1 the effect of additional symptoms on the spectrum of diagnoses considered is illustrated. This figure is not comprehensive and clearly varies with different age-groups. It does, however, indicate the way in which the interpretation of the presenting symptom is modified by elucidating other symptoms.

Examination and investigation

The examination and investigation which are undertaken are related to the patient's problem.

In babies and children, an initial assessment of the general health of the child should be made. Is this an ill baby, or a child who is failing to thrive? The general appearance of the child in terms of complexion, liveliness, response to the examiner and to the mother may be supplemented by measurement of height and weight in relation to normal standards. Inspection of the abdomen will identify abdominal distension and the presence of visible peristalsis, and rectal examination will determine the character of the anal sphincter, and the presence or absence of faeces in the rectum.

In young adult life the onset of constipation in the absence of other symptoms is often due to a change in diet or habits, pregnancy or drug therapy. Occasionally, it may complicate a painful anal lesion which will not be spontaneously complained of. Only rarely will examination add anything of diagnostic value, but abdominal and rectal examination should be carried out, not only to identify the relatively rare organic lesions, but to reassure the patient who has an underlying anxiety about serious organic disease.

In middle or old age the probability that constipation indicates serious disease is much greater than in the younger age-groups. An initial and conscious assessment of the patient's general appearance should precede local examination. If the doctor is familiar with the patient he may identify evidence of depressive illness with a slowing down of normal reactions, a general pathetic countenance, a readiness to tears or a paranoid response to the world around. There may be evidence of weight gain, a coarsening of features, and hair loss, suggesting a diagnosis of myxoedema. There may be obvious signs of weight loss with ill-fitting clothes or objective evidence of weight loss by comparison with previous records. This general examination should be followed by examination of the abdomen for distension, visible peristalsis, tenderness or masses. Finally, a rectal examination should be conducted. In this age-group organic disease such as carcinoma of the large bowel should be suspected, and in most cases further examination will be desirable. This will usually be most quickly achieved by referral to a surgeon who will carry out sigmoidoscopy and a barium enema. The latter examination must not be regarded as any substitute for the former. They are complementary and, unless the general practitioner can undertake both, he should refer the patient.

In the very elderly, constipation may result from a general loss of muscle tone, leading to faecal impaction. In these cases the diagnosis of a full rectum by rectal examination should be followed by treatment with manual removal or enema. If normal bowel function then returns, no further investigation may be necessary.

Only rarely will other investigations be necessary in the diagnosis of the cause of constipation. A test for faecal occult blood may be helpful in confirming or eliminating an organic lesion, which may also be accompanied by a fall in haemoglobin value. In rare cases, a small-bowel barium meal may be necessary to identify regional ileo-colitis or rare causes of small-bowel obstruction. Very rarely, inflammatory disease of the small bowel or colon may present with constipation in the absence of other symptoms when an erythrocyte sedimentation rate, white blood count or positive tuberculin test may give the clue to the cause.

Management

Infants and children.- The parent of a constipated infant probably needs dietetic advice. In a baby fed with cow's milk or cow's milk substitute, the addition of extra sugar will often resolve the problem. If the child becomes constipated the insertion of vaseline on a finger into the anal canal will often prevent a painful struggle before the infant can open the bowels. In hot weather extra fluids in the form of fruit juice will often relieve the situation. In the rare cases in which Hirschsprung's disease or megacolon is suspected specialist advice is required.

In older children it is important to relate parental expectations of bowel action to the normal distribution of this activity. Constipation may be held responsible for a variety of symptoms to which it does not contribute, and unless the doctor is prepared to evaluate such symptoms rather than treat the child, the patient may be condemned to a lifetime of laxatives. As an occasional laxative in childhood Dioctyl paediatric syrup may be useful, or lactulose syrup 5 ml twice daily.

In young adults.- Management usually consists of appropriate dietetic advice. The lack of bulk in modern western diets has been held responsible for a variety of disorders, and there is evidence that coarse bran[3] both reduces transit time and reduces intra-luminal pressures in the colon. An apple (or orange) a day, carrots, brussels sprouts, wholemeal bread and bran may still be among the most effective methods of treating constipation and none of these substances requires a prescription. Patients with the irritable-bowel syndrome will be helped by any explanation of their problem and efforts to resolve tension in their lives. The symptoms may be relieved by the use of a bulking agent, e.g. Isogel, and when diarrhoea is a problem by the use of codeine phosphate. When pain is a prominent factor, mebeverine hydrochloride (Colofac) may be useful in reducing colonic spasm.

In the middle-aged or elderly. — Management must be directed to the cause of the disorder. In some cases this will consist of major surgery, in others the treatment of myxoedema or depression or the modification of analgesic therapy. There will, however, be many middle-aged and elderly patients whose bowels not only move at long intervals of time, but who experience painful and difficult defaecation as a result. Dietetic advice will often be helpful and the regular 'pint' at the local is not inappropriate in this context. When laxatives are necessary the first line of treatment should be the prescription of bulk laxatives. Methylcellulose may be prescribed as tablets, granules or liquid but is often rather unpalatable. Preparations containing isphagula husk, e.g. Fybogel taken as one sachet in water twice daily, are more acceptable. As an alternative an osmotic laxative, e.g. lactulose 15 ml twice daily may be valuable.

There are some special circumstances which demand the prescription of laxatives. In the treatment of haemorrhoids and following haemorrhoidectomy and in the treatment of fissure-in-ano faecal softeners are indicated and dioctyl tablets 100 mg or syrup may be used. In the management of terminal illness where morphine derivatives are being used, constipation may become a major problem and a stimulant laxative, e.g. sodium picosulphate, may be combined with an osmotic or bulk laxative.

In cases in which faecal impaction has occurred, relief may be provided by the use of suppositories, enema or in extreme cases, manual removal.

References

[1] Dunnell, K. and Cartwright, A. (1972): *Medicine Takers, Prescribers and Hoarders*. London: Routledge and Kegan Paul.

[2] Cornell, A.M., Hilton, C., Irwin, R., Lennard-Jones, J.E., and Misiewicz, J.J. (1965): *British Medical Journal*, *2*, 1095.

[3] Kirwan, T.O., Smith, A.N., McConnell, A.A., Mitchell, W.D., and Eastwood, M.A. (1974): *British Medical Journal*, *4*, 187.

3.48
Rectal bleeding and pain

J.S.K. Stevenson

Rectal bleeding is a common symptom that can occasionally herald life-threatening disease. The bleeding is often ignored by the patient or is erroneously self treated. Even when the patient does report the symptom, his doctor can be lulled into a sense of false security by assuming that the bleeding is due to piles. He may therefore begin treatment without adequate history taking and examination. This assumption, and the resultant delay, can be dangerous.

In a random sample of adults in the London Boroughs of Bermondsey and Southwark,[1] 2.4 per cent of those interviewed admitted to having passed blood with their stools within the previous 14 days: just over a third of them (37.5 per cent) had consulted their doctor about it, and 8.3 per cent had treated themselves – often inappropriately. If these figures were representative of all patients in the United Kingdom, then a general practitioner, with an average sized list of patients, could expect to have about 50 with some rectal bleeding during any two-week period: 31 of these patients would not consult their general practitioner (though five would treat themselves) and only 19 would seek their doctor's advice. In fact, studies of symptoms presented in general practice suggest than an even smaller proportion of patients actually consult their doctor about this symptom.

According to the Registrar General's statistics for England and Wales and for Scotland, 18,316 patients died as a result of carcinoma of the colon or rectum in 1983. The figures for 1973 and 1963 were 17,962 and 16,236, respectively. A majority of these patients would have had some degree of rectal bleeding as one of their earliest presenting symptoms.

As there is ample evidence that earlier diagnosis and treatment improve the prognosis, there is good reason for teaching patients about the importance of seeking early advice when they have rectal bleeding. As Aylett[2] points out, however, there is little point in this unless at the same time medical delay in diagnosis is eliminated. In two studies of patients suffering from cancer of the colon and rectum, one conducted in 1949 and the other in

1965, he examined two factors causing delay in diagnosing these conditions and starting appropriate treatment. The first he called 'patient delay' and the second 'medical delay'. He found that there had been no reduction in either category during the sixteen years between the two studies. In the 1965 group, medical delay averaging 10.3 months occurred in 22 per cent of patients with cancer of the rectum (a quarter at hospital level) and in the same proportion of patients with cancer of the colon, averaging 7.8 months (two-thirds at hospital level).

The general practitioner has therefore an important part to play in reducing the time that is allowed to elapse between the patient reporting his rectal bleeding and the discovery and treatment of its cause. He should seldom misdiagnose serious disease, provided he takes a careful history, makes a thorough examination, refers the patient for any necessary specialist investigation and always considers carcinoma of the colon or rectum to be the cause until proven otherwise. He must keep this diagnosis in mind even for patients under the age of 40, for, although bowel cancer is more common in both men and women over this age, it is not unknown in younger patients.

Presentation of the complaint

Bleeding from the rectum can occur at any age. It is usually painless and can vary in amount, from a slight staining of the underclothes, to haemorrhage requiring urgent treatment. It occurs almost equally in both sexes, with a slight preponderance in males. It is usually noticed when the patient is cleaning himself after defaecation.

Some patients appear to be reluctant to report rectal bleeding and may, in fact, not complain until symptoms of chronic blood loss appear. They may thus present with breathlessness, ankle oedema, loss of energy or even myocardial ischaemia, without mentioning rectal bleeding unless prompted to do so.

Causes of rectal bleeding

Rectal bleeding in young children is not uncommon, but is rarely serious. If accompanied by pain and constipation the cause is usually simple anal abrasions. If painless, the child may have a rectal prolapse or a small rectal polyp which tends to disappear quite spontaneously if left untreated. Special care should be taken to remember any child in the practice with a family history of polyposis coli and the child's records should be suitably flagged to jog the memory. Rectal bleeding may also accompany an infective diarrhoea, and the classical red currant jelly stool, associated with intussusception, should be remembered in any acutely ill child with symptoms of intestinal obstruction.

In adults, rectal bleeding is most often due to piles, or if accompanied by pain, to anal fissures, but the most serious cause is undoubtedly carcinoma of the large bowel, which must never be overlooked in the older patient, even when there is a history of piles or rectal polyp. Diverticular disease of the colon and proctitis are other common causes of bleeding in older age-groups, while ulcerative colitis, Crohn's disease and fistulae can give rise to rectal bleeding at an earlier age. Occasionally rectal bleeding can be due to drugs, for example anticoagulants, and rapid bleeding from a duodenal or gastric ulcer can sometimes cause frank rectal blood loss.

Tropical causes of rectal bleeding should always be remembered by those doctors looking after immigrant patients. Amoebiasis is fairly common while schistosomiasis and hookworm, although less common, should also be considered.

History taking

Many patients find it difficult to describe rectal or anal symptoms and care must be taken by the doctor when interpreting what the patient says. In any patient presenting with rectal bleeding, however, the importance of taking an adequate history cannot be over-emphasized. Even in the busiest consulting session this should not be overlooked. All the relevant details can be obtained in a matter of minutes. If each area of questioning is remembered, the doctor should have a good idea of his likely subsequent management before he even examines the patient.

For example, if the doctor elicits a history of the blood being dark, mixed with faeces and associated with the passage of mucus, he will probably have already decided to refer the patient for specialist examination, whether or not his own subsequent examination is negative. On the other hand, if the patient complains of passing fresh red blood, the doctor should be particularly thorough with his digital examination of the rectum.

The questions to be put to the patient may therefore be listed as follows:

1. *What colour is the blood?* Bright red bleeding indicates that the source is low in the rectum and is most commonly piles,

when it frequently spatters the sides of the lavatory pan. It could, however, be due to a rectal carcinoma or, if accompanied by pain, to an anal fissure. Less commonly, fresh bleeding may be due to a rectal polyp or to proctitis. If the blood is dark in colour it probably comes from above the pile-bearing areas and signifies a possible lesion of the colon, or pelvi-rectal junction, which must be excluded by specialist investigation.

2. *Is the blood mixed with the stool or sticking to it?* Such blood is unlikely to have come from piles or an anal fissure and necessitates full investigation.

3. *Are there any clots associated with the bleeding?* Clotted blood passed rectally indicates the presence of a serious lesion of the rectum or colon and warrants full investigation. The only simple lesion of the area associated with bleeding and clotted blood is a peri-anal haematoma which is always of sudden onset, painful and easily recognizable at the anal margin.

4. *Is there any mucus or slime passed with the stool or mixed with the blood?* The passage of mucus per rectum often indicates a serious lesion. If passed alone, it may be missed by the patient, or not mentioned by him: a fact which prompted a prominent Scottish surgeon to remark: ‘I wish mucus were tartan’.

5. *Is there any alteration in normal bowel habit?* Even slight changes may be significant. More dramatic upset in bowel habit, such as alternating constipation and diarrhoea, usually indicates more advanced disease with incipient intestinal obstruction. If diarrhoea, rather than bleeding, is the major symptom, the diagnosis is most likely to be ulcerative colitis or Crohn’s disease. On the other hand, patients with anal fissure have extreme pain and may develop constipation simply because defaecation is so uncomfortable. Some patients may deny constipation but admit to an increasing use of aperients. The patient should also be questioned about any abdominal discomfort or colic, a feeling of incomplete rectal emptying after defaecation, or the passing of pencil-like stools. All of these may indicate serious causes, if accompanied by rectal bleeding.

6. The final questions should be related to the patient’s feeling of well-being. The doctor should be thinking of such things as tiredness, anorexia, loss of weight, dyspnoea, ankle oedema, or myocardial ischaemia. Positive answers to any of these questions may give him some clue as to the amount of blood loss or its cause. If, for instance, the patient feels relatively well, is putting on weight, and has a good appetite, it is most likely that his rectal bleeding will be due to piles or to some form of diverticular disease, although confirmation of this latter condition must be

sought. It is also worth while asking the patient if he had travelled abroad recently.

Examination

The general practitioner is often in the fortunate position of having known the patient over a period of years and is therefore more likely to notice changes in the patient's appearance or demeanour than is a doctor who is not responsible for providing continuing care. If the patient complains of symptoms such as breathlessness, ankle oedema, or tightness in the chest, which could be caused by anaemia, secondary to rectal blood loss, then appropriate differential diagnosis of such symptoms must be considered when examining the patient. For the purpose of this chapter, however, only the examination of patients presenting solely with rectal bleeding will be considered.

The patient should first of all lie flat on the bed or couch and the abdomen should be inspected for any signs of distension. If this is present, intestinal obstruction should be suspected. Should this be the case subsequent percussion is likely to be hyper-resonant, especially over the caecum but, since obstruction is a late sign of chronic intestinal disease, more often than not inspection of the abdomen will be negative. It should then be gently palpated in all areas for signs of tenderness or the presence of an intra-abdominal mass.

In most patients these signs will be negative. The patient should then be asked to lie over on his side with his buttocks at the edge of the couch and with the knees drawn up as high as possible. The anal margin should be inspected for any peri-anal haematoma (thrombosed external piles), the sentinel pile associated with anal fissure, or peri-anal warts. The patient should then be asked to strain down, while the doctor looks for any prolapse of piles, polyp or rectal mucosa. This is followed by a careful digital examination with the gloved index finger in the rectum and with the other hand pressing gently on the lower abdomen. If a cancer is present in the rectum it should be easily felt as either a firm mass or as an ulcer (it is reckoned that over 95 per cent of rectal cancers are palpable on digital rectal examination). After the examination, any blood on the glove or finger cot should be noted. If apparently normal coloured faeces are present, the sample on the glove or finger cot should always be tested for occult blood. A negative test, in the absence of any other positive finding, can be reassuring. If the digital examination is difficult, or even impossible because of discomfort, an anal fissure is the most likely cause.

With the patient still in the lateral position, a lubricated proctoscope should be passed to the limit of its length and then slowly withdrawn as the patient strains and the observer looks down the instrument. In this way sources of bleeding can be visualized; for example, piles which protrude and balloon into the instrument, simple proctitis, rectal polyp or low rectal carcinoma.

The patient should then have his wieght taken and compared with any previous recording. Blood should next be taken and examined for evidence of hypochromic iron-deficiency anaemia and an erythrocyte sedimentation rate (E.S.R.) determined. A high E.S.R. can be a useful pointer to the presence of serious disease, but a normal, or marginally raised sedimentation rate, should not be taken as excluding it.

Having thus completed his part of the examination, the general practitioner may, or may not, have made a diagnosis, but he should have confirmed or excluded a rectal or anal cause of his patient's bleeding. Sigmoidoscopy and barium enema may still require to be done to exclude higher lesions beyond the reach of either the examining finger or the proctoscope. It is strongly recommended that the patient be referred to a specialist for these further investigations. Although many general practitioners have open access to contrast-media radiology, few have the necessary skill and experience to use a sigmoidoscope effectively. Most surgeons perform a sigmoidoscopy before asking for a barium enema, and it is helpful for the findings of the sigmoidoscopic examination to be made available to the radiologist who is asked to perform the barium enema examination.

Management

In patients under the age of 40, it is reasonable for the general practitioner to treat simple causes of rectal bleeding, such as piles or anal fissure, without referring the patients for specialist opinion. In older age-groups, however, if there is any doubt at all about the findings, it is wise to arrange for sigmoidoscopy and a barium enema. When the general practitioner takes the responsibility for treating rectal bleeding himself, he must ensure that his treatment has been effective. Patients should therefore always be urged to report if the symptom remains or recurs.

Simple piles may be treated with bismuth subgallate compound suppositories, B.P.C. and if, accompanied by pruritus ani, the peri-anal region can be sparingly lubricated with 1 per cent hydrocortisone acetate ointment, B.P. before the suppository is inserted. Most proprietary brands of suppositories contain some form of local anaesthetic and should therefore be avoided as this may cause sensitivity to the skin around the anal margin. Injections of 3 to 5 ml of oily phenol injection, B.P.C. to the base of each of the three pile sites, may be safely undertaken by the general practitioner who has been instructed in this technique. Patients with prolapsing bleeding piles should be referred for haemorrhoidectomy.

Small anal fissures may be successfully treated with simple applications of lignocaine gel or ointment and by making sure the stools remain soft. Those resistant to such simple measures should be referred for more radical treatment. The pain associated with anal fissures often prevents adequate initial examination. This should always be carried out once the pain subsides.

The pain and misery of a peri-anal haematoma may be easily and simply relieved by incision and evacuation. The patient's grateful thanks is more than ample reward for the little time that the procedure takes. Infiltration of the skin surface, overlying the haematoma, with 1 or 2 per cent lignocaine, followed by a small incision, usually allows the clot to be expelled easily with immediate relief of discomfort. If the overlying skin is thin and tense a local anaesthetic may not be needed. Simple hygienic measures, with soap and water, and dressing pads, to protect the underclothes from any subsequent bleeding are all that is required.

The management of patients with rectal bleeding associated with ulcerative colitis, Crohn's disease, diverticular disease, intussusception, peptic ulceration and tropical diseases is beyond the scope of this chapter. For the management and treatment of these conditions, reference should be made to standard textbooks of medical and surgical treatment.

There is one further aspect of the management of the patient presenting with rectal bleeding that deserves mention. A small number of patients will inevitably be found to have cancer of the colon or rectum requiring surgical treatment. Such patients may well be left with a permanent colostomy. If this is thought to be a possibility, the general practitioner should set aside the time to explain to the patient what this means, before he undergoes surgery. Ideally, such explanations should be given jointly, in association with the surgeon responsible for the operation, but, whatever happens, care must be taken to avoid the situation of the patient awakening after the operation and finding that he has a colostomy that no-one had warned him about. It is therefore good practice to ensure that the patient returns to the general practitioner after the initial consultation with the surgeon so that the findings may be discussed.

Conclusion

Much is known about the causes of rectal bleeding, yet despite the many advances in medical science and technology over the past forty years, there has been little or no improvement in prognosis for those whose rectal bleeding stems from serious organic disease. Programmes of health education aimed at encouraging patients to report this symptom whenever it occurs, will only improve the situation if, at the same time, this is matched with a greater awareness among doctors that life-threatening causes of rectal bleeding must always be excluded by diligent history taking, examination and appropriate investigations.

References

[1] Wadsworth, M.E.J., Butterfield, W.J.H. and Blaney, R. (1971): *Health and Sickness: the Choice of Treatment.* London: Tavistock Publications

[2] Aylett, S.O. (1968): Rectal Bleeding with Special Reference to Cancer of the Large Intestine. *British Medical Journal, 3,* 103–106

3.49 Jaundice

Mairi G.B. Scott

Presentation

Jaundice is rarely presented to the general practitioner. In a population of 1,000 persons, the annual episode rate for infective hepatitis is 0.5, and for (unspecified) jaundice is 1.0. Most of the causes of jaundice can be identified within general practice, and treated without referral to hospital.

The presentation is variable. Either the patient or someone close to him may have noticed a change in appearance. The skin or sclera may appear yellow; the urine may have become dark or the bowel motions pale and putty-like. Sometimes it is the doctor himself who first notices the change in appearance. The changes may be looked for when the patient presents with a history of vague malaise or nausea or anorexia or when there are other symptoms suggestive of liver or gall-bladder disease, or the possibility of hepatic metasteses. Most often the cause of the jaundice will be suggested by the history.

Causes and history

The causes of jaundice can be divided into three main groups: haemolytic, hepato-cellular and obstructive; these are summarized in Table I. The initial questioning is directed to determine the mode of onset, the duration and the presence of any other symptoms.

The commonest cause of jaundice is viral hepatitis and this may occur within a few days of a flu-like illness. A history of anorexia, a distaste for smoking, and pale stools or dark urine are all suggestive. If the jaundice has developed painlessly and slowly it may be due to a malignant process. If the onset has been sudden with associated pain, gall-stones are the most likely cause.

The depth of jaundice may be helpful in making the diagnosis. It is usually mild in haemolytic disease, more pronounced in viral hepatitis, and most pronounced with gall-stones. It can also be severe in carcinoma of the head of pancreas where, because the

A	*Hepato-cellular jaundice*		
1.	Acute hepatitis	Viruses	(a) Infectious (epidemic) hepatitis (IHA)
			(b) Serum hepatitis (IHB, Australia antigen)
			(c) Infectious mononucleosis
			(d) Cytomegalovirus
		Bacteria	(a) Leptospirosis, syphilis
			(b) Septicaemia
		Toxins	(a) Alcohol
			(b) Drugs
			(c) Poisons
2.	Chronic hepatitis		(a) Chronic aggressive (active, progressive) hepatitis
			(b) Alcohol, drug-induced hepatitis
			(c) Portal cirrhosis
3.	Congestive heart failure and pulmonary infarcts		
B.	*Obstructive jaundice*		
1.	Intrahepatic		(a) Drugs: phenothiazines, oral contraceptives
			(b) Malignancy: metastatic carcinoma, lymphoma
			(c) Primary biliary cirrhosis
2.	Extrahepatic		(a) Gall-stones
			(b) Carcinoma, metastatic, or primary in pancreas
C.	*Haemolytic anaemia with jaundice*		
1.	Congenital		(a) Hereditary spherocytosis
			(b) Haemoglobinopathy
2.	Infection		(a) *Mycoplasma pneumonia*
			(b) Malaria
3.	Drugs, poisons		
4.	Auto-immune disease		Systemic lupus erythematosus

Table I. Classification of jaundice

(after Manners, B.T.B. in *Practice*, Instalment 4)

liver may be preserved, it may be accompanied by few or no associated symptoms.

A history of pain is important. It is rare in haemolytic disease, but can also be absent even when the cause is gall-stones. In most cases of gall-stone obstruction, there is severe pain (not colicky, despite the misnomer 'biliary colic') and the pain can be associated with fever and rigors. Carcinoma of the head of pancreas is initially painless, but where pain develops it is constant and can be very severe.

Itching is unusual in haemolytic, may be present in hepato-cellular, and is common in obstructive jaundice. The relationship between symptoms and causes are summarized in Table II.

1. *Pain in the right upper abdomen*
   If colicky consider gall-stones
   Constant pain may be found in infective hepatitis, but also occurs with gallstones

2. *History of anorexia, dark urine, fever, rigors*
   Viral Hepatitis
   Alcoholic liver disease
   Cholecystitis

3. *Raised temperature*
   Gall-Stones (if pain is present)
   Viral hepatitis

4. *Nausea and vomiting (especially in the morning)*
   Alcoholic liver disease

5. *Weight loss*
   Malignancy
   Malabsorption with cholestasis

6. *Pruritus*
   Cholestasis

Table II. Symptoms and commoner causes

In addition to taking a careful history of the development of events associated with the jaundice, the past history including medication, the family history, smoking and alcohol habits, and an occupational history can all provide important clues. A past or family history of gall-bladder disease may be present. Spherocytosis is familial, and the patient may well be more aware of the possible diagnosis than the doctor. It is unlikely that the patient with already known alcohol-related hepatic cirrhosis will present for the first time with jaundice. But with a new patient who presents with jaundice and dyspepsia, particularly if there are associated stigmata of social neglect, a careful history of alcohol consumption may provide the vital clue.

1.	*Dose – dependent hepatotoxicity*	
	Paracetamol	
	Salicylates	
	Tetracycline	
	Antineoplastic and immuno-suppressive agents	
2.	*Dose – independent hepatotoxicity*	
	Antidepressants and tranquillizers	MAOI Tricyclics Benzodiazepines
	Antimicrobials	Antituberculous Sulphonamides Erythromycin
	Anticonvulsants	
	Anti-inflammatory drugs	Indomethacin Penicillamine Gold
	Anaesthetics	
	Antithyroid drugs	
	Cardiovascular drugs	Methyldopa Hydralazine
	Hypoglycaemic drugs	Chlorpropamide Glibenclamide

Table III. Medication and hepatotoxicity

A number of commonly prescribed drugs may be associated with hepatic damage, and these are summarized in Table III.
The increasing incidence of drug abuse by injection can cause a rapid spread of serum hepatitis, which can also spread through sexual contact. Recent foreign travel in areas where serum hepatitis is endemic may also provide an important clue to the cause.
Jaundice in the new born is commonly physiological, and may be more pronounced in premature babies. The jaundice fades in the first two or three weeks. This can be alarming to the mother and careful explanation and reassurance are important.

Examination

Pallor may occur with mild jaundice and, with spenomegaly, may be indicative of haemolytic anaemia. In cholestatic jaundice there may be scratch marks and pigmentation. In hepato-cellular jaundice the patient may have ascites, oedema, palmar erythema, spider naevae and a flapping tremor. The forearms should be inspected for signs of needle injections.

The abdomen should be examined to determine the presence of a palpable or percussable liver edge. A small liver indicates severe hepatitis or end-stage cirrhosis. An enlarged, smooth, tender liver suggests hepatitis. An enlarged, irregular liver suggests metastases. The gall-bladder should be palpated to determine tenderness as in cholelithiasis, or enlargement, which would suggest pancreatic cancer.

If malignancy is suspected the patient should be examined for lymphadenopathy; the breasts in women should be examined and the chest examined fully, and a chest X-ray should be arranged. A rectal examination will be important, to search for rectal or prostatic tumours.

In young patients the possibility of infectious mononucleosis should be borne in mind, particularly if the history suggests this. The findings of typical changes in the throat and associated lymphadenopathy will also be helpful.

Investigations

In almost all cases of jaundice it is advisable to exclude serum hepatitis before any other laboratory tests are undertaken. A full blood count should be performed to exclude anaemia. A high MCV may indicate alcohol abuse and target cells can be seen on the film. The haematologist is often able to suggest the presence of liver disease. Liver function tests are poor indicators of liver function as they are affected by many factors within and outwith the liver. However, they may give guidance to the cause of the jaundice.

Bilirubin: (0–25 umol/1) levels over 200 indicate obstruction and in hepatitis they can be very high early in the disease.

Aspartate Aminotransferase or AST: (5–40 IU) this is a very helpful indicator of hepato-cellular damage. In the early stages of acute viral or drug-induced hepatitis the AST can reach levels as high as 1000IU/1 and will fall very rapidly. It is important to remember that elevation may also be seen in heart failure or myocardial infarction with hepatic congestion.

Alanine Aminotransferase or ALT: (5–40 IU) this enzyme is specific to the liver and it will be elevated in line with AST. Some hospitals, however, do not routinely measure this enzyme.

Alkaline Phosphatase: (30–110 IU/1) high levels will be found in obstructive jaundice. Elevation is also seen in bone growth, Paget's disease and pregnancy. Isoenzyme studies can be carried out to determine whether this finding relates to liver disease.

Gamma Glutamyl Transferase: (men 0–65 IU/1 women 0–40 IU/1)

this enzyme is more specific for hepato-cellular damage and is very sensitive to alcohol abuse.
Serum Albumin: (35–50g/1) this is synthesized in the liver. After liver damage has become established this will begin to fall. There is an associated rise in globulin.
Prothrombin Time: (10–14 Seconds) this will be increased in liver disease.
Radiology: a straight X-ray of the abdomen may be helpful in supporting a diagnosis of gall-stones (10 per cent of these stones are radio-opaque), but unhelpful in excluding it. An abdominal ultrasound is more useful, and some general practitioners now have access to this investigation.

Management

The management is dependent on the nature of the diagnosis and the degree of confidence which the doctor has in it.
Almost all patients with hepatitis A or B have a self-limiting illness from which they recover spontaneously. It is important to protect contacts of the patients and careful explanation of the mode of transmission should be given. Immunoglobulin should be given as soon as possible to close contacts.
Patients with hepatitis A are non-infectious after the appearance of jaundice but contact with faeces should be regarded as hazardous for up to ten days after the jaundice appears. Bed-rest is not needed and the diet need not be restricted. The patient will usually show signs of improvement within 2–3 weeks, but should be feeling well and have normal liver function tests before being advised to return to work. Alcohol should be avoided for three months. Relapses, which are usually mild and need little action, occur in 5–10 per cent of patients.
Drug-induced and alcohol-related liver damage is best treated by withdrawing, or attempting to withdraw, the causal agent.
If obstructive jaundice is present the patient should almost always be referred to hospital and, where the patient is very unwell or the onset has been very rapid, this referral is urgent.
Specific symptoms may require symptomatic treatment — for example, pruritus can be treated with cholestyramine. However, the doctor should bear in mind that many drugs useful in the symptomatic treatment of pain, anxiety and nausea are themselves hepatotoxic.
Finally, particular care must be taken when a patient on long-term medication with drugs which are hepatotoxic, or which are excreted by the liver, develops jaundice. The dose of such drugs as anticoagulants, digoxin, diuretics, some antibiotics and anticonvulsants will need to be adjusted, and the help of a clinical pharmacologist may be indicated.

3.50
Lumps in the groin

F.M.Hull

This symptom, though common in surgical outpatients, has a very different incidence in general practice. The Third National Morbidity Survey[1] gives a figure of 6.0 episodes per thousand for males, 1.0 for females and 3.3 for the total population for hernias alone. Morrell and his colleagues[2] make no specific mention of groin lumps, simply listing them under other swellings and Dunnell and Cartwright[3] include them with other symptoms. In a survey of 5,936 presenting symptoms in six different practices Hull[4] included two cases presenting as hernia and six hernias among 141 patients presenting with unspecified lumps, giving a rate of 0.13 per thousand. In addition to these, there may have been a few other patients presenting with groin lumps other than hernia which cannot be extracted from those data; these are likely to be no more than the hernias and probably less. In our practice, where three doctors look after 7,500 patients, 7,757 new diagnoses were recorded in the diagnostic index in one year. There were 3,334 diagnoses for men which included nine hernias and 4,423 diagnoses for females including one hernia. These figures give rates of 2.7 per thousand for males, 0.2 per thousand for females and 1.2 per thousand for the total population.

Thus hernia, which is probably the commonest of the many causes of a lump in the groin, is a rare presenting symptom in general practice.

Presentation

Hernia is predominantly found in the male, in whom it is a condition of middle age. When it does occur in women it often affects the extremes of life. Because of an association with physical work it is somewhat commoner in the Registrar General's lower social classes.

With the exception of malignancy most of these conditions respond to treatment. Prognosis in the lymphomas has improved recently and here early diagnosis may allow several years of active life.

Cause	*Groups of patients likely to present*
Maldescent of testis Congenital abnormalities of spermatic cord Congenital inguinal hernias	Infants and pre-school boys
Local furunculosis Local lymphadenopathy Generalized lymphadenopathy	Younger age-groups
Trauma due to sports or other injury	Teenagers and young adults
Inguinal hernia	Middle-aged men
Femoral hernia	Older women
Vascular abnormalities Saphena varix Femoral aneurysm	Old people
Benign tumours of skin or deeper tissue, e.g. papilloma, lipoma, neurofibroma	Any age or sex
Serious causes	
Psoas abscess	Young adults
Obstructed hernias	The very young and the old
Neoplasms: Primary Sarcoma Lymphoma	Young adults
Secondary Melanoma Carcinoma	Middle-aged and over

Table I. – Common causes of lumps in the groin

Causes

Common conditions

In *maldescent of the testis* the appropriate side of the scrotum is empty, the lump is firm (though not so firm as a normal testis) localized and slightly tender; it is often peculiarly elusive and may be felt at any site below the inguinal canal.

Cysts of the cord may be difficult to distinguish from hernias but will sometimes transilluminate.

In young children *congenital hernia* must be borne in mind since this is often not observed by mother and may present as a screaming baby not as a groin lump.

Infective lesions are common, especially in children and young adults. *Local furunculosis* is obvious but the portal of entry in *infected glands* may not be. Here the cause may be secondary infection in pre-existing skin disease; for example, tinea pedis. Single inflamed glands may be present in *cat-scratch fever* (less of a novelty than might be supposed) or glands may be enlarged as part of a *general viral* or even *spirochaetal infection.*

Local trauma is usually suggested by the history but in sexual assault or *non-accidental* injury of children this may be withheld. In such cases local bruising may be present and the behaviour of the patient or his parents may provide clues.

Probably the commonest groin lump is a *hernia* most often seen in middle-aged men and usually inguinal. In women femoral hernia is commoner but distinction between these hernias is often difficult, particularly in the obese, and may not be made until operation.

Vascular abnormalities arise in older age-groups. *Femoral aneurysms* pulsate but a *saphena varix* may provide a difficult differential diagnosis from hernia since both fill from above, may be easily reducible and have a cough impulse.

Benign tumours may require histological examination for diagnosis.

Serious and treatable conditions

Psoas abscess, now mercifully rare, may cause diagnostic difficulty unless the lumbar spine is examined where tenderness or the typical angular kyphosis of Pott's disease may be present.

Very important is the diagnosis of *obstruction* of a hernia associated with pain, irreducibility, and tenderness. If there is vomiting, abdominal distension and constipation urgent admission to hospital is demanded.

Neoplasms can give rise to difficulty, particularly early in their natural history. Although a *sarcoma* arising from the femur carries so severe a prognosis that by the time it presents it is often inoperable, any fusiform bony mass demands urgent investigation.

Lymphomas, on the other hand, may be more treatable and early diagnosis is important. *Melanomatosis* should be considered; this may be secondary to a lesion in the leg and by the time glands are involved carries a grave prognosis. *Secondary carcinoma* may occur from any primary site, of which the penis is perhaps the commonest.

History

Although history taking is traditionally taught as preceding examination, in certain cases the experienced practitioner takes much of his history during the course of physical examination. This is often so with groin lumps, where, especially with common groin lumps, examination often provides the diagnosis immediately. Only in more obscure causes is a detailed history essential. Before examination the doctor needs to know the occupation of the patient, the duration of the symptom and any history of trauma. An assessment should be made as to the patient's general health and if he is in pain. With this information one can rearrange the list of differential diagnoses on a probablistic basis and further history taking may become necessary during the course of examination.

Examination

Examination is usually simple. The patient should be stripped from the waist down and examined standing and lying. Inspection is often more rewarding than palpation. The patient's general condition is noted; most will appear well but obvious illness will suggest more serious causes of the lump. The legs should be examined for vascular, traumatic or inflammatory changes. The lump may or may not be visible; if it is, its anatomical position should be considered especially in relation to the inguinal ligament and the genitals. Visible physical signs such as induration, discoloration, oedema or pulsation may provide clues.

In palpating the lump one should elicit tenderness, temperature change and consistency. Is the mass pulsating and if so is this direct or transmitted pulsation? The lump may have a cough impulse. It may be possible to feel the lump in the inguinal canal by invaginating the scrotum. Lymph glands are usually discrete and multiple. Tenderness over the inguinal canal may indicate that muscular strain has occurred which may later result in a hernia.

Finally, more general examination may be needed. The appropriate limb should be searched for a portal of entry of infection;

this is often found in the interdigital clefts. Similarly the genitals should be searched for scrotal or labial infection (including pediculi) since this may give rise to lymphadenopathy. Testicular abnormality, which may cause para-aortic lymphadenopathy, will not affect groin glands. Examination of the abdomen including the rectum is important when there is suggestion of intestinal obstruction due to strangulation of a hernia or when there may be intra-abdominal malignancy or the splenomegaly associated with lymphoma. Cardiovascular examination may be necessary to exclude general arterial disease if there is a femoral aneurysm. Chest examination may reveal a bronchogenic carcinoma as the primary cause of generalized secondary lymphadenopathy. The finding of a neurofibroma will indicate a neurological examination.

Investigation

Once the primary diagnosis is made few lumps in the groin need investigation. Infections may require bacteriological investigation, and generalized lymphadenopathy requires haematological investigation with possibly the inclusion of the Paul Bunnell reaction to distinguish between the infective and lymphomatous causes. In all but a few the diagnosis of groin lumps depends on clinical observation.

Management

Maldescent of the testes may respond to gonadotrophin injections but usually requires surgical correction. If bilateral, failure of descent may give rise to sterility; the often quoted increased risk of malignancy is now disputed but there is a greater danger of trauma or torsion.

Hernia is best treated surgically, and when obstructed this is imperative. With a simple hernia in the old and debilitated where surgery is contraindicated or where long delay before operation is anticipated a truss may be helpful.

Bacterial infection often requires antibiotics. When there is general lymphadenopathy from mononucleosis or *viraemia* antibiotics should be avoided.

Vascular abnormalities are often best ignored unless giving rise to peripheral symptoms. *Femoral aneurysm* is usually part of general

vascular degeneration and rarely large enough to be dangerous.
Local benign tumours may be removed for cosmetic reasons or the certainty of histological diagnosis.
Psoas abscess requires supervision by an orthopaedic surgeon and will require general anti-tuberculous therapy.

The management of lymphoma should be undertaken only by those specialized in the field. The down-hill course of generalized malignant disease requires the full medical, social and psychological support of terminal care.

References

[1] Royal College of General Practitioners, Office of Population Censuses and Surveys, Department of Health and Social Security (1986): *Morbidity Statistics from General Practice 1981–82*. HMSO Series MB5 No. 1

[2] Morrell, D.C., Gage, H.G., and Robinson, N.A. (1971): Symptoms in General Practice. *Journal of Royal College of General Practitioners*, *21* 32

[3] Dunnell, K., and Cartwright, A. (1972): *Medicine Takers, Prescribers and Hoarders.* London: Routledge and Kegan Paul

[4] Hull, F.M. (1972): Diagnostic Pathways in General Practice. *Journal of Royal College of General Practitioners*, *22*, 241

3.51
The patient complaining of difficulty in passing urine

David Morrell

The patient experiencing a disturbance of micturition may present to the doctor with such symptoms as pain on passing urine, frequency of micturition, difficulty or inability to start micturition, terminal dribbling, incontinence on coughing or laughing, or the passage of blood in the urine. In children and the elderly, but rarely in the intervening years, the patient may complain of incontinence of urine unassociated with stress.

The annual incidence of new symptoms suggestive of a disturbance of micturition in general practice is about 20 per thousand patients at risk.[1] These symptoms are three times as common in women as in men. Of the symptoms mentioned the combination of frequency and dysuria is by far the most common with an incidence of about 14 per thousand patients, and a female preponderance of five to one. With the exception of enuresis, disturbances of micturition are uncommon in children. Frequency and dysuria are most common in women aged 15 to 44 years and are encountered four times as often in sexually active women. The symptoms of difficulty in initiating micturition along with increase in frequency with advancing years are most common in men. The symptom of incontinence of urine in response to stress occurs most often in postmenopausal women.

Presentation

The most common presenting symptoms of patients suffering from a disturbance of micturition are burning or scalding pain on passing urine, or increased frequency of micturition. In young adults, usually women, the symptoms are often combined and of sudden onset, and may be accompanied by systemic upset and occasionally loin or abdominal pain. Sometimes haematuria may be reported in addition. In the elderly, usually men, these symptoms and in particular frequency of micturition may have been present for a long time, and only brought to the doctor when they become a social inconvenience or disturb sleep. Problems associated with stress incontinence of urine are often tolerated for years before they are presented to the doctor, and in many cases only come to light when the doctor initiates an enquiry in response to his own olfactory senses. The sudden onset of retention of urine usually presents in men as an acute abdominal emergency in which pain is the presenting symptom. Haematuria with or without other symptoms usually seriously alarms the patient, and is presented as an emergency.

Causes

Children. — Most children have good bladder control by day and night by the age of 3 to 4 years, although the proportion of children who are still wet at night by the age of 5 years is as high as 10 per cent. Rarely delay in bladder control may be due to some organic lesion such as spina bifida or congenital polycystic kidneys or hydronephrosis. Most commonly delay is simply due to slow maturation which is sometimes hereditary. Occasionally, secondary enuresis may occur as a result of urinary infection; more often as a result of an emotional upset. Unfortunately, urinary infections frequently occur in children without presenting symptoms suggestive of urinary-tract disease. Vague attacks of abdominal pain or pyrexia may indicate a urinary infection. It is extremely important to identify these infections as this is the stage at which the kidneys are growing and are particularly vulnerable to infection, and the general practitioner must constantly bear this in mind.

Young adults. — In men symptoms of a disorder of micturition often indicate either gonorrhoea or non-specific urethritis. They may rarely be due to a non-venereal urinary infection and occasionally are the presenting symptoms of a sexual problem.

In women these symptoms are extremely common. Their rarity in women in the absence of sexual activity clearly indicates the relevance of sexual intercourse to these symptoms. It seems probable that potential pathogens are present on the female perineum, and that sexual intercourse is sufficient to massage them into the bladder. There remain, however, a large number of women experiencing disturbances of micturition in whom there is no bacteriological evidence of a urinary infection. This is often referred to as the urethral syndrome.[2] It may in some cases be due to a virus infection of the urethra, and in others to urethral trauma resulting from sexual intercourse, or hypersensitivity to deodorants or bubble baths. In a significant minority of patients who present to the general practitioner with symptoms suggesting a disorder of micturition the main problem is a psycho-sexual one such as dyspareunia or failure to experience orgasm. The general practitioner should be aware of this possibility.

Post-menopausal women. — The most common cause of a disturbance of micturition in this group is uterovaginal prolapse leading to urinary incontinence. Other less common causes are urethral caruncle which may produce pain on micturition, and dyspareunia and atrophic vaginitis which again may cause both dyspareunia and urinary symptoms. Haematuria in this age-group may be caused by tumours in the kidney or bladder.

Elderly men. — The most common cause of disturbance of micturition in elderly men is prostatic hypertrophy. This may present as frequency of micturition, dribbling incontinence or in rare instances acute retention of urine. Symptoms due to obstruction of the urinary tract caused by prostatic hypertrophy may be brought to the patient's and doctor's attention by a superadded infection, always likely to occur when the patient has a significant amount of residual urine.

Haematuria. — Haematuria is always an alarming symptom to the patient. The commonest cause in general practice is probably a simple urinary infection, when it may be accompanied by dysuria and frequency. In the absence of this it should lead to full investigation by a urologist. In patients presenting with painless haematuria there are many advantages in referring them immediately for cystoscopy in the hope that the source of the bleeding may be identified at once. So often haematuria is intermittent and if the patient waits a few days for an appointment it may have ceased and the opportunity to identify the source may be lost. Causes include papilloma of the bladder, ruptured prostatic veins and tumours of the kidney. These are all in the province of the urological specialist. Haematuria in the presence of unilateral abdominal or loin pain suggests a ureteric calculus.

History and examination

The history-taking and examination of patients presenting with disturbances of micturition vary with the age and sex of the patients complaining of these symptoms. In this it is a classical example of the way the general practitioner's approach to his patient is influenced by the diagnostic probabilities learned from epidemiological studies (Chapter 1.3).

Children. — In the child presenting with enuresis the doctor will be concerned to establish whether the patient has been enuretic from birth or whether this has developed following a period of bladder control. He will enquire about the age at which bladder control was established in the parents. In cases of secondary enuresis he will take a detailed history of the family circumstances: the arrival of a new baby or marital conflict may lead to regression in a child's bladder control. The sudden onset of wetting by day and/or night may be the only indication of a urinary infection, and the examination and investigations will be designed to exclude this possibility.

Young adult. — In the young adult disturbances of micturition are uncommon in the male. They suggest a venereal infection, either gonorrhoea or non-specific urethritis. The history-taking and examination will therefore focus on venereal contact and the presence or absence of a urethral discharge.

Disturbances of micturition are common in women in the reproductive years, and particularly in those having sexual intercourse. Less than half the patients complaining of dysuria or frequency of micturition have a bacteriologically proven infection. The anatomical position of the female urethra in relation to the vagina not only exposes it to trauma during sexual intercourse, but also by virtue of its short length predisposes it to the passage of pathogenic bacteria into the bladder. Disturbances of micturition in a sexually active woman may therefore indicate bacterial infection or trauma to the urethra, or both. History-taking must explore the relationship between symptoms and sexual intercourse and will particularly enquire about any difficulties in sexual intercourse. These symptoms not uncommonly indicate a physical or psycho-sexual problem which can only be exposed by tactful history-taking. For this reason the examination of the abdomen for renal enlargement should be followed by a vaginal examination (Chapter 3.59).

Bacteriological examination of the urine has been greatly facilitated by the development of the dip inoculum technique. To carry this out the patient is asked to pass a mid-stream specimen of urine into a clean container; a slide made of culture media is then dipped into the specimen of urine. Any excess urine is shaken from the dip slide and this is then sealed in a container and can be transmitted, if necessary by post, to the laboratory. This avoids the problem of bacterial multiplication in specimens of urine during the time taken to transmit them from the general practitioner's surgery to the bacteriology laboratory. Patients with recurrent bacteriologically proven urinary infections should be investigated by intravenous pyelogram to exclude any major abnormality in the urinary tract. Micturating cysto-urethrography should be carried out in those in whom the excretion urogram demonstrates renal scars or a dilated ureter.

Women who develop pyelonephritis during pregnancy should always be followed up by careful investigation in the postnatal period. Excretion urography carried out after the pyelographic changes of pregnancy have settled (six months must be allowed for this) shows that between 20 and 50 per cent of them have radiological abnormalities. Persistent or recurrent bacteriuria is found in about 25 per cent.[3]

Post-menopausal women. — Disturbances of micturition are rarely complained of in post-menopausal women and yet a large number of women in this age-group are troubled by stress incontinence. Not uncommonly, the doctor will become aware of this from the smell of stale urine noted when examining a patient in this age-group for other complaints. Women are extremely tolerant of urinary incontinence and a specific enquiry about this symptom should always be made at the post-natal examination. It should also be raised specifically in post-menopausal women suffering from chronic respiratory disease and chronic cough. A vaginal examination should be carried out in patients complaining of this symptom, and will often reveal vaginal prolapse amenable to surgical intervention.

Elderly men. — Disturbances of micturition are common in men over the age of 60 years. These are nearly always due to prostatic enlargement which may be complicated by infection of residual urine. History-taking should include enquiry about the frequency of micturition by day and by night, difficulty in initiating the act of micturition, dribbling incontinence following the act, and the quality of the stream produced on micturition. Abdominal examination should be carried out to detect renal enlargement and to exclude significant retention of urine. Rectal examination will indicate the size of the prostate and bacteriological examination of the urine the presence of complicating infection. In history-taking it is important to establish not only the objective findings concerning the frequency of micturition, but also the way in which these are disturbing the life of the individual patient. Blood urea and/or creatinine examination should also be carried out in order to evaluate the effect of obstruction on renal function. If carcinoma of the prostate is suspected the plasma acid phosphatase level should be measured, but the specimen should not be taken immediately after rectal examination. In the elderly the sudden onset of urinary incontinence should always be looked at critically. It may be simply due to a urinary infection, or it may be caused by increasing disability which makes it more difficult for the individual to micturate, or to dementia, making the individual less conscious of his bodily needs. It should never be attributed simply to senility without investigation.

At any age, frequency of micturition, particularly if accompanied by excessive thirst, should lead to examination of the urine for sugar.

Management

Enuresis in children. — Most children have become dry by day and night by the age of 3 to 4 years although one child in 10 is still enuretic at the age of 5 years, and one in 20 at the age of 10. There is, thus, wide variation in the age at which a child achieves bladder control, and this does appear to be related to the age at which the parents achieved control. Primary enuresis, i.e. the child has never been dry, is extremely tiresome to mothers, who have to wash the sheets each day, but it rarely responds to treatment and should not be made an issue until about the age of 5 years. If the parents have themselves been late in bladder control this may help them to understand the problem, but they will doubtless need support and explanation. When treatment is instituted the co-operation of the child should always be sought. The possibility of infection must always be excluded. The child should then be encouraged to keep a record of the nights on which he is dry or wet. Fluid intake should be encouraged during the day, during which the child should be told to empty its bladder as infrequently as possible. Excessive fluid intake is avoided during the evening, and the child empties his bladder before retiring. Imipramine, 25 mg, is given as a syrup on retiring and four weeks later the child should return to the doctor with his chart recording the results of treatment. If an improvement has occurred the treatment should be continued for a further four weeks. If there is no improvement the dose if imipramine should be increased to 50 mg and in due course to a maximum of 75 mg. When the child becomes dry every night treatment should gradually be withdrawn. Equally good results have been reported with the use of Viloxazine (Vivalan) which is less toxic and has fewer side-effects.[4] In children who fail to respond to this treatment a 'bell and buzzer' should be tried. This is an electrical device in which two electrodes are placed with the bed sheet between them so that when the sheet becomes wet the circuit is completed and a buzzer sounds. The child roused by the buzzer stops micturating, turns off the device and empties his bladder. If this treatment fails it is probably wise to stop all treatment for a year or so and allow further maturation of the nervous system. In rare cases in which there are other neurological abnormalities such as spina bifida specialist advice should be sought.

Secondary enuresis in which the previously dry child has started bed wetting is almost always due to a urinary infection or some emotional disturbance in the family. Refusal to use the potty is not uncommon in children aged 2 to 3 years. This is part of the negativism which occurs at this age. It should be ignored by the parents and will usually quickly resolve. If attention is focused on it, it may be reinforced and so become a major problem. Likewise, enuresis occurring following the birth of a new baby should not cause concern, but should indicate to the parents the need to give affection to the older sibling and to try to share the new baby with the older child. Major marital disharmony may also lead to secondary enuresis in a child.

In secondary enuresis a urinary infection should always be excluded. The management of urinary infection in children is extremely important. Initial treatment should be with the appropriate antimicrobial, usually trimethoprim. The child should be carefully followed up with urine cultures at monthly intervals for a year. Any recurrence should be referred to a paediatrician and full urological investigation carried out. It is highly probable that recurrent infection in childhood when the kidneys are growing is a major precursor in the development of chronic pyelonephritis. This can probably be prevented by close follow-up of urinary infections, often over a period of 10 to 12 years.

Urinary symptoms in young adults. — In young men presenting with symptoms of dysuria or frequency of micturition, examination should be conducted to confirm or eliminate urethritis. In the presence of urethral discharge, referral to a venereologist is desirable. In the absence of this a mid-stream specimen of urine should be examined bacteriologically. Frequency of micturition in the absence of bacteriuria or glycosuria should raise a possibility of tuberculosis of the renal tract; it is rare today but may be particularly suspected in immigrants. Occasionally sexual difficulties in the male can be presented as symptoms of urinary disorders. A question about sexual behaviour and satisfaction should therefore be included in the management of men presenting with these symptoms.

The symptoms of dysuria and frequency of micturition are extremely common in young women. No more than 50 per cent of women presenting in general practice with dysuria and frequency of micturition will have significant bacteriuria, i.e. a colony count of more than 100,000 per cubic millilitre of urine. Of these, 70 to 80 per cent will have an *E. coli* infection, the majority of which will be sensitive to trimethoprim or cotrimoxazole. The initial treatment of patients presenting with these symptoms in this age-group usually consists of the prescription of trimethoprim or co-trimoxazole. Recent studies[6, 7] (see appendix to this chapter) have indicated that many episodes of urinary tract infection respond to a very short course of antibiotic agents — either by a single large dose, or a 3 day course at conventional doses. Culture of a mid-stream specimen on presentation is not always necessary, but patients should be followed up a week to 10 days after the initial episode at which time a mid-stream specimen or dip slide should be collected to confirm bacteriological cure. If the symptoms are very distressing the prescription of a mixture of potassium citrate and hyoscyamus does appear to provide symptomatic relief, although the pharmacological explanation of this is poorly understood. Patients should also be encouraged to increase their fluid intake to three litres per day while symptoms persist; this is approximately one full tumbler hourly while awake. Even in the absence of bacteriologically proven infection many patients appear to improve with this treatment.

Many women in this age-group experience recurrent urinary infection. It is probable that these are promoted by retrograde infection along the urethra which is facilitated by sexual intercourse and may also occur after bathing. Such patients should be advised as follows:

1. To empty the bladder at regular intervals during the day
2. To empty the bladder after sexual intercourse
3. To empty the bladder after taking a bath
4. To clean themselves from the front backwards after defaecation.

If in spite of these precautions infections recur, the ingestion of a single dose of antibiotic following sexual intercourse may prevent further infections.[5]

Despite these precautions some patients will continue to have symptomatic recurrences, and in these long-term therapy with, for instance, co-trimoxazole, one tablet at night, may prevent recurrences. Asymptomatic bacteriuria is present in about 4 per cent of women in this age-group. There is no evidence that these women are more vulnerable to chronic pyelonephritis and hypertension and no evidence that making the urine sterile confers any advantage.

About 6 per cent of women have bacteriuria in the antenatal booking clinic. These patients are more likely to develop acute pyelonephritis during the pregnancy and should be treated vigorously. Evidence is still equivocal as to whether bacteriuria alone in pregnancy increases the incidence of toxaemia or hypertension, or whether it enhances the risks of prematurity, neonatal death or still birth. These patients should all be followed up carefully after pregnancy and excretion urography undertaken six months later.

Post-menopausal women. — In the presence of uterine prolapse the presenting symptom may be urgency or incontinence, and this is particularly so in the elderly. The onset of incontinence should therefore always lead to bacteriological examination of the urine and treatment with appropriate antibiotics.

Women in this age-group also present simply with stress incontinence. This may be confirmed by vaginal examination and a cystocele may be demonstrated. The problems caused by this are likely to become worse with increasing age and early surgical intervention is desirable. The patient should therefore be referred to a gynaecologist. In the occasional very old patient, or one who is a poor surgical risk, the condition may be treated symptomatically by the use of a ring pessary. Occasionally, dysuria or dyspareunia in the elderly may be caused by a urethral caruncle. This responds to surgical treatment and the patient should be referred to a gynaecologist. Atrophic vaginitis may in some cases lead to symptoms of urinary infection in this age-group, although more commonly the presentation is one of dyspareunia. This condition responds dramatically to intermittent courses of small doses of oestrogens administered systemically, or the local application of topical oestrogens.

Elderly males. — From the age of 50 years men may begin to get symptoms caused by prostatic enlargement, usually presenting initially as frequency of micturition. The bladder-neck obstruction leads to incomplete bladder emptying, and this predisposes to infection. The management of urinary infection in men in this age-group must therefore consist not simply of treating the infection but also looking for an underlying cause. Rectal examination will confirm prostatic enlargement, and excretion urography will give some indication of the amount of obstruction present and the amount of residual urine. In the absence of urinary infection prostatic symptoms may develop slowly over many years, and the doctor should not rush his patient into surgery. The features likely to prompt referral to a urologist include disturbances of sleep and social constraints caused by the symptoms, terminal incontinence of urine which may become a social embarrassment and acute retention of urine. This last event may be provoked by the doctor himself prescribing ephedrine or a similar drug, tricyclic anti-depressants or diuretics to a patient who already has bladder-neck obstruction. Prostatic surgery on the whole is very successful, and can be undertaken in very elderly men, who should not be left to a life of misery for fear of operation. Selection of patients for surgery will not, however, depend entirely on the social inconvenience of their symptoms. Objective tests of renal function and urinary infection should be carried out before reaching a decision.

Urinary incontinence in the elderly

This should never be accepted as an inevitable result of ageing. If it develops suddenly it may be due to infection of the urinary tract, infection elsewhere causing mental confusion, or faecal impaction. These possibilities must be explored and treated appropriately. It is also wise to review the patient's drug therapy. The introduction of a diuretic or of a sedative may lead suddenly to incontinence and the importance of this may be missed unless specifically looked for.

Many elderly patients become incontinent because their mobility is impaired and they cannot get to the toilet in time or on arrival cannot use the toilet. A variety of walking aids, the use of a commode or adjustments to the toilet furniture may solve such problems. If the patient or a relative keeps an incontinence chart this may provide a lead to the patient's main problem.

Occasionally incontinence in the aged may be due to detrusor hyper-activity. In these cases anticholinergic drugs, such as emepronium bromide 200 mg t.d.s. or imipramine 25 mg t.d.s. or at night, may be helpful but their side-effects on the heart or in glaucoma must be considered.

Once incontinence which is not amenable to curative treatment is established, the main problems are concerned with preventing bed sores and keeping the patient socially acceptable. In males, there is a choice between the use of a penile clamp, well tolerated by a few, or condom drainage, which often leads to irritation of the penis. An in-dwelling catheter may be required when the skin is threatened. This requires changing about every three months and regular irrigation to prevent the accretion of debris. Chronic bacteriuria is almost inevitable but should probably be treated only if it presents symptoms.

Special clothing is available for the chronically incontinent patient, such as Kanga pants which have a pouch for disposable, absorbent pads which contain not only a hydrophilic agent but also deodorants. A variety of services can be made available by the general practitioner to the incontinent patient. Social services departments may be able to arrange for modifications to the toilet facilities, such as raising toilet seats or providing supporting bars. They or the British Red Cross Society will also supply commodes and some social services provide an incontinence laundry service. Catheters, bags and sheaths may be obtained on prescription as also may some of the sophisticated appliances for patients suffering from incontinence. Instrument and appliance suppliers will usually provide personal advice and equipment, much of which may be prescribed, and are almost always both knowledgeable and helpful.

Conclusion

In this chapter the common causes of disturbances of micturition have been considered. There are many conditions which rarely occur in general practice, and which may present with these symptoms. These include congenital anomalies of the genito-urinary tract, some uncommonly acquired infections such as tuberculosis, the rare complications of infection such as urethral stricture and tumours of the bladder and kidneys. The general practitioner should be alert to the possibility of these causes of disturbances of micturition, but in most cases will not be concerned in their detailed investigation or management. His role is to identify and treat the common causes of disturbance of micturition, and to identify and promptly refer those problems which are outwith his competence.

References

[1] Mond, N.C., Percival, A., Williams, J.D. and Brumfitt, W. (1965): Presentation, Diagnosis and Treatment of Urinary Tract Infections in General Practice. *Lancet*, *i*, 514

[2] O'Dowd, T.C., Smail, J.E. and West, R.R. (1984): Clinical judgement in the diagnosis and management of frequency and dysuria in general practice. *British Medical Journal 288*, 1347

[3] Wing, A.J. and Morrell, D.C. (1972): Infections of the Urinary Tract. *Medicine, 22*, 1333

[4] Altenburrow, A.A., Stanley, T.V. and Holland, R.P.C. (1984): Nocturnal enuresis; a study. *Practitioner*, *228*, 99

[5] Wing, A.J. (1970): Infections of the Urinary Tract. *British Medical Journal*, *4*, 35

[6] Charlton, C.A.C., Crowther, A., Davies, J.G., Dynes, J., Haward, M.W.A., Mann, P.G. and Rye, S. (1976): Three-day and Ten-day Chemotherapy for Urinary Tract Infections in General Practice. *British Medical Journal*, *1*, 124

[7] Jones, R.H. (1982): Single dose and seven day trimethoprim and cotrimoxazole in the treatment of urinary tract infection. *Journal of the Royal College of General Practitioners*, *33*, 585

Appendix

Developing a practice policy for the treatment of acute urinary tract infection

Explanation

This appendix describes the steps which were taken by a general practitioner who was asked by his partners to establish a practice policy for the treatment of acute urinary tract infection.

In developing this policy, the doctor searched recent publications on this subject and decided to use the research published by Dr R.H. Jones in the *Journal of the Royal College of General Practitioners* as his major resource[1]. He selected this paper for the following reasons:

—The study was undertaken in general practice within the last year.

—The patients entering the study were clearly defined.

—The diagnosis of urinary tract infection was described in terms of symptoms, bacteriological examination of the urine and microscopy.

—A questionnaire was used at the beginning of the episode and at the end which enquired not only about symptoms of urinary tract infection, but also about the possible side-effects of treatment.

—The study design was of a double blind randomized controlled trial of conventional therapy as compared with a single dose of an antibiotic.

—The outcome measures were clearly defined in terms of immediate bacteriological outcome and a longer term review of the records for recurrence.

—Simple but appropriate statistical tests were used to measure the significance of the findings.

The report of the study contained a useful list of references, two of which were to recent studies in general practice[2,3], but neither was as carefully designed as Dr Jones' paper although both supported the general thesis that short term therapy for urinary tract infection was as good as longer term therapy.

Results of the study

The population studied was mainly of women of average age 41 years. Sixty-seven per cent of the 94 patients presenting with dysuria and frequency of micturition had significant bacteriuria and pyuria. This is higher than figures reported in other studies, but this may, in part, be due to different criteria applied by different research workers.

The organisms isolated in the study, in the 74 patients who had significant bacteriuria, were *E. Coli* 44 (60 per cent), *Staphylococci* 8 (11 per cent), other Coli-forms 6 (8 per cent), *Strep. Faecalis* 6 (8 per cent). Of the 74 patients with significant bacteriuria, 15 had organisms resistant to sulphonamides, 10 resistant to ampicillin and 5 resistant to cotrimoxazole.

The patients were randomly allocated to 4 different regimes:

(1) A single dose of 400mg of trimethoprim.
(2) A single dose of 2g of cotrimoxazole.
(3) A 7 day course of trimethoprim — 200mg twice daily.
(4) A 7 day course of cotrimoxazole — 1g twice daily.

Bacteriological cure occurred in the 4 groups in all but 2 patients. Symptomatic cure occurred in between 85–92 per cent and there was no significant difference between the groups. Eight patients suffered a recurrence within 6 weeks, but there was no significant difference between the groups.

Side-effects of treatment were recorded in 21 patients. There were important differences between the groups in that only 1 patient on a single dose of trimethoprim developed side-effects whereas 5 or 6 in the other groups recorded symptoms such as anorexia, nausea and dyspepsia.

Evaluation of the literature review

The study by Jones was carefully designed. Its one weakness is concerned with the sample size. A bigger sample might have revealed significant differences in treatment outcome, but clearly these are not important as the overall results are so good. On the other hand, important differences in side-effects and recurrence of infection might well have been statistically significant if a larger sample had been studied.

Another study[2] compared the results of treatment with a single dose of ampicillin, cotrimoxazole or trimethoprim: cure rates of 87–95 per cent were recorded. A weakness of this study was that only 64 of 206 patients presenting were admitted to the study, there was no long term follow-up and no routine enquiry about side-effects.

Another study[3] compared a 3 day course of cotrimoxazole with a variety of other treatment regimes and revealed that a 95 per cent bacteriological cure rate in both groups occurred. The study design was not clearly described and there was no record of side-effects.

Relevance of the research findings to the practice

The average age of patients treated in Dr Jones' trial was 41 years and this compares closely with the average age of patients in this practice presenting with symptoms of urinary tract infection. The social class of patients in Dr Jones' practice is likely to be higher than in our practice, but this would affect particularly compliance with therapy which is a greater problem with patients in the lower social classes and would therefore favour single dose therapy. The bacteriology of the urine specimens examined in Dr Jones' practice differs in some ways from the most recent figures published by the Department of Microbiology from our district hospital. Of specimens submitted by general practitioners they found that 70 per cent showing significant bacteriuria grew *E. coli* and that 75 per cent of those were sensitive to sulphonamides, 66 per cent to ampicillin and 95 per cent to cotrimoxazole or trimethoprim.

One important difference between our practice and that of Dr Jones is that 67 per cent of his patients with frequency and dysuria had significant bacteriuria while the figure in our practice is 45 per cent. Should we be looking for causes of frequency and dysuria other than bacteriuria in our practice which is derived from lower social classes? Reports from some venereal disease clinics suggest that *Chlamydia trachomatis* is an important pathogen. Studies in a general practice very similar to ours do not substantiate this for patients seen in general practice[4].

Practice policy

(1) Female patients presenting with dysuria and/or frequency of micturition in the age group 16–70 years should be treated with a single dose of 400mg of trimethoprim.

(2) Little is gained by examining a mid-stream specimen of urine bacteriologically at the time of presentation because 95 per cent of the infecting organisms will be sensitive to the drug and even those patients who do not have significant bacteriuria appear to recover when treated.

(3) Patients should be seen one week later when a mid-stream specimen of urine should be collected to ensure bacteriological cure.

Effect of practice policy

The need to carry out diagnostic culture of a mid-stream specimen of urine is not supported on the basis of the research data, thus saving both general practitioner time and laboratory resources.

A single dose of 400mg of trimethoprim costs 57p, compared with £1.49 for a 7 day course of treatment, and a single dose of cotrimoxazole costs 86p as compared with a 7 day course costing £3.62 (1984 figures).

References

[1] Jones, R.H. (1982): Single dose and seven day trimethoprim and cotrimoxazole in the treatment of urinary tract infection. *Journal of the Royal College of General Practitioners*, *33*, 585–589

[2] Harboard, R.B., Gruneberg, R.N. (1981): Treatment of urinary tract infection with a single dose of amoxycillin, cotrimoxazole or trimethoprim. *British Medical Journal*, *283*, 1301–1302

[3] Rapoport, J., Rees, G.A., Willmott, N.J. et al. (1981): Treatment of acute urinary infection with three doses of cotrimoxazole. *British Medical Journal*, *283*, 1302–1303

[4] Burney, P., Marson, W., Evans, M., Forsey T. (1983): *Chlamydia trachomatis* and lower urinary tract symptoms among women in one general practice. *British Medical Journal*, *286*, 1550–1552

3.52
Penile problems

F. M. Hull

The commonest penile problems are those relating to disorders of psychosexual function and these are dealt with elsewhere. They are briefly mentioned in this chapter to show that they are two or three times commoner than any other problem relating to the penis. Neither Morrell and his colleagues[1] nor Dunnell and Cartwright[2] make specific mention of penile problems. The National Morbidity Survey[3] lists 1.7 episodes per 1,000 males for malignant neoplasms of the urinary and genital tract, less than one episode per 1,000 for non-specific urethritis, for venereal warts or for syphilis and gonorrhea, and 2.5 for 'other diseases of the male genitalia'. In the survey of 5,936 presenting symptoms in our practice[4] there were 35 cases of symptoms relating to the male genitalia (out of a total of 2,624 men) of which 28 were penile problems and seven related to the scrotum and testes. This gives a rate per 1,000 males of 10.7. Of the 28 penile problems 10 were due to anxiety, marital or sexual problems.

History

The history varies with age since history of sexual contact becomes so important after puberty. The usual complaints are discharge, injury, swelling, ulceration or pain. In children the problems are nearly always mechanical and little is gained by taking a detailed history. In adults history-taking requires more care. The duration, character and associated problems of micturition are important in the presence of a discharge as is the history of sexual exposure. Details of the sexual partner's health may help, but often women are either asymptomatic or no details are known. Injury is frequently sustained in sports, the zip fastener is commonly involved and bizarre injuries due to biting or ligature may occur sexually. Swelling of the penis, which may be considerable, may occur with infection, insect stings, allergy or as part of the generalized oedema of heart failure or nephrosis; these points should be looked for in the history. Acute ulceration suggests viral or spirochaetal disease and in the latter sexual history must be explored. Herpetic ulceration may be recurrent. Penile pain is relatively rare, except as dyspareunia, due to mechanical problems of erection, vaginal dryness or sometimes to intra-uterine contraceptives. Carcinoma should be suspected in older men.

Causes and investigation

The causes to be borne in mind are listed in table I.
Primary diagnosis requires testing of any discharge by bacteriological swabs in transport medium. In such cases the possibility of latent syphilis should be excluded by serial serology. Ulcers of the penis require treponemal examination, often most conveniently arranged by referral to a Special Clinic. Any suspicious chronic lesion of the penis in older men requires biopsy and the rare vascular conditions or problems of erection need haematological investigation.
Congenital abnormalities such as *epispadias* or *hypospadias* are usually obvious. *Phimosis* and *paraphimosis* which may be congenital or acquired are equally obvious. Collections of *smegma* under the foreskin may be missed if the foreskin is not retracted sufficiently. Balanitis in small boys produces preputial oedema and ballooning with pus; occasionally little boys may produce a similar state of affairs by inserting *foreign bodies* into the foreskin or even urethra. The presence of balanitis in older patients suggests *diabetes mellitus* and testing the urine is important. Urethral discharge should always be cultured by sending a swab in transport medium to the laboratory. Trichomonas does not transport well to the laboratory: the organisms show up better if fixed on a slide. This will prove (or disprove) *gonorrhoea* or *trichomonal* infection but will be unhelpful in *Reiter's syndrome, non-specific* and *viral discharge.* In any case in which sexually transmitted disease is likely the possibility of *latent syphilis* must be remembered. *Trauma* is diagnosed on the history but again in *sexual* and *non-accidental* injury of children may be denied. In such cases the nature of the injuries and lack of history may be suggestive. Allergic problems are diagnosed on a history of contact and lack of other cause. *Vascular* problems such as thrombosis of the dorsal vein or of the coronal vein are uncommon but easily palpable. They may be secondary to infection, trauma or generalized disease.

Carcinoma of the penis should be suspected in all chronic lesions of the penis. It is rare below the age of 40 and consultation for penile problems over 50 is also rare. Thus all older men consulting for this reason should be suspected of having carcinoma. There

Cause	*Groups likely to present*
Epi- or hypo-spadias	Should be spotted at neonatal examination
Phimosis and paraphimosis	Boys and young men at periods of great sexual activity. Occasionally old men
Smegma	Children
Problems of size	Usually teenagers, or those about to marry
Balanitis, acute or monilial	The very young and the diabetic
V.D., viral, gonorrhoea, syphilis, N.S.U., *Trichonomas vaginalis*	The years of most active sex drive
Reiter's syndrome (urethritis, conjunctivitis, arthritis)	The years of most active sex drive
Trauma: e.g. sport, bizarre sexual activity, zips	Young men
Allergy, often due to contraceptive, but also clothes	
Vascular problems: e.g. thrombosis of coronal or dorsal veins	
Benign tumours (papillomas)	
Serious	
Carcinoma of penis	Old men, Asiatics (very rare in Jews)
Chordee (bent erection) and priapism – associated with blood dyscrasia; i.e. leukaemia, sickle cell disease	

Table I. – Common causes of penile problems

may be a history of precancerous conditions of the glans. Because of its undramatic early symptoms presentation may be late.

Chordee and *priapism* are usually dramatic enough to require little diagnostic acumen but underlying causes must be suspected.

Examination

The penis should be inspected in a good light, examining both dorsal and ventral surfaces and retracting the foreskin to allow thorough inspection of the glans, coronal sulcus and meatus. The skin should be checked for ulcers, herpes or eczematous changes. The foreskin should be retracted to exclude phimosis and paraphimosis. Parents of infants should be encouraged to tolerate the adherent non retractable foreskin. The habit of forceful retraction in the name of hygiene should be discouraged since this can cause trauma, scarring and later true phimosis.

The position of the meatus is noted and milking of the urethra may be necessary to exclude discharge. Discharge in gonorrhoea is profuse, purulent and full of gram-negative intracellular diplococci. In non-specific urethritis the discharge is scanty and glairy; *Trichomonas vaginalis* infection is often symptomless in the male but should be treated presumptively in the sexual partners of women with the infection. The eyes and joints should be examined if the history suggests Reiter's syndrome.

Ulceration of the penis, if acute, suggests a chancre but, if of longer standing, may be due to carcinoma. Carcinoma may be fungating and foul smelling but sometimes presents as a sclerosing dry lesion of the glans (balanitis xerotica obliterans or Paget's disease of the penis). Presentation is often delayed and in many cases there will be involvement of the inguinal lymph nodes. If carcinoma is suspected a general examination will be necessary to exclude pulmonary or intra-abdominal spread.

General examination may also be necessary when the penis is unduly small since this may be due to various endocrine disorders affecting the testis, the suprarenals or pituitary. When the rare conditions, chordee or priapism, are present general examination is required since these may be presenting symptoms in blood dyscrasias such as leukaemia or a sickle cell crisis.

Management

Congenital lesions should be referred to a urologist since they may predispose to urinary-tract infection and may be associated with covert congenital abnormality of the renal tract.

Paraphimosis and *phimosis* are usually an indication for circumcision as is *balanitis* in young boys. These are probably the only surgical indications for circumcision though there may be many cultural, religious or superstitious reasons for requesting this operation; unless there are serious cultural reasons the practitioner should discourage such unnecessary surgery. *Paraphimosis* may present as an emergency with gross oedema of the glans. If seen early this can sometimes be reduced manually, but it often requires a dorsal slit to release the constricting band.

Hygiene problems respond to soap and water and advice to parents on retraction of the foreskin.

Problems of size are often more imagined than real, and may well be the expression of some sexual anxieties or uncertainties that require further explanation (see Chapter 3.61).

Infections of the glans, particularly if monilial, may suggest diabetes mellitus but when this is absent they rarely require more than hygiene. Suspicion of *venereal disease* should lead to referral for treatment, exclusion of syphilis, adequate follow-up and tracing of contacts.

Trauma and allergic conditions rarely require more than conservative management apart from severe injuries, such as traumatic amputation. Zip fasteners cause much trouble; I have had to use general anaesthesia to sort out three zip fastener injuries. A zip can sometimes be removed by cutting below and undoing it upwards.

Carcinoma of the penis requires referral to a urologist for surgery and radiotherapy.

References

[1] Morrell, D.C., Gage, H.C. and Robinson, N.A. (1971): Symptoms in General Practice. *Journal of Royal College of General Practitioners, 21,* 32

[2] Dunnell, K, and Cartwright, A., (1972): *Medicine Takers, Prescribers and Hoarders.* London: Routledge and Kegan Paul

[3] Royal College of General Practitioners, Office of Population Censuses and Surveys, Department of Health and Social Security (1986): *Morbidity Statistics from General Practice 1981–82*. HMSO Series MB5 No. 1

[4] Hull, F.M. (1972): Diagnostic Pathways in General Practice *Journal of the Royal College of General Practitioners 22,* 241

3.53
Swellings in the scrotum

F.M. Hull

Swellings in the scrotum are remarkably uncommon. The National Morbidity Survey[1] records 1.2 episodes per thousand for hydrocoele and 2.0 for orchitis and epididymitis; a few more may be be included in 'other diseases of the male genital organs 2.5'. In the survey of 5,936 symptoms in our practice[2] there were seven patients presenting among 2,624 men with scrotal swellings, giving a rate of 2.7 per thousand episodes, a figure similar to the National Morbidity episode rate. Some scrotal swellings are commoner at certain ages; e.g. varicocoele is commonest between 15 and 35; of malignant tumours the rarer teratoma occurs most commonly in the third decade while seminoma occurs more often in the fourth decade.
while seminoma occurs more often in the fourth decade.
Although inguinal hernia often presents as a scrotal swelling, no further reference will be made to this condition which is considered in Chapter 3.50.

History

In most cases nothing more than a simple history relating to duration of the symptom, to pain and systemic symptoms is required initially. When other history is needed this will be elicited during examination. Since mumps is a common cause of orchitis a history of contact should be sought. Epididymo-orchitis may be due to a number of organisms including *E. coli*, the gonococcus, staphylococcus, proteus or even trichomonas.
Torsion of the testis may present as an acute emergency with sudden agonizing groin and lower abdominal pain which may be associated with vomiting. It may present difficulties of differential diagnosis from orchitis which has a less dramatic and sudden onset. Torsion is a vascular accident and as such must be treated within four hours or the testis will become necrotic.
A relevant history will usually be volunteered if there is a traumatic cause of the swelling but, as with other groin trauma, sexual injury or child battering must be considered. Varicocoele

and hydrocoele usually present with a history of slow painless enlargement and, when the hydrocoele is secondary to underlying testicular or epididymal disease (e.g. neoplasm, or acute or chronic infection), the history may relate to the primary cause.

Of the more serious causes tuberculous epididymitis presents with pain and a hard lump in the scrotum. There may be haemospermia, usually reported as blood in a condom. Neoplasms are usually undramatic unless far advanced; the patients complain of painless enlargement. Since the growth is painless it is often unnoticed until minor trauma causes self-examination, the lump subsequently being attributed to the trauma.

Causes and investigation

The more important causes to be borne in mind are listed in table I.

As with other symptoms below the belt there may be little indication for investigation. The possibility of gonococcal orchitis

Cause	*Groups of patients likely to present*
Epididymitis/orchitis	Young adults
Torsion	Teenagers
Trauma	Young adults
Hydrocoele	
Congenital	Children
Acquired (1° or 2°)	Elderly
Serious causes	
Chronic epididymitis, tuberculosis	Age 20-30
Teratoma	Age 20-30
Seminoma	Age 30-40
Treatable causes	
Almost all with the exception of generalized malignant disease	

Table I. – Common causes of scrotal swelling

should be considered and any penile discharge should be cultured. In older men a full urological investigation should be carried out since infection may be secondary to other genito-urinary disease. When the history suggests venereal infection serological examination for syphilis should be undertaken. When hydrocoele fluid is tapped this should be sent for bacteriological and cytological examination for evidence of acute or chronic infection or of malignancy.
When tuberculosis is suspected a chest X-ray should be requested and examination made of three early morning specimens of urine and possibly of seminal fluid and sputum (if present) for acid-fast bacilli. Suspicion of malignancy also requires chest X-rays and a full blood count.

Acute infections are of less sudden onset than *torsion* with which they may be confused. There is sometimes a history of contact with mumps, and when this is the cause there will often be a constitutional disturbance. Since *torsion of the testis* rapidly leads to necrosis, if there is doubt immediate admission to hospital should be sought. Diagnosis can be even more difficult if the testis is *imperfectly descended*; here there may be confusion with a *strangulated hernia* but since both conditions require urgent surgery this diagnostic problem is best passed swiftly to a surgeon. A sign which may help distinction between acute infection and torsion depends on the pain of infection being relieved by elevation of the scrotum whereas that of torsion is made worse.

Varicocoele usually presents little diagnostic difficulty and *hydrocoele* only that of missing a serious underlying cause. *Trauma* is an equally easy diagnostic problem, but one should beware of minor trauma drawing the patient's attention to pre-existing tumours. Early *tuberculous epididymitis* may be difficult to distinguish from *simple cysts* of the epididymis or *spermatocoele* which the patient usually discovers on self-examination. Later tuberculous lesions are painful and have a hard localized nature. A similar lesion increasingly often felt nowadays in the scrotum is the tied end of the vas following vasectomy.

Formerly, *neoplasms* of the testicle required differentiation from gummas which also cause painless enlargement. A *gumma* is extremely hard, a sign so commonly associated with malignancy as to mislead. Nowadays gummas are rare. Any enlarging, non-tender testis requires surgical opinion to exclude neoplasm.

Examination

Examination of the scrotal contents consists of systematic identification of the anatomical structures in order to determine the site of the lesion. The first requirement is to determine if the lump originates in the scrotum, in which case the examining finger can get above it. If this is not the case then one is dealing with a hernia descending into the scrotum. In acutely tender lesions such as epididymo-orchitis or torsion this differentiation by examination can be difficult. An acutely tender testicle with dramatic onset of symptoms, especially in a teenager, should be regarded as torsion until proved otherwise. Varicocoele has a characteristic varicose appearance and the affected side of the scrotum hangs lower than normal. Palpation of a varicocele gives the impression of feeling a bag of worms. Hydrocoeles vary in size and when very big are easily diagnosed though they effectively mask any underlying cause to which they are secondary. Hydrocoeles are fluctuant and brilliantly transilluminable. When large, aspiration is necessary before the underlying cause, such as infection or tumour, can be determined.

Tuberculous epididymitis gives rise to a craggy moderately tender enlargement of the epididymis with or without secondary hydrocoele. The cord may be thickened and rectal examination may reveal enlargement of the seminal vesicles, but these are rare late signs. General examination is indicated with all the more serious causes of scrotal swellings to exclude generalized disease.

Neoplasms are painless swellings of the testis. In the teratoma this may be nodular due to complexity and differentiation of the tissue producing cartilage, lymphatic tissue and even hair and teeth. In seminomas the swelling is usually smooth and uniform. In both cases the tumour is firm and rubbery rather than rock hard; a haematoma may give rise to similar signs and lead to confusion. Examination includes abdominal palpation and auscultation of the chest. Lymphatic spread is into the para-aortic glands and only if the scrotum becomes involved is there spread to the inguinal glands.

Management

Epididymo-orchitis usually responds to rest, scrotal support and analgesics. When there is proven gonorrhoea a full course of penicillin (600 mg benzylpenicillin thrice daily for five days) should be given. Otherwise antibiotics have little place. Trauma, unless severe, settles with rest and analgesics, but where severe penetrating wounds occur hospital admission may be indicated. Hydrocoele may be aspirated in the surgery and indeed should be as a diagnostic procedure since the fluid may obscure underlying pathology. Neoplasms, tuberculosis and torsion all require surgical referral, torsion urgently.

References

[1] Royal College of General Practitioners, Office of Population Censuses and Surveys, Department of Health and Social Security (1986): *Morbidity Statistics from General Practice 1981–82*. HMSO Series MB5 No. 1

[2] Hull, F.M. (1972): Diagnostic Pathways in General Practice. *Journal of Royal College of General Practitioners*, *22*, 241

3.54 Lumps in the breast

M.E. Preston-Whyte

The significance of a lump in the breast to the patient and doctor depends on whether it is a benign or malignant lesion. Cancer of the breast is the most common neoplasm of females and is the cause of one-fifth of all deaths from malignant disease. More than 21,000 new cases are registered annually and the deaths from mammary cancer in England totalled 12,672 in 1983. From the Morbidity Statistics from General Practice[1] it is possible to make the following observations:

The consultation rate for malignant disease of the breast increases with age but can occur from the age of 25 onwards.

Benign neoplasms are more common in the years preceding the menopause and this trend is even more prominent in breast disease which includes cystic change.

Male cancer of the breast is uncommon, and lumps in the male breast other than neoplasm, so-called 'physiological mastitis', occur most commonly at puberty.

Hodgkin[2] in his practice records an incidence of 1.0 to 1.2 per 1,000 NHS patients per year for carcinoma of breast and an incidence of 0.3 to 0.5 for breast abscess.

Presentation

A study[3] of 300 patients presenting with breast lumps at a London hospital revealed that 85 per cent had been found by the patients themselves. The remainder were discovered as an incidental finding during an examination at a hospital clinic; only one was found by a general practitioner on routine examination.

The commonest presenting symptom is usually a lump or lumps which have been discovered accidentally by the patient while washing or because minor trauma or discomfort has initiated examination of the breast and the finding of a pre-existing lump. Discharge from the nipple, particularly if bloodstained, may be the presenting complaint, but is much less common than the symptomless lump.

Discomfort and pain are uncommon accompanying symptoms of cancer unless it is advanced and encroaching on other structures. They are, however, often the presenting symptoms of benign conditions: for example, premenstrual breast engorgement,

dysplasia (chronic mastitis) or breast abscess.
Elderly patients may not present until the odour of their advanced necrotic cancer is obvious to others and medical help is then sought on their behalf.

Causes

The lesions encountered can be divided into three groups.[4]
Common breast disorders
Dysplasia
Fibroadenoma
Cyst
Carcinoma
Abscess
Less common disorders
Mammary duct ectasia type of dysplasia
Duct papilloma
Fat necrosis
Galactocoele
Lipoma
Paget's disease of the nipple
Sarcoma
Rare disorders
Tuberculosis
Hydatid disease of the breast.

Dysplasia (synonyms: chronic mastitis, fibroadenosis, fibrocystic disease) consists of an abnormal increase in fibrous and glandular tissue, as well as epitheliosis which is an increase in the thickness of the epithelial-cell lining of the ducts — causing obstruction and subsequent cyst formation proximal to the obstruction. Its cause is thought to be hormonal and therefore it tends to be a dynamic condition varying with the menstrual cycle and the taking of oral contraceptives and is often improved by pregnancy, although it may recur afterwards. It is usually distinguished clinically by being undetected by the flat of the hand and *presenting as multiple granular or nodular areas*, usually bilateral. A persisting solitary area of dysplasia, however, even though impalpable by the flat hand, should be excised, for it has been shown that the incidence of breast cancer in association with dysplasia is four times that of the general female population of equivalent age.

A *fibroadenoma* is a solitary, well-defined, benign lump derived from epithelial and connective tissue of the breast, its consistency depending on the ratio of cells to stroma. It is typically described as a 'breast mouse' because of its discreteness and mobility within the breast tissue.

Cysts may be single or multiple formed following obstruction of a mammary duct, and may occur in association with dysplasia or with an intraduct papilloma. It is this latter association which is important to remember in the treatment for cystic disease of the breast by aspiration.

Breast cancer is always an adenocarcinoma which may vary histologically from the well-differentiated or scirrhous type to the extremely anaplastic or medullary type of growth. The scirrhous is the slower growing and produces the typical skin tethering, peau d'orange and nipple retraction which, in association with lymphadenopathy, is pathognomonic of a malignant growth. The prognosis will depend on the stage of the disease and the histology of the tumour. The Manchester Classification of Breast Cancer describes four stages:

Stage I. Growth confined to the breast

Stage II. Stage I plus affected mobile lymph nodes in axilla

Stage III. (a) Skin involvement larger than tumour and/or
(b) Lymph nodes fixed and/or
(c) Tumour fixed to pectoral muscle and/or
(d) Affected lymph nodes in supraclavicular fossa

Stage IV. Stage III plus distant metastases.

The International Union against Cancer has developed the T (Tumour) N (Nodes) M (Metastases) Classification which is becoming more widely used.

Four factors[5] are known to increase the risk of developing breast cancer. They are:

1. The age at first pregnancy: women whose first pregnancy occurs after the age of 35 are twice as likely to develop cancer of the breast as women whose first pregnancy occurs before the age of 20;
2. Nulliparity;
3. A family history of malignant disease, particularly breast cancer;[3]
4. A history of previous breast cancer.

The role of viruses in the etiology of breast cancer has not been established but recent work suggests that endocrine factors play a major role in that the oestrogen profile in the decade following puberty may be different in those women who do and those who do not develop breast cancer later. Factors which do not appear to affect the risk are previous breast feeding and taking the oral contraceptive pill.[6]

Carcinoma of the male breast, although uncommon, is usually fatal as the patient does not present until the disease is well advanced for the comparative lack of breast tissue means more rapid spread to adjacent structures.

Adolescent boys may occasionally present with an unilateral small subareolar nodule which is due to the physiological effect of puberty. Regression, even of marked mammary enlargement, generally occurs within one or two years.

An *abscess* presents typically with signs of an acute infection and causes few problems of diagnosis. Rarely a lactating carcinoma may mimic an abscess.

Mammary duct ectasia is usually found around the time of the menopause and is usually bilateral. Clinically it may be confused with carcinoma if apparently localized. The diagnosis will probably only be made after operation.

A *duct papilloma* characteristically gives rise to a bloody discharge from the nipple. It is a precancerous condition and should therefore be excised. A cyst may occur in association with it.

Fat necrosis is distinguished by the history of a recent blow to the breast but an elderly person may not recall such an incident and a diagnosis of carcinoma may be made as the condition presents as a solitary lump often attached to the skin. Again diagnosis will usually follow operation.

History

The history taking should include the following specific questions:

1. How long has the lump been present?
2. Does it fluctuate in size?
3. What is its relationship to the menstrual cycle and, if relevant, to oral contraceptives, pregnancy, puberty, menopause?
4. Is there discomfort, pain or tenderness?
5. Is there discharge from the nipple?
6. What is the general health of the patient, particularly with regard to weight loss or back pain?
7. Is there past history of disease, particularly of the breast?
8. What is the previous obstetric history?
9. Is there a family history of malignant disease?

Examination

Clinical examination of breast lumps should be meticulously carried out. It must be performed systematically with the patient undressed to the waist. A stamp outline of the breast is useful in recording the findings at the initial examination and on subsequent occasions.

Inspection. — With the patient seated the breasts should be inspected first from in front, both with the patient's arms at her side and raised above her head. Asymmetry, a visible lump, skin tethering or fixation of the breast may be noted. Particular attention is paid to the nipples, retraction, altered axis or excoriation suggesting malignancy.

Breast palpation. — This is best carried out with the patient lying down. A small pillow placed under each shoulder in turn allows the breast to 'flow' over the chest wall. Before starting palpation the patient should be asked to point to any suspected lump. Each quadrant of the breast is palpated in turn with the flat of the hand, initially with the patient's arm at the side and then tucked under the head. Any lump thus detected can then be delineated by palpation with the finger and thumb to test for mobility and consistency. Finally, the areola is compressed 'around the clock' to detect a latent discharge.

Lymph node palpation. — With the patient seated and the hands placed on the shoulders of the examiner, both axillae can be simultaneously palpated. The pectoral nodes can be palpated by curving the fingers around the lateral edge of the pectoralis major muscle, which is relaxed by supporting the arm in 90° flexion. The subscapular nodes are palpated from behind as are the supraclavicular fossae. If a lump or lumps be present, certain other features, e.g. size, contour, consistency, overlying skin changes or fixation should be looked for.

Finally, if the history suggests that metastatic spread may have occurred a general examination is indicated, particularly of the abdomen for liver enlargement, the chest and spine.

In a hospital series of 144 histologically proven carcinomas of breast, clinical examination correctly diagnosed 123 preoperatively: an accuracy of 85 per cent; 88 per cent of benign lesions were also correctly diagnosed.[7] Although small, the error of diagnosis is such that one cannot rely solely on clinical examination for an accurate diagnosis of carcinoma.

Management

A patient who presents with a lump in the breast which has any or all of the characteristics of a malignant tumour should be immediately referred to a surgeon. She should not have to wait more than a week for an appointment, for the vast majority of women once their suspicions are aroused are extremely anxious and apprehensive not only because of the fear of malignancy but also because of the fear of mutilation. Reassurance can only be given once a diagnosis is established. No patient with a lump in the breast should be reassured that there is 'nothing wrong' until either the lump disappears on aspiration and does not recur, or the lump is removed and is shown to be benign.

A patient who presents with a lump which has none of the characteristics of a malignant tumour, but which is still palpable a week after the period in a premenopausal woman or a fortnight after the initial examination in a postmenopausal woman, should also be referred for further investigation. A lump which fluctuates in size with the menstrual cycle is probably benign but most general practitioners in these circumstances would prefer the reassurance of a second opinion.

When the decision to refer is made, the patient may wish to know what this will entail with regard to further investigation. It is likely that aspiration may be attempted by the surgeon to determine whether a 'doubtful' lump is cystic or solid. Recently this has been shown to be a satisfactory method of treatment of cysts of the breast particularly when these tend to be multiple, but it is only safe provided the cyst does not refill, the fluid withdrawn is not bloodstained and histological examination does not reveal malignant cells and there is no residual lump after aspiration.

Mammography or soft-tissue X-ray is particularly useful when the breast is large and palpation difficult and the only complaint is of discomfort or pain often not easily localized. In women under 40, however, the dense architecture of the breast impedes satisfactory definition of abnormal masses and xeroradiography, which is a development of the image recording process in photocopying documents, produces better definition in these women and requires a lower dose of radiation than mammography.

The patient may not mention spontaneously her fear of a mutilating operation. It is wise, indeed essential, to explore this fear with her and positively reassure her that, in the event of the breast being removed, she would be advised about the various cosmetic aids available which could be fitted before her discharge from hospital. In special circumstances, such as a carcinoma being removed at a very early stage, surgeons are now implanting silastic prostheses at the time of mastectomy. In the letter of referral to the consultant the particularly apprehensive patient should be identified and close liaison between consultant and general practitioner should be aimed at to ensure satisfactory management.

The treatment of an *abscess* should be initially with antibiotics but, if after 48 hours, inflammation fails to subside, the area should be incised and drained.

There remains the problem of *dysplasia*, in which the main complaint is of tenderness and often diffuse lumpiness of the breasts in relation to the menstrual cycle. There is no satisfactory treatment for this condition but symptomatic help can be given in the form of a diuretic or a mild analgesic. Counselling may be indicated when a woman seems to be using her symptoms in order to escape from some intolerable situation, usually an unsatisfactory sexual relationship. The appearance of a persisting lump, however, even when there is a long history of dysplasia, should be managed as though the patient were presenting for the first time with a lump in the breast.

Treatment

The fact that the mortality from breast cancer has not altered significantly over the past 20 years largely explains why the majority of British surgeons now prefer a simple mastectomy plus or minus radiotherapy instead of the more mutilating radical mastectomy. Advanced breast cancer may be hormone dependent and the type of dependence will be related to whether the patient is pre- or post-menopausal. Tumours which present before the menopause and for some five years afterwards appear to be oestrogen dependent and are therefore inhibited by the removal of the sources of oestrogens or by the administration of androgens. In the older age-group the reverse is true and inhibition can be obtained by the administration of oestrogens.

Screening

In a long-term investigation[8] to determine whether periodic breast cancer screening with clinical examination and mammography leads to lowered breast cancer mortality, the results in a random sample of 31,000 women in New York aged 40 to 64 years offered screening examination were compared with the results obtained in a similarly constituted control group. The mortality at the 3½ year stage of the screened group was 18.1 per cent, compared with 33.7 per cent in the unscreened group. A significant factor was that 70 per cent of the breast cancers detected did not have evidence of axillary node involvement. The authors of the screening programme state that ten years' follow-up is needed to establish whether the effect of the screening programme is short or long term. The evidence (see Table I) that local disease offers a better prognosis than disseminated disease, however, must surely emphasize the necessity for early diagnosis.

Stage when first diagnosed	*Recurrence-free rate*
Stage I	68 per cent
Stage II	40 per cent
Stage III	15 per cent
Stage IV	2 per cent

Table I. — Recurrence-free rates five years after all forms of treatment for carcinoma of breast at the Royal Marsden Hospital.

Women should therefore be encouraged and taught to examine their own breasts. A film strip entitled 'Self-Examination of the Breasts' available from the Health Education Council could be used by practice health visitors as part of a health education programme.

Women who form the high-risk group (that is, those whose age at first pregnancy was over 35 years, those with a previous history of breast cancer and those with a family history of malignancy) could be recorded in an At Risk Register. This entails recording elderly primigravida (information available from the practice antenatal clinic and the health visitor's 'Infants at Risk Register'), and recording all patients with a known history of breast carcinoma together with their female relatives who belong to the practice. Screening of this 'At Risk' population can then be carried out annually. This should include mammography as well as clinical examination if such facilities are available.

Whatever the arguments for and against screening for breast cancer, it seems sensible to suggest that, whenever the general practitioner examines a woman's chest, he should also take the opportunity of making an examination of the breasts.

References

[1] Royal College of General Practitioners, Office of Population Censuses and Surveys, Department of Health and Social Security (1986): *Morbidity Statistics from General Practice 1981–82*. HMSO Series MB5 No. 1

[2] Hodgkin, K. (1973): *Towards Earlier Diagnosis.* 3rd ed. Edinburgh: Churchill Livingstone

[3] George, P. and Chalstrey, L.J. (1969): Factors in the diagnosis of breast disease. *British Journal of Surgery*, *56*, 337

[4] Scott, P.R. (1971): *An Aid to Clinical Surgery.* Edinburgh: Churchill Livingstone

[5] Cole, P. (1974): Epidemiology of human breast cancer. *Journal of Investigative Dermatology*, *63*, 1133

[6] Vessey, M.P., Doll, R. and Sutton, P.M. (1971): Investigation of the possible relationship between oral contraceptives and benign and malignant breast disease. *Cancer*, *28*, 1395

[7] Stewart, H.J., Gravelle, I.H. and Apsimon, H.T. (1969): Five years' experience with mammography. *British Journal of Surgery*, *56*, 341

[8] Shapiro, S., Strax, P. and Venet, L. (1971): Periodic breast cancer screening in reducing mortality from breast cancer. *Journal of the American Medical Association*, *215*, 1777

3.55

Other breast problems

Pauline A. McAvoy

Morbidity statistics from general practice[1] have shown that for every 1,000 consultations with females of all ages, 10.8 are for diseases of the breast other than neoplasm. The figure in the 25–45 age group is 22 per 1,000. The overall figure for males is 1.5 per 1,000.

Fear of cancer may be a precipitating factor in many consultations but of course the breasts are susceptible to many other problems not least because of their function as organs of lactation, sexual attraction and feminine identity.

In this chapter it is proposed to discuss under the following broad headings, some of the problems, other than cancer, for which a person may consult his or her general practitioner:

1. Developmental concerns of the female breast
2. Gynaecomastia
3. Concerns around breast feeding
4. Breast pain
5. Discharge from the nipple
6. Skin problems

1. Developmental concerns of the female breast

Physiological abnormalities

Failure of breast development. — At puberty the breasts increase in size due to deposition of fat around the mammary lobules and the nipples also enlarge. The usual age of onset of puberty is 12–14 years and is influenced by heredity, environment, nutrition and socio-economic status. If puberty has not occurred by the age of 16 it is considered delayed and if a girl is seen at this stage then a general examination to exclude gross endocrinological upset and a pelvic examination to exclude major congenital defect is all that is indicated. Intensive investigation should not be undertaken before the age of 18 years and at this stage most general practitioners would refer either to an endocrinologist or gynaecologist.

When the breast fails entirely to develop at the normal age of puberty it may be due to ovarian agenesis. This, associated with webbed neck and short stature, was described by Turner as a characteristic of the syndrome that now bears his name. The incidence of Turner's syndrome is 1 per 2,000 live female births. Another cause of failure of development is congenital adrenal hyperplasia. One particular variant of this is not usually diagnosed until after puberty, with amenorrhoea, absence of secondary sexual characteristics, hypertension, hypokalaemia and osteoporosis being the main features. Haagensen[2] describes a larger group of young women in whom development of the breasts is delayed beyond normal puberty. Menstruation may begin late and stop after a few cycles, the patient then experiencing menopausal symptoms. This is due to a relative ovarian deficiency.

Treatment with oestrogens may allow some degree of breast development to take place and, in the case of adrenal hyperplasia, supplement therapy with appropriate steroids is indicated.

Most of the girls who are seen with concerns about breast development do not have any underlying pathology and are developing normally, but perhaps at a rate which compares unfavourably with their peers or with their mothers' ideas of normality.

Precocious development. — This is usually seen as part of the syndrome of precocious puberty, this relating to puberty which occurs before the age of eight or nine years. Although this is sometimes seen as the result of the endocrine effect of various ovarian tumours, e.g. granulosa-cell tumour, more commonly no demonstrable causative lesion is found and the girl's adolescence although premature is normal.

Adolescent hypertrophy. — This type of hypertrophy occurs at or soon after puberty in otherwise normal girls. The breasts continue to enlarge in both stroma and glandular tisssue often to such a degree that they cause real physical and of course psychological distress. Occasionally the hypertrophy is asymmetrical. As there is no natural regression reduction mammoplasty is usually indicated.

Asymmetry. — This is present to a small degree in all women and can be regarded as normal. In some cases however the asymmetry is very marked and indeed there may even be a total lack of development of one breast. The cause for this is unknown and treatment with oestrogen is usually ineffective. These patients may be helped by the insertion of a prosthesis on the affected side.

Perceived abnormalities

In our society where the breasts are organs of sexual attraction as well as of lactation, it is perhaps difficult to remember Gregory's statement in *A Father's Legacy to His Daughters*, 'The finest bosom in nature is not so fine as what imagination forms', when the 'perfect' bosom confronts us from the pages of popular magazines and newspapers. Small wonder then that some individuals are unhappy with their lot.

Among the requests to alter in some way the shape of the breasts will be those from women who have carefully considered the problem with regard to their own attractiveness and self-esteem, others who are reflecting the opinion of their partners and others again who blame the inadequacies and failures in their lives on this particular anatomical or perceived variation.

Obviously it is important before referring a patient for a plastic procedure that the reasons behind the request are clearly understood and some assessment made of the patient's psycho-sexual make-up.

Reduction mammoplasty usually involves hospitalization for a few days. There are of course residual scars beneath and lateral to the breast but the reduction in breast size which can be achieved, will probably make this an acceptable side-effect.

Augmentation involves the insertion of an implant either made of silicone gel or, more recently, various plastic materials, anterior to the pectoralis muscle sheath thus allowing the normal breast tissue to overlie the implant and effectively increase the breast size.

There is no evidence as yet that there is an increased incidence of breast cancer in women who have undergone this procedure.

2. Gynaecomastia

Gynaecomastia is extremely common. The degree of breast enlargement is very variable and ranges from a small button-like swelling to the size of the adult female breast. There is often associated breast tenderness. The causes are numerous but bearing in mind the probable underlying disorder in oestrogen/androgen balance it is helpful to think of these in terms of physiological, pathological and pharmacological problems.

Physiological problems

Gynaecomastia is seen in the neonate as a result of the action of placental oestrogens. It is a transient condition usually disappearing soon after birth.

It is seen again at puberty when it is extremely common, being present in some degree in 50 per cent of boys.[3] It can be a source of great concern to boy and parent and, of course, embarrassment to the former. The majority do however resolve spontaneously in 6–18 months.

Rarely the hypertrophy progresses to resemble the female breast, in some cases asymmetrically, and at this stage surgical intervention is generally justified.

A similar hypertrophy occurs in older men — the so-called senile gynaecomastia. This is presumably due to a reduction in testosterone production.

There is no evidence to date that hypertrophy in this age-group predisposes to carcinoma.

The main differential diagnoses of gynaecomastia are tumour and simple obesity.

Pathological problems

The list of possibilities here is long. The basic disorders however appear to be due to increased oestrogen production either at the target organ or by some failure in the androgen-to-oestrogen conversion, reduced androgen production by the testes or testicular feminization, where there is a normal level of testosterone but oestrogens are able to act unopposed.

Causes:

Bronchial carcinoma
Tumours of adrenal or testis
Cirrhosis
Hyperthyroidism
Acromegaly
Testicular atrophy
Klinefelter's syndrome
Hermaphroditism and pseudohermaphroditism
Malnutrition
Paraplegia
Generalized skin disease

Pharmacological problems

Both oestrogen and androgen therapy may produce gynaecomastia. The most frequently seen example of the former is the effect of treatment of carcinoma of the prostate with stilboestrol. Other drugs, by binding to oestrogen receptors, have also been associated with gynaecomastia, e.g. digoxin and griseofulvin.

Spironolactone, which has an anti-androgen effect, and the phenothiazines, methyl-dopa, cimetidine and reserpine, which appear to act by disturbing control of gonadotrophin/prolactin production, may occasionally cause gynaecomastia.

Treatment. — In general no treatment is required. Where there is a low level of androgens, testosterone therapy may be tried. Obviously in drug-induced gynaecomastia, the side-effect has to be balanced against the therapeutic value of the drug and if necessary the drug changed or discontinued. Surgical intervention is usually indicated when the degree of breast enlargement is intolerable to the patient.

3. Concerns around breast feeding

Although currently there is an upward trend in the number of mothers wishing to breast feed, the figures available do not suggest that this is the preferred method of infant feeding.

A national study carried out by the DHSS in 1975–6[4] revealed that half the mothers in the sample wanted to breast feed and that one-quarter had heard no mention let alone discussion of infant feeding at any time during attendance at antenatal clinics, surgeries or classes. Of the 50 per cent who started to breast feed, over one-third had given up by the time they left hospital.

Concerns and misconceptions around breast feeding are numerous and if we believe that breast is indeed best we should be giving clear and sensible advice and encouragement throughout pregnancy.

Questions are often raised about breast size in relation to ability to provide an adequate milk supply. This of course is one factor which has no bearing on the success of breast feeding.

Very little is required in the way of preparation of the breasts during pregnancy. As there is an increase in breast size a well-fitting, supportive brassiere will be of help from the point of view of comfort. Daily washing of the nipples with warm water will remove any crusts of colostrum which have formed. Nipples which are flat or retracted may be helped by gentle massage and pulling between the thumb and fore-finger and if necessary nipple shells can be worn in the later stages of pregnancy to encourage protraction.

Many women give up breast feeding in the first few days when they learn that the baby is losing weight, fearing that their milk supply is inadequate. These fears can be anticipated and the mother prepared for the event with the knowledge that, until the fourth day, colostrum only is produced which will give the baby some nourishment until the milk comes in and that weight loss, in the early days, is a normal event.

Milk supply is not established for a couple of weeks and indeed may fall off if the mother is very active and becomes overtired and anxious. It is for the health visitor and general practitioner to advise on adequate diet, fluid intake and rest so that a milk supply once established has the chance of being maintained.

Breast engorgement may occur around the third or fourth day of the puerperium. If possible feeding should be continued with the added measures of adequate analgesia, good breast support and fluid restriction. Sometimes, however, the breast is so distended that the infant is unable to fix on the nipple. It may be necessary to express some milk either manually or with a pump before feeding to soften the breast and afterwards to empty it.

Feeding should initially be for a couple of minutes at each breast, gradually increasing this to between ten and fifteen minutes. This together with ensuring that the baby is well fixed to the breast and not sucking on the nipple alone can help to avoid cracked nipples. This can be a very painful complication of breast feeding and indeed may cause the mother to give up altogether. The use of lanolin or a spray such as Rotersept seems to offer some protection to the nipples if used regularly after feeding. If the problem should arise then twenty-four hours' rest from suckling on the affected side and firm support is usually all that is required.

Cracked or abraded nipples are of course a source of entry of infection which may result in mastitis and breast abscess. These two are very difficult to distinguish. Hodgkin reports the incidence of breast abscess in his practice as 0.3 to 0.5 per 1,000 NHS patients per year. This is equivalent to 1.0 per 50 pregnancies.[5]

The patient will usually complain of severe pain in the breast and of feverishness. Examination reveals a hard, acutely tender, red area on the breast.

These conditions used to be considered indications to stop breast feeding. The tendency now, however, is to encourage the mother to continue feeding on the unaffected side. Should engorgement occur, this is more comfortably relieved using a pump as manual expression may be extremely painful.

As the causative organism is usually *Staphylococcus aureus*, treatment should be with cloxacillin or flucloxacillin to avoid problems with penicillin resistance. Analgesia and breast support will also be necessary.

Weaning is best carried out over a period of weeks gradually substituting a bottle feed for a breast feed until the changeover is complete. In this way little breast discomfort is experienced. The 10 p.m. and 6 a.m. feeds are usually last to be substituted for the convenience and comfort of both mother and baby. It is possible of course to discontinue breast feeding immediately and in this situation as there may be a degree of engorgement, fluid restriction, support and analgesia may be required. Drug suppression of lactation is seldom required but if indicated bromocriptine (Parlodel) 2.5 mg b.d. or t.i.d. for fourteen days is effective and has largely superseded oestrogens for this purpose.

4. Breast pain

Although frequently complained of, breast pain or mastalgia has received little attention or sympathy from the medical profession. No obvious physical cause being found it is readily attributed to psychological causes with the suggestion[6] that it is most commonly seen in frustrated unhappy nulliparous women of late middle age. More recently, however, the setting up of specialist clinics dealing with breast problems has afforded the opportunity to look more closely at the problems and an attempt made to define aetiological factors and relevant treatment.
Six specific causative factors have been identified,[7] in some cases by mammography or histology.

(i). Cyclical mastalgia. — A mild degree of breast tenderness in mid-cycle and premenstrually is a normal finding. Mastalgia is distinguished from this either by its intensity or duration — the pain may last for most of the cycle but usually has a premenstrual exacerbation. The discomfort is often described by the woman as a fullness or heaviness in the breast and is generalized rather than localized. On palpation the breasts are often diffusely nodular. The underlying pathology is usually fibroadenosis or fibrocystic disease.

(ii). Duct ectasia. — There is no relationship here to the menstrual cycle although as with many conditions a pre-menstrual exacerbation may be reported and the pain is more readily localized to the nipple area or inner quadrant. Cold weather may aggravate the pain. Mammography shows areas of calcification or evidence of periductal mastitis.

(iii). Tieze's syndrome or costochondritis is often described by patients as breast pain but on examination tenderness and swelling are found over a costochondral junction.

(iv). Trauma. — Apart from pain resulting from an injury to the breast this refers to pain at the site of a previous surgical procedure, e.g. at the point of drainage of a cyst or abscess or biopsy.

(v). Sclerosing adenosis. — In this condition pain is usually present at the site of pathology. There may also be cyst formation, large enough to be palpable. The diagnosis of sclerosing adenosis is a difficult one to make both clinically and histologically as the overgrowth of fibrous stroma may so distort the glandular pattern that it resembles an infiltrative carcinoma. There is a four-fold increase in breast cancer in women with this condition.

(vi). Cancer. — Pain is an infrequent presenting symptom of breast cancer but nevertheless should be considered not least because fear

of cancer is more than likely the reason why the patient has consulted.

Mastalgia may be a symptom in juvenile fibroadenoma which is a soft rapidly growing tumour in adolescents and in the fibro-adenoma or 'breast-mouse' which occurs in the adult woman usually before the age of 40. Breast tenderness is also of course one of the earliest symptoms of pregnancy.

Treatment is dependent on the underlying condition. Women suffering from cyclical mastalgia who are on the oral contraceptive may find an improvement in their symptoms on discontinuing this. Danazol, the antigonadotrophin agent, has proved successful in relieving symptoms in many patients. Surgical excision of a wedge in duct ectasia has been successful in some cases. Treatment of sclerosing adenosis by surgical excision is unpredictable. Pain related to carcinoma is usually relieved by the treatment of the cancer itself which is discussed in Chapter 3.54.

5. Discharge from the nipple

This is not a common symptom, but as it may be a sign of an underlying carcinoma should certainly not be ignored. According to Haagensen[8], discharge which has to be expressed from the nipple, that is, does not escape spontaneously, is usually not of pathological significance: the nature of the discharge may give a clue to the underlying disorder.

Serous. — This is a thin, yellowish discharge which may be first noticed as a stain on the brassiere or nightgown. It is usually due to an intraductal papilloma. Rarely it is associated with carcinoma. It has also been reported with long-term use of oral contraceptives.

Blood-stained. — The presence of blood has no particular significance with regard to carcinoma but more commonly is secondary to the proliferation of intraductal epithelium seen in intraductal papilloma. Rarely intraductal carcinoma is present.

Milky (galactorrhoea). — Lactation not associated with pregnancy has been reported with oral contraceptive use. Other drugs which may occasionally induce this symptom are the phenothiazines, reserpine and methyl-dopa. Pathological causes include pituitary adenoma, pituitary necrosis as in Sheeham's syndrome, hypothyroidism and trauma to the chest wall, which, by stimulating the thoracic nerves, activates the hypothalamic–pituitary mechanism.

Nipple discharge of physiological origin has been reported in the last months of pregnancy being blood-stained in nature and resolving spontaneously in the puerperium, and in middle-aged women the nipples when squeezed may produce a thick greyish material. This comes from the terminal ectatic ducts, and is harmless.

Because of the difficulty in establishing the cause of the discharge from the nipple on purely clinical grounds, it is frequently necessary to refer such patients for further investigation, e.g. mammography or surgical exploration.

6. Skin problems

Obviously the breasts may be involved in any generalized skin disease, infection or infestation and are just as susceptible as any other part of the body surface to sebaceous cysts, seborrhoeic warts, etc.

Intertrigo of the submammary region can be a problem in obese women. Drying the area carefully after washing and dusting with talcum powder are measures which can be taken in prevention. Secondary infection with *Candida albicans* may occur forming a bright red glazed erythema with a well-demarcated edge which may exude serum. In severe cases psoriasiform lesions may appear on the trunk as a sensitization reaction and make the differential diagnosis from flexural psoriasis or seborrhoeic eczema very difficult. It is probably worthwhile checking a urine sample for sugar in these patients as diabetes mellitus is a predisposing factor to *Candida* infection.

Topical treatment with nystatin or a combination of nystatin and hydrocortisone is indicated.

Paget's disease of the breast is a specialized form of intraductal carcinoma that arises in the main excretory ducts of the breast and extends to involve the skin of the nipple and areola.[9] The changes in the nipple and areola have the appearance of dermatitis and indeed this is often why delay in diagnosis occurs. Any unilateral chronic eczema of the nipple and areola should always be suspect. Final diagnosis depends on histological examination.

Conclusion

In recent years there has been much publicity about breast self-examination and early detection of cancer. This increased awareness may have caused many women with breast problems to consult their doctor hoping for reassurance that they do not have cancer. It is often not possible to give this reassurance on clinical grounds and referral for further investigation may be indicated, to allay the anxieties of both doctor and patient.

Because in our society the breasts are organs of sexual attraction and identity, concerns about the breast may be an expression of underlying anxieties regarding sexuality. An awareness of this may allow the doctor to offer the patient more than mere assurance that nothing is physically wrong.

References

1 Royal College of General Practitioners, Office of Population Censuses and Surveys, Department of Health and Social Security (1986): *Morbidity Statistics from General Practice 1981–82*. HMSO Series MB5 No. 1

2 Haagensen, C. D. (1971): *Diseases of the Breast*, 2nd ed. Philadelphia: Saunders

3 Large, D. M. and Anderson, D. C. (1978): The Breast. *Medicine*, *10*, 459

4 Office of Population Censuses and Surveys (1978): *Infant Feeding: Attitudes and Practice in England and Wales.* London: HMSO

5 Hodgkin, K. (1973): *Towards Earlier Diagnosis*, 3rd ed. Edinburgh: Churchill Livingstone

6 Jeffcoate, N. (1975): *Principles of Gynaecology*. London: Butterworth

7 Preece, P. E., Mansel, R. E., Bolton, P. M., Hughes, L. E., Baum, M. and Gravelle, I. H. (1976): Clinical Syndromes of Mastalgia. *Lancet ii*, 670

8 Haagensen, C. D. (1971): *Diseases of the Breast*, 2nd ed., p. 102. Philadelphia: Saunders

9 Robbins, S. L. (1968): *Pathology*, 3rd ed. Philadelphia: Saunders

3.56
The patient with painful periods

John McEwan

Perception and interpretation of painful stimuli from viscera vary greatly in different individuals. Pain and discomfort related to menstrual periods arise from two sources:

1. Contraction of uterine muscle
2. Tissue responses to changing hormone levels.

Symptoms from 1. can be broadly described as *dysmenorrhoea*; those from 2. as *premenstrual tension*.

It is rare for either of these syndromes to be caused by disease but as complaints in general practice they arise commonly. Consultations for dysmenorrhoea in the 1981–82 National Morbidity Survey showed an annual average rate of over 42 per 1,000 in women aged 15 to 24 years, with an average of 4.9 episodes.[1] In the higher reproductive age-group (25 to 44) the consultation rates per 1,000 women came down to just under half of these for women in the younger decade.

Little is likely to be gained for the younger patient by specialist referral or elaborate investigations, but all these patients require a sympathetic hearing and therapeutic endeavour on the doctor's part. Women developing painful periods later in life, i.e. *secondary dysmenorrhoea*, may well benefit from full gynaecological assessment as the symptoms can be caused by the presence of uterine or other pathology such as endometriosis, recurrent pelvic inflammatory disease or, occasionally, fibroids.

The perception of pain or discomfort is greatly affected by psychological states and it is important for the practitioner to be aware of tension and depression in the patient and to discover, if possible, the causes.

In a sense dysmenorrhoea is linked with the premenstrual syndrome because the sudden fall in progesterone just before menstrual flow begins, combined with the steady rise, from a low level, of oestrogens in the blood stream, probably makes the myometrium more sensitive to the prostaglandins released locally during the process of menstruation. Contractions of the non-pregnant uterus occur at all times and are usually pain-free between periods. At or just before menstruation, they may be felt by the woman as severe colicky pains in the central lower abdomen with even some reflex autonomic radiation causing nausea, vomiting or faintness. Backache may occur, possibly referred from the uterine cervix, as may pain in the iliac fossae due to spasm of the fallopian tubes and pains in the anterior thighs and groins referred from the ovaries.

The majority of women between the menarche and the menopause are aware of some discomfort during menstruation, particularly the non-parous, but for most it does not interfere with their lives in any way nor do they even take simple analgesics. A large group take medicines obtained without prescription, such as aspirin, paracetamol or combinations of these and other drugs. Only a very small proportion ask the doctor for help and of these only a very few need time off work or school, or need to retire to bed. Equally a proportion of women go through life without ever experiencing symptoms of dysmenorrhoea.

Similar factors apply to the prevalence of symptoms of premenstrual tension (PMT). The majority of women will feel some difference in their bodily sensations in the few days before a period begins. A great deal of work has been done on changes in behaviour occurring at this time, with the implication that the hormonal changes are reflected by altered reactions in the central nervous system.[2] Suicide, violence, crime, marital disruption, car accidents, epileptic attacks and migraine have all been said to occur more often in the premenstruum and authorities have related this to current hormonal status. Symptoms more specifically associated with premenstrual tension are related to local tissue swelling probably caused by fluid retention. This can produce a distinct and regular aching pain anywhere, e.g. from gums or teeth, to the lower spine or ankle joints, together with a weight increase of a few pounds and sometimes dependent oedema. A characteristic symptom is a heavy feeling in the lower abdomen known as 'bloating' and the waist-line can enlarge. Usually all these discomforts disappear at menstruation or at the most within a day or two after its onset.

Presentation

What makes a patient come to the doctor? Serious interference with everyday living is probably the commonest reason, but there may also be anxiety that something is physically wrong. There is also the expectation of relief from medical treatment. Attitudes and early experiences of menstruation may set a pattern, which the perceptive doctor can help to prevent by suitably advising the young teenager and her mother. Psychiatric presentations are probably the commonest: those patients who become unbearably depressed or tense, sometimes for more than a week each month. Direct presentation of dysmenorrhoea *per se* is less common: most women just 'get on with it', but occasionally there will be a younger woman who needs a certificate to be off work for a day, or whose symptoms are severe enough to require strong analgesics. They may also be causing her to feel anxious about herself. Women with migraine often have their attacks in the premenstrual week but will probably need specific treatment for the migraine as well as attention to any other PMT symptoms.

History and examination

With dysmenorrhoea the history is usually clear enough to make a firm diagnosis. Just occasionally a pre-menarchal girl may present with cyclical pain and not understand that this is a kind of dysmenorrhoea. The rare occurrence of haematocolpos must not be forgotten in such a case. Further information required to identify the patient's problem will be centred round the question of what the symptoms mean to the patient and how they affect her with a view to deciding on appropriate treatment.

With premenstrual tension the picture is much more varied. The periodicity of symptoms is suggestive, but it may not strike either patient or doctor at first, especially if the symptom is unusual such as, for example, pain in the shoulder. Keeping a diary card recording symptoms and menstrual flow will be helpful in such cases. The range of symptoms is wide and all those experienced by a patient should be elicited, as this may be helpful in treatment. For instance, if there is ankle oedema a diuretic (e.g. bendrofluazide 5 mg every morning for the premenstrual week) may be indicated rather than a hormone analogue or a tranquillizer.

The extent of physical examination depends on the symptoms. In simple dysmenorrhoea gynaecological examination is not necessarily indicated unless there are associated genital tract symptoms, or if treatment with ovarian steroids is contemplated. If the occurrence of dysmenorrhoea is unusual — for example coming on severely for the first time in an older woman — it may have arisen in association with a pathological process within the pelvis, endometriosis, fibroids, changes from pelvic inflammatory disease, such as hydrosalpinx or pyosalpinx, or even from neoplasia. A full gynaecological assessment may then be indicated, including cytology, curettage and laparoscopy. Ultrasonic scan may play a useful part in the diagnosis of fibroids or ovarian tumours.

Management

Neither dysmenorrhoea nor premenstrual tension is a disease in the pathological sense. They are discomforts related to normal physiological change. It is important therefore that neither doctor nor patient should regard them as diseases. If there is a tendency for the patient to adopt a 'sick role' the doctor must find out why and, if possible, try to prevent its establishment.

Analgesic prescriptions should be kept as simple as possible: for example, soluble aspirin or paracetamol should be pushed to the fullest extent. Substances interfering with prostaglandin activity may be specifically helpful.[3] Aspirin is one of these; some of the drugs used in arthritis are prostaglandin synthetase inhibitors and can also be used in dysmenorrhoea: e.g. mefenamic acid (Ponstan), or ketoprofen (Orudis) which is recommended in a dose of 50 mg eight-hourly.

Diazepam is often given in small doses, such as 2 mg once or twice daily, in addition to analgesics. Its effect is probably entirely psychotropic, in reducing mental tension. The patient should be warned that it can become habit forming. Addictive drugs such as barbiturates, opiates, amphetamines, pentazocine, pethidine and dipipanone should not be used.

Symptoms of premenstrual tension respond to similar analgesics if there is distinct pain. Diuretics are often helpful while symptoms last, such as bendrofluazide, 5 to 10 mg each morning. In severe depression affecting behaviour and relationships, tricyclic drugs taken at night may be helpful: e.g. amitriptyline, 25 mg or 50 mg at 9 p.m. Some authorities recommend progesterone which produces good results in some very severe cases. Criteria for use are a clear-cut diagnosis, severe disturbance of living and willingness to make regular use of vaginal pessaries, rectal suppositories or intramuscular injections. Progesterone is not absorbed reliably by mouth: pessaries or suppositories should be inserted daily (200 mg) for seven to ten days before menstruation is expected. A similar effect is obtained by an intramuscular injection of hydroxy-progesterone caproate, 250 mg in oil given on day 18 of a 28-day cycle (or on days 15 and 22 if a single injection is not effective). Side-effects of these steroids are not dangerous but there may be weight increase and some hirsutism. Often treatment for three to six months is effective in breaking a pattern and the hormone can then be discontinued. On the whole, synthetic progestogens have proved disappointing and may even produce symptoms of premenstrual tension. Some authorities however recommend dydrogesterone 10 mg twice daily for two weeks before the expected onset of the next period.

The question of contraceptive method often arises in the treatment of dysmenorrhoea and premenstrual tension. Both disappear in most cases if patients take the combined oestrogen-progestogen contraceptive pill. In cases of very severe dysmenorrhoea, provided there are no contraindications, a combined pill can be prescribed even if not required for fertility control. In these cases it is best to start with a pill having a fairly high level of progestogenic activity such as Gynovlar (ethinyloestradiol 50 micrograms with norethisterone acetate 3,000 micrograms) or a pill containing norgestrel such as Ovran or Eugynon 50 (ethinyloestradiol 50 micrograms with levonorgestrel 250 micrograms).[4] Unfortunately, the results of giving oral progestogens alone are disappointing.

Patients using intra-uterine devices are liable to experience an increase in dysmenorrhoea. This can be treated with analgesics or, if it is severe, may require removal of the device and trial of an alternative IUD or a completely different method of fertility control.

Over the years doctors have tended to advise patients consulting about dysmenorrhoea that it will improve at various times of change in the life cycle: e.g. 'when you get married' or 'when you have a baby'. This type of prognostication is unwise as both dysmenorrhoea and premenstrual tension depend on such a complex of individual variables, both organic and psychological. If there is some psychosocial stress or maladjustment then it is important for the doctor to find out about it and try to help the patient towards a better balance. Naturally, major events such as childbirth will have a profound effect by resetting all the variables, physical and mental. Probably sexual adjustment is as important a factor as any. Lack of normal sexual response and failure of experience to reach expectation, for example lack of orgasm, may well be important factors. The practitioner must be prepared to assess the importance of sexual functioning in relation to the aetiology in any particular individual. If there are problems in this area he should be able to assist with counselling advice or refer the couple to a suitable alternative agency, such as those provided in some hospital departments in family planning clinics or by social work agencies.

References

[1] Royal College of General Practitioners, Office of Population Censuses and Surveys, Department of Health and Social Security (1986): *Morbidity Statistics from General Practice 1981–82*. HMSO Series MB5 No. 1

[2] Dalton, K. (1964): *The Premenstrual Syndrome*. London: Heinemann

[3] Goldberg, V.J. and Ramwell, P.W. (1975): Role of prostaglandins in reproduction. *Physiological Reviews*, *55*, 325

[4] Cullberg, J. (1972): Mood changes and menstrual symptoms with different gestagen/estrogen combinations. *Acta Psychiatrica Scandinavica*, Supplementum 236, 1–86

3.57 The patient complaining of abnormal periods

John McEwan

Menstrual loss lacks an easy reliable method of measurement and so complaints of abnormality can only be subjective. They therefore require careful assessment of the complaint by the practitioner. The symptom may essentially be a change of pattern which is not really abnormal. On the other hand, the patient feels that things are not right and this feeling also needs to be assessed. Periods can be too heavy, too light, too short or too long: the thresholds of tolerance both of the patient and the doctor further complicate the diagnostic issue.

Methods of measurement are being developed and may eventually become practicable as a routine. Duration and frequency of menstrual periods can be recorded conveniently on diary cards such as those available from the Royal College of General Practitioners. Total amounts of iron lost can be measured by eluting haemoglobin from tampons or pads and estimating it by the alkaline haematin method.

Disturbances of menstruation present as symptoms in 2·8 per cent of all complaints annually in an average urban practice and form almost two-fifths of those for genito-urinary diseases found in women, being responsible for 3 to 4 consultations per week from a practice population of 4,455.[1,2] Naturally, the incidence of complaints will vary not only with the characteristics of the practice population, but also with the age, sex and special interests of the doctor. Menorrhagia and irregular periods produce high consultation rates in the 25–44 age-group (a national average of 64.4 per thousand in 1981–82) reducing to about half this rate in the age-group 15 to 24. Over 44 the rate probably rises considerably in the pre-menopausal group.[3]

Causes

These divide naturally into the causes of reduced or absent menstrual loss, and of excessive loss.

The commonest physical causes of menorrhagia are probably

fibroids and the presence of an intra-uterine device (IUD). Occasionally users of hormonal contraceptives also have menorrhagia: some from combined oestrogen-progestogen pills but more often those using low-dose progestogen-only pills or depot injections of medroxyprogesterone acetate. A change of formula is needed to correct this, or even a change of method. With the IUD the menorrhagia may be tolerated once there is reassurance that nothing is going wrong; alternatively a change of device may improve bleeding after a further three to four months.
A cause of prolonged bleeding, not necessarily heavy, is a missed abortion or retained products of conception. The uterus is likely to feel bulky, may be tender and in some cases the cervical os is open.
Chronic non-specific pelvic inflammatory disease is a further cause of menorrhagia and may occur following septic abortion in the past or an attack of gonorrhoea with tubal involvement. It can also present as an insidious process with no clear-cut causal episode.
Tuberculous endometritis is a rare cause nowadays but may at the same time cause infertility.
Carcinoma of the uterus, either of the body or the cervix, may have led to menorrhagia or prolonged periods, particularly when there is a change in menstrual pattern. For this reason nearly all patients complaining of excessive loss should have an endometrial curettage at some time during the assessment stage. Conditions such as adenomyosis, possibly a pre-cancerous stage, can be a cause, also endometriosis, metropathia haemorrhagica, and polyposis of the endometrium. Menorrhagia may also be a feature of thyroid disease.
The amount of blood loss is said to depend on the fibrin system operating in the uterine cavity.[4] Any disorder affecting this can lead to menorrhagia, as also can platelet deficiency and the use of anticoagulant drugs.
Finally, there will be a large proportion of patients complaining of excessive menstrual loss for whom no physical cause can be discovered. It seems likely that hormonal imbalance can play a part, although an exact mechanism has not been worked out. This may be connected, through alterations in release of pituitary gonadotrophins, with psychological causes. Depression, anxiety states, stress, all seem able to affect menstrual patterns, and equally require the general practitioner's attention.
In the same way, presumably, psychological factors can lead to amenorrhoea, scanty or reduced periods usually associated with failure of ovulation. This is common in young women who leave home for university or travel abroad. There is also the group who suffer from anorexia nervosa. Pregnancy immediately comes to mind, however, as the chief cause of amenorrhoea. There may be scanty losses at monthly intervals for several months which makes

the dating of gestation difficult. A delayed period with a reduced loss may be due to a threatened spontaneous abortion and in this connection ectopic gestation should always be kept in mind. Pregnancy tests are not helpful when an abortion is in the process of occurring. Lactation is another physiological cause of amenorrhoea about which a patient may be ignorant.

When the combined contraceptive pill is used ovulation is intentionally suppressed but 'interval losses' occur between packs of pills. These may cease in some women, particularly on the low-dose combined pills, and cause anxiety. More serious difficulties are caused by failure of spontaneous menstruation after stopping the pill, particularly if a pregnancy is wanted. Periods are often irregular for up to three months. In about 0.5 per cent of women taking combined pills there is amenorrhoea for six months or longer. If conception is desired, early referral to a specialized centre for induction of ovulation is indicated. Women who have a past history of amenorrhoea or oligomenorrhoea are probably more likely than others to develop 'post-pill amenorrhoea'.

Endocrine abnormalities can cause scanty or absent periods, such as cystic ovaries, pituitary tumours, diabetes mellitus, hypogonadism, and the Stein-Leventhal syndrome which in some patients is also manifested by hirsutism. Hypothyroidism may accompany anovular amenorrhoea but in less severe cases there may be menorrhagia. Thyrotoxicosis may cause oligomenorrhoea or amenorrhoea. Acute psychotic breakdown is a further cause of amenorrhoea; this is common in schizophrenia for example, and it also occurs in the debilitated states found in severe drug addiction.

Failure to menstruate 'adequately' can have a marked subjective effect on the patient. Many women believe that menstruation eliminates harmful substances from the body. Alternatively, they may expect thrombotic disease as 'the blood goes somewhere else and clots'. These beliefs are part of our tradition and are common throughout the world. Passing clotted menstrual blood can also distress women unless this is their usual pattern. Again there may be an anxious association with intravascular clotting.

History and examination

Having defined the nature of the complaint itself, information about related and associated functions is required. Age and parity are obviously important, previous menstrual problems of any kind, the outcome and sequel of previous pregnancies, general medical conditions, use of drugs, gynaecological conditions including infections and operations and sexual activity: these may all be relevant as well as a consideration of environmental stress and psychological problems.

It is useful at this stage to assess the patient's feelings about her complaint and in particular to distinguish whether the presentation of genital dysfunction overlies a need for psychosexual counselling or advice on fertility control measures. Poor sexual responsiveness may be affecting the relationship with her husband and thereby threatening her marriage. Fear of pregnancy may be contributing to the malaise. Many women in the older age-group of reproductive life find difficulty in initiating discussion with the doctor about contraception in case they are thought to be 'silly'. There is also the prospect of the menopause about which many women are afraid, as well as the inevitable fear of developing cancer. With patients complaining primarily of excessive menstrual loss – that is, menorrhagia – there may be an underlying anxiety about hysterectomy being the final outcome of their complaint to the doctor. It is best to elicit this if it is present – not otherwise – at an early stage, so that it can be faced as rationally as possible. Many women regard hysterectomy as a kind of castration: some even think they will automatically lose their ovaries and their sexual responsiveness. This is not physiologically necessary but all too often becomes a psychogenic reality.

Another field of anxiety céntres round the question of pregnancy. It is important for the doctor to find out in the case of a patient complaining of scanty, short, absent or delayed menstruation, whether they think they might be pregnant and what their reaction would be if they were. This may lead to consideration of sub-fertility, or, on the other hand, the need for adequate birth-control measures. This consultation may also be the prelude to a discussion on induced abortion. The reason for presenting at a particular time is probably more important than the symptom itself.

Physical examination is straightforward: a bimanual pelvic examination followed by speculum examination of the cervix and vagina, and cervical cytology. If there is evidence of inflammation in the genital tract, bacterial swabs should be taken from the vagina and cervical canal. They should be sent to the laboratory in a transport medium (e.g. Stuart's medium). If there is suspicion of gonorrhoea, a swab of the urethra should be taken, and possibly an additional one from the rectum, and a specific request made for appropriate anaerobic culture designed to isolate Neisseria.

Many doctors would also examine the breasts as a convenient screening exercise, take the blood pressure and test the urine for albumin and glucose.

Further investigation may include a urine test for pregnancy, a haemoglobin estimation and blood count. Patients with menorrhagia for several months often become iron deficient and a serum iron estimation may be indicated.

Management

The need for psychological assessment and support against anxious fears has already been mentioned. This applies to the whole range of menstrual symptoms.

In many of the causes outlined, particularly organic factors, treatment depends on dealing with the underlying pathology, which is often the task of a gynaecological specialist. Fibroids, retained products, neoplasms and distinct hormonal disorders need specialist investigation and treatment. Very often the general practitioner will be required to explain what is happening to the patient and help her towards reasonable choices, if there are any.

This leaves a hard core of patients with continuing menorrhagia for whom hysterectomy is being considered, not to treat an underlying cause but to stop the excessive blood loss. It is a serious operation both in physical and psychological terms and should only be decided upon if there is no alternative. The first question is whether there is indeed excessive blood loss and whether this is merely a nuisance — and it can interfere considerably with a woman's life — or whether it is undermining her physical health: e.g. by causing chronic iron deficiency. Secondly, family intentions must be carefully considered, owing to the factor of irrevocable sterilization. This in itself can cause a psychological aftermath.

The question of chronic loss should be dealt with by six to twelve months of observation with regular estimations of haemoglobin levels and serum iron. Any existing anaemia is corrected, a diary card is kept and the practical feasibility of living with the condition, or not, will become apparent.

For this type of patient with menorrhagia hormone therapy can be helpful. The principle is to reduce endometrial bleeding by giving progestogens: e.g. norethisterone tablets, 5 to 15 mg daily, for the last 10 to 14 days of the cycle. This substance can also be used in acute haemorrhagic menorrhagia, when an injection of 15 mg of norethisterone intramuscularly, followed up with tablets, will sometimes save hospital admission. Another useful progestogen in this connection is dydrogesterone: it can be given similarly in a dose of 10 mg b.d. The anti-gonadotrophin, danazol, has been found helpful in resistant cases but should be used cautiously because of side-effects, e.g. permanent voice changes.

In that nearly all menorrhagic patients require diagnostic curettage at some time to exclude intra-uterine disease, it is necessary for the general practitioner to work in close collaboration with the gynaecologist. Similarly the final decision to carry out hysterectomy must be made a matter of consensus between the two doctors and their patient.

In patients with amenorrhoea or scanty losses, management depends largely on tracing out the physiological events. Sometimes specialist treatment is indicated; sometimes nothing specific. One point can be made with certainty: it is futile to induce uterine bleeding artificially by giving ovarian steroid hormones or their analogues. If there is failure of pituitary function, this will make it worse: if the woman is pregnant the compounds may affect foetal development: and any sense of security gained by the patient is totally false.

References

[1] Morrell, D.C., Gage, H.G. and Robinson, N.A. (1971): Symptoms in general practice. *Journal of the Royal College of General Practitioners*, *21*, 32

[2] Morrell, D.C., Gage, H.G. and Robinson, N.A. (1970): Patterns of demand in general practice. *Journal of the Royal College of General Practitioners*, *19*, 331

[3] Royal College of General Practitioners, Office of Population Censuses and Surveys, Department of Health and Social Security (1986): *Morbidity Statistics from General Practice 1981–82*. HMSO Series MB5 No. 1

[4] Nilsson, L. and Rybo, G. (1971): The treatment of menorrhagia. *American Journal of Obstetrics and Gynecology*, *110*, 713

3.58 Unscheduled vaginal bleeding

John McEwan

The doctor's approach to the complaint of vaginal bleeding when it is not 'meant' to occur depends a great deal on the stage in the patient's life cycle at which it is presented. There is a spectrum of causes with varying frequencies between infancy and old age. Each of these therefore varies in significance. Often the patient, or her relatives, sees the bleeding as likely to indicate severe disease and it may cause anxiety both to patient and doctor. This factor needs to be considered when weighing the subjective evidence.

It is important to discover exactly what is happening and when. The doctor may be able to classify the bleeding as a normal variation of menstruation: for example, in a young teenager whose cycle varies between 24 and 32 days between the first days of menstrual bleeding. He may similarly be able to reassure a woman in her first trimester of pregnancy who gets a small amount of painless bleeding at eight weeks after the last menstrual period, that this is likely to be bleeding from the uninvolved part of the endometrium (a 'decidual loss') rather than a threatened spontaneous abortion.

Anxiety about unscheduled vaginal bleeding has been modified in recent years by the frequency with which it occurs in women of reproductive age who are using either hormonal contraceptives or intra-uterine devices. Bleeding between periods is common with both methods, but the likelihood of the unusual loss being due to the method or to some other cause needs to be carefully assessed in each individual case.

In an urban practice caring for a population of 4,455, age-specific consultation rates for diseases of the genito-urinary tract are high in women of fertile age, varying between 300 and 600 annual consultations per 1,000 people at risk. Of the presenting symptoms, one-quarter were described as bleeding and abnormal discharges (1·9 per cent of symptoms in all women) and almost two-fifths as disorders of menstruation (2·8 per cent of symptoms in all women). Unscheduled vaginal bleeding could come into either category and so represents a significant proportion of a general practitioner's work-load.[1,2]

In terms of mortality the most serious causes are neoplastic, most commonly carcinoma of the uterine cervix. In 1985 this showed a mortality rate in England and Wales of 75 per million for all age-groups (compared with 526 per million in women for breast cancer, 155 for stomach and 384 for lung cancer, both also in women). Age-specific rates are shown in table I, from which it is clear that cervical cancer is a relatively important cause of death in women over 35 and it commonly presents with unscheduled vaginal bleeding.

	All ages	15-24	25-34	35-44	45-54	55-64	65-74	75-84	Over 84
Neoplasms of cervix uteri	75	1	32	66	92	152	192	196	210

Table I.–Age-specific mortality rates for carcinoma of the cervix uteri: England and Wales 1985, per million population[3]

Causes

Probably the commonest type of unscheduled vaginal bleeding is a brief mid-cycle loss occurring at ovulation time and caused by the sudden change in ovarian steroid hormone levels. This can be diagnosed on the history and the absence of abnormalities on examination. Most women experience this event at some time in their lives between the menarche and the menopause. Reassurance can be given in an isolated instance. Suspicion of a pathological cause may be aroused by persistence of the symptom in further cycles without adequate alternative explanation.

Bleeding from the endometrium is increased by the presence of an intra-uterine contraceptive device. This applies to mid-cycle losses which may start to occur for the first time after an intra-uterine device (IUD) is fitted. Reassurance can be given in nearly all cases, but if a woman has worn an IUD for several years and the unscheduled bleeding is entirely new, it may indicate a new underlying cause.

Intermenstrual bleeding or spotting is also common in women taking oral contraceptive pills. Combined oestrogen-progestogen pills can produce this, particularly in the first few cycles on a pill containing only a small dose of progestogen (e.g. Minovlar or Norinyl-l). With the low-dose continuous progestogen-only pills (or depot progestogen injection) irregular bleeding and spotting are common. 'Break-through bleeding' is the term often applied to these types of intermenstrual bleeding. There is some evidence that it is more likely to occur in a woman under emotional stress and it is well worth enquiring about stress factors if such bleeding has newly arisen.

Outside the reproductive age-groups, hormonal changes can cause uterine bleeding either from physiological causes, such as in the newborn in whom it may be due to withdrawal from the influence of maternal oestrogens, or as a result of treatment. In the early postmenopausal time or in the elderly, oestrogens may be used to prevent osteoporosis or to control discomforts such as sweating and flushing. Such women often have unscheduled vaginal bleeding.[4] The difficulty is to be certain whether it is caused by the treatment alone or whether there is an underlying neoplasm of the uterine body or cervix, or a condition of the endometrium such as adenomyosis which may predispose to neoplasia. A diagnostic curettage, perhaps of aspiration type, should be carried out in most cases. Some drugs can also cause uterine bleeding in post-menopausal women such as levodopa used to treat Parkinson's disease.[5]

Rarely, endocrine abnormalities can give rise to uterine bleeding: for example, 'precocious puberty' in young children with steroid-secreting ovarian tumours.

Inflammation of the cervix combined with trauma is a common cause of post-coital bleeding in the reproductive years, including during pregnancy the so-called 'infected erosion'. This can bleed at other times, too, and may be associated with pain and dyspareunia due to inflammation in the structures around the uterus. An associated vaginal discharge would support this diagnosis. Sometimes a similar picture is found due to a cervical polyp which may be sessile or pedunculated. In the latter case the polyp can often be avulsed by twisting, although the patient should be carefully followed up in case there are further polyps in the uterine cavity or an underlying neoplasm.

Trauma is a cause of vaginal bleeding and the practitioner should find out if the injury was intended and how it arose, as intervention in the social situation may be needed. Foreign bodies in the vagina may cause bleeding also, such as a forgotten tampon or a small pebble or marble put inside experimentally by a child. In all these situations there may be important psychosocial factors needing careful attention. This may also be the case if there is the suspicion of sexually transmitted infections, such as gonorrhoea or trichomoniasis. Candidiasis of the vagina, not always sexually transmitted, is common, particularly so in glycosuria due to diabetes mellitus.

Carcinoma of the genital tract has already been mentioned as a cause of vaginal bleeding. It is obviously important since early discovery may improve the chances of successful treatment. The commonest is cervical carcinoma, in one-half to two-thirds of which the disease is rapidly invasive.[6] Appearances of the vaginal portion of the cervix are not particularly helpful in early diagnosis. Early experience of coitus, childbirth and multiple sexual partners are considered to be predisposing factors.[7] Carcinoma of the body of the uterus may present only as some bleeding abnormality with no apparent signs. In the non-parous this is a more likely cause than cervical cancer.

Vaginal bleeding during pregnancy can occur at any time but it is commonest in the first trimester. If there is associated abdominal pain and it is not at the time of decidual bleeding, it is reasonable to diagnose a threatened abortion. Many authorities now believe that spontaneous abortions, not arising from uterine abnormalities, are the result of non-viable embryonic maldevelopment. The difficulty for general practitioners in the early stages is to be sure whether or not the bleeding is from this cause.

At a later stage of pregnancy – in the middle trimester – bleeding may give warning of a spontaneous abortion due to cervical incompetence. This should be treated by immediate admission to hospital with a view to suture. In the last trimester bleeding is known as 'ante-partum haemorrhage' and may be due to placenta praevia or it may constitute a revealed accidental haemorrhage, bleeding from the placental attachment. These are dangerous for both mother and baby and accidental haemorrhage is associated with pre-eclampsia. Admission to hospital is required urgently, although prior resuscitation of the mother may have to be considered. A small bleed, of course, may herald the onset of normal labour.

Finally, there are cases of unscheduled vaginal bleeding, usually during the reproductive part of the life cycle when there is no apparent cause. This is then usually labelled as part of the 'dysfunctional uterine bleeding' syndrome. It may be hormonally determined although there is no direct proof of this as yet. Hormone output from the ovaries is controlled by the pituitary gonadotrophins which are in turn stimulated or released by hormones from the hypothalamus. At this point there is a connecting link between the neural centres controlling mood and other vegetative functions, and also with the sensorium generally, through the basal ganglia and the cerebral cortex. It is probable that many patients with this kind of disorder of uterine bleeding are suffering from stresses in the environment or psychic changes that affect the pituitary-ovarian axis. Certainly the practitioner should try to assess the patient in psychological and social terms as well as the purely physical: this may reveal factors that need specific attention whether or not there is an organic condition present.

History and examination

To find out exactly what is being described by the patient the doctor will need to ask about the duration, frequency and regularity of the bleeding and for how long over-all the abnormality has been noticed. The amount of blood loss may be important in certain cases: for example during pregnancy. Associations and concomitant symptoms need also to be elicited: for example bleeding after coitus, and the presence of pain or vaginal discharge. A history of drug therapy, such as with sex hormones or similar compounds, or with anticoagulants, may also be relevant. The exact source of blood loss may be in some doubt, particularly if the amount is slight. In sexually active women, placing a tampon in the vagina may clear up the question of whether the blood is from the vagina or uterus on the one hand, or from the vulva, urethra or anus on the other. (A midstream urine specimen will contain red cells or haemoglobin if the origin is in the urinary tract.) In infants and the elderly careful inspection on different occasions may be the only way to find out whether the blood is coming from the uterus or vagina.

Other features of the examination involve the principle that it should be as extensive as the significance of the symptom merits. In a baby with a small vulval abrasion there may be no need to go further than inspection. On the other hand, a profuse blood-stained discharge may suggest the rare occurrence of neoplasia and indicate the need for referral to a gynaecologist for a full examination under general anaesthesia. The same type of assessment may be relevant in an 80-year-old with vaginal atrophy, in whom a full vaginal examination, with passage of a speculum to look at the cervix and take a smear, could be unduly painful. In the common presentations in the fertile age-groups, bimanual vaginal examination with inspection through a speculum and cytological testing of the cervix should never be omitted. During pregnancy it may be wisest to carry this out in hospital (and therefore may in some cases require specialist referral) if there is any chance that the examination will cause further and heavy bleeding. In the third trimester, for example, an antepartum haemorrhage may be due to placenta praevia. In cases of threatened spontaneous abortion, it is sometimes valuable to carry out an immediate one-finger vaginal palpation

very gently to determine the size and direction of the uterus and whether or not the cervical os is open. The findings may well determine the next decision in management, such as whether hospital admission is indicated.
The examination of other parts of the body may be important in some cases. For example, hypertension, anaemia and blood dyscrasias may predispose to vaginal bleeding. In a woman over 35 it might be considered reasonable routinely to examine the breasts as well for screening purposes. Apart from cervical cytology, investigations may include haemoglobin estimation and blood count, urinalysis, pregnancy testing of the urine to detect early pregnancy if the symptoms suggest this, examination of vaginal and cervical secretions directly under the microscope and culture (using a transport medium) to detect microbial infection. If gonorrhoea is suspected, anaerobic culture for Neisseria should be specifically requested. Suction curettage of the endometrium and punch biopsy of the vaginal portion of the cervix may be considered by those practitioners with specialized experience in gynaecology. For the most part, however, the importance of excluding neoplastic disease as a cause of unscheduled vaginal bleeding in susceptible age-groups entails a high rate of referral to the gynaecological specialist with a view to examination under anaesthesia, curettage of the uterus and adequate biopsy of the cervix.

Management

Every patient complaining of unscheduled vaginal bleeding is likely to have anxiety about the cause, as in the public mind the symptom is associated very much with cancer. The doctor may also react anxiously and it is important that he be aware from the beginning of the possible feelings he and the patient may have. It is all too easy to feel duty-bound to refer such a patient without facing the worries openly. Yet some relief for her feelings may be what the patient needs most. In the case of a pregnancy the woman often fears an abnormality in the baby, which may be well-grounded, but in that case the conceptus is likely to be unviable.
From the gynaecological point of view an important part of management is the adequate diagnostic process which has been indicated in previous sections. When there is a serious organic condition further treatment is likely to be in the hands of the specialist. In the case of minor organic conditions the specialist is likely to have picked these up and treated them also.
Any bleeding which is a threat to life clearly needs hospital care and chronic excessive loss needs attention to the possible iron deficiency.

In the case of patients regularly worried by intermenstrual bleeding, in whom organic conditions have been reasonably excluded, cyclical hormone therapy should be tried, using either combinations of oestrogen and progestogen such as are used for contraceptive pills, or progestogen alone in higher dosage: for example, norethisterone acetate, 5 mg daily from day 10 to day 28 of a 28-day cycle.

With perimenopausal patients who bleed with oestrogen replacement therapy, some authorities recommend regular intervals in the medication, say of one week in six, so that predicted – and therefore 'scheduled' – bleeding can occur. Others have suggested using additional progestogens in combinations similar to the contraceptive pill, but these have not yet been fully evaluated, either in their effectiveness or in their liability to cause adverse effects. A reasonable regime for oestrogens alone would be ethinyloestradiol, 10 micrograms daily for 35 consecutive days in every 42.

For patients using intra-uterine devices who suffer from intermenstrual bleeding there is no rational treatment. On the other hand, they may become reassured if the doctor shows that he is not worried about it. In some women in whom bleeding is heavy, irregular, prolonged and associated with menorrhagia, the device may be wrongly positioned. This can be corrected by removing the IUD and inserting a fresh device.

References

1 Morrell, D.C., Gage, H.G. and Robinson, N.A. (1970): Patterns of Demand in General Practice. *Journal of the Royal College of General Practitioners, 19,* 331

2 Morrell, D.C., Gage, H.G. and Robinson, N.A. (1971): Symptoms in General Practice. *Journal of the Royal College of General Practitioners, 21,* 32

3 Registrar General's Statistical Review for England and Wales: Mortality Tables for 1972. HMSO

4 Marshall, B.R. (1974): Post-menopausal vaginal bleeding during oestrogen therapy. *Journal of the American Medical Association, 227,* 76

5 Procope, B.J. (1971): Aetiology of post-menopausal bleeding. *Acta obstetrica et gynaecologica scandinavica, 50,* 311

6 Lewis, T.L.T. (1974): Cancer of the uterus, including the importance of pelvic examination as well as cervical screening. *Health Trends, 6,* 52

7 Martin, C.E. (1967): Marital and Coital Factors in cervical cancer. *American Journal of Public Health, 57,* 803. See also Rotkin, I.D. (1967): *ibid,* pp. 815–829

3.59 Vaginal swellings, discharge and soreness

John McEwan

This chapter will deal with a wide variety of conditions producing symptoms and signs in the vagina or vulva. Although interrelated, the three groups in the chapter heading will be taken separately, as such classification divides the topics into manageable sections. In the clinical evaluation of these conditions in general practice, two important generalizations can be made: the physiological norm must be fully understood by the doctor and he must be sure that his patient shares this information; and secondly, the doctor should not only take an adequate history of what the presenting symptoms really comprise, but he should always make a careful examination of the vulva, vagina and cervix with good lighting in order to be able to inspect and if possible palpate any lesion that may be causing the symptoms. If these two rules are observed, management becomes at once simpler and more successful.

Swellings

Cysts, trauma, inflammation, prolapse and warts are the commonest causes of swellings in the vulva and vagina. Boils are often seen in and around the pubic region and perineum, particularly if the patient is excreting *Staphylococcus aureus* from the gut, and it is important to distinguish them from perirectal lesions, such as ischio-rectal abscesses and fistula-in-ano when they are pointing near the perineal body. In the region of the labia majora such a swelling may be a *cyst* of a *Bartholin's gland* or, if infected, a Bartholin's abscess. The former soon becomes the latter and the abscess must be treated surgically, by marsupialization. Further inside the vaginal introitus a cystic swelling on the lateral aspect may be a *lateral wall cyst* of the vagina, formed from embryonic duct tissue. These do not become infected and can be left alone unless they are causing discomfort or obstruction in coitus. In the fourchette of the vaginal introitus near the mid-line posteriorly, a cystic swelling can follow perineal repair after childbirth: this may be a *haematoma*, a *stitch abscess* or, later on, an *inclusion dermoid*.

Perineorrhaphy scars sometimes also lead to soreness. Smaller swellings of the area include *sebaceous cysts*, *genital warts*, and *urethral caruncles*. Caruncles often cause dysuria and require referral to a surgeon. Warts are frequently the source of uncomfortable itching and are usually transmitted by sexual contact. They can be treated by the application of 1 per cent podophyllin paint but it is wise to smear paraffin ointment on the skin around the warts first as a protection. If genital warts do not easily respond to such treatment they will require cauterization. *Carunculae myrtiformes*, the tag-like remnants of the hymen, can appear as swellings of the vaginal mucosa in inflammation due to infections such as candidiasis.

Inside the vagina, *uterovaginal prolapse* can be found as a swelling or bulge in the vaginal wall, either anteriorly (urethrocoele, cystocoele) or posteriorly (rectocoele). The bulging is often accompanied by descent of the cervix into the vaginal space on coughing or straining.

Anterior wall prolapse may cause associated urinary symptoms with incomplete bladder emptying and a consequent tendency to infection. Such a condition will require specialist referral for assessment and treatment. In other cases, much depends on the time in the life cycle. If family building is completed, referral for surgical repair or suspension of the uterus may be necessary. Moderate degrees of prolapse between pregnancies can be treated with an intravaginal pessary, such as a polythene ring (see NHS Drug Tariff), together with a course of exercises to strengthen the pelvic floor muscles and increase their postural tone. Again, in very elderly women for whom an operation under general anaesthesia presents serious risks, it may be better for the general practitioner to use one of the various pessaries designed to keep the uterus in place. Such a patient may present with a *complete procidentia* with the vagina everted and most of the uterus outside the vulva. In this case immediate referral to hospital is required.

The cervix uteri often presents to the examining finger as if there were abnormal swellings on the vaginal portion. These are usually normal findings, however, due to Nabothian follicles which are harmless, or irregularities of the cervical lips following childbirth. Occasionally, bands of fibrous tissue may be present across the vagina in the upper third, sometimes involving the cervix. These need surgical division.

Finally, *trauma* can be a cause of genital swellings. Typically, bruising of the vulva may be presented in a child who has fallen astride an object; spontaneous resolution is usually the rule in such provided the urethra is not obstructed and there is no laceration. In either of these conditions, the child should be referred to hospital. Trauma can occur in relation to sexual behaviour, sometimes self-inflicted. In these cases there is likely to be a psychosexual problem that needs attention. Otherwise genital damage may result from marital violence, but serious damage to the genital tract is fortunately uncommon in such cases. Haematoma may require surgical drainage and lacerations may need repair.

Vaginal discharge

It is important to be aware of the variation in secretion of vaginal fluid among individuals. The source of this is twofold: the cervical mucus which flows out of the cervical canal quite profusely in some women at mid-cycle, and vaginal secretion proper which is a transudate through the mucosal lining of the vaginal walls. To these fluids are added the desquamated keratinized material from the vaginal epithelium. The origin of the vaginal fluid is the blood supplying this tissue and the amount produced depends to some extent on the amount of vascular flow. In response to sexual stimulation, for example, quite a large amount of watery fluid is normally produced at an early stage. It is possible that conditions leading to chronic congestion of pelvic veins may lead to the production of extravaginal fluid. It may be necessary to explain this aspect of physiology to a woman complaining of vaginal discharge that she considers abnormal, when in reality she may be showing a variation of the normal range. Changes in the amount of secretion may occur in women taking combined oestrogen-progestogen pills for contraception.

A further complication can arise if a woman feels unduly ashamed of her apparently excessive secretion and sets about trying to eliminate it by 'being cleaner'. This usually involves excessive washing with soap and water, to which a strongly irritant disinfectant may have been added. Such activities will probably cause irritation of the vulva and may induce a vaginal discharge in response to chemical irritation, particularly if frequent vaginal douching is also carried out. For this reason treatment by douche is usually discouraged nowadays in this country, and it is clearly important that the attitude of such patients to their own bodily secretions be changed to a more rational view.

Pathologically, vaginal discharges can be caused by conditions in the vaginal structures themselves or from abnormalities higher up the genital tract. The squamous epithelium of the vaginal wall or the vaginal portion of the cervix may become inflamed: a *vaginitis* or *cervicitis*. These tissues then appear bright red instead of pink, with sometimes a fine network of dilated blood vessels. There may be an exudate, typically like white wet blotting paper in *vaginal candidiasis*, with roughening of the normally glistening smooth surface. The material in the vaginal lumen may be yellow and creamy, or frothy and muco-purulent. These appearances are more characteristic of *trichomoniasis* or gardnerella vaginalis. The latter has a strongly fishy odour. These are common conditions and diagnosis should be confirmed by sampling with a charcoal-impregnated swab and transferring this into Stuart's medium for transporting to the laboratory. *Trichomonas vaginalis* is easy to identify under direct microscopy in a drop of normal saline. Treatment should be started with topical nystatin or clotrimazole (Canesten) if the presence of *Candida albicans* is suspected, or by oral metronidazole for trichomonas or gardnerella (nystatin pessaries, one inserted at night for 15 days or Canesten vaginal tablets 200 mg, one inserted nightly for three nights; metronidazole tablets, 200 mg three times a day, for seven days). Patients taking metronidazole should be warned not to take alcohol concurrently as the combination can cause disulfiram-type reactions. Candidiasis, trichomoniasis and gardnerella have been called sexually transmitted infections but they are not invariably contracted through intercourse with an infected partner. These organisms can remain dormant in a male partner and reinfect the patient when medication ceases. It is often advisable therefore to treat both partners simultaneously. In the case of candidiasis topical nystatin ointment can be applied once daily to the penis.

There has been a marked increase in the incidence of vaginal and vulval candidiasis in recent years. Broad-spectrum antibiotics have probably played a major part in causing this, as *Candida albicans* can overgrow in the intestinal flora of a person taking ampicillin or one of the tetracyclines. Vaginal candidiasis is also common in pregnancy and some authorities believe that taking the combined oestrogen-progestogen contraceptive pills causes a similar tendency. In a small number of patients with recurring severe infections resistant to treatment, it may ultimately be necessary to change to another method of contraception. In some patients all manoeuvres seem to fail to prevent symptoms recurring and in such cases the following regime may be helpful: two pessaries of nystatin should be inserted and kept in place with a tampon for 24 hours. Thereafter two pessaries should be inserted night and morning for six weeks (including the duration of any period), with a tampon worn in the daytime. Nystatin cream should be used on the vulva and the patient's partner should also use nystatin cream. Both parties should also take one tablet of oral nystatin (500,000 units) six hourly for ten days in an attempt to eliminate candida from the bowel. Patients should be advised not to wear tights and to boil underwear or wash it in a clothes washing machine. Daily baths should be taken in warm water, using bland soap only.

The results of bacteriological culture from vaginal swabs often report coliform bacilli, haemophilus, or anaerobic streptococci. The role of these organisms in causing vaginal discharge is uncertain but, if it is thought to be due to bacteria, an application such as a sulphonamide vaginal cream (Sultrin) can be used. A useful alternative is to prescribe a phosphate buffer jelly (Aci-jel) with the object of restoring and preserving the relatively acid pH inside the vagina. This discourages pathogens and promotes the normal flora.

Cervical erosions are essentially outgrowths of columnar epithelium from the canal on to the vaginal portion of the cervix. This occurs particularly after childbirth and is affected by hormonal changes. There is nothing abnormal in such a finding. Some erosions become 'infected', however, the tissues around them become inflamed, e.g. parametritis, and this can give rise to vaginal discharge. The soft-tissue inflammation will respond to broad-spectrum antibiotics. Occasionally the cervix will be improved by electric cautery: to be effective this usually needs to be done very thoroughly under general anaesthesia. Alternatives are cryocautery or touching with silver nitrate which can be done without an anaesthetic.

Fistula into the vagina causes persistent vaginitis and consequent vaginal discharge. These cases, fortunately rare, are usually difficult to detect on simple speculum examination. Vesico-vaginal fistula usually arises as an unfortunate sequel to instrumental delivery or pelvic surgery. It is usually easy to determine that urine is flowing from the vagina. Recto-vaginal fistula is more difficult to diagnose. Faecal material may be seen in the vagina but it may be necessary to use a dye to detect and locate the fistula. This is a complication of chronic proctitis, diverticulitis or ulcerative colitis. Referral to a specialist is necessary for treatment of these conditions.

A mild vaginitis and vaginal discharge can be set up by a *foreign body* inside the vagina, left in the vagina for more than a day or two: for example, a mislaid tampon, or sometimes, in children, stones or other objects placed in the vagina experimentally.

Vaginal discharges are common in association with lesions in the *upper genital tract. Carcinoma of the cervix* or the uterine *body*, may present as a complaint of vaginal discharge. *Endometritis* or *salpingitis*, usually of the chronic or subacute type, will usually lead to a muco-purulent discharge from the cervical canal. In these patients the vaginal mucosa will appear normal but the discharge may be heavy and smell unpleasant. A bacterial swab should be taken from the canal, as well as from the vaginal fluid. Inflammation of this kind may be associated with intra-uterine contraceptive devices (IUD). In the early stages, treatment with antibiotics is effective, leaving the device in the uterus. If symptoms

and signs persist for more than three days, the IUD must be removed.
Gonorrhoea is often symptomless in women. It can lead to chronic tubal inflammation with a persisting discharge. If this condition is suspected, as it should be in every case of persistent discharge, swabs should be taken from the cervical canal, the urethra and the rectum using transport medium, and special anaerobic culture for Neisseria requested. *Herpes genitalis* can affect the cervix causing discharge. It produces a typical vesicular lesion on the vaginal portion of the cervix.

Vulval and vaginal soreness

The group of symptoms included in this heading relate to the vulva and lower third of the vagina: itching, irritation and various kinds of pain. Here again, it is important to know the wide variations of normal appearances. For example, the relative sizes of different parts of the vulva vary and a woman may have marked reddening of the skin of the labia majora, but yet there may be no discomfort of any kind. There may also be disturbed sensation but no outward appearance of any abnormality. Patients with sexual difficulties can present with complaints of introital soreness on coital penetration, although tolerating digital examination fairly easily, as in moderate vaginismus. It is important to make sure of the exact nature of the presenting complaint.
Visible abnormalities causing soreness can be divided into specifically genital conditions: those arising as part of a skin disorder, which may be localized to the vulva or perineum; and those which are caused by a disease primarily of another system. An example of this last kind is the *vulvitis*, usually a candidal infection, associated with the glycosuria of *diabetes mellitus*. Another is the local dysuria and soreness caused by *chronic urinary-tract infection*, particularly if there is incontinence due, for example, to a neurological disorder such as multiple sclerosis, or in an elderly person with loss of sphincter control. Routine testing of the urine for sugar and albumen is an important investigation when assessing vulval or vaginal lesions.
One common cause of soreness in the genital area, often leading to entry dyspareunia after childbirth, is the painful episiotomy scar. The doctor should always ask about this at post-natal examination and find out digitally if it is tender. There is often a small reddened punched out linear depression in the centre of the scar at the fourchette. Simple advice such as regular nightly massage with chlorhexidine ointment or a simple cosmetic cream will quickly correct the disorder. But all too often it is not elicited by the doctor who pronounced the woman 'quite all right' after having her baby.

When coitus proves acutely painful, a situation can be set up in a marriage which can lead to serious discord over the ensuing months.

Skin conditions affecting the vulva commonly seen in general practice include *psoriasis*, *fungal infections*, *contact dermatitis* (e.g. from soaps or detergents), or much less commonly exanthemata such as *chickenpox*, *molluscum contagiosum*, *lichen planus*, *atopic eczema*. Treatment depends on recognizing the condition in this situation and treating accordingly. Referral to a dermatologist may be indicated in resistant cases, for confirmation of diagnosis and further advice.

Specifically genital lesions are usually infective, but also include the age change following falling oestrogen levels, e.g. *atrophic vulvovaginitis*, in post-menopausal women. The effect of this is very variable. Many women show an atrophic appearance, but only a minority feel intense irritation and itching with discharge. The condition responds well to oestrogen therapy either locally as, for example, dienoestrol cream applied at first twice daily, tailing off, as symptoms improve, to once weekly. Some clinicians prefer oral hormone replacement therapy, such as ethinyloestradiol, 10 micrograms once or twice daily, provided there are no contraindications to systemic oestrogen supplements.

Kraurosis vulvae, possibly a severe degree of atrophic vulvitis, sometimes causes irritation. There is reddening and keratinous thickening of parts of the vulva. *Leukoplakia* is rare but has a similar appearance. *Carcinoma of the vulva* is sometimes painful and will present either as a warty growth or an ulcer with rolled edge, fortunately not often seen in general practice. Patients with these conditions should clearly be referred to a gynaecologist for confirmatory opinion and treatment.

Sexually transmitted infections affect the vulva, such as *chancroid* and *syphilitic chancre*, fortunately rarely seen today in general practice in the United Kingdom, but always to be borne in mind. The latter is characterized by associated inguinal lymph node enlargement but is not usually painful.

Trichomoniasis is common and probably not exclusively transmitted by sexual activity. Irritation and dysuria are common: treatment is with oral metronidazole.

Candidiasis is also common and often causes intense itching.

Herpes genitalis gives intense burning pain and the appearance of the vulva can be very alarming. Although self-limiting with time, this condition is difficult to relieve by treatment. Cold normal saline soaks may help. Idoxuridine paint may help persistent lesions.

Genital warts (condylomata acuminata) are often transmitted by sexual contact; so is *pediculosis pubis*: infestation with pubic lice or 'crabs'. This is easily treated with application of gamma benzene hexachloride.

Gonorrhoea in women is usually symptomless but there may be vulvovaginitis with irritation and discharge, or dysuria for a few days due to the urethritis. Cowper's glands may be red and enlarged, and a bead of pus may appear at the urethral meatus with digital pressure forwards along the anterior wall of the vagina. Referral to a venereologist should be arranged for full diagnosis and treatment.

Miscellaneous conditions causing vulval symptoms include *Behcet's syndrome*, rarely seen, consisting of vulval ulcers associated with ocular inflammation; *aphthous ulceration* associated with stomatitis, and *lichen sclerosus et atrophicus. Varicose veins* in the labia majora may be painful or cause skin irritation during late pregnancy.

As with vaginal discharges, so also in patients with vulval soreness the attitude of the patient to her condition may be very important. A great deal of vigorous cleansing with soap or disinfectants may have preceded the consultation. It is vital to advise against further activities of this kind. Vaginal deodorants in aerosol sprays may have been used and may well have produced a florid contact dermatitis themselves, and bubble baths can be particularly irritant. A constantly worn sanitary towel attempting to control a vaginal discharge may induce vulval soreness. Finally there is often the fear at the back of the patient's mind that she has either a venereal disease, or cancer. These anxieties should be brought out into the open and discussed sensibly and sympathetically. Patients often feel they have been silly to have such feelings and they may not easily admit to them in front of a doctor.

Although some specific treatments have been mentioned, there may well be none that is applicable to a patient with vulval discomfort and it may be necessary to prescribe in order to alleviate the symptoms. Itching may require oral medication, especially overnight, with an antipruritic such as trimeprazine tablets (Vallergan), 10 to 20 mg taken on going to bed. Pain may require analgesics such as soluble codeine compound tablets, or Coproxamol, one or two tablets six hourly. Besides the local preparations already mentioned, calamine lotion may relieve perineal rashes but is very desiccating on the vulva itself. A corticosteroid application, such as 1 per cent hydrocortisone ointment, is often helpful if there is a marked inflammatory reaction, e.g. in contact dermatitis, or this may be combined with an antifungal agent, e.g. nystatin and hydrocortisone.

Finally there is the importance of the doctor himself. He must listen to the complaints carefully and appear unhurried; in particular, he must be willing to carry out a careful genital and pelvic examination. He must then also be willing to try persistently to relieve the patient's distress. All too often, on account of the psychosomatic connotation of the sexual organs, such patients fail to receive the attention that is their due.

Further Reading

Friend, J.R. (1970): Vaginal discharge. *Update*, *2*, 841

Novak, E.R. and Woodruff, J.D. (1974): *Gynaecologic and Obstetric Pathology.* 7th ed., pp. 1–69. London: W.B. Saunders

Rook, A., Wilkinson, D.S. and Ebling, F.J. (1968): *Textbook of Dermatology*, pp. 1547–1563. Oxford: Blackwell

3.60
The woman complaining of menopausal symptoms

Deborah Sharp

The word menopause is derived from the Greek words *men* month and *pausis* halt and simply means the end of menstruation. The word climacteric, again from the Greek, more accurately describes the whole transitional phase during which ovarian function diminishes and symptoms of oestrogen deficiency amongst others may be experienced.

The mean age for the menopause in western countries is just over 50 (range 40–57 years) but a woman does not know she has reached the menopause until it is passed. Amenorrhoea for over a year is the usual criterion. Before the beginning of this century it was unusual for many women to live beyond the age of 50 but now most will reach this age and in the developed world, live another 30 years. Thus most women will live one third of their life in the post-menopausal state of oestrogen deficiency. It is not known from the literature as to how many women actually experience menopausal symptoms nor what percentage of women consult their doctor specifically for them. Possibly 75% of women will experience the symptom 'hot flushes', but only one quarter will seek help from their doctor[1]. However the accuracy of any consultation figures for perimenopausal women is suspect and the term 'change of life' may well be appropriate and an aid to remembering that there are many alterations to a woman's life at around the age of 50, not all of them due to diminishing ovarian function. Transient depression, loss of confidence, emotional lability and minor neurotic illness are all common around this time and to label the reason for consultation as being due to the menopause may be misleading.

Hormonal changes

The exact mechanism responsible for triggering the endocrine changes of the climacteric has still not been established. It is clear that the menopause is not a sudden hormonal event but rather a series of gradual changes occurring over a period of years. The decline in ovarian function towards the end of the fifth decade produces falling levels of oestrogens, in particular oestradiol. In response to this removal of the negative feedback effect of oestradiol on the anterior pituitary, levels of the gonadotrophins, luteinizing hormone (LH) and follicle stimulating hormone (FSH) rise dramatically.

The LH level is increased to three to four times the pre-menopausal level in the year after the last menstrual period and the FSH level to some 15–20 times. Oestradiol levels fall to approximately one-tenth of those found at the lowest level in the menstrual cycle. The high levels of gonadotrophins presumably represent an attempt by the pituitary to stimulate the failing ovary which still has significant numbers of primordial follicles with normal oocytes present inside them. The hormone imbalance that these changes induce probably accounts for the irregularities seen in the menstrual cycle — variations in blood loss and cycle length and an increased incidence of anovular cycles. Thus symptoms of oestrogen deficiency may appear before menstruation has ceased completely. The post-menopausal ovary continues to secrete small amounts of oestrogens and androgens for many years after the menopause and the adrenal gland also contributes to the hormonal pool. This is most important when considering those women who have a surgical menopause, i.e. have both ovaries removed and will thus experience a sudden fall in oestrogen levels and also lose a major source of post-menopausal hormones.

Physical changes

The falling hormone levels produce obvious changes in the oestrogen-dependent structures of the body. Atrophic changes occur in the vagina and vulva. The vaginal mucosa becomes thin, dry and atrophic, causing the vagina to narrow and the vault to become continuous with the cervix. There is a loss of glycogen and Doederlein's bacilli; the pH rises and this can lead to superimposed infection by pathogenic organisms. The urethral changes may give rise to dysuria and frequency, and atrophy of the bladder mucosa of the trigone may be responsible for the urge incontinence that some women experience. The body skin loses its collagen and this leads to wrinkling. The breasts undergo similar changes causing them to lose their contours and decrease in size.

The most important long term consequence of oestrogen depletion is on the bones. Oestrogen acts as an anti-parathyroid hormone, preventing loss of calcium from the skeleton into the urine. While both men and women lose bone mass after the age of 40, the rate of mineral loss by post-menopausal women is about 3 times that in men, falling at a mean rate of 1% per annum so that by the age of 70 a 30% reduction in skeletal mass will have occurred. This post-

menopausal osteoporosis which is due to the increase in bone resorption leads to an increase in fractures of trabecular bone, i.e. of the vertebral bones, upper femur and lower radius. There is good evidence to support a causal relationship between loss of ovarian function and osteoporosis. Although exogenous oestrogen administration cannot reverse already established osteoporosis, it can retard its further progress. Placebo controlled trials in menopausal women have shown a benefit for oestrogen therapy in terms of prophylaxis against further bone loss. Osteoporotic fractures are a serious cause of morbidity and mortality in older women and fractured neck of femur in particular results in a substantial cost to the NHS in England. The use of long term oestrogen administration in post-menopausal women in an effort to prevent many of them developing osteoporosis and thereby reduce the number of fractures, is now gaining more widespread acceptance.
Coronary artery disease is very uncommon in pre-menopausal women who appear to be protected during their reproductive life by their oestrogens. After the menopause, the death rates from ischaemic heart disease increase very rapidly in women, more rapidly than in men of a similar age, and this has posed the suggestion that exogenous oestrogen administration might be used to prevent this increase in cardiovascular morbidity. However there is no conclusive evidence from the studies so far performed that oestrogen therapy has a role in the prevention of heart disease in post-menopausal women, the risks outweighing the benefits in this particular instance.

Presentation of problem

The evaluation of the clinical features thought to be entirely due to the menopause is difficult. There has been an unfortunate tendency amongst both doctors and patients to attribute all complaints of middle-aged women to this single cause. Some menopausal symptoms are certainly related to falling hormone levels — the vasomotor instability causing hot flushes or sweats and atrophic changes in the vagina and urethra. The later metabolic effects such as osteoporosis also have a hormonal basis. However, whether the host of psychological symptoms that occur at this time are causally or casually related to declining ovarian function is still the subject of much controversy.

Hot flushes and sweats

The hot flush (or flash as it is called in the USA) often followed by profuse sweating, is the commonest symptom experienced by menopausal women and that which most often compels them to seek medical advice. This vasomotor phenomenon, directly related to falling oestrogen levels, is often experienced before menstruation has ceased completely. It causes sudden dilatation of skin blood vessels, resulting in flushing of the skin, and a rise in skin temperature followed by perspiration and in many cases palpitations. The exact cause of the hot flush is unknown but some degree of disturbance of thermo-regulatory control is thought likely, possibly at the level of the hypothalamus. There is a great variation in susceptibility to hot flushes despite the fact that all women go through the same hormone changes. However the most intense symptoms do tend to occur when the hormone levels fall sharply such as after surgical removal of the ovaries. The symptoms respond well to oestrogen replacement therapy although why this is so is not clear and the symptoms do remit spontaneously with time as the body readjusts to the new low hormone levels. Hot flushes occur at any time of day or night, but as they tend to be more severe at night they may be responsible for some of the secondary or psychological symptoms such as insomnia, fatigue, irritability and depression. Thus relief of hot flushes, ensuring a good night's sleep, may greatly improve a woman's general well-being.

Genito-urinary symptoms

Irregular periods in the years leading up to the menopause are normal and the variations in cycle length enormous. In addition, heavy bleeding, pelvic pain and inter-menstrual bleeding are not uncommon and may require investigation. This will always be required if a woman presents with post-menopausal bleeding — vaginal bleeding after one year's amenorrhoea. Atrophy of the vaginal mucosa leads to narrowing of the vagina and reduced secretions, both of which predispose towards dyspareunia. In addition the change in pH may create a more favourable environment for pathogenic micro-organisms. As well as a feeling of dryness, women often complain of soreness or itching and may have a discharge or even bleeding.

Similar changes in the urethra may lead to the symptoms of the 'urethral syndrome' with frequency and dysuria, often in the absence of infection. Urge incontinence due to trigonitis may also be a problem due to atrophic changes in the oestrogen sensitive bladder mucosa.

Musculo-skeletal

Aches and pains are commonly reported by women at this time and this may be due to the increased laxity of ligaments and reduced muscular strength that occurs after ovarian failure. These generalized aches and pains should be distinguished from arthritis and psychological illnesses both of which commonly appear around this time and which may co-exist with other menopausal symptoms.

Psychological and psychosexual symptoms

There have been considerable differences of opinion about the significance of emotional symptoms occurring at the time of the menopause and their relationship, if any, to hormonal changes at this time. Common complaints are of tiredness, insomnia, depression, irritability, inexplicable mood swings and anxiety. It is possible to link some of these indirectly with hormonal changes (e.g. tiredness to disturbance of sleep by night sweats) but it would appear that the prevalence of psychiatric disorder in women in this age group is more likely to be a function of age rather than the onset of the menopause itself. Changes in role and lifestyle are the norm for most 50-year-old women — children leaving home, parents becoming ill and dying, the prospect of retirement, both their own and their spouses', are just some of the life stresses which may be present.

In particular, a decrease in self-esteem and self-confidence due to her changing physical appearance and perceived loss of sexual attractiveness, may make a woman particularly vulnerable to the simultaneously declining sexual interest of her husband. He may try to attract the attention of a younger woman with whom he can prove his (waning) potency. A daughter, whose attractiveness and sexuality are increasing, may suddenly be seen as a competitor for the affections of male friends, neighbours and relations.

Community studies have not shown a clear association between depression and the menopause; in fact results seem to favour an increase in psychiatric disturbance *before* the menopause, related to age rather than cessation of periods[2]. Certainly there is no good evidence implicating oestrogen levels with depressive symptomatology and the results of treatment trials with oestrogen have been disappointing. It is probably wisest to treat depressed menopausal patients with methods appropriate to depression at any other time of life.

The climacteric affects sexual relations both emotionally and physically. Some of the problems are related to both partners. For the woman, dyspareunia often results from the narrowing and dryness of the vagina and this discomfort results in less enjoyment of intercourse and a loss of libido. Men who may be experiencing erectile difficulties and feeling inadequate themselves can have further difficulties if their partner does not seem responsive to their sexual advances. Sexual activity, particularly intercourse, does decrease with age — but at a time when a woman may most need support and attention from her partner, a continuing and satisfying sex life may well help to promote her self-confidence and re-vitalize a marriage after many years building a home and bringing up children.

Diagnosis

The diagnosis of the climacteric is usually quite straightforward in post-menopausal women of previously good mental health and with symptoms of recent onset. The findings of hot flushes and sweats are virtually diagnostic and vaginal dryness is also a strong indicator. These characteristic symptoms together with loss of libido, loss of energy, headaches and irritability make the diagnosis almost certain to be one of the climacteric. It is not always quite so easy, especially if a woman is still menstruating or has had a hysterectomy. In these instances, it may be necessary to measure hormone levels and the most useful are gonadotrophins. An FSH level of greater than 15 iu/l is diagnostic.

It is important not to overlook other diagnoses. A woman who complains only of tiredness and lethargy may have anaemia from menorrhagia. Thyroid function tests may be useful, again if menorrhagia is present together with lethargy and weight gain. The diagnosis of a primary psychological illness should also be considered.

Management

In any woman who presents with symptoms attributable to the climacteric and in whom treatment is contemplated, a pelvic examination, including a cervical smear, a breast examination, blood pressure and weight check should be performed. A complaint of abnormal bleeding may require a curettage to exclude endometrial carcinoma, especially if hormonal treatment is required.

Treatment should be tailored to the problem: if depression is the major complaint, an anti-depressant may be given; if a psychosexual problem is apparent, seeing the couple together or referral to a specialist agency might be appropriate. However most climacteric symptoms respond well to hormone replacement therapy with oestrogens and this may well be what the patient will request, having heard so much about it in the media and in women's magazines.

Hormone replacement therapy

Modern hormone replacement therapy is extremely effective in treating physical menopausal symptoms and, as long as certain checks are made, is very safe. The scares in the early 1970s due to reports from the USA of an association between oestrogen therapy and endometrial cancer, made some doctors wary of its use. However, more recent studies have shown that there is no risk of endometrial cancer if a progestogen is added to the oestrogen for at least seven days of each cycle[3]. There are however certain contraindications to oestrogen therapy which can be seen in Table 1.

Absolute	*Relative*
Breast carcinoma	Hypertension
Endometrial carcinoma/hyperplasia	Thromboembolic disease
Ovarian carcinoma	Myocardial infarction
Acute liver disease	Cerebrovascular accident
Chronic impaired liver function	Benign breast disease
	Obesity
	Heavy smoking
	Oestrogen-dependent pelvic disease
	Abnormal lipid profile

Table 1. — Absolute and relative contra-indications to oestrogen therapy

Women receiving the usual doses of post menopausal oestrogen replacement therapy show some laboratory evidence of abnormal changes in their blood clotting mechanisms. However, no studies have demonstrated an increased risk of clinical thrombo-embolic events; neither stroke nor myocardial infarction. There is, however, an increased incidence of hypertension in women receiving oestrogens, but for most individuals the rise in blood pressure is not clinically significant. It should be remembered that the usual doses of oestrogen in replacement therapy are less than half those used in the oral contraceptive pill.

A large variety of hormone preparations, mainly oestrogens with or without progestogen and also testosterone, are available for treating menopausal symptoms. It is most important to choose the right preparation for each woman so that both risks and side-effects are minimized.

In women with an intact uterus it is most unwise to prescribe unopposed oestrogens due to the risk of endometrial hyperplasia which may progress to adenocarcinoma. Unopposed oestrogens should only be used in women who have had a hysterectomy or who cannot tolerate progestogenic side-effects. There is some evidence, albeit very slight, that because the oestrogen receptors in the breast are very similar to those in the endometrium, there may be a slightly increased risk of developing breast cancer when oestrogens alone are prescribed. Therefore in practice, it is usual to recommend that all women requiring hormone replacement therapy should have a combined oestrogen and progestogen preparation.

The decision as to whether continuous or cyclical treatment should be given depends largely on whether a progestogen is deemed necessary by both doctor and patient. If in a woman who has had a hysterectomy, oestrogen alone is prescribed, then continuous therapy is more usual since a cyclical regimen is only required to allow shedding of the endometrium. If a combined preparation is to be used, oestrogens may still be given continuously (28 days) with the progestogen being added in for the final 10 to 13 days of the cycle. It is more usual however, to prescribe a preparation which gives a tablet-free week, with oestrogens being taken for 21 out of 28 days and progestogens for the latter 7 to 10 days — this is called sequential therapy.

For women who have not yet stopped menstruating, the vaginal bleeding in the week off therapy will be quite acceptable and should be light and painless. However, for post-menopausal women the return to regular periods may encourage them to request an oestrogen only preparation and GPs should be prepared to explain fully the reason for using preparations that cause a withdrawal bleed.

The various oestrogen or oestrogen/progestogen preparations have little to choose between them but in general, natural oestrogens rather than the synthetic ones used in contraceptive pills are to be preferred, as they are less likely to be associated with thromboembolic disease. As well as different types and doses of oestrogens, different progestogens are available in the various combination packs and sometimes if side-effects are a problem, e.g. breast tenderness, then changing to a pill with a different progestogen may be helpful. Table 2 shows the types of oral hormone replacement therapy available.

Oestrogen vaginal creams are particularly useful if the only problem is atrophic vaginitis. It is important to remember that it is possible to achieve the same blood levels of oestrogen using the vaginal route as by the oral route if administration is not supervised carefully. This should be used sparingly and infrequently, perhaps after an initial course of daily use.

Hormone implants have recently gained increasing favour. This method of hormone replacement therapy is particularly useful in the woman who has had a hysterectomy, perhaps quite early in life. As well as implanting 100 mg of oestradiol subcutaneously, a testosterone implant can be inserted simultaneously. Testosterone, which is not very safe when taken orally, particularly helps the problem of loss of libido that young women who have a

Preparation	*Daily dose*	*Schedule*
Oral oestrogens (to be used alone in women without a uterus or in combination with a progestogen)		
Ethinyl oestradiol	0.01 mg	once/twice daily
Piperazine oestrone sulphate (Harmogen)	1.5/3 mg	once/twice daily
Oestradiol valerate (Progynova)	1/2 mg	once daily
Conjugated equine oestrogens (Premarin)	0.625/1.25/2.5 mg	once daily
Oral progestogens (to be added to oestrogens for the last 7 to 10 days of the cycle or used alone where oestrogens are contra-indicated)		
Norethisterone (Primolut N)	5 mg	one/three daily
Medroxyprogestrone acetate (Provera)	5 mg	daily

Combined oestrogens and progestogens
(the preferred treatment for most women)

Proprietary name	*Oestrogen*	*Days*	*Progestogen*	*Days*
Cycloprogynova	Oestradiol valerate 1/2 mg	21	Levonorgestrel 0.25 mg	10
Prempak	Conjugated equine oestrogens 0.625/1.25 mg	21	Norgestrel 0.5 mg	7
Prempak C	Conjugated equine oestrogens 0.625/1.25 mg	28	Norgestrel 0.15 mg	12
Menophase	Mestranol 20–50 μg	28	Norethisterone 0.75/1.5 mg	13
Trisequens	Oestradiol 1/2 mg Oestriol 0.5/1 mg	28	Norethisterone acetate 1 mg	10

Table 2. Hormone replacement therapy

premature menopause (for whatever reason) complain of, and which is not improved by oestrogens alone. If an implant is used in a woman with an intact uterus, then oral progestogens should be given for 7 to 10 days each month to induce a withdrawal bleed. A woman receiving hormone replacement therapy should be closely monitored — the surveillance should be similar to that given to women on the contraceptive pill. She should be seen about every six months for blood pressure, weight and breast check and to enquire about any irregular bleeding. Cervical smears are only necessary every three years unless otherwise indicated. Any irregular bleeding should be investigated by endometrial biopsy

and some specialists recommend that any women taking unopposed oestrogens should have yearly biopsies.
It is not clear for how long therapy should be continued, but the rule of giving the lowest effective dose for the shortest possible time is a good one to adhere to. The duration of symptoms is so variable that it is usually necessary to stop therapy (gradually) and then assess whether the symptoms return.

Non-hormonal therapy

Although in general non-hormonal treatments are less effective than oestrogens, for those women in whom there are absolute contraindications to hormone replacement therapy and in those women who do not wish to be treated with hormones there are some useful alternatives. Oral progestogens alone are rarely prescribed but can relieve the hot flushes and night sweats. The two progestogens used in this way are norethisterone (5 mg daily) and medroxyprogesterone acetate (5 mg daily). Clonidine (Dixarit) and a mixture of phenobarbitone, ergotamine and belladona alkaloids (Bellergal) may also be used to control hot flushes. Both of these have some sedative properties and therefore may also help in relieving sleeplessness.

Counselling

Many women who present to the doctor with climacteric symptoms do not require any drug treatment at all. For women who have more complex psychosocial problems, traditional counselling or brief psychotherapy may be required. Many of the complaints and problems that present at this time of life have nothing to do with the climacteric and are age-related rather than 'disease' related. The doctor should not be too quick to reach for his prescription pad — a listening ear and reassurance of the normality of the patient's symptoms may be all that is required.

References

[1] Dewhurst, C.J. (1976): In: *The Management of the Menopause and Post-Menopausal Years*. ed. Stuart Campbell, Lancaster: MTP
[2] Osborn, M. (1984): Depression at the Menopause. *British Journal of Hospital Medicine*, 126–129
[3] Studd, J.W.W., et al. (1980): *The Prevention and Treatment of Endometrial Pathology in Post-Menopausal Women Receiving Exogenous Oestrogens*. In: *The Menopause and Post-Menopause*. ed. N. Pasetto et al. p 127. Lancaster: MTP

3.61 Difficulties with sexual intercourse

Michael Courtenay

Although direct complaints of difficulties in sexual intercourse to general practitioners seemed to be rare at the beginning of the 1970s (less than 0.2% in a study of symptoms brought to a general practice in Lambeth[1]), there is an impression that in the second half of the 1980s they are becoming more common. On the other hand symptoms which often mask some difficulty with sexual intercourse accounted for more than 10% in this study and included disturbances of sleep, anxiety, depression, pain in the abdomen, back and genital organs, as well as the ill-defined symptoms of lack of energy. It is probable that sexual function in almost all people is subject to occasional difficulty over time, but that most problems are dealt with by those concerned in their own way.

Presentation of complaint

As has been indicated, overt symptoms of sexual problems are less often presented in general practice. It therefore usually falls to the general practitioner to identify the patient's problem when faced with such general complaints as depression, the need for a tonic, tiredness, backache, pelvic pain or menstrual irregularities.

The most common problems in men are premature ejaculation, erectile impotence and occasionally non-ejaculation. Shapiro[2] distinguished two groups of patients presenting with premature ejaculation. The first are young men who have good erections, but from the start of their erectile awareness have experienced rapid ejaculation. The second group are older men who, after years of normal ejaculation, find themselves ejaculating quickly, often associated with erectile problems. Three types of erectile impotence may be encountered. In the first, the man may fail completely to obtain an erection. In the second, an erection is obtained but it is not sufficient to permit easy penetration. Thirdly, there are those men who attain a normal erection, but this collapses before it can be used. Non-ejaculation, which is much less common, may rarely occur in young men, or rather more commonly in elderly men after years of normal sexual function.

In women, the most commonly encountered problems are pain on sexual intercourse (dyspareunia), an inability to permit penile entry to the vagina (vaginismus) and failure to achieve orgasm. Some women totally fail to achieve orgasm. Others may achieve orgasm in response to direct clitoral stimulation, but not in response to penile penetration of the vagina.

All the problems identified may be primary or secondary, i.e. they may have been present from the start of the individual's sexually active life or they may develop after a period of normal sexual functioning.

While difficulties individually experienced by men and women almost invariably affect the sexual union, one problem may occur in either sex and this is loss of libido. This may stem from any of the problems described, but can also develop in the course of what has previously been a satisfying relationship.

Causes

Communications. — Many of the difficulties with sexual intercourse encountered in general practice result from lack of understanding or lack of consideration for the needs of the sexual partner. This can be, and very frequently is complicated by poor communication between the partners, which may result from shyness, lack of a suitable vocabulary or, in some cases, a self-centred approach to intercourse, which may be seen more as an athletic pursuit than an act of love. Any illness which reduces the general well-being of an individual will almost inevitably reduce his or her sexual performance and this may be a mental illness, e.g., depression, or chronic physical problems. Overwork and alcohol are two other potent sources of reduced sexual desire and performance.

Ageing. — The effect of ageing on sexual intercourse is also important to consider. In males, from about the sixth decade, the amount of stimulation required to produce an erection is greatly increased as is the time taken to achieve it. This may lead some men to feel that they are becoming impotent. As a result they become anxious and this, in turn, may lead to further difficulties and to a vicious circle, sometimes described as anxiety impotence. In fact, in older men, once erection is achieved it may persist for a longer time and ejaculation is often delayed. This altered pattern carries with it as many gains as losses from the female view point. In women the menopause brings with it a fall in the amount of circulating oestrogen. This sometimes leads to vaginal dryness and dyspareunia. It may also lead to changes in the skin and breasts which make the female feel less sexually attractive, and her confidence may be undermined, particularly if her partner seems to continue to attract the opposite sex.

Psychological. — The individual's attitude to sexuality is inevitably conditioned by the circumstances in which he or she has matured. Individuals brought up in families in which emotional succour is lacking, or where parents have been at enmity with each other, are unlikely to be sufficiently secure to give themselves in a loving relationship to another. Specific traumatic sexual experience in childhood, either observed or experienced, may equally deform the individual's sexual development. An attitude to sexuality, which associates the sexual organs with something unclean, can hardly encourage a healthy sexual relationship in later life. An association during sexual development of pain with sexual pleasure, may also lead to problems in developing a loving relationship. These sexual factors may present as primary impotence, premature ejaculation, vaginismus or lack of libido.

Secondary impotence. — This is a very common problem and has been reviewed in some detail by Jeffcote[3]. Conventional views on impotence are based on whether it is 'organic' or 'psychogenic', yet for most men the aetiology is mixed. Even if the initial erectile failure has organic causes the reactions of the man and his partner may determine the outcome. Too hasty a labelling of the symptom as 'organic' or 'psychogenic' may determine its management either by sympathetic nihilism or referral to a psychiatrist. The distinction is often based on inadequate grounds, as very little is currently known of the mechanisms of erection and erectile failure. Clearly blood flow into the corpora cavernosa will be impaired if arteriosclerotic changes have reduced the maximum arterial supply; reduced elasticity of the microvalves within them may make erection become more difficult (and also to persist longer), while reduced sensation in the genitalia would block the afferent limb of the excitatory reflex carried by the pudendal nerves when reflex stimulation becomes increasingly important with increasing age. Erection may be induced by stimulation of the sympathetic erectile or inhibition of the sympathetic anti-erectile fibres which run together from the hypogastric plexus. Studies on men with traumatic lesions of the spinal cord indicate that the parasympathetic system is essential for reflex erection but that psychogenic and sleep erection may be mediated by either pathway[4]. Little is known of the neurotransmitters concerned. Vasoactive intestinal polypeptide (VIP) almost certainly plays a part since it is present in the nerve fibres of the corpora cavernosa, and decrease of VIP has been demonstrated in the penises of impotent men[5]. Because so little is known, it is as difficult to exclude organic factors contributing to erectile failure in 'psychogenic' cases as it is wrong to ignore psychological factors in those which are 'organic'. If nocturnal penile tumescence is absent, considerably reduced, or short lived, erectile failure is likely to have at least some organic component.

The chances are increased if there is concomitant evidence of peripheral or autonomic neuropathy, peripheral vascular or cardiovascular disease, diabetes (especially with retinopathy) or excessive alcohol consumption. If nocturnal tumescence is normal the problem is usually assumed to be essentially psychogenic, but this interpretation must be made with caution since nocturnal penile tumescence tests only one aspect of the erectile mechanism. All this sounds very daunting to the general practitioner consulting in his surgery, but in practice there is much room for manoeuvre.

Premature ejaculation. — In younger men, unassociated with erectile problems, this is thought to be due to a lack of conscious awareness of the sensations which precede ejaculation. This awareness can, in many cases, be increased by behavioural therapy. As with impotence, however, the causes are multifactorial and in some cases serious psychological difficulties may contribute to the problem.

Dyspareunia. — This is frequently associated with local lesions in the female genital tract. These may vary from an imperforate hymen to senile vaginitis and include inflammatory conditions of the female pelvis, and endometriosis. A tender episiotomy scar is a common cause.

History and examination

In identifying a sexual problem, the first task is to define the nature of the complaint. In the case of impotence, for instance, is the man really complaining of erectile failure, and is it he who is complaining? The history may suggest gross social and psychological derangement, a debilitating or painful disease or depression. A medical examination will establish the presence or otherwise of normal genitalia, neuropathy, and peripheral vascular disease. Drugs may be incriminated, especially those used in the treatment of hypertension. A second interview can be arranged for a more detailed conversation with the man, and if possible, with his sexual partner.

The same principles can be used whatever the symptom of sexual difficulty presented. When it comes to taking a sexual history it is helpful to assume a bold strategy and not to rely on tentative questions which may allow the patient to hide behind a screen of embarrassment. It is wisest to assume that the patient has been and wishes to continue to be sexually active. Thus it is probably best to ask how often sexual activity occurs rather than ask when it occurs. If such activity is in doubt a question about the method of birth control used may encourage a shy patient to speak the truth. The amount and nature of sexual activity in the past may also be elicited by relaxed enquiry, not relying on direct questions more than is absolutely necessary. A detailed account of the nature of the sexual difficulty is essential. This may best be left to the second consultation suggested above.

Examination of the female genitalia will establish the diagnosis of vaginismus, as such an examination will be resisted. It is also useful in diagnosing the cause of dyspareunia by identifying possible infections, urethral caruncle, post-menopausal vaginitis, post-episiotomy syndrome, deep pelvic conditions including endometriosis, and cervical lesions. Orgasmic problems are not usually helped by examination, though a dry vagina may indicate lack of vaginal transudate production which is considered by many workers to be the female counterpart of a male erection. However, a professionally privileged examination is also a time when the feelings of the woman about sexuality can be explored with greater ease than when sitting and talking in the consulting room.

Management

Many patients presenting with difficulties in sexual intercourse are not suffering from major physical or psychological problems, but have difficulties in communicating with each other about their sexual relationships. They are not able to tell each other how or where they like to be touched or kissed, and as a result frustration and bitterness are engendered. Such problems can very easily be defused by a three-way consultation in which the doctor acts as a catalyst to promote communication between sexual partners. This is probably the most common and therapeutically most successful situation which the general practitioner encounters in his management of sexual problems.

Anxiety impotence is probably the next most common problem. In this, the usually middle aged man has, on one occasion, failed to achieve an erection or has ejaculated prematurely. On the next occasion, he becomes acutely aware and anxious about his performance and predictably fails again. A vicious circle of anxiety and failure is now being built up. Meanwhile, his wife may suspect that his failure with her is due to extra-marital affairs and the situation is ripe for severe marital disharmony. In this type of case, there is an urgent need for a careful assessment of the problem in a consultation involving the doctor, the husband and the wife. This should then lead on to a new approach to sexual relationships in which performance is set on one side, and feelings become paramount. This is the basis of the 'sensate focus technique'. In this, the couple are encouraged to revert to their feelings for each other in their courtship days. They are advised to abstain from sexual intercourse and from direct sexual stimulation for a period of time, but to re-live the joys of touching each other and being touched in a non-sexually directive way. In carefully controlled stages, they are then permitted to indulge in direct sexual stimulation and, in due course, to proceed to sexual intercourse. In the management of impotence, and in some cases of orgasmic failure in women, this behavioural therapy is very successful. With erectile failure of organic origin, there is no place for androgens, gonadotrophins, luteinizing hormone or dopamine receptor agonists in the absence of a defined endocrine abnormality. There are, however, some surgical options which should, perhaps, be more widely adopted in Britain than they are at present, although all implants do is to make the penis stand up. Very careful selection of patients is essential, but on the other hand, high satisfaction rates have been reported[6]. Non-ejaculation is a very difficult symptom to treat, except in the context of the ageing man.

Premature ejaculation may be treated by the 'squeeze technique' first described by Semans and developed by Masters and Johnson. This technique is used in the context of the behavioural treatment they advocate. Initially, the couple are instructed in the sensate focus technique. This provides a series of exercises in which the couple are encouraged to re-learn their mode of physical communication, first in a relatively unerotic manner and then in a more erotic one until the specific technique of encouraging erection and then discouraging ejaculation by pressing the penis below the glans to inhibit the reflex. When ejaculatory control has been achieved in terms of manual stimulation, then introduction of the penis into the vagina, with the woman astride the man, forms the next stage with inhibition of ejaculation being undertaken when the man feels it approaching. When control has been achieved in this position, any position can be adopted. This method is set out by Kaplan[7]. Clomipramine 10 mgm or more at night may help in those cases where the partner will not help or the squeeze technique fails.

The treatment of vaginismus is concerned with helping the patient to become familiar with her own body and to enjoy self-examination and stimulation. The technique for treatment of this condition is described by Tunnadine[8]. Dyspareunia should be treated by applying remedies to the cause whether it be treating an infection, dealing with some pelvic pathology or applying hormones to the post-menopausal vaginitis. The application of a local anaesthetic to a tender episiotomy scar, together with stretching the introitus, by the patient herself until comfortable introduction of 3 fingers is possible, will assure her that penile intromission will no longer be painful. This technique is most easily taught in the surgery setting. Treatment of orgasmal difficulties in the female may also be approached by use of the sensate focus technique. In the course of using this, it may become apparent that there are some major psychological problems and counselling by doctors working with the Institute of Psychosexual Medicine[9], may be helpful.

Conclusion

Sexual difficulties are common, often camouflaged, and of all grades of severity. Many are simple and within the competence of a general practitioner without specialized training to treat. Some extra time will need to be spent but not necessarily more than can be accommodated in the surgery consultation. What is required is a little bit of science and a lot of sensitivity.

References

[1] Morrell, D.C., Gage, H.G. and Robinson, N.A. (1971): Symptoms in General Practice. *Journal of the Royal College of General Practitioners*, *21*, 32

[2] Shapiro, P. (1943): Premature ejaculation. Review of 1,130 cases. *Journal of Urology*, *50*, 374–379

[3] Jeffcote, W.J. (1986): Impotence: Science and Sciencibility. *British Medical Journal*, *292*, 783–84

[4] Brindley, G.S. (1985): *Pathophysiology of erection and ejaculation*. In: Whitfield, H.N., Hendry, W.F. eds. *Textbook of Genito-Urinary Surgery*, Vol 2, pp 1083–94. Edinburgh: Churchill Livingstone

[5] Gu, J., Lazarides, M. and Prior, J.P. (1984): Decrease of Vasoactive Intestinal Polypetide (VIP) in the Penises from Impotent Men. *The Lancet*, *2*, 315–317

[6] Whitehead, E.D. and Leiter, E. (1982): New frontiers in alloplastic genito-urinary prostheses II. The Surgical Management of Erectile Impotence. *NY State J Med*, *82*, 1806–11

[7] Kaplan, H.S. (1981): *The Illustrated Manual of Sex Therapy*. London: Granada Publishing Ltd

[8] Tunnadine, P. (1970): *Contraception and Sexual Life*. London: Tavistock Publications

[9] Institute of Psychosexual Medicine, 10 Chandos Street, London W1

3.62
The infertile couple

John McEwan

In a society in which families are small and some couples, a greatly increasing number, choose not to have children at all, the plight of those unable to have children when they want them becomes increasingly hard. This is accentuated by the difficulty in finding a child for adoption, now that fewer unwanted pregnancies are carried to term. The current prevalence of involuntary sterility cannot be determined exactly until demographers can look back on the present generation, when its capacity for reproduction will have passed.

It is believed that about 10 per cent of couples of child-bearing age cannot conceive. A larger proportion seeks advice and many achieve conception before any conscious medical treatment has been applied. Some conceive in spite of a negative prognosis or when the treatment applied could not have been expected to be operative. These factors lead to confusion over the determination of the incidence of infertility. Criteria for seeking advice vary, some couples waiting several years before coming to their general practitioner; others will attend anxiously after lack of success in the first month or two. The doctor's attitude is very important. On the one hand, practitioners should encourage patients who are worried about their fertility to attend early in case treatment is needed. On the other, it is futile to initiate time-consuming and expensive investigations or procedures when it is reasonably likely that the couple will conceive in a few months without medical intervention.

Physiological conception of pregnancy depends on:

1. An adequate number of normal spermatozoa in a normal seminal fluid,
2. Adequate insemination – that is contact between normal semen and normal cervical mucus – near to the time of ovulation,
3. Normal ovulation, normal tube transport of gametes and fertilized ovum, with synchronized endometrial maturation, to produce normal secretion in a normal uterine cavity,
4. Relatively quiescent uterine muscle,
5. Normal hormone production to support the early blastocyst.

It will be seen that these criteria depend on factors in the genital tracts of male and female as well as on aspects of sexual behaviour and the mechanics of coitus. The general practitioner can establish whether most of these factors are operating normally. Correction of faults in reproductive physiology in the male or the female is on the whole complex and requires specialized investigations and treatment which may be surgical or endocrinological. But a great deal can be done to help most couples before such intervention is indicated.

Presentation

When a couple comes complaining of infertility or delay in conceiving there are several items of information needed by the doctor to decide on a plan of management.

For a couple with normal physiology and average coital frequency it usually takes up to three or four months for the woman to become pregnant. If they have had no success after six months it is worth taking action to find out whether anything is wrong, bearing in mind that many such couples will conceive spontaneously soon anyway. The value of early action lies in helping the morale of the couple and in treating conditions such as post-pill anovulation as early as possible.

History

Once he has decided to act the doctor should take a careful history of gynaecological conditions in the woman and details of any previous pregnancies, being careful not to omit pregnancy with a previous partner. He must go over the medical history of both and the history of their sexual relationship. It is not unusual for couples to attend a specialist clinic for complex investigations only to find that there cannot be adequate insemination because of a sexual problem, such as very infrequent coitus or even failure to achieve penetration. Some couples may not even want a pregnancy but have reached the clinic because they have been unable to express their sexual difficulties in any other way than by complaining of inability of conceive. The interview with the general practitioner obviously plays a vital part in identifying and initiating a correct plan of management for such patients.

Regarding coital frequency, the woman should be highly fertile for two days either side of ovulation. It follows that a coital frequency of two to three times a week evenly spaced will ensure insemination at the right time.

A record of the woman's menstrual pattern gives useful information. Menstrual diary cards, such as those available from the Royal College of General Practitioners, are most helpful and their use may be combined with that of a Basal Body Temperature Chart. A chart showing regular cycles of about four weeks with an average menstrual loss requiring at least two changes of sanitary protection daily for three days or more implies regular ovulation. If there is variation in the duration or amount of blood loss from cycle to cycle, this may suggest irregular ovulation, accounting for the delay in conceiving. Periods that are always scanty or occur at intervals of 42 days or more suggest failure of ovulation, as do very short cycles of less than 21 days. In these cases probably it is best to refer straight away to a specialist unit for further investigation. The presence of galactorrhoea may indicate hyperprolactinaemia which, in some cases, could be due to pituitary adenoma. The condition can also occur with combined oral contraceptives and with phenothiazine medication.

Hypothyroidism can also lead to oligomenorrhoea but it may be part of a wider endocrine dysfunction, such as Simmond's (or Sheehan's) syndrome of hypopituitarism after a past experience of post-partum haemorrhage. Previous episodes of amenorrhoea or oligomenorrhoea, often associated with slimming diets, travelling or stress, may indicate an underlying weakness of ovulatory function. This may come to light after stopping combined oral contraceptive pills in order to become pregnant. Basal Body Temperature Charts are helpful for checking whether or when ovulation is occurring. Charts are available from Family Practitioner Committees (intended to be used for rhythm contraception) and a fertility thermometer can be prescribed on FPIO. It is important that the couple understand exactly how to use the thermometer and the chart. After three or four months the pattern of ovulation can be picked out from the chart.

A history of unremitting and severe dysmenorrhoea during menstruation may indicate endometriosis or chronic pelvic inflammation. Usually there is also deep dyspareunia and there may be similar episodes of pain between periods.

A history of previous pregnancy and its outcome, previous difficulty in conceiving and previous use of contraception are all important in assessing the causes of present failure to conceive. If there have been pregnancies on either side with a previous partner, this is helpful evidence. A history of sexually transmitted infections such as gonorrhoea is also clearly very important and if it has occurred in the man may indicate seminal fluid analysis as the first step.

At this stage, some practitioners will prefer to refer the couple to an infertility clinic for specialist investigation or, where such a clinic is not available, to refer the woman to a gynaecologist and the man to a urologist. It is best for both to be referred together as there may be factors on both sides and it is important for their relationship that the focus of 'blame' should not fall on either individually. The couple is 'the patient'.

Examination

If the general practitioner chooses to initiate the investigations himself – which is usually more helpful for the couple as the problems may require relatively simple remedies – he should start with a *post-coital test*. This is easily done if an ordinary microscope is available. At the same visit a bimanual pelvic examination of the woman can be done with speculum examination of cervix and vagina, cervical smears and bacterial swabs from the cervix and urethra to ascertain whether an infection is present. Routine urine testing and a blood count can also be done at this stage. The post-coital test is carried out as near as possible to the time of ovulation. The couple are required to have sexual intercourse 12 to 18 hours before the test. A portion of cervical mucus is aspirated and placed on a warm slide. Its physical characteristics are noted and it is examined under the microscope. If insemination is adequate there will be large numbers of actively mobile and progressing spermatozoa, obvious even in a low power field. Any other result is abnormal, and is due either to poor spermatogenesis, blocked vasa deferentia, abnormal mucus, unsatisfactory coitus or coital mechanics; or various combinations of these. Rarely there may apparently be a 'hostile' reaction to spermatozoa which some authorities consider to be an immune process. At this stage it is worth making sure that vaginal deodorants or heavily scented or deodorant-containing soaps are not used as any of these may have a spermicidal action.

Sperm production and transport in the male can be tested by a *seminal fluid analysis* which is best done by a suitable laboratory. Counts below 10 million mobile sperm per ml are associated with subfertility. A high proportion of abnormal forms may also indicate the need for treatment.

The quality of the *cervical mucus* can be assessed in several ways. Under the influence of oestrogen at the time of ovulation it should be profuse, clear and glistening with the capacity to be drawn out into threads of 10-15 cm between two points of attachment ('spinnbarkeit' or 'spinnability'). Under the microscope it should be clear rather than cellular and when the slide is allowed to dry slowly crystals are produced in an elegant branching pattern ('ferning'). If any of these features are deficient or absent, the mucus may be abnormal enough to prevent sperm transport up the cervical canal. It is important to be sure of the timing of the test in relation to ovulation, otherwise it is easy to draw false conclusions.

Management

If the post-coital test is normal and ovulation has been confirmed it is possible that there is a disorder of the uterus or fallopian tubes requiring specialist treatment. The prognosis is not good even with modern micro-surgical techniques if there is tubal obstruction. In such cases there may be hope in the future if the success of Steptoe and Edwards in achieving extra-corporeal fertilization with reimplantation into the uterine cavity can become a routine service procedure. At present the feasibility of a regular success rate is unproven.

The outlook for men with blocked vasa is a little better, the pregnancy rate after vasovasostomy being about 25-30 per cent in expert hands. The prognosis is better after mechanical obstruction, such as a contraceptive vasectomy, than if the block is the result of infection such as gonorrhoea. Deficient sperm production is becoming more amenable to treatment. Endocrine control of spermatogenesis is complex involving four separate hormones. Some patients respond to androgens, such as mesterolone, or to pituitary hormones, but treatment should be advised by a specialist who may need to carry out testicular biopsy.

One simple factor affecting sperm production is hyperthermia due to a varicocoele, tight clothing or excessive hot baths. It is always worthwhile for the general practitioner to go into this factor if the sperm count is low. A history of orchitis, such as in mumps, may lead to azoospermia if both testes have been affected. If in doubt careful examination of the testes may indicate atrophy with normal androgenic effects. Just occasionally a degree of hypospadias may be evident, which could effect insemination adversely.

If there is a problem of ovulatory failure and he is satisfied that all else is normal, it may be helpful for the general practitioner to try the effect of clomiphene therapy, which can be used at low dosage levels without laboratory control. The first stage is to give 50mg of clomiphene as an oral tablet once daily for five days, starting on the first day of a period, if these occur. Ovulation is expected to occur on the eighth day and if there is no conception a period will follow on about the 22nd day. If there is no bleeding, the woman may be pregnant. In this case the pregnancy test on urine will be positive by the 36th day after beginning the clomiphene treatment. If not, repeat the five days of clomiphene using 100mg daily. The Basal Body Temperature Chart should be used to monitor the procedure. If there are no signs of ovulation, the couple should be referred for endocrinological studies without further therapeutic trials.

If the cervical mucus remains poor and it is strongly suspected that ovulation is occurring normally, then it is worth giving a very small dose of oestrogen by mouth for three days in the pre-ovulatory phase, on days 10, 11 and 12 in a 28-day cycle. The dose is 10 micrograms of ethinyloestradiol daily for these three days. Such treatment over three months may improve the mucus without inhibiting ovulation.

Artificial insemination

If insemination is poor due to a problem of coital mechanics not easily corrected or if there is a relatively low sperm count, the couple may be advised to try artificial insemination using the husband's semen (A.I.H.). The couple may want to discuss this with their general practitioner and he can do a great deal to relieve anxiety, give correct information and reassure them. They may need to ventilate anxiety and irrational fears. Discussing these with a sympathetic family doctor can do much to prevent misunderstanding and tension in the future. The general practitioner can virtually take charge at this stage and give full instruction on the use of the Rocket Cup (obtainable from Rocket of London Ltd, Imperial Way, Watford, Herts.) for example. With this technique the woman inserts into her vagina a plastic cup with a tube attached centrally to lie against her cervix. The tube will project from the vulva. The husband produces seminal fluid by manual masturbation. A 20ml plastic syringe is required into which 10ml of air is first drawn and then the seminal fluid is aspirated. The syringe is applied to the Rocket Cup tube and the seminal fluid blown gently down the tube into the Cup against the woman's cervix. It is a simple method which can be carried out by the couple in privacy once they have become familiar with the apparatus.

The emotional problems may need more attention if the husband's semen is infertile and the couple are considering donor insemination (A.I.D.) This is an increasingly popular solution and is now available at several regional centres. It is obviously important that both man and woman have clear information about what is happening, have considered the implications in the long-term future and are in complete agreement over this policy of management. Others may prefer to adopt a child.

Adoption

Adoption will be considered as a solution also if some condition in the woman prevents conception, or if both have factors combining to make fertility unlikely or resistant to treatment. Adoption procedures are well organized and supervized by local authorities through the social service departments. The family doctor may be asked for advice and should be prepared to discuss the procedures and implications with the couple together or separately. He may have to give them support during the difficult time of social assessment and waiting for an offer. He should encourage them to attend one of the many groups of intending adopters which are now being organized in many areas. He may have to advise on the medical implications of accepting a child with an abnormality, such as a talipes or a minor congenital heart lesion. He will probably be required to examine the couple, or the prospective child for adoption, and give a report on their health. Sometimes the general practitioner is urged to act as guardian *ad litem,* that is to be legally in charge of the child's welfare during the trial period. As a general rule this is probably better avoided as it could put the doctor in a position of divided loyalty.

Patients' organization

Sometimes great help and support is obtained by people with medical problems if they are in touch with an association of patients in a similar situation. The National Association for the Childless (318, Summer Lane, Birmingham 19. Tel: 021-359 4887) provides a regular newsletter and holds twice-yearly meetings. There is an opportunity for social contact, particularly at festival times when other people tend to be with their families. Reliable medical information is also provided and clear explanations given about physiological processes concerned with reproduction.

Conclusion

The active involvement of the general practitioner during all these stages of investigation, treatment and counselling can give immediate help to infertile couples and in the long term can do much to prevent strains and tensions that may arise from disorders of fertility.

Further reading

Cooke, I.D. (1974): The Management of Infertility in Clinics in *Obstetrics and Gynaecology, 1(2).* London: W.B. Saunders

Davidson, H.A. (1968): The post-coital test, *The Practitioner, 201,* 467

Steptoe, P.C. and Edwards, R.G. (1978): Lancet, *2,* 366 (Letter)

See also Whittingham D.G. (1979): In vito fertilization, embryo transfer and storage, *British Medical Bulletin, 35,* 105-111

The author wishes to acknowledge the kind help of Dr Ruth Curson of King's College Hospital, London.

3.63 The patient complaining of rheumatism

J.D.E. Knox

Aches and pains apparently related to muscles and joints are relatively common symptoms in the adult population of the United Kingdom. Most studies of morbidity in UK general practice reveal 'rheumatism' to be among the top five symptom groups in the frequency with which they present. The Third National Morbidity Survey,[1] based on a population of around a third of a million studied for one year, showed that episodes of musculo-skeletal and connective tissue disorders comprised a substantial proportion of all morbidity brought to the family doctor. This study indicated the range and extent of these problems (Table I). In terms of work load, a general practitioner with a practice of 2,000 patients might expect those suffering from some of the more clearly defined entities to give rise to the number of consultations set out in Table II, with backache the most common cause.

Condition	***Rate***
Backache	31.1
Osteoarthrosis and allied conditions	24.8
OA spine (including cervical spondylosis)	16.3
Intervertebral disc lesions	10.7
Shoulder syndromes	6.6

Table I. – Rheumatic complaints in general practice, 1981–82. Episode rate per 1,000 population (Source: 3rd National Morbidity Study, 1981–82)

'Rheumatism', loosely defined, is age-related:[1] rare in children, it increases in frequency with age until among those aged 75 years and over it is almost universal. In the elderly, such complaints may be accepted by the victims as inevitable; this and the increased effort required to move around undoubtedly reduce patient-initiated demands on general practitioners which the symptoms might otherwise cause.[2]

Condition	*Consultations*
Osteoarthrosis & allied conditions	106
Backache	95
OA spine (including cervical spondylosis)	53
Rheumatoid arthritis & allied conditions	35
Shoulder syndromes	23

Table II. – Approximate numbers of consultations associated with some components of the group 'rheumatic complaints' in one year in a practice list of 2,000 (Source: 3rd National Morbidity Study, 1981–82)

Presentation

Many problems commonly encountered in general practice are such tnat no label may be applied: the label does not exist. Diagnosis is further complicated by the evanescent self-limiting nature of many illnesses seen by the doctor of first contact as well as the minor nature of the deviations from an ill-defined range of normality.

Group	*Episode rate per 1,000 Population*
Back troubles	45.7
OA/RA	30.7
Cervical spine syndrome	12.1
Shoulder syndromes	6.6

Table III. – 'Rheumatic' conditions in broad groups (Source: 3rd National Morbidity Study, 1981–82)

Rheumatology is at an early stage of development, and in most patients the underlying cause or causes of their diseases are not understood. This means that such diagnostic labels as exist do not convey clearly ideas concerning specific pathological changes, aetiologies or even prognoses. Therapy, too, cannot generally be regarded as specific; it is still largely symptomatic. Because of this, it may be more appropriate to classify the various conditions into four broad groups as in Table III, which indicates the order of frequency with which they may present to the general practitioner.

In the face of such facts, the general practitioner may be reluctant to embark too readily on a series of investigations which may cause greater disturbance to the patient than the condition from which he evidently suffers and which do not really help the doctor to assess the problem. Again, the general practitioner is concerned not only to attempt to diagnose what the condition may be, he must occasionally be exercised to know what the condition must not be if his patient is to enjoy good health. Common strategies in defining problems of rheumatism include the following:

1. *Pattern recognition.* – This strategy may remain at a fairly superficial level. 'I don't know what causes this, but I've seen this before and it will follow such-and-such a course.' Wry neck in children is one example.
2. *Traditional diagnosis.* – This involves the gathering of information, analysing it in relation to known 'diagnoses', allocating the result to a suitable 'pigeon hole' and taking the appropriate action. The firm diagnosis of rheumatoid arthritis usually involves this approach.
3. *Symptom-to-treatment.* – Because of the factors already described, the strategy outlined in 2. is commonly not possible. The doctor has then to move from a consideration of symptoms directly to management without the sustained effort sometimes necessary to formulate a diagnosis in pathological terms. Most of the common minor 'fibrositic' aches and pains are in this category.
4. *'Pay-off'.* – The diagnosis is not immediately clear, but the patient's response to some line of therapy suggests the nature of the rheumatic condition. Examples might include the prompt amelioration of the pain of acute mono-arthritis by indomethacin, suggesting gout, or the easing of vague muscle aches and stiffness by thyroxine in myxoedema.

Despite these uncertainties, it is worth while to make an appropriate effort to formulate as clear a diagnosis in physical terms as circumstances will allow. Not only does this indicate to an increasingly knowledgeable patient that his complaint is being given due attention, it is also possible sometimes to classify arthralgias and arthropathies in ways which assist prognosis, allay or avoid raising unnecessary anxieties in the patient's mind and help towards a more rational approach to drug therapy.

In such an ill-defined field, problem definition in general practice is heavily dependent on 'probability diagnosis', assessment of associated clinical features and observation of the patient over a period of time, in addition to the more familiar clinical findings and laboratory investigations of hospital-based medicine.

Causes

Non-articular rheumatism. – Musculo-skeletal pain not apparently related to joints is a common presentation of many different underlying conditions. It is customary to consider such non-articular rheumatism apart from the arthropathies, but the distinction is not always clear cut. Aches and pains not specifically related to joints and of short duration may accompany febrile illnesses such as influenza, or may follow unaccustomed exercise (post-exertion myalgia) or be due to muscular strain or tension secondary to anxiety.

Although the term 'fibrositis' has now been discarded by rheumatologists it remains a useful non-specific word for explaining to patients the cause of localized pain due to reflex muscle spasm, provided the use of the term does not lull the doctor himself into a false sense of security. 'Fibrositis' is a label and not a diagnosis; as a label it has a valid use as a shorthand description of symptoms but if symptoms fail to resolve after a short period of time, further effort is needed to reach a diagnosis.

Among the causes to be considered when faced with aches and pains of weeks' or months' duration, even when these do not directly appear to relate to joints, are rheumatoid disease, polymyalgia rheumatica, depressive illness, neoplasia and metabolic bone disease.

Patients with joint pains. – Pain is usually associated with other symptoms, the commonest of which is limitation of movement of the joint: if pain is unrelated to movement then the joint as such is unlikely to be involved, but the differentation is not always easy, especially in the presence of febrile illnesses like influenza.

Age can afford a helpful pointer because diagnostic probabilities differ with each group. Parents may bring toddlers and pre-school children complaining of pain in elbow, knee or hip. Trauma is the likely factor, and the possibility of non-accidental violence should be considered. Joint pains in the school child may suggest the possibility of acute rheumatic fever or Still's disease (juvenile rheumatoid arthritis). While these hypotheses should be entertained because of their prognostic significance, the conditions are rare in general practice. More probable diagnoses include arthralgia associated with virus infections, Henoch-Schonlein purpura and allergic conditions (including adverse responses to drugs). In adolescents also trauma is a likely cause and the differential diagnosis between traumatic synovitis and haemarthrosis can be a challenge. Later still, rheumatoid disease with its numerous variants and related conditions, becomes a possibility to be considered. The forties and fifties age-group present osteoarthrosis and, much less likely, gout. In the elderly, possibilities include osteoarthrosis, depressive illness, polymyalgia rheumatica and rheumatic manifestations of organic non-rheumatic diseases such as neoplasia, Paget's disease and metabolic bone diseases.

The sex of the patient is another pointer. Women, especially in the 30 to 40 age-group, present with joint pains of rheumatoid disease more often than men, in whom degenerative disease (especially osteoarthrosis) is a more frequent presentation. Men present more commonly with ankylosing spondylitis, Reiter's syndrome (in young adults) and gout (in middle age).

Other information about the patient may occasionally provide cues for the general practitioner. Families may show a predisposition among their members to exhibit similar patterns of symptoms, including joint pains. Sometimes this is more a manifestation of 'family myths' ('our womenfolk always get rheumatics at the change') rather than a true genetic predisposition; yet there is evidence, for example, that the prevalence of rheumatic fever is significantly greater among the children of parents who have had the disease than that in the general population.[3] In general, however, this is a much weaker diagnostic pointer than either age or sex of the patient. Occupation may also point the way, the link most commonly being trauma (e.g. the footballer's knee, gamekeeper's hip).

The patient's history: present and past

A history of trauma will usually be reasonably clear; yet there is always a risk in accepting too readily this explanation by the patient. Most people will seek a cause for their discomfort, and 'injury' in some degree is an every-day occurrence. The time relationship between the two is important: e.g. the immediate swelling of the knee after injury assists to differentiate haemarthrosis from traumatic synovitis which develops more gradually over a period of hours or a day.

The site of the symptoms may assist in diagnosis; indeed some clinicians classify joint pains according to whether the condition is a monoarthritis or a polyarthritis and whether it is acute or chronic. Such distinctions probably have greater validity for the hospital-based doctor than they have for the doctor of first contact. The unilateral painful knee, however, with a history of recent trauma presents a different clinical picture from the same joint symptom associated with pain and swelling in the fingers, or with a stiff back, worse on rising in the morning. The red, swollen, hot, painful metatarso-phalangeal joint of itself should suggest acute gout, but the condition is so readily confused with 'cellulitis' or 'injury' that the true diagnosis may be missed.

Duration of symptoms depends on many factors, including the

personality of the patient as well as the intensity of the disease process. There has to be a starting point for chronic as well as acute disease, and it does not necessarily follow that the duration before seeking medical help from the family doctor will be long in one and short in the other. In general, however, joint symptoms of weeks or months are likely to be associated with osteoarthrosis and rheumatoid disease while symptoms of shorter duration suggest trauma, infection (local or a joint manifestation of systemic illness) or anaphylaxis. When the symptom is a repeat of a previous complaint or one in a series of related phenomena, more likely possibilities include rheumatoid disease and gout.

The presence of malaise and generalized stiffness are important diagnostic pointers, which support such hypotheses as rheumatoid disease (and related conditions) and systemic illness which could include tuberculosis or brucellosis, rare in general practice, yet important because of their implication for prognosis and therapy.

The three cardinal symptoms of joint disease are pain, stiffness and weakness.[4] The character of joint *pain* is of a deeply aching quality, like toothache, which can be distinguished from the tingling quality of nerve pain. Joint pain is often referred; referred tenderness and muscle spasm (analogous to abdominal guarding in peritonitis) can also be present, but the true site of the pain can be distinguished by its being much more sharply tender than the site of referral.

The *stiffness* experienced, especially on waking and in the early morning, is characteristic of active inflammatory joint disease (rheumatoid arthritis, ankylosing spondylitis and polymyalgia rheumatica) whereas in osteoarthrosis and ordinary disc degeneration such stiffness is not a feature.

Weakness, especially of hand grip and/or quadriceps, again helps to differentiate rheumatoid disease from osteoarthrosis, being present in the former and not in the latter. Weakness predominates over pain in the rare primary muscle diseases such as polymyositis and the myopathies.

Clearly, many factors in addition to those already mentioned influence the doctor's approach to the patient complaining of such rheumatic aches and pains: e.g. the doctor's previous knowledge of the patient as a person, of his family, of the morbidity prevalent in the practice area and so on. One convenient starting point might be the duration of the patient's symptoms. Complaints of one or two days' duration, especially associated with features such as unaccustomed exercise, negative physical findings or a normal erythrocyte sedimentation rate (ESR) will raise a set of hypotheses rather different from those generated by a long history with evidence of systemic upset. Simplified flow charts (figures 2, 3) illustrate this approach to problem definition. These are not intended to dictate the pathway which must be taken; rather they are intended to stimulate the family doctor to construct such flow charts for himself.

Clinical examination

Some of the less common rheumatic diseases are associated with involvement of other bodily systems in addition to the locomotor system. When a patient first presents with such systemic disease, it may not always be easy for the doctor to distinguish, on history and local examination alone, this disease from the welter of common minor and self-limiting conditions. In theory, then, it could be argued that most, if not all, patients presenting with rheumatic complaints should be subjected to a complete physical examination – and such is the teaching of hospital specialists. This teaching completely ignores certain considerations especially relevant to general practice, such as:

1. The low yield of helpful information which the indiscriminate application of such a policy will give in primary care, however much it may be the rule in the selected cases of the hospital clinic.
2. The time taken up in unhelpful activity oft repeated (because rheumatic conditions are common in general practice) limits the time available for other patients: i.e. it is an inefficient way to deliver primary medical care.
3. The possibility of using time as an instrument to assess the nature of the underlying process, and the degree of impairment, disability and handicap. This useful diagnostic instrument is more readily available to the general practitioner than to the specialist. Not only can he follow up his patient by a home visit or at a return consultation, but also he often already knows his patient, and thus has a base line against which to evaluate the new rheumatic symptoms.

Most of us soon learn to cope with the realities of primary care by developing further the skills of selective examination which all clinicians in fact practise – whatever they preach.

How extensive an examination? Often when the patient's main complaint is related to local abnormalities such as Heberden's nodes, or the uncommon fibro-fatty pads on the knuckles (so-called 'Garrod's pads'), local inspection may be all that is required. In most patients complaining of backache the information needed to formulate the problem may be obtained without having the patient undress. Yet, there are certain indicators which alert the family doctor to select a different approach. The middle-aged or elderly man who hitherto has been an infrequent attender and who presents with 'my rheumatics, doctor' may warrant fuller examination, as will the patient whom he has never met before. Evidence of systemic upset, weight loss, fever, or a general appearance of being unwell should likewise alert us. Multiple joint involvement, and a history of morning stiffness, (suggestive of rheumatoid disease), the sudden onset of joint pain after an operation, or the association of rheumatics and oral diuretics (which might suggest gout) will indicate not only that a systems examination should be carried out, but also that blood should be taken for estimation of the erythrocyte sedimentation rate, serum uric acid and rheumatoid factor as well. The single episode of 'rheumatics' which fails to respond to simple analgesics and observation, or frequently repeated episodes of 'rheumatics' are other indications for a fuller reappraisal of the situation.

The most important physical signs of joint disease are swelling, limitation of joint mobility and muscle wasting. The 'feel' of any *swelling* is important – a boggy feel indicates the synovial thickening which occurs in rheumatoid arthritis, and local warmth suggests underlying inflammation. Tenderness over a swelling, if severe, points to the presence of infection, crystal deposition or blood – such a joint should be aspirated. The sites of such swelling can be helpful diagnostically, as for instance the proximal interphalangeal joints typically affected in rheumatoid disease. Very localized tenderness, however, if limited to a small area of joint margin, more usually indicates some form of tendonitis.

Joint mobility is assessed by putting the joint passively through its full range of movements, noting when there is pain or limitation; it is sometimes difficult to ensure that only the joint in question is moved during the examination – it is important, for example, to immobilize the pelvis when examining the hip, the scapula and elbow when examining the shoulder and the subtalar joint when examining the forefoot. The presence of crepitus is strongly suggestive of osteoarthrosis.

The importance of examining for *muscle wasting* is that definite absence of such wasting usually rules out inflammatory disease. The deltoids waste quickly in shoulder disease, the erector spinae in ankylosing spondylitis, the outer side of the upper thighs in inflammatory hip disease and the vastus medialis in disease affecting the knee.

Principles of management

While there are obviously individual differences in the detailed management of rheumatic diseases, the basic objectives are:

1. relief of pain and stiffness,
2. reduction of inflammation,
3. preservation of function.

Specific treatment in the sense of removing the cause is usually not possible. Any treatment is largely symptomatic and depends heavily on analgesics. Commercial drug firms make much of the anti-inflammatory properties of drugs. Aspirin possesses this property to the same extent as many more expensive and more toxic preparations and it remains the drug of first choice.

The effective dosage of aspirin is 3-5G/day (10-16 tablets) and it is best prescribed in soluble form and taken with or immediately after food. Gastrointestinal side effects are unfortunately common: if such side effects are mild, buffered or enteric-coated aspirin should be tried. However, if gastrointestinal side-effects are severe all aspirin preparations should be avoided because of the risk of a serious bleed.[5]

Aspirin in full doses may cause tinnitus (especially in the elderly) and reducing the dose by 1-2 tablets per day may effectively remedy this.

Indomethacin in doses of 25-50 mg four times a day is a useful alternative to aspirin and may be combined with it – an evening dose to lessen morning stiffness may be given orally or as a suppository – although gastrointestinal side effects may occur even when the rectal route is used.

If the patient has a peptic ulcer or severe dyspepsia or if intolerance develops to aspirin and/or indomethacin, then a trial of one of the many other so-called non-steroidal anti-inflammatory drugs (NSAID) is indicated. The choice of these is bewildering and it is recognized that there are much greater differences between patients' responses to these drugs than differences between the drugs themselves. It has been suggested[6] that a system involving the patient himself in the assessment of the drugs and his response to them may help to tailor therapy to the needs of the individual. In this system a standardized proforma is used and the patient given prescriptions for sufficient tablets for a five-day course of each of four different preparations. Detailed instructions are given and after three weeks the position is reviewed. The system can, of course, be adapted to include other drugs and different dosage schemes. An example of such a 'patient observation sheet' is shown in Figure 1.

Many patients (especially those with osteoarthrosis) need to supplement their anti-inflammatory drugs with an analgesic which has no anti-inflammatory action – such as paracetamol, dihydrocodeine or dextropropoxyphene.

Non-analgesic drugs used in the treatment of rheumatoid disease – antimalarials, gold, penicillamine (and, in some cases, steroids) may be needed when response to analgesic drugs is poor. These are drugs, however, which will rarely if ever be prescribed without specialist advice and review, because of their considerable potential toxicity.

In addition to pain relief, the following principles may help to guide approaches to therapy:

1. Not only may perception of pain be influenced by analgesics, but the patient's (and family's) reaction to pain may be affected by 'morale'. Understanding of the patient and communicating that understanding may be as important as prescribing drugs.
2. Relief of pain can also be achieved by physical measures. Rest, both to the part and to the patient, is helpful. Warmth and massage appropriately applied as part of a planned regime can reinforce other measures. The patient and his family can be encouraged to take responsibility for such physical treatment; occasionally more may be achieved by readily available and accessible professional help. The National Health Service has lagged far behind some other countries in ensuring the provision of such help to patients outside hospital.
3. The local injection of steroids and local anaesthetics is an integral part of general-practice management of common periarticular conditions, e.g. 'tennis elbow', and is as free from problems in this setting as it is in hospital.
4. The patient's views on management should be taken into account. Failure to pay sufficient attention to this point has allowed such practices as manipulation to pass largely out of trained medical hands.
5. The social implications of the more chronic rheumatic complaints are sufficiently numerous and complex to warrant a closer link between social workers and the primary care team. This is enhanced by attachment of social workers to group practices and to health centres.
6. More attention needs to be paid to improving communications between the general practitioner and the rheumatic clinic – and vice versa. The general practitioner could assume a greater responsibility for follow-up of the patient referred to hospital: the regular communication of progress reports to hospital colleagues would make for more efficient long-term care, relieving the clinic of an escalating commitment and the patient of unnecessarily tedious and time-consuming journeys.
7. The routine follow-up and home visiting of patients with chronic rheumatic diseases can, and should be shared by appropriate members of the primary health care team: especially the nursing sister and the health visitor.
8. Patients should be encouraged to assume as much responsibility for the management and prevention of disease as they can. It is true that in the absence of knowledge of causation specific prevention is not possible, but the link between obesity and

osteoarthrosis is clear, and failure to maintain efficient quadriceps muscle action can lead to problems with the unstable knee. Aspirin is an appropriate analgesic in most instances, in the absence of specific contraindications, and it is readily available. The infra-red and ordinary heat rays are produced as effectively by a domestic electric fire as by sophisticated equipment in a physiotherapy department.

9. The resources of the hospital specialist team can be deployed most effectively if they are used selectively. Among the principles governing referral are the following:
   (a) Doubt about the nature of the underlying process, especially if the patient's disability is marked
   (b) Failure of the condition to follow the course predicted
   (c) For confirmation of suspected diagnosis of 'major' disease
   (d) The provision of therapeutic measures not readily available outside hospital
   (e) Desire of the patient, and sometimes of relatives, for a second opinion for whatever reason
   (f) To facilitate insurance, legal or pension cases.

References

[1] Royal College of General Practitioners, Office of Population Censuses and Surveys, Department of Health and Social Security (1986): *Morbidity Statistics from General Practice 1981–82*. HMSO Series MB5 No. 1

[2] Williamson, J., Stokoe, I.H., Gray, S., Fisher, M., Smith, A., McGhee, A., Stephenson, E. (1964): Old People at Home, *Lancet, i,* 1117

[3] Knox, J.D.E., and Kuenssberg, E.V. (1964): Rheumatic and other locomotor diseases, *Medical World, 100,* 456

[4] Balme, H.W. (1978): Diagnostic difficulties in joint disease. *Practitioner, 1315,* 8-34

[5] Drug and Therapeutics Bulletin (1975): Choice of drugs in rheumatoid arthritis in adults: *13,* 57-59

[6] Gumpel, J.M., (1978): Which anti-inflammatory drugs in rheumatoid arthritis? *British Medical Journal, 2,* 256

Medication		Ibuprofen 400 mg ONE to be taken at breakfast, lunch and evening meal					Naproxen 250 mg ONE to be taken at breakfast, and ONE at night with a drink and biscuit					Benorylate 750 mg TWO to be taken at breakfast, lunch and evening meal					Diclofenac 25 mg ONE to be taken at breakfast, lunch and evening meal				
Day		1	2	3	4	5	6	7	8	9	10	11	12	13	14	15	16	17	18	19	20
Duration of morning stiffness (in hours)		1	0	½	1	½	¼	½	½	½	½	2	3	2	2	1	1	1	2	2	1
Pain during day (please tick appropriate box)	None	✓																			
	Mild		✓	✓		✓	✓	✓			✓						✓	✓	✓	✓	
	Moderate				✓				✓	✓		✓	✓		✓	✓					✓
	Severe													✓							
Do these tablets/ capsules suit you?	Yes	✓	✓	✓	✓	✓											✓	✓	✓	✓	✓
	No						✓	✓	✓	✓	✓	✓	✓	✓	✓	✓					
Any Comments?																					

Figure 1 – Patient observation form

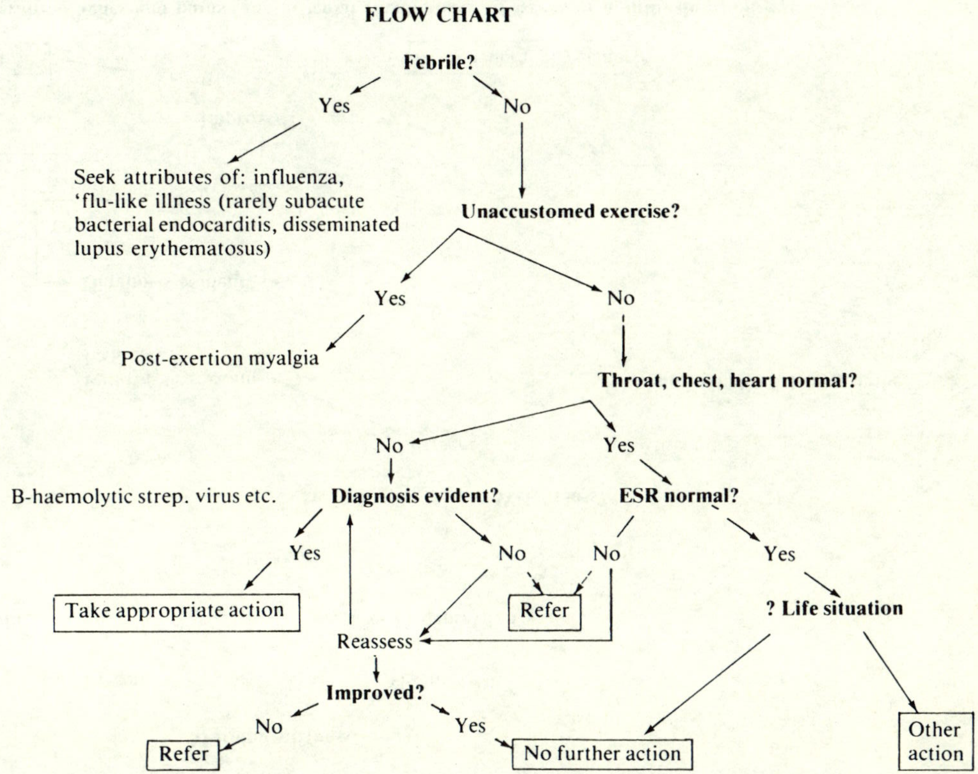

Figure 2 – Patients with generalized aches and pains (non-articular rheumatism) of short (less than 2 to 3 days) duration

FLOW CHART

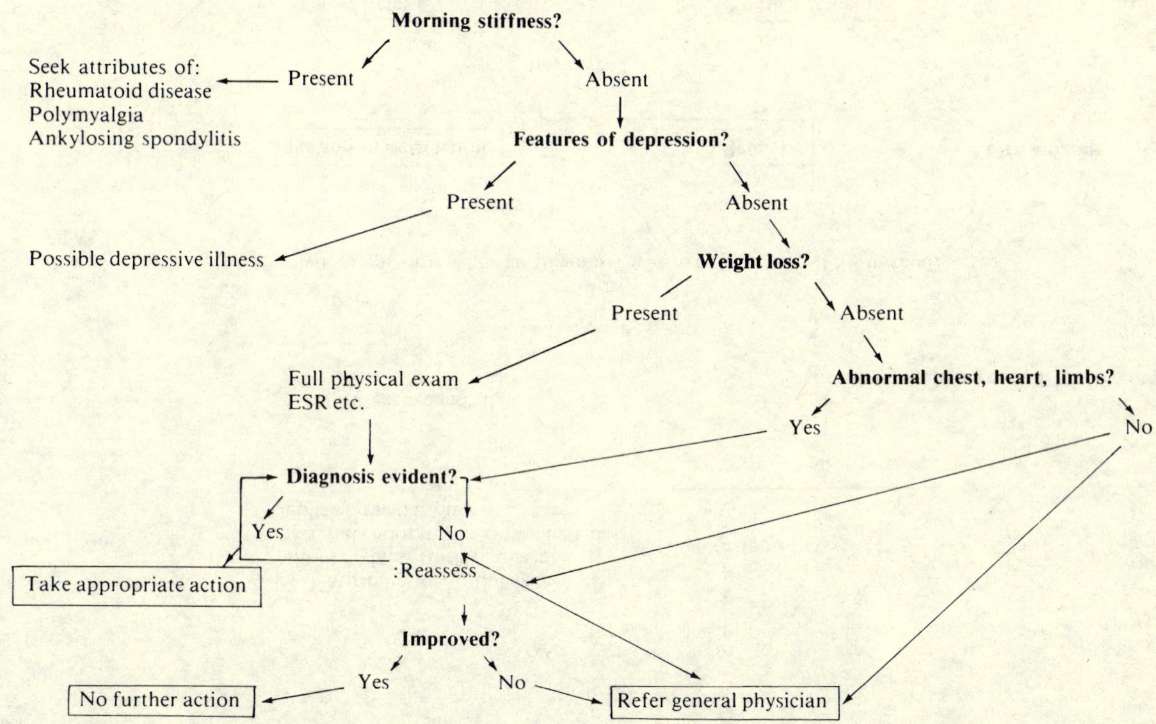

Figure 3 – Patients with generalized aches and pains (non-articular rheumatism) of weeks or months duration

3.64
Shoulder problems

J.D.E. Knox

Rheumatic conditions affecting the shoulder are relatively common, and present a diagnostic challenge both to general practitioners and to specialists. Many of the conditions run a short course and are not associated with florid clinical signs, beyond pain, stiffness and limitation of movement. Whilst trauma is often implicated and in such instances is the likely cause of symptoms, more often the symptoms appear to arise for no obvious reason. Usually symptoms are felt in one or other shoulder region, but the less common bilateral involvement suggests that the underlying condition may be cervical spondylosis, rheumatoid disease, or polymyalgia rheumatica. An estimate of the frequency with which various conditions occur is set out in Table I.

Condition	*Frequency*
Simple non-articular rheumatism	8
Trauma	
Sprains	6
Fracture/dislocation	1
Referred pain	
Cervical spondylosis	6
Ischaemic heart disease	1
Other	<1
Rotator cuff	
E.g. Supraspinatus lesions	2
Adhesive capsulitis	
Frozen shoulder	2
Miscellaneous	
Rheumatoid disease)	
Polymyalgia rheumatica)	
Carcinoma)	<1
Herpes zoster)	
Bicipital tendonitis)	
Shoulder-hand syndrome)	

Table I.– Some presenting conditions affecting the shoulder region with estimated frequency of occurrence in one year in a practice of 2,000 patients

Presentations and causes

Injury includes sprains, fractures and dislocations. The nature of the condition will usually be evident from the history, the commonest being a fall, either on the outstretched hand or on the point of the shoulder. Recurrence of dislocation may occur apparently spontaneously or in association with minor injury and the patient will usually make his own diagnosis. Fracture of the clavicle is usually associated with pain, tenderness and swelling over the junction of the middle and outer thirds of the bone.

Non-articular rheumatism of the shoulder region is suggested by pain, stiffness and limitation of movement arising without a history of injury immediately preceding the onset. There may be no other abnormality, no localized tenderness or other associated feature, and the transient nature of the condition, which usually clears within a week, makes definitive diagnosis impossible. Such a picture may also be seen during the prodromal phase of herpes zoster afflicting the middle cervical root ganglia, though some degree of hyperaesthesia may be found (if looked for) before the characteristic vesicles appear two to three days later.

By careful consideration of clinical features as they unfold over a period of time, it is possible to recognize more discrete entities in about half of the presentations of pain and stiffness in the shoulder. Such conditions include adhesive capsulitis (the 'frozen shoulder'), subacromial bursitis, tears and calcification of the supraspinatus tendon, and other lesions of the so-called 'rotator cuff'. The glenohumeral joint is surrounded by a complex of tendons merging with one another: those of subscapularis, supraspinatus, infraspinatus and teres minor. This cuff moves within the superficial structures – e.g. acromion and coracoid processes – and may be the site of tears and degenerative changes. Sufferers from all such conditions are usually middle-aged or older, and men and women are affected in roughly equal proportions. A history of myocardial infarction (or cerebrovascular accident or trauma) some weeks before the onset of the shoulder pain is given by some patients suffering from frozen shoulder (and the less common shoulder-hand syndrome). All shoulder movements become restricted and the condition persists for several months – or even longer – before the shoulder 'thaws'. Lesions of the rotator cuff give rise to pain which is aggravated by certain movements: the restriction is selective, and physical examination reveals more characteristic evidence of disturbed function of the joint.

Disability associated with the rare 'shoulder-hand syndrome' is even greater. Its onset is usually gradual and sometimes follows a myocardial infarction or a cerebrovascular accident. The sufferer's attention is concentrated on the painful limb which is carefully protected from injury. The hand may become swollen, the fingers stiff and the skin shiny and atrophic. The etiology of the syndrome is not well understood, but it is thought to be due to a complex autonomic disturbance.

When such ill-defined 'rheumatism' persists, and is associated with subjective complaints, or objective evidence, of constitutional upset (such as loss of weight) the possibility of neoplastic disease, especially bronchogenic carcinoma, must be considered and the patient should be referred for chest X-ray.

Persistent 'fibrositis' or 'muscular rheumatism' of the shoulder girdle in the elderly is one way in which polymyalgia rheumatica may present. This condition is associated with weakness of the proximal muscles and there may be a characteristic history of inability to comb the hair or raise the arms above shoulder level because of pain, a feeling of heaviness, and stiffness which is especially marked in the morning.

Involvement of the shoulders in pain apparently radiating downwards from the neck and aggravated by neck movements is a feature of cervical spondylosis. There is sometimes a previous history of similar symptoms, occasionally having their origin in some episode of injury, such as the whip-lash trauma of a road traffic accident. Pain may radiate into either shoulder from, and even be the presenting symptom of, the carpal-tunnel syndrome, although usually the peripheral symptoms predominate (see Chapter 3.66, Wrist and hand problems).

The discomfort experienced in most of these conditions is rather diffuse and has a dull aching quality, in contradistinction to that felt in the referred pain of diaphragmatic irritation, in which the pain is localized to the tip of the shoulder, is sharp in character, and exacerbated by inspiration. Shoulder tip pain is usually a secondary phenomenon, part of a clinical picture in which the features of the underlying cause predominate, but occasionally it may be the presenting feature, as in some cases of spontaneous pneumothorax. The referred pain of myocardial ischaemia involving the left shoulder should be borne in mind.

Pain and tenderness in the anterior aspect of the upper arm, aggravated by flexing the elbow, suggest bicipital tendonitis. This condition is associated with partial tear of the long head of biceps, usually as it lies in the bicipital groove on the anterior surface of the humerus.

Examination and investigation

If the patient has a full range of movement in the shoulder, the joint is most unlikely to be the seat of the cause of the symptoms: pain referred from structures such as the neck or cervical spine, from the heart or great vessels, or from the pleura should be considered and appropriate confirmatory evidence sought.

The patient should be asked to raise both arms above his head and lower them sideways. Pain during part of this maneouvre, sometimes associated with the sudden dropping of the arm to the side, is evidence of the 'painful arc' seen in rotator cuff lesions.

With his arm by his side, the patient is asked to flex his elbow, and then swing his hand outwards. External rotation of the shoulder can thereby be assessed: it is characteristically restricted early in the evolution of the frozen shoulder. Internal rotation is tested by asking the patient to put his arm behind his back and reach with his hand for the opposite shoulder blade.

The patient is then asked to abduct the arm: supraspinatus tendon lesions typically result in upward displacement of the head of the humerus in a shrugging movement instead of a smooth outward swing, although the arm may be actively held in abduction after being assisted passively through the first 30° or so.

The patient should be examined stripped to the waist and the shoulder movements repeated, while attention is focused on the scapula. Moderate ranges of shoulder movement are still possible even with a fixed scapulo-humeral joint because the scapula moves on the posterior chest wall.

Wasting of muscles around the shoulder gives it a sharper appearance: such evidence is found in capsulitis and long-continued affections. If symptoms persist, the erythrocyte sedimentation rate (ESR) should be estimated. Abnormal values suggest such conditions as rheumatoid disease or polymyalgia rheumatica, infections, such as tuberculosis, or bronchogenic carcinoma, and indicate referral for fuller investigation. X-ray examination of the shoulder joint is not likely to yield information of use to the general practitioner in the common run-of-the-mill shoulder affections encountered in primary care. Indications for this investigation include the persistence of symptoms for weeks, the suspicion (for whatever reason) of neoplasm, or an associated raised ESR. When shoulder pain appears to be part of cervical spondylosis, neck movements should be tested: normally full flexion allows the chin to touch the chest, full lateral rotation allows the chin to touch the shoulder and full lateral flexion allows the ear to touch the shoulder. Cervical spondylosis is associated with restriction, especially of lateral rotation, though all neck movements may be limited. Evidence of nerve root irritation (diminution or loss of tendon reflexes, hypoaesthesia in appropriate dermatomes and possibly wasting of small muscles of the hand) should be sought.

Management

Principles of management of painful shoulder conditions in general practice consist of rest, analgesics, early active mobilization supplemented by appropriate physical measures such as heat in various forms, and, in certain circumstances, infiltration with local anaesthetics or hydrocortisone.

Sprains and 'fibrositis' may benefit in the early stages from resting the affected arm in a sling, either collar-and-cuff or triangular bandage. The arm is supported with the elbow flexed and adducted so that the hand points to the opposite shoulder.

Treatment of fractures of the clavicle will usually be initiated at hospital with the application of a figure-of-eight bandage holding the shoulders braced. Management is continued by regularly re-assessing progress and tightening the bandage twice weekly for four to six weeks.

Since dislocation of the shoulder usually requires an X-ray (to ensure, among other things, that there is no associated fracture) reduction is usually carried out in hospital. Rest in a collar-and-cuff sling is continued for several days thereafter, following which the patient is encouraged to carry out active exercises. As an early move towards this, he should be instructed to carry out assisted movements. This can conveniently be arranged in the home by using a clothes rope thrown over an open door: the patient grasps one end in the 'good' hand and, holding the other end in the hand of the affected side assists elevation to above shoulder level. He should be encouraged to carry out a programme of such movements thrice daily, gradually increasing the number of elevations to 20 to 30 at a session. This may be followed by active exercises in which the patient stands a little less than arm's length from the wall and 'walks' his fingers up it as far as possible without undue pain. The session may be finished off by attempts to obtain full circumduction, swinging the arm round 10 to 20 times — the patient should be advised to bend forward at the waist so as to let the arm hang free and then to swing the arm round in ever widening circles (as if stirring a pudding).

Such efforts at home physiotherapy are most likely to succeed if a relative can be involved in supervising the session, which may begin with a gentle 'rub' using warm olive oil or other appropriate lubricant. Heat from an electric pad, an electric fire or a warm bath are useful adjuvants. Such a programme may be prescribed for most of the so-called rheumatic afflictions of the shoulder region, but the key factor in management is pain relief. The emphasis should be on the prescription of adequate and appropriate doses of simple analgesics — aspirin or paracetamol — and the patient is the important decision maker rather than the doctor, whose conventional 'take two tablets thrice daily' may be utterly inadequate.

Infiltration of the shoulder joint can provide some relief in rotator cuff lesions and can be carried out in general practice provided appropriate aseptic precautions are taken. For frozen shoulder or synovitis the best approach is the anterior one (see Figure 1). The patient sits comfortably, with the arm loosely by the side and the space between the glenoid cup and the head of the humerus is identified, about 1 cm below the coracoid process. The skin is swabbed with spirit and anaesthetized with an intradermal injection of local anaesthetic. A 21 G 1½ inch needle should be inserted in a slightly medial direction and 25 to 50 mg hydrocortisone injected.

For the painful arc syndrome the lateral approach should be used. The lateral tip of the acromium is identified and the needle inserted medially in a slightly downward direction, until the tip reaches the head of the humerus. The needle is then gradually withdrawn with gentle pressure on the plunger — when a sudden decrease in resistance is felt (indicating that the subacromial bursa has been entered) after first aspirating any fluid to determine that pus is not present, 50 mg of hydrocortisone is injected.

In some of the conditions mentioned, the course runs on for weeks and months: e.g. frozen shoulder, shoulder-hand syndrome. Management in such instances is eased by sharing it with skilled colleagues in hospital; yet much can be achieved by the judicious application of the simple measures described. By encouraging patients to take more responsibility for the management of their conditions the overload on rheumatic and orthopaedic clinics will be lessened, and, where the common shoulder conditions of general practice are concerned, the outcome, in cost benefit and other terms, is likely to be as good.

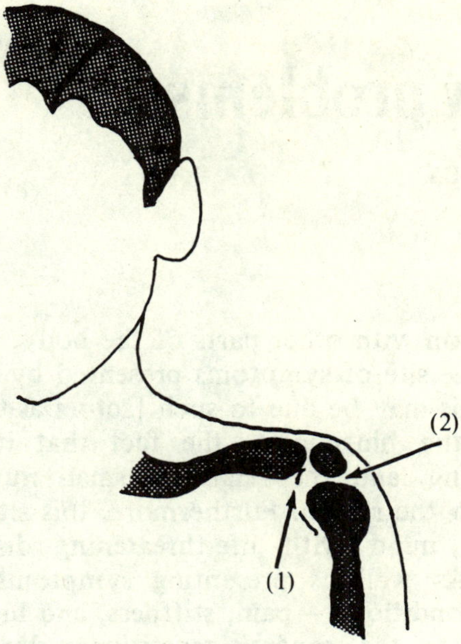

Figure 1. Sites for (1) anterior and (2) lateral injections of the shoulder

3.65
Elbow problems

J.D.E. Knox

In comparison with other parts of the body, the elbow is much less often the site of symptoms presented by patients in general practice. This may be due to such factors as the relatively stable nature of the hinge-joint, the fact that it is not normally weight-bearing, and the relatively small number of different structures in the region. Furthermore, this site is not associated in the lay mind with life-threatening disease or crippling disability. As well as presenting symptoms characteristic of rheumatic conditions – pain, stiffness, and limitation – patients may also cue the general practitioner by the presence of swellings, subcutaneous nodules and skin conditions: such phenomena are not usually 'presented' and may have to be sought. Table I sets out a list of commoner conditions affecting the elbow together with an estimate of numbers of episodes likely to be encountered in an 'average' general practice.

Condition	*Estimated number*
Trauma: Sprains (including 'pulled elbow')	4
Fracture/dislocation	<1
Tennis elbow/Golfer's elbow	5
Non-articular 'fibrositis'	1
Olecranon bursitis: acute	1
chronic	<1
Articular: Rheumatoid arthritis	2
Osteoarthrosis	<1
Miscellaneous: Subcutaneous nodules (rheumatoid arthritis)	<1
Referred pain	4 to 8

Table I.– Some conditions affecting the elbow region, and estimated frequency with which they may present in one year in a practice of 2,000 patients

Presentation

Symptoms (usually pain) in the region of the elbow are most commonly part of a more widespread symptomatology. Pain of ischaemic heart disease may sometimes present as discomfort in the left elbow ('the restless elbow'): when the patient is describing his chest pain, he may occasionally convey his message non-verbally by holding or rubbing his left elbow. Less often, pain may be felt as a deep ache in the elbow as part of the radiculopathy of cervical spondylosis, brachial neuritis and thoracic inlet syndromes. The pain in these conditions radiates into the elbow from above. Sometimes pain radiates into the elbow from the wrist and forearm: such may be the presentation of the carpal tunnel syndrome (see Chapter 3.66, Wrist and hand problems).

Of the small number of cases of trauma, apart from dislocations and fractures, the greater proportion are soft tissue injury such as sprains, including pulled elbow in young children. The presentation is usually pain, but in babies it may be crying, irritability and failure to move the affected arm. Both fracture and dislocation are usually associated with deformity and a recent history of violence, either direct or indirect.

Non-articular rheumatism affecting the elbow is characteristically seen as so-called 'tennis elbow'. The sufferer, likely to be more middle-aged and non-athletic than the name of the condition would suggest, presents with pain and tenderness localized to the region of the lateral epicondyle of the humerus. The condition has usually been present for a few days before the patient comes to the general practitioner. A similar clinical picture may occasionally be encountered affecting the tissues on the medial aspect of the elbow ('golfer's elbow'). Other forms of soft-tissue rheumatism include bursitis, of which the commonest is olecranon bursitis. The acute form – sometimes known as student's elbow – may be seen in young adults who present with a painful tender swelling of the point of the elbow. Olecranon bursitis may also prompt the practitioner to consider the presence of other disease such as gout or rheumatoid arthritis, although in these contexts the condition is more often a secondary phenomenon and chronic, rather than primary and acute.

Causes

The commonest causes of elbow symptoms are traumatic. With tennis elbow or golfer's elbow, while there is often no obvious precipitating cause, a history is sometimes elicited of preceding activities involving unaccustomed rotatory movements of the arm, as with screw-driving or wringing wet clothes. Acute olecranon bursitis is usually ascribed to excessive prolonged pressure on the elbow as may occur when reading a heavy book upon the table with the head supported (less charitably, the object supported is traditionally a heavy beer mug).

History and examination

Traumatic causes for the various elbow conditions will usually be evident from the history and circumstances. Caution needs to be exercised in cases of some rheumatic conditions to avoid accepting too readily patients' attempts to ease their own perplexity (and sometimes their doctor's) with facile explanations: '... must have strained it'. Sometimes parents may not have observed the traumatic incident in a child or, as in some cases of child abuse, they may deliberately mislead the doctor. For most general practitioners, clinical distinctions between supracondylar fracture and dislocation are of less relevance because any patient with pain and deformity requires x-ray examination and hospital specialist treatment.

The presence of tenderness localized to the muscle attachments to the lateral epicondyle is characteristic of tennis elbow. Symptoms are aggravated by extension of the elbow, pronation of the forearm and palmar flexion of the wrist. In other forms of soft-tissue rheumatism there may be no objective evidence of abnormality. Diagnosis may then depend upon the history, the self-limiting course of the condition and absence of features of other conditions. A tender fluctuant swelling over the olecranon, sometimes with redness of the overlying skin, suggests an acute bursitis, whilst chronic bursitis may be painless and not associated with clinical evidence of inflammation.

Firm subcutaneous swellings in the region of the olecranon are seen in some patients with rheumatoid disease. Such nodules are not usually tender and are situated more distally than the point of the elbow. The early appearance of nodules in the course of rheumatoid arthritis is one factor suggesting a poor prognosis. The olecranon is also a site of the much less common subcutaneous nodule of rheumatic fever: this nodule is much smaller and may be more easily felt than seen.

The skin of the posterior elbow region may be a site affected by psoriasis, and afford a clue to the nature of a polyarthritis (which may affect the elbow joint).

The elbow joint may be the site of arthritis, as evidenced by pain, limitation of movements and even swelling. Such clinical evidence of joint disease may be seen as an isolated phenomenon, but it is more likely to be part of a polyarthritis of rheumatoid type. Osteoarthrosis of the elbow does occur but it is a relatively uncommon condition in general practice and is usually part of a more widespread osteoarthrosis.

Management

Sprains of the elbow joint are managed by immobilization of the joint in a sling, and simple analgesics such as aspirin or paracetamol in appropriate dose and at suitable intervals decided by the patient. Resting the elbow on a pillow at night may allow the patient to sleep more comfortably. Cold compresses and 'rubs' of various types have the merit of providing a channel for therapeutic activity by the patient and relatives, but objective evidence of their value is minimal. Early active movement is to be encouraged: some patients may require persuasion to relinquish the sling which serves as a badge of their disability, and an excuse for avoiding responsibilities.

The 'pulled elbow' is usually dealt with in general practice and without an anaesthetic. The pronated forearm is flexed, supinated and passively extended, with the manipulator's thumb over the radial head. Resolution is sometimes accompanied by an audible click (and a surprised cry from the patient) as the radial head is felt to slip into position.[1]

The course of tennis elbow can be shortened by the injection, with appropriate aseptic precautions, of 1 ml of hydrocortisone. This procedure, which may be carried out in a suitably equipped treatment room, is occasionally followed within twelve hours by an exacerbation of the pain. The patient should be warned of this possibility before the procedure is undertaken. Symptoms usually then settle completely in the next twenty-four to forty-eight hours, but they may recur.

Acute bursitis is managed in the same way as a sprain, by a sling and analgesics, and the course may be shortened by aspirating the fluid and sending the aspirate for culture if infection is suspected. The presence of marked degrees of tenderness, redness and regional lymphadenopathy (e.g. tender enlargement of epitrochlear lymph glands) suggest that the bursitis is infective in nature. Oral phenoxymethylpenicillin, 250 mg four times daily before meals, may then be given, and the condition reviewed next day. Failure of this condition to respond promptly warrants surgical drainage.

Chronic bursitis usually causes little discomfort. Definitive management entails surgical excision. The patient and doctor will be guided by such factors as the degree of disability and length of history.
Whilst rheumatoid nodules may be excised, their removal sometimes involves a much more extensive surgical procedure than was envisaged, and they are best left alone.

Reference

1 Illingworth, Cynthia M. (1975): Pulled Elbow. A Study of 100 Patients. *British Medical Journal, 2,* 672

3.66
Wrist and hand problems

J.D.E. Knox and J.J.C. Cormack

As it is in large measure through the use of our hands that we control our environment (it is from the Latin word for hand that we derive 'manipulate') conditions affecting the functioning of the hands have peculiar importance in affecting work and activities of daily life. This section deals with the commoner 'rheumatic', infective and traumatic conditions usually presenting with pain, stiffness and swelling.

The hands and wrists are particularly vulnerable in forward falls where the impact tends to be on the hand outstretched reflexly to break the fall. Fractures of the radius and/or ulna (including Colles' fractures) accounted for 1.5 episodes per 1,000 patients at risk per year in the National Morbidity Survey (although such figures may not represent the total incidence of such fractures as a proportion may bypass the general practitioner). Hodgkin (1973) reports the incidence of fractured scaphoid to be 0.4 per 1,000 patients per year. Figures are not readily available for fractured metacarpals or phalanges. The incidence of sprains of the thumb or fingers was 3.9 per 1,000 patients per year in Hodgkin's study and sprains of the wrist and forearm 2.5 per 1,000 patients per year. These figures may also be underestimates as Hodgkin points out that many cases are never reported. Infections of the fingers and hands can lead to considerable pain and in some cases serious diminution of function. Hodgkin reports an incidence of 11.5+ per 1,000 patients per year consulting on account of whitlow or paronychia. Web space or palmar space infections are less common, but important to treat adequately.

Pain, stiffness and swelling of the hands and wrists may be early manifestations of rheumatoid disease, and the terminal interphalangeal joints (especially in elderly women) are quite commonly the subject of osteoarthritic changes although this results less in disability than unsightly swelling. Pain and tenderness at the base of the thumb may be another manifestation of osteoarthrosis. Other conditions of the hands and wrist which will be considered here (with Hodgkin's figures for incidence per

1,000 patients per year) are tenosynovitis and tendovaginitis (5.6), ganglia (2.0), carpal tunnel syndrome (0.9) and Dupuytren's contracture (0.3).
Extrapolating from the figures given, the number of patients likely to present in a practice of 2,000 patients with various wrist and hand problems are shown in table I (no figures are available for fractured metacarpals or phalanges, palmar or web space infections or rheumatoid arthritis or osteoarthrosis specifically affecting the wrist or hand).

Whitlow or paronychia	23
Tenosynovitis or tendovaginitis of wrist	11
Sprains of thumb or fingers	8
Sprains of wrist or forearm	5
Fractures of radius and/or ulna	4
Ganglia	4
Carpal tunnel syndrome	2
Dupuytren's contracture	1
Fractured scaphoid	1

Table I.– Number of patients likely to present in one year in a practice of 2,000 patients with certain wrist or hand problems.

Presentation

In *paronychia,* throbbing pain is the common manifestation of an infection in the region of the nail fold: the tissue around the nail cuticle becomes red and irritable and in its later stages, if untreated, pus may collect at the base of the nail.
A *whitlow* is a pulp space infection causing extreme throbbing pain at the tip of the finger with some redness and swelling but usually little palpable fluctuation because of the confined space in the terminal pulp compartment.
Palmar and web space infections are characterized by the development of the pain in the fingers and hand, stiffness and loss of grip, and tenderness over the affected areas.
All these infections may be accompanied by lymphadenitis and/or lymphangitis.
Tenosynovitis presents as pain along the line of the affected tendon, especially associated with movement and sometimes accompanied by palpable or audible crepitus. Sometimes a circumscribed sausage-shaped swelling may be felt in the region of the affected tendon.

The presentation of *tendovaginitis* is more localized, with pain in the region of the radial styloid on movement of the thumb, often becoming more widespread up the forearm if initial treatment has been delayed or ineffective.

Sprains present with a history of injury associated with pain at rest, aggravated by movement, especially against resistance, and sometimes with associated swelling.

Almost all *fractures* and sprains present with a fairly obvious history of recent severe trauma together with pain, tenderness, loss of function and sometimes deformity (as in the characteristic 'dinner fork' appearance of a Colles' fracture).

Ganglia have often been present for some considerable time before a doctor is consulted (indeed they are typically presented as an extra 'while I'm here, doctor' syndrome at the end of a consultation about something else). They are small lumps, usually painless, with a characteristic firm consistency. The patient is often simply concerned to know what the lump is without seeking any active treatment.

The *carpal tunnel syndrome* presents with burning pain and pins and needles in the fingers, especially the middle fingers, typically occurring at night and sometimes waking the patient. The pain may involve the whole forearm and the condition is commoner in women than men.

Dupuytren's contracture presents as a flexion deformity of the little and ring fingers, with the patient having difficulty in fully extending the fingers. In its early stages there is some puckering at the base of the two fingers while in the fully developed condition the fingers can contract to such an extent that they cannot be extended and the finger nails excoriate the palms.

The presentation of *rheumatoid disease* with pain and stiffness (especially in the mornings) of the affected joints and general systemic disturbance, is characterized in the hands and wrists by the development of 'spindling' of the fingers – fusiform swellings at the proximal interphalangeal joints – and (in more advanced disease) 'ulnar drift' and palmar flexion at the wrist and metacarpo-phalangeal joints. A less common presentation is the carpal tunnel syndrome. Although rheumatoid disease does not usually present for the first time with 'trigger finger' this not uncommon complication occurs when the affected digit can be flexed easily, but only with difficulty can the patient extend it, sometimes with the accompaniment of an audible click or snap.

Osteoarthrosis may affect the wrists, with pain and stiffness especially at the radial aspect. Commonly in elderly patients the interphalangeal joints may be affected with the typical nodular swellings (Heberden's nodes) which give rise to a gnarled appearance on the back of the fingers.

Causes

Paronychia and whitlow are usually caused by infection with *Staphylococcus aureus,* introduced by minor trauma in the form of small abrasions or pricks. *Palmar and web space infections* are caused similarly. More chronic low-grade paronychia is caused by *Candida albicans* infection.

Tenosynovitis is a reaction to mechanical insult: sometimes direct injury, but more commonly overuse in unaccustomed circumstances. *Tendovaginitis* has similar primary causes but results in thickening of the fibrous sheath of the thumb tendons over the groove of the radial styloid.

Sprains and fractures are the result of trauma.

Ganglia usually arise from degenerative changes in a tendon sheath or joint capsule, but the underlying pathogenesis is still not clear.

Carpal tunnel syndrome is caused by constriction of the median nerve beneath the flexor retinaculum on the anterior aspect of the wrist. Oedema of the tendon sheaths (often occurring at night when the tendons are immobile), sometimes associated with 'physiological' fluid retention as in pregnancy, at the menopause or premenstrual phase of menstruation, rheumatoid tenosynovitis or myxoedematous thickening, are amongst other conditions which precipitate the development of the syndrome.

Dupuytren's contracture is associated with abnormal thickening and contracture of the palmar fascia, the basic cause of which is not known, though it may be associated with trauma and there is a hereditary predisposition. Sometimes the condition is associated with similar fibrous thickening over the knuckles: so-called 'Garrod's pads'.

Rheumatoid arthritis continues to present one of the major etiological puzzles still facing medicine and the reader is referred to Chapter 3.63 on The patient complaining of rheumatism, for further consideration of both the causes and management of rheumatoid disease and of *osteoarthrosis*.

History and examination

The history of infective lesions of the hands and fingers is commonly a short one and usually fairly typical. Paronychia develop as a painful lesion of the nail fold sometimes associated with a history of previous trauma (as with a 'rag nail') or a small scratch or prick in the region of the nail base (though often no such injury can be recollected). A longer history may be given of a chronic low-grade infection of the nail fold in patients involved in wet work with the hands (e.g. housewives). Examination consists of inspection of the lesion and palpation to detect any fluctuation. If there is any discharge a swab may be helpful.

With pulp-space infection (*whitlow*) there is a similarly short history of pain, often very severe and throbbing, in the tip of the finger. There may sometimes be a preceding history of a prick (e.g. with a thorn) and inspection reveals an inflamed swelling of the terminal pulp space with acute tenderness on palpation. Pus obtained after incision of the abcess should be cultured as a guide to further antibiotic management if drainage proves to be inadequate.

In *palmar and web-space infections* there is a similar fairly short history of pain and stiffness of the hand and fingers. Inspection often shows a red swelling on the dorsum of the hand but careful examination with gentle palpation (using the point of a pencil) to elicit tenderness will show the source of the infection to be on the palmar aspect.

Symptoms suggestive of *tenosynovitis or tendovaginitis* should lead to an attempt to elicit any preceding history of unaccustomed use of the wrist (hedge cutting and typewriting being two common pursuits implicated). There is usually no abnormality to be detected on simple inspection, and tenderness is not common but palpation may reveal crepitus on movement of the affected tendon. In tendovaginitis the fibrous tendon sheath may be felt in the region of the radial styloid. In tendovaginitis of the long extensors of the thumb, pain is aggravated when the patient adducts the wrist while grasping the thumb in the affected hand.

Differentiation between *sprains and fractures*, especially around the wrist, may be difficult on clinical grounds alone. A clear history of the injury may give a clue, direct violence being the most usual cause of fractures. A history of a fall on an outstretched hand should lead to a careful examination for tenderness over the distal ends of the radius and ulna (even in the absence of an obvious 'dinner fork' deformity) and, especially in younger patients, for tenderness in the anatomical snuff box which may indicate a fractured scaphoid. In most cases of direct trauma to the hands or wrists x-ray examination will be indicated at the outset, and in *all* patients whose symptoms fail to subside within a few days.

The history of a *ganglion* is that of the gradual development of a small swelling, usually on the wrist, occasionally causing mild discomfort. Inspection and palpation confirm the presence of a non-inflamed and often slightly mobile firm lump. Given the characteristic site, consistency and lack of inflammation no further examination or investigation is needed.

Symptoms suggesting the *carpal tunnel syndrome* include the distribution and time relationship of the pain (typically disturbing the sleep at night), methods of relief adopted by the patient (many find that exercising the fingers or shaking the hands in the air or pressing them on a cold surface help to relieve the pain), any association with the menstrual cycle, and symptoms and signs of pregnancy, myxoedema or rheumatoid disease. Local examination is generally unrewarding, but in advanced cases there may be wasting of the thenar eminence and loss of sensory perception in the distribution of the median nerve: palmar aspect of the thumb, index and middle fingers – especially the tips of these digits.

Dupuytren's contracture develops gradually and, while there is rarely any contributory antecedent history, occasionally trauma may predispose and there is also a hereditary tendency. Diagnostic features include puckering of the skin at the base of the ring and little fingers, the late development of flexural deformities and eventually inability to extend the fingers.

When *rheumatoid arthritis* is suspected enquiry should be made about the time relationship of maximum pain and stiffness (characteristically worst in the mornings), symptoms in other joints, manifestations of systemic disease (undue tiredness, breathlessness) or symptoms of neuropathies – such as the carpal tunnel syndrome, or tendon involvement – such as trigger finger and family history of arthropathies. Inspection and palpation of the affected joints and observation of ranges of movement should be supplemented by x-rays of the affected joints (on both sides, for the purposes of comparison), chest x-ray, a blood count (for anaemia), erythrocyte sedimentation rate (as a measure of disease activity) and latex rheumatoid test (Rose Waaler or equivalent).

A similar scheme of history taking and examination is suitable when *osteoarthrosis* appears likely. A history of preceding injury in the far past is mainly of academic interest and unlikely to influence substantially either further investigation or management. Some patients, however, are encouraged by the thought that their symptoms are not the non-specific result of advancing years, but are associated with a specific (if incompletely understood) degenerative process.

Management

Paronychia in the early stages can be treated with local applications of antibiotics such as fucidic acid or neomycin and bacitracin. If the presence of *Candida albicans* is suspected or confirmed, nystatin is indicated. If the lesion is very moist, painting with povidone-iodine or 1 per cent gentian violet, may be helpful. Where there is any fluctuation indicating the presence of pus, incision is indicated. This should be performed under ring block anaesthesia with a longitudinal incision from the base of the nail bed just proximal to the nail fold extended distally to join with the straight edge of the nail (Figure 1). It is essential to check that the lignocaine used for the ring block is *plain* and does not contain adrenaline. Pus should be evacuated by gentle squeezing and a firm dressing applied and changed twice a day for the next two or three days.

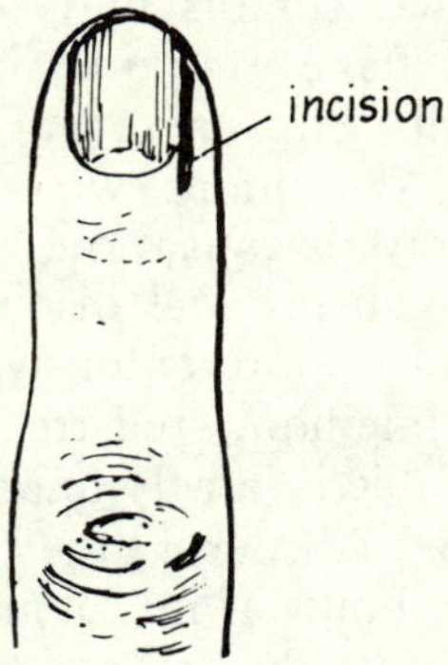

Figure 1 – Incision for paronychia

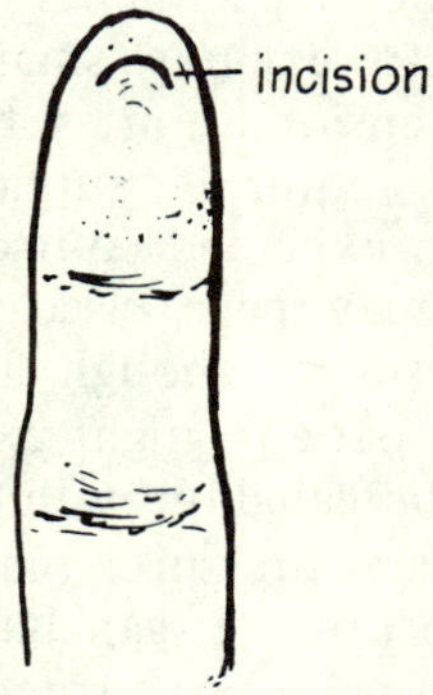

Figure 2 – Incision for whitlow

A *whitlow* seen within the first twenty-four hours may also be dealt with in the general practitioner's surgery or treatment room. Temporizing by prescribing antibiotics or using poultices alone is unwise because the condition readily develops into osteomyelitis. In this case the incision should be made transversely over the point of maximum tenderness (Figure 2). If symptoms have been present for longer than twenty-four hours it is likely that slough will be beginning to form and treatment is best undertaken (as a matter of urgency) by a surgeon.

Palmar and web space infections are similarly best treated at a hospital accident and emergency department.

Stiffness and swelling are common concomitants of hand infections and injuries. They may be minimized by elevation (resting the hand on a pillow at night) and early *active* exercises to hasten rehabilitation.

Tenosynovitis can be treated by partial immobilization in Elastoplast strapping for a week or ten days followed by two or three weeks with a 'tubigrip' support. Alternatively, counter-irritation by firm massaging with iodine ointment, B.P. twice a day for a fortnight has been reported to be effective treatment.

Tendovaginitis may be treated initially by an injection of 100 mg of hydrocortisone acetate into the swollen tendon sheath (felt over the radial styloid). If this fails referral for formal division of the sheath is indicated.

The sprained wrist is treated by immobilization in an adhesive bandage applied from the mid-forearm and extending to the metacarpal heads. For patients known to have skin sensitivity to the adhesive, the bandage can be applied with the sticky side out: dusting with talc once the bandage is applied removes the stickiness.

Fractures are in the main best dealt with initially in accident and emergency departments and suspected sprains may also need referral to exclude small crack or flake fractures or (as in hyperextension injuries to the thumb) rupture of a collateral ligament requiring surgical repair. All sprains which fail to follow an expected course require x-ray investigation.

Ganglia may be excised if they are causing real discomfort or embarrassment, though this may involve more extensive surgery than the patient might expect. The time-honoured treatment of hitting the ganglion with the family Bible is largely impractical – but direct pressure may sometimes disperse the ganglion. A proportion of ganglia (possibly about 1 in 3) may settle spontaneously. Recurrence after various treatments (including surgery) is not uncommon.

The management of severely disabling and persistent *carpal tunnel syndrome* is also surgical. Longitudinal division of the flexor retinaculum almost invariably relieves symptoms successfully and permanently. If the symptoms are not too severe a short trial of diuretic treatment may be worth while and often this is all that is required. The condition is usually mild when it is associated with pregnancy, and it clears spontaneously during the puerperium. If symptoms are sufficiently disabling they may warrant consideration of steroid injection and/or splinting but this may be only a temporary measure pending surgery.

The management of *rheumatoid arthritis* and *osteoarthrosis* is considered in chapter 3.63 on The patient complaining of rheumatism. One of the general practitioner's most useful roles in the management of the arthropathies, especially when affecting the hands, is that of advising or obtaining advice on suitable aids to daily living, such as enlarged grips for cutlery or pens, gadgets for turning taps and unscrewing lids, 'velcro' fastenings in place of buttons on clothes, and so on.

Conclusion

The diagnosis of most hand problems seen in general practice presents few difficulties and adequate history and simple examination **will usually suffice,** with X-rays in cases of injury and some **simple blood tests when rheumatoid disease is suspected. Management of some of these problems is surgical, and here the general practitioner has an important role in suggesting the initial diagnosis and in reinforcing advice in the vital process of rehabilitation, especially by encouraging maximum mobilization to prevent the development of chronic or even permanently disabling stiffness.**

Further reading

Bailey, H. (1956): *Pye's Surgical Handicraft*. 17th ed. Bristol: John Wright & Sons

Ellis, M. (1970): *The Casualty Officer's Handbook*. 3rd ed. Longman: Butterworths

Hodgkin, K. (1973): *Towards Earlier Diagnosis*. 3rd ed. Edinburgh: Churchill Livingstone

Royal College of General Practitioners, Office of Population Censuses and Surveys, Department of Health and Social Security (1986): *Morbidity Statistics from General Practice 1981–82*. HMSO Series MB5 No. 1

3.67
Hip problems
J.D.E. Knox

Before considering the hip problems common in general practice, some generalizations can be made about clinical features — especially pain — of patients with conditions relating to the hip region.

Pain associated with abnormality in the hip joint is usually described as aching, aggravated by movement and felt in the groin and antero-medial aspect of the upper thigh. Sometimes, however, it may be felt in the knee and if the knee should also be the site of osteoarthrosis, the hip lesion may easily be missed. Some patients with osteoarthrosis of the hip experience pain in the low back and buttock and some patients with conditions of the lumbo-sacral spine may present with pain in the hip region. As the adductor muscles are stronger than abductors, when the hip is in spasm, the leg tends to take up a position of adduction, external rotation, and flexion. This may lead to apparent shortening as the patient tilts the pelvis to realign the leg. A limp is a frequent accompaniment and if the patient uses a walking-stick, he may have found greater help from holding the stick in the hand of the side opposite to that of the affected hip.

Epidemiological considerations

Pain in the region of the hip is not a common complaint in general practice: in a personal series of 300 consecutive patients presenting any painful condition at a first consultation, less than ten were related to the hip region. Table I lists some of the more common encountered in general practice.

Causes

Osteoarthrosis of the hip joint is the commonest of the conditions in which a definitive diagnosis is possible. The etiology is still not fully understood, but factors include pre-existing underlying conditions, such as congenital subluxation of the hip, developmental conditions like Perthe's disease or slipped epiphysis, and trauma. Obesity is an associated factor and one which is linked with other painful hip conditions, the causes of which remain obscure: these include slipped femoral epiphysis, and non-articular rheumatism ('fibrositis'). In Perthe's disease, the nature of the condition is an osteochondritis of the femoral head, but why this should occur remains unclear.

History and presentations

Among commoner presentations is the middle-aged or elderly patient (more often male than female) who complains of a boring pain, worse towards the end of the day, relieved by lying down and aggravated by standing. This is suggestive of osteoarthrosis. Having to stand around for long periods at social functions becomes an ordeal. Pain may also be accompanied by stiffness which, unlike the pain, may be more marked after a spell of rest, and eased after movement. In some patients, it is the stiffness, deformity and limp which become the main features, pain taking second place. Such presentations of osteoarthrosis may also be associated with past episodes of acute pain associated with relatively minor trauma but giving rise to several weeks' incapacity at a time.

Bruises and muscle strains and other trauma	8
'Non-articular' rheumatism (mainly in gluteal muscles)	8
Osteoarthrosis of hip/spine	4
Sciatica (not associated with lumbago)	3
Fractured neck of femur	2
Paget's disease (pelvis and femur)	1 in 2 years
Acute painful hip in children	1 in 5 years
Perthe's disease	1 in 5 years
Slipped epiphysis	1 in 5 years

Table I. — Commoner hip conditions
Number of episodes in one year in a practice of 2,000

Pain in and around the hip region may be encountered as a transient phenomenon, especially in middle-aged obese women. There is no clear history of injury or strain, and, apart from local tenderness in the soft tissues of the affected region, there is little to be found on examination. Such a condition, settling usually within about ten days, is likely to have been a manifestation of non-articular rheumatism. These ill-defined conditions are relatively common, yet the underlying cause is not understood.

In painful lesions of the hip region, and especially in the elderly, the possibility of fracture of the neck of the femur may be raised. The history of injury, characteristically a fall (such as falling out of bed), will usually be forthcoming. The immobility of the affected leg because of pain on movement will be evident, and the foot will be seen to be everted.

The child, 2 to 5 years of age, brought by parents anxious because of a newly developed limp, raises different possibilities. If the condition is associated with obvious pain, limitation of hip movements and some systemic disturbance, acute transient arthritis of the hip is one possibility. The onset of acute osteomyelitis, though much less common, is another. Acute transient arthritis usually settles spontaneously within one week. The child presenting with a limp may also suggest the possibility of trauma — accidental or non-accidental.

The older child, 5 to 10 years, may present with a complaint of aching pain, worse on walking and associated with a slight limp. There is usually no clear-cut history of injury and the child is obviously in good health. Such a presentation raises the possibility of osteochondritis (Perthe's disease). A similar history in a rather older child, around the age of puberty, might suggest slipped epiphysis, especially if the patient is overweight.

When the complaint of pain persists, and does not appear to respond to analgesics or is associated with other signs and symptoms, such as loss of weight, less common possibilities need to be considered; these include malignant disease with secondary deposits in bone, Paget's disease, or metabolic bone diseases.

Examination

Before attention is directed to the hip, observation of the patient and the setting may provide useful diagnostic information. The elderly patient lying in bed with the leg externally rotated is a clinical pointer to fractured neck of femur. The patient who walks with the leg adducted and the foot externally rotated, using a stick as already described, is likely to be suffering from osteoarthrosis.

While the detailed examination of the hip described in undergraduate textbooks is not likely to give the general practitioner a high yield of diagnostic information, attention should be paid to the following points, especially at a first consultation for the complaint.

The patient should strip, leaving on only the pants. The way he undresses will give some indication of any restriction of movements of the hip joints and spine.

The gluteal muscles and thighs are examined for wasting, which may be a feature of osteoarthrosis. Bruising may be looked for in cases of suspected injury.

The patient is asked to stand on one leg, and supporting himself on the back of a chair, swings the other leg round in a circle: circumduction is impaired in many hip conditions, especially osteoarthrosis. With the patient lying relaxed on the couch, the leg should be rolled from side to side: limitation of internal and external rotation are early signs of osteoarthrosis, but as the disease progresses adduction, abduction, flexion and extension all become limited.

If the question of shortening needs to be settled, it is worth while measuring both legs from fixed points, such as the distance from anterior superior iliac spine to medial malleolus.

In most consultations, the information derived from the history and examination, augmented by the family doctor's pre-existing knowledge of the patient and his circumstances, will usually allow the problem to be formulated. Occasionally, however, additional investigation is necessary, such as estimation of the erythrocyte sedimentation rate (ESR) and X-ray of the hips. While a normal ESR does not exclude malignant disease, it makes it less likely and is in keeping with such diagnoses as non-articular rheumatism, trauma and osteoarthrosis. Before ordering an x-ray of hips in a woman of childbearing age, the possibility of early pregnancy must be excluded. Most X-ray request forms now include a section for information about the last menstrual period.

Management

As in most consultations in general practice the patient wants to know the following:

— What the doctor thinks is the matter
— Whether or not it is serious
— What is likely to happen
— What he needs to do to alleviate the symptoms
— What can be done to prevent future similar trouble
— Must he stay off work.

For the relief of pain in the hip aspirin in simple or soluble form in a dosage of two 300 mg tablets three or four times a day is often the drug of choice. (In extreme cases, especially of rheumatoid disease, the dose may be pushed as high as 12 to 16 tablets a day.) For patients with peptic ulceration or known intolerance to aspirin for other reasons, 500 mg tablets of paracetamol, though perhaps marginally less effective, are adequate substitutes. Severe exacerbations of pain may be treated by short courses of indomethacin 25 mg three times daily and nocturnal pain may be controlled by the use of indomethacin suppositories.

A stout walking-stick, used on the unaffected side, is a simple and sensible aid to mobility. Elderly patients are sometimes reluctant to resort to the use of a stick and may need a great deal of encouragement: it can be helpful to point out that other devices such as spectacles, dentures and even hearing aids are often used without embarrassment, and that the use of a walking-stick should be viewed in this way.

Patients who are overweight should be encouraged to lose weight. The prospect of some relief from discomfort provides an incentive which can make the control of obesity a much more purposeful exercise than is often the case.

Physiotherapy in the form of deep heat and exercises can be useful in selected cases, especially of osteoarthrosis. The more self-reliant patients will welcome instruction on exercises which can be carried out at home. It is useful to keep a supply of written or printed instructions which can be given to such patients. An example of such a set of hip exercises is as follows:

> Lying on a firm bed, either flat with one pillow, or half propped-up with two or three pillows, whichever is more comfortable, first of all tighten and then slowly relax your seat muscles.
>
> Next, stretch one leg out to the side of the bed keeping the knee straight, and bring it across the other leg and then down: repeat this with the other leg.
>
> Finally, with your legs straight together, turn one foot in towards the centre and then roll it over as far as you can to the side: do this three times with each foot.
>
> This set of exercises should be carried out for ten to fifteen minutes daily.

In addition it is helpful in preventing a flexion deformity to lie prone on a firm surface for up to half an hour daily when this is possible. It may be done while watching television or reading. Long periods of standing should be avoided but walking within moderation helps to retain mobility.

Referral

In those episodes in which the diagnosis is in doubt, and especially where fractured neck of femur is suspected, referral for x-ray and consultant opinion will usually be indicated.

The condition of osteoarthrosis of the hip has received more attention in recent years partly because of increasing success of surgical management. Among the operative treatments available are the following:

— The hanging hip procedure, in which pain relief can be obtained by reducing mechanical pressure through the hip joint. Operation involves 'releasing' the adductor muscles, gluteus medius and minimus and psoas. This is a palliative procedure for bed-ridden patients. Another soft-tissue procedure involves cutting the adductor tendons, and the operation can help elderly women whose bilateral hip joint disease causes difficulties with personal hygiene.
— Osteotomy has been employed in a variety of ways, the principle being to attempt to improve alignment and the distribution of weight by correcting rotational flexion and

adduction deformities. This operation has the disadvantage of a prolonged postoperative spell of incapacity, with up to three months or longer before weight bearing is permitted.

— The operative procedure of choice today is the total hip replacement in which the acetabulum is relined and the head of the femur replaced. The materials used for the prostheses and the glue employed to cement these into place are constantly being improved and because of this the long-term prognosis is continually improving so that modern hip replacements may be expected to last at least 15 years. This has encouraged surgeons to operate on younger patients. Surgeons are however reluctant to undertake a total replacement on patients under the age of about 55 years and in these cases some specialists favour a surface arthroplasty in which the head of the femur is retained but re-covered and the acetabulum is relined. The relatively short experience of this operation and the rapid changes in materials used make it difficult to forecast how long these hips will last. The major advantage of the procedure is that it can always be converted later into a total hip replacement.

Convalescence after arthroplasty is much quicker than after osteotomy. Patients can be expected to be walking on crutches within a week, with sticks in six weeks and with full weight bearing in three months. Full weight bearing is usually possible much earlier but some surgeons believe that the long-term prognosis is improved, particularly in surface arthroplasties, if it is delayed to this time.

In the meantime active physiotherapy is necessary to build up the muscles around the hip joint.

As with all major surgery, hip replacement carries an immediate mortality due usually to pulmonary embolus. The most important complication is infection in the new joint causing recurrence of pain and loosening of the prosthesis. There also appears to be an increased risk of late infection and many surgeons recommend that patients should take antibiotics before procedures, e.g. dental care, which may cause a bacteraemia, or in treating infections in which a bacteraemia is likely to occur.

The general practitioner's main role in the management of osteoarthrosis of the hips is in deciding when the patient should be referred for surgery, bearing in mind the waiting lists which exist in most hospitals. In making this decision it may be assumed that about 90 per cent of operations will be very successful in terms of pain relief, but about 5 per cent may be disastrous. Two useful guides in making a decision are the extent to which pain disturbs sleep and the extent to which it interferes with the individual's occupation or, in older patients, threatens social intercourse.

3.68
Knee problems

J.D.E. Knox

When one considers the stresses to which the knee joints are exposed and the apparent lack of strong supporting structures in comparison with other joints, knee problems might be expected to be commonly encountered in general practice. Precise and detailed information on this point is not available, but personal experience suggests that patients present with symptoms referable to the knee much less often than, say, with backache. If all knee conditions are taken together, some 30 to 40 episodes may be expected to be encountered in a year in a practice of 2,000 patients. The commoner presenting symptoms include, in order of frequency, pain, stiffness, swelling, clicking and locking. A limp is a frequent accompaniment; as a presenting symptom, it is more usually encountered in children.

Pain may be of various kinds, varying from an agonizing stabbing associated with locking (when a loose body becomes entrapped between joint surfaces) to a dull ache worse after walking (as in osteoarthrosis). The possibility of pain apparently related to the knee but in reality arising from the hip joint has already been mentioned (Chapter 3.67).

Commoner conditions and causes

In table I are listed some commoner conditions, with an estimate of the frequency with which they occur.

Trauma is a relatively frequent factor and may be responsible for a variety of clinical pictures. Among the commonest are simple bruising arising from falls, and seen more often in boys and elderly ladies (sometimes associated with 'drop attacks'). Here the trauma is of a direct nature. More extreme violence (as in a road traffic accident) may be associated with fractures of the patella or articular surfaces.

Strains and bruises	16
Osteoarthrosis	8
Prepatellar bursitis	4
Internal derangements (mainly tears of cartilage)	2
Genu valgum and genu varum	2
Traumatic synovitis	2
Miscellaneous	6–8
including – bursae around the knee synovitis and arthritis part of a polyarthritis.	

Table I. – Estimate of frequency of some commoner conditions in a practice of 2,000 patients in one year

Indirect injuries, usually resulting from rotation of the body with the knee in flexion, may be the start of tears of the semilunar cartilages. Both direct and indirect injury may be associated with a transient painful stiffness and swelling, the result of traumatic synovitis.

Low-grade trauma of repeated or continuous nature, such as frequent kneeling, may give rise to prepatellar bursitis: the traditional housemaid's knee. A knee which has been the site of past trouble affecting internal structures is especially liable to instability and osteoarthritic changes. Osteoarthrosis may arise for no obvious reason, and although both joints are usually affected, attention is commonly fixed on one.

Genu valgum and varum in children. – A degree of valgus ('knock knee') is normal, and in children it may reach such marked proportions as to create considerable anxiety in the parents. It is important for the doctor to appreciate that this 'deformity', if unaccompanied by other features, is almost always an extreme example at the upper end of the normal range. Left to itself, the condition resolves spontaneously. If the intermalleolar gap (measured with the child lying flat with his knees together and patellae facing forward) is more than 9 to 10 cm (3½ to 4 inches), it may be wise to seek an orthopaedic opinion.

Genu varum is much less common and may also be a transient developmental phenomenon. Both postural 'abnormalities' may of course be associated with a variety of pathologies, from metabolic bone disease to osteitis deformans, and the reader is referred to the appropriate specialist textbooks for further information.

Osgood-Schlatter's disease. – Prepubertal children (most commonly boys) occasionally present with pain and tenderness over one or both tibial tuberosities, due to osteochondritis (Osgood-Schlatter's disease). The only physical signs are some enlargement and acutely localized tenderness of the affected tuberosity and the condition can be confirmed by X-ray examination. This is generally a self-limiting condition and the only treatment usually recommended is abstinence from active sports for a period of some months, although occasionally immobilization of the joint in a plaster of Paris splint may be indicated.

Presentation

The history of trauma will usually be clear, though care may be needed in the elderly. The consternation of relatives and the doctor's concern to exclude a cerebrovascular cause of a drop attack can divert attention away from knee injuries which may not be complained about by the old person now confined to bed. The twisting injury, with subsequent inability to straighten the leg fully, commonly sustained in an athletic setting, suggests the possibility of a cartilage tear. The pain is often localized by the patient to a point medial (or lateral) to the patellar ligament in the line of the joint. A stiff, rather painful, slightly swollen knee, with the stiffness and swelling developing some hours after the injury are more characteristic of traumatic synovitis. Swelling and stiffness of rapid onset (within the hour) following injury, suggest the possibility of haemarthrosis – a possibility which calls for speedy referral to hospital. Swelling which has gradually become apparent over a period of days, and confined to the lower aspect of the patella, is characteristic of 'housemaid's knee'. Although the relationship to trauma is usually obvious, the condition may apparently arise spontaneously.

Pain, swelling and stiffness of the knee may be a manifestation of systemic conditions such as rheumatoid arthritis, sarcoidosis or rheumatic fever, to mention but a few. Knee involvement in rheumatoid arthritis is relatively common, though not usually a presenting feature.

A history of a knee that gives way, and occasionally locks, dating from an athletic injury, suggests an established tear of one of the cartilages, but a similar history may be given by the patient with a loose body in the joint. In both conditions the patient may complain of clicks.

Some otherwise normal people are plagued by knees that emit loud clicks, especially on climbing stairs. The cause is not clearly understood, and the condition, which may run in families, is of no pathological significance.

Examination

In general practice, the combination of the history and simple inspection of the joint will usually afford enough information for the problem to be defined with sufficient clarity for action to be recommended.

If the diagnosis is not immediately clear, fuller examination, with both thighs exposed and all movements tested, including hip movements, is called for. Tenderness on the medial side in the line of the joint and a positive McMurray's sign confirm the suspicion of a torn medial meniscus. The McMurray test is carried out as follows. With the patient lying on a couch, the doctor places one hand over the front of the affected knee. With the other he grasps the ankle and controls rotation of the tibia on the femur. Gently rotating the leg, first medially and then laterally, he straightens the patient's flexed knee, keeping a steady pressure on the hand over the knee. Pain, spasm and a click indicate the presence of a tear.

Effusion can usually be determined by the presence of a swelling bulging out above and at the sides of the patella. If the patella is held fixed with one hand pressing from above, the fluid may be displaced laterally or medially by appropriate pressure from the other hand. The eliciting of a 'tap' by pressing the fixed patella back on the surface of the femur is not now considered to be a useful sign.

In long-standing conditions, it is worth while to assess the state of the quadriceps muscles by feeling the tone and measuring the circumference of the thighs at equal points above the tibial tuberosity. Any degree of wasting calls for careful monitoring and advice on quadriceps exercises, as set out in the appendix.

More detailed examination will be indicated in the diagnosis of other conditions, suspicion of which will of itself indicate referral for specialist help in diagnosis and/or management.

Further investigation

Theoretically a long list of investigations could be drawn up, but in practice if further tests are required, they can usually be confined to the erythrocyte sedimentation rate (ESR) and X-ray. Elevation of the ESR helps to confirm a suspicion of more widespread disease than the swollen painful joint might indicate: e.g., rheumatoid disease. X-rays can help in providing base-line data for later comparison as well as assisting in the diagnosis of individual conditions such as osteoarthrosis.

Some principles of management

As with many other conditions affecting the locomotor system, management of common sprains or arthralgias consists of heat and support to the affected part, and analgesics. Securing adequate rest is not always easy, especially when the patient is a mother of young children, or an unskilled worker in an area of high unemployment. The ideal of complete non-weight bearing may occasionally have to be modified to instruction to the patient to rest as much as possible. The knee may be supported and its movements restricted by the application of a Jones' bandage: an elastic non-adhesive bandage is applied round the joint, and several pads of cotton wool (about the size of the hand) are incorporated into the windings so that firm pressure is fairly evenly applied around the joint.

As part of this initial management, the patient should be instructed to perform isometric quadriceps exercises (Appendix (a)) even while resting in bed, with the aim of preserving the strength and tone of the muscles on which stability of the joint largely depends. These may be combined with other exercises (appendix (b)) as convalescence proceeds.

Heat in the form of the hot water bottle or electric pad can be a soothing form of treatment: some patients find that massage with warm olive oil alleviates pain and stiffness.

The choice of analgesic should be governed by simplicity, effectiveness and cost, and the patient is usually given the responsibility of judging and adjusting dose and frequency of administration. For most conditions, aspirin and paracetamol suffice, but indomethacin can be a more effective drug for acute exacerbations of osteoarthrosis.

Some special considerations

The patient with exacerbations of either rheumatoid arthritis or osteoarthrosis can be helped by intermittent injections of hydrocortisone. There are no reasons why this should not be performed under suitable conditions in general practice: indeed the knee is one of the most accessible joints in the body, and the procedure is straightforward.

The patient sits on the edge of a high couch with the knee flexed over the side. The doctor sits facing the patient in a well-lighted room. The line of the joint lateral to the patella ligament is identified by palpation. The skin is cleaned, sterilized and anaesthetized with a small intra-cutaneous injection of local anaesthetic which is then continued more deeply into the capsule of the joint. A larger bore needle is then substituted and aimed to enter the joint obliquely behind the lateral edge of the patellar ligament. It is worth while aspirating any effusion and sending a specimen for appropriate bacteriological, biochemical and other analysis, before injecting 1 to 2 ml hydrocortisone. There may be an initial increase in pain over the next twenty-four hours before relief is experienced.

Prepatellar bursitis. – This condition may subside spontaneously, if the patient avoids activities such as kneeling. If there has been no improvement after ten days of rest and support, the bursa may be aspirated under conditions similar to those described above for intra-articular injection. A Jones' bandage or 'tubigrip' bandage is then applied and the support is maintained for a week.

Cartilage problems. – Once a firm diagnosis has been made that a tear has occurred, it is probably wise to obtain an early surgical opinion because of the high frequency with which exacerbations occur. Often, however, the evidence is not clear-cut, or the patient may be reluctant to accept referral. In these circumstances, a combination of local support to the knee and self-help physiotherapy along the lines set out in the Appendix (a) and (b) may suffice.

Control of obesity. – Any measures likely to ease the strain on locomotor structures of the lower limb should be considered in the management of patients suffering from painful chronic or recurrent conditions of the knee. Control of obesity, so rarely achieved in the absence of good motivation, may be attempted with a greater sense of purpose and the reader is referred to Chapter 3.41.

Appendix

Self-help physiotherapy

(a) *Quadriceps exercises*

1. Sit on a low stool and then stand up and sit down again without using your hands.
2. Sitting on a chair, put a weight of one or two pounds over your ankle (a plastic bag with some sand or soil will do) and then lift your leg until it is horizontal and then gently lower it.
3. Sitting on a chair, tighten up the muscles of your thighs and then slowly relax them again.

Do each of these exercises six to eight times every two hours.

(b) *Knee exercises*

1. Press backs of knees on to bed and tighten thigh muscles (i.e. quadriceps contraction), then relax.
2. Bend one knee up until the heel is level with the opposite knee: repeat with other knee.
3. Lift leg straight off bed, hold it, then lower slowly down: repeat with other leg.

The exercises should be done three times. The routine should be performed daily. The exercises should be carried out on a firm bed either in the half-lying position supported by two or three pillows or lying flat with one pillow.

3.69 Ankle and foot problems

J.D.E. Knox and J.J.C. Cormack

Problems involving the ankle or the foot seldom give rise to much diagnostic difficulty in general practice, although decisions about management may present a greater challenge. Osteoarthrosis affecting the ankle or foot is relatively rare, and while all the distal joints may be involved in rheumatoid disease, the foot and ankle do not appear to give rise to symptoms as often as the hand and wrist. A sizeable proportion of foot and ankle problems arise from the wearing of unsuitable (if fashionable) footwear: a situation which the medical profession seems to be singularly powerless to prevent.

The conditions which will be considered in this chapter are:

- Ankle sprains
- Ankle fractures
- Achilles tendon injuries
- Ingrowing toenails
- Verrucae
- Bunions
- Gout
- Fractures of the small bones of the foot
- Flat feet.

Figures relating to the epidemiology of ankle and foot problems are incomplete. Table I gives an estimate (derived from the National Morbidity Survey[1] and Hodgkin's studies[2]) of the number of episodes likely to present in one year in a practice of 2,000 patients.

Ankle sprains and fractures

Patients presenting with trauma to the ankle usually give a history of an inversion injury causing a sprain of the lateral ligaments. Those patients with the much rarer eversion injuries will usually require to be x-rayed to exclude fractures of the fibula and/or tibia. In the case of a fall from a height, fracture of the calcaneus (and possibly compression fractures of vertebral bodies) should be looked for.

Ankle sprains	14
Ingrowing toenails	9
Bunions	4
Gout	6
Fractures of the small bones of the foot	3
Flat feet	2
Ankle fractures	2

Table I. – Estimated number of episodes of ankle and foot problems presenting in one year in a practice of 2,000

If the history is clearly one of an inversion injury, the ankle should be examined for swelling and tenderness which usually occur in front of, and either over or below, the external malleolus. If there is swelling over the internal malleolus, it is wise to refer for an x-ray, to exclude tibial or fibular fracture. If, however, the practitioner is satisfied on clinical examination that the injury is a simple sprain of the lateral ligaments, treatment can be undertaken without radiology at this stage.

The immediate treatment of a sprained ankle consists of firm support by means of elastic adhesive strapping (reversed in known cases of allergy). With the foot in the neutral position, at right angles to the leg, a stirrup of strapping is applied from half way up the medial side of the leg, round the heel to half way up the lateral side of the leg. A long strip of adhesive bandage is then wound round from a line just proximal to the toes up to and including the free ends of the stirrup. The patient should be encouraged to rest with the foot elevated during the next twenty-four hours, and the use of simple analgesics can be recommended. Symptoms may be alleviated with contrast bathing during this time, by immersing the ankle alternately in hot and cold water (about 20 seconds, in each) for about 5 minutes every 3 to 4 hours, and then thoroughly drying the strapping. After the first twenty-four hours the patient should be encouraged to carry out non-weight-bearing exercises, plantar and dorsi-flexing the foot as fully as possible.

After three to four days the situation should be reviewed. If the strapping is loose, it will need to be reapplied. If at this stage there is tenderness over one or other malleolus, it may be wise to obtain an x-ray, but provided progress is being maintained (that is swelling, pain and tenderness decreasing) active weight bearing should now be encouraged. After the first week the adhesive bandage should be replaced by a non-adhesive support (such as 'tubigrip'). Full pain-free function should normally be achieved in about two to three weeks.

Occasionally an ankle sprain will be associated with avulsion of the base of the fifth metatarsal. The treatment here is the same as that for a simple ligamentous sprain but full recovery may take longer: usually about 4 to 5 weeks. Fractures of the long bones should be treated in an Accident and Emergency or an Orthopaedic Department.

Achilles (calcaneus) tendonitis and rupture

Achilles (calcaneus) tendon injuries tend to occur in the active and athletic. Tendonitis presents as a diffuse pain over the entire length of the tendon, worsened by plantar flexion: there is often a history of preceding unaccustomed running or a long walk. Examination reveals tenderness and sometimes palpable crepitus over the tendon when the foot is moved. Treatment is rest with the ankle supported with elastic adhesive strapping. Hydrocortisone injections are now thought to be contraindicated because of a liability to predispose to later tendon rupture.

Rupture (either partial or complete) of the tendon presents with sudden pain typically described as the feeling of being suddenly struck from behind while walking or running. If the rupture is incomplete, the partial integrity of the tendon can be demonstrated by lying the patient prone and gripping the calf muscles which will cause a small degree of plantar flexion of the foot. If a diagnosis of tendon rupture is made, the patient should be referred for specialist treatment which will consist of immobilization of the ankle in plaster of Paris with the foot held in extreme plantar flexion if the rupture is partial. The treatment of complete rupture is open surgical repair.

Ingrowing toenails

Ingrowing toenails are apt to be considered among the trivia of medical practice, but they can cause significant pain and disability. The symptom usually presented is one of pain at one or other side of the nail of the big toe, caused by inflammation secondary to the irritation of the skin-fold by the pressure of the growing margin of the nail. The treatment for this is time-consuming, involving repeated attendances for dressings (usually best carried out by a nurse). The infection in most cases will settle with the application of a local antibiotic (such as fucidic acid) or antiseptic (such as povidone-iodine), with overlying tulle dressings. If cellulitis is present, a course of systemic flucloxacillin or erythromycin should be prescribed.

Once the initial infection is controlled, the angle of the nail should be packed with a wisp of chiropody wool to diminish the pressure of the growing nail on the skin-fold, while distal growth proceeds. A 'v'-shaped cut in the middle of the growing edge of the nail may help to relieve pressure. If conservative measures fail, the patient should be referred to a chiropodist, or in very resistant cases to a surgeon for avulsion of the offending nail, or excision of the nail bed.

An undramatic but important piece of health education to prevent the occurrence of ingrowing, is the instruction to patients that they should always cut their toenails straight across rather than shaping them down at the edges.

Verrucae

Verrucae or plantar warts may be symptomless but noticed by a child's parents as flat lesions on the plantar aspect of the foot or a toe, peppered with small black spots which are in fact tiny localized thromboses. Verrucae occurring on the weight-bearing surfaces of the forefoot or heel can give rise to discomfort or pain. The condition is one that affects children and young adults almost exclusively. The responsible virus appears to be spread by the use of communal changing facilities and areas surrounding swimming pools.

Many forms of treatment are advocated (indicating that none is entirely satisfactory) but one of the simplest regimes, as effective as any, is as follows. The area around the wart is first swabbed with ether, to dry the skin and encourage the adhesion of plaster. The healthy skin surrounding the verruca should be protected by a smear of vaseline. A drop of podophyllin compound paint is placed on the verruca and lightly injected in with the tip of a hypodermic needle. A piece of waterproof plastic adhesive strapping is then placed over the lesion and the patient instructed to replace this if it comes off with similar waterproof strapping, emphasizing that the adhesive should come into direct contact with the verruca, so that a dressing should not be used. This procedure is repeated, after scraping the lesion with a clean blade or rubbing with a pumice stone or emery board, at intervals of seven to ten days, and in the majority of cases three or four such applications will lead to total removal of the verruca. Alternative methods are described in Chapter 3.38.

On the vexed question of whether or not to allow the child to continue to go to swimming baths while the verruca (or verrucae, as they are often multiple) is being treated, it would seem illogical to prohibit such healthy recreation — especially in the light of the number of apparently symptomless and untreated lesions which can be observed on the feet of swimmers by any observant doctor who frequents swimming baths — so long as the lesion being treated is covered either with plastic socks, which can be purchased at some of the larger pools or in sports shops, or by simply applying waterproof strapping covering the lesion and encircling the foot.

Bunions

Bunions present as swellings overlying bony prominences on the foot. They are thickened bursae, which may become infected and cause pain. They are uncommon before the fifth decade and women are far more often affected than men. The commonest position for a bunion is overlying the metatarsophalangeal joint of the big toe, especially if there is a degree of hallux valgus.

Apart from dealing with infections occurring in bunions, which falls within the province of the general practitioner, the long-term management of these lesions is properly the responsibility of the chiropodist or the surgeon. Chiropody can ameliorate the symptoms by relieving the pressure of footware by means of pads or rings. A more radical approach involving excision of the underlying bone and arthrodesis can give lasting relief. Judgment is required in deciding which course will be the more appropriate for the individual. Factors such as the patient's wishes, the patient's age, state of general health and mobility will influence the choice.

Gout

Gout is a condition which affects men predominantly and it usually manifests itself clinically after the age of 40. It most commonly begins as an acute monoarthropathy, classically affecting the metatarsophalangeal joint of the big toe, although it may involve the ankle and occasionally the fingers, wrists or elbows. Although sometimes preceded by a vague malaise, the onset is sudden, the patient waking with an acutely painful, red and tender joint for which he is unable to account. The acute onset is the most characteristic diagnostic feature in the history. Examination reveals a hot, red, swollen tender area over the affected joint. The first metatarsophalangeal joint is characteristically affected; yet it is all too easy to dismiss the lesion as a 'cellulitis' or to accept the patient's explanation: 'I must have strained it'. A raised serum uric acid should clinch the diagnosis.

Gout is an inborn error of purine metabolism. It is a hereditary disease but may be precipitated by diuretic drug therapy. The pathology is associated with the liberation of inflammatory agents from leucocytes which have ingested precipitated urates in the affected articular and peri-articular tissues. As the disease becomes chronic, deposition of uric acid may occur in the cartilages of ear or eyelid or elsewhere ('tophi').

While referral to a specialist is not essential, this is often useful to establish the suspected diagnosis, to provide base-line information for judging future moves and for motivating the patient to comply with long-term drug therapy which does not appear to him to offer immediate benefit.

Treatment falls into two phases: the initial treatment of the acute attack and subsequent preventive treatment. For the acute episode indomethacin 50 or 100 mg every four to six hours for the first 48 to 72 hours will usually relieve the pain. The dosage can be reduced as the pain comes under control.

The two most commonly used agents for the long-term preventive treatment of gout are allopurinol and probenecid (Benemid). Allopurinol, usually given in a dose of 300 mg daily, taken after food, blocks the metabolic production of uric acid by inhibiting the action of the enzyme xanthine oxidase. Probenecid (250 mg twice a day after food, increasing stepwise if necessary to 2 g daily in divided doses) increases the excretion of uric acid.

Paradoxically, the initial reduction in serum uric acid levels sometimes itself leads to an exacerbation of acute symptoms. For this reason long term treatment should never be started during an acute attack of gout and colchicine (0.5 mg three times a day) or an anti-inflammatory analgesic is usually additionally prescribed as a prophylactic measure in the initial few months of the introduction of allopurinol or probenecid, until the hyperuricaemia has been corrected.

Although dietary factors are not now thought to play a large part in the pathogenesis of gout, it is reasonable to advise patients to avoid purine-rich foods such as game and offal. A high fluid intake is also desirable in an attempt to prevent the development of uric acid renal calculi.

Exacerbations may be precipitated by alcoholic excesses, or by surgical operations, and patients should be advised accordingly. If the condition is associated with diuretic therapy, appropriate specialist advice may be needed in the management of this more complex (and increasingly prevalent) situation.

Fractures of the metatarsals and phalanges

While as already indicated an avulsion fracture of the base of the fifth metatarsal can occur in severe ankle sprains, most metatarsal and phalangeal fractures are caused by direct trauma. An exception to this is the stress fracture (or 'march fracture') usually involving the 2nd or 3rd metatarsal, occurring after long-distance walking. Tenderness and swelling at the site of the fracture are the two main symptoms, and X-rays are not usually necessary if the history is clear (although they may be desirable for medico-legal purposes, especially if any question of compensation is likely to arise). Small bone fractures heal in two to three weeks and the only treatment required is the wearing of strong footwear, although sometimes a metatarsal support relieves the pressure on the affected metatarsal head and gives some symptomatic relief. Extremely severe pain can be an indication for the application of a below-knee walking plaster.

Flat feet

Flat feet or 'fallen arches' appear largely to have gone the way of septic foci: that is, a condition once thought real and treatable by the medical profession and now generally relegated to the diagnostic dustbin, (although an exception must be made for the rare condition of rigid flat feet, which require specialist orthopaedic management). Flat feet do, however, worry patients, or more accurately patients' parents. The rate of development of the longitudinal arch in the foot varies – all babies' feet are flat and by adolescence, given normal activity, the arches will have formed. The treatment of flat feet is, therefore, the imparting of this knowledge to the parents. If the parents' (or the doctor's) tolerance of therapeutic nihilism is low, a recommendation that the child's shoes are fitted with $\frac{1}{8}$ inch medial inner-raisers may be of at least psychological benefit.

3.70
The patient complaining of discomfort in the legs

J.J.C. Cormack

The symptoms of discomfort or pains in the legs may be due to trauma, musculo-skeletal or rheumatic problems (see Chapters 3.67, 3.68, 3.69), varicose veins (Chapter 3.40) or to intermittent claudication, night cramps or the restless legs syndrome. These last three conditions will be considered in this chapter.

Intermittent claudication was reported by Hodgkin[1] to be presented by 2 patients per 1,000 per year and muscle cramps (bracketed with restless legs) by 5 patients per 1,000 per year.

Intermittent claudication occurs almost exclusively in patients over the age of 50 and predominantly in males. There is frequently a close association with cigarette smoking and the symptom is quite commonly a complication of diabetes. Nocturnal leg cramps tend to occur in the elderly and in a substantial proportion of pregnant women in the third trimester. The epidemiology of the restless legs syndrome, first described by Ekbom[2], is not clearly established, but it is considerably less common than the other conditions considered here. There is some evidence of a familial pattern in the incidence of the syndrome.

Presentation

Intermittent claudication consists of cramp-like pains produced by exercise, promptly relieved by rest. The patient will often be able to detail quite accurately the remarkably constant distance he can walk before being halted by the pain. Although the pathological changes are usually present in both legs symptoms commonly occur on one side only. The pain of intermittent claudication usually occurs in the calf, less often in the foot or gluteal muscles.

Cramp is experienced as a sudden painful and involuntary contraction of a muscle or group of muscles. The cramp can occur in the calf, foot or thigh and typically wakes the patient from sleep.

The restless leg syndrome is characterized by deep, ill-defined disagreeable sensations in the lower legs and an irresistible urge to move them[3]. Patients often have difficulty in describing the symptoms and tend to use such terms as 'funny', 'heavy' (or 'light') or 'fidgety'. Mild cases may last from ten to 30 minutes, but in more severely affected patients the symptoms may persist much of the night and seriously interfere with sleep.

Causes

The pain of intermittent claudication is due to relative ischaemia in the muscles. The underlying pathology is that of atherosclerosis obliterans: atheromatous plaques partially occluding particularly the popliteal and distal arteries. Predisposing conditions include cigarette smoking, diabetes and obesity.
The cause of nocturnal cramps is not well understood, although they are thought to be due to the accumulation of metabolites and oxygen debt in the affected muscles.
The etiology of the restless legs syndrome is even less clear, although it has been proposed that it may be due to primary dysfunction of the reticular system.

History and examination

The history elicited from patients suffering from intermittent claudication is typically of pain in one (or occasionally both) legs, usually in the region of the calf muscles, brought on by walking a fixed distance and quickly relieved by rest. Additional points which should be looked for include cigarette smoking and other symptoms of generalized atherosclerotic disease (chest pains or cerebrovascular symptoms).
History taking from patients suffering from night cramps is similarly straightforward: the description of the symptoms of cramp in the legs waking the patient at night is unlikely to be confused with any other condition.
With patients suffering from the restless legs syndrome the important points to note are the distress caused by the condition accompanied by difficulty in putting into words the actual nature of the discomforts experienced.
The examination of all patients with leg discomforts is mainly concentrated on the lower limbs. The legs should be inspected for varicose veins or skin discoloration or the signs of localized skin infection (such as tinea pedis, which should be vigorously treated). The legs should be palpated to detect any temperature difference between the two limbs and pulsation should be felt for in the peripheral arteries (dorsalis pedis and posterior tibial). It is a characteristic of atherosclerosis obliterans that pulsation is lost in one or more of the peripheral arteries, and bruits may be heard over the larger arteries if they are partially obstructed. The patient's weight should be noted and his blood pressure measured

and signs of cardiac failure should be looked for.

Patients with nocturnal cramps and the restless legs syndrome are unlikely to have any positive physical signs, and if such are present the diagnosis may need to be revised. Very occasionally a patient will be seen actually suffering from cramp, when the 'knotted' muscle or muscle group may be palpable.

The only investigation usually indicated is an examination of the urine for sugar, in view of the frequent association of intermittent claudication with diabetes.

Management

Patients with severe or increasing intermittent claudication or with signs of skin discoloration or temperature changes or a bruit should be referred to a specialist in peripheral vascular diseases. Further investigation may include arteriography or ultrasound with a view to consideration of arterial surgery — grafting or bypass procedures.

Less severely affected patients should be advised about the care of the legs emphasizing warm clothing and footwear (gloves are also important to avoid reflex spasm), careful attention to cleanliness and expert help with chiropody. Diabetes should be treated, obesity avoided (or dietary advice given if the patient is already overweight), and smoking should be strongly discouraged. Vasodilator drugs have not been proved of any value in intermittent claudication and the most important therapeutic advice is the prescription of graduated exercise with the aim of encouraging the formation of collateral vessels. A programme of modified Buerger's exercises[4] may be advised, such as those detailed in Table I.

Lying:	1. Pull ankles up and down, then round in a circle.
	2. Raise straight leg for count of three and slowly lower; repeat for other leg.
	3. Bend and straighten alternate legs quickly.
Sitting:	4. On dining-room chair, with arms folded, slowly stand then sit.
Standing:	5. On tiptoe, with support, slowly bend knees and sit on heels, then stand up.

Each of these exercises should be done ten times, once or twice daily. In addition, a walk of at least half an hour should be taken every day.

Table I. Exercises to improve the circulation in the legs

Patients consulting about night cramps will almost invariably have tried massage, stretching of the affected muscles by vigorous contraction of the opposing muscle groups, or standing on a cold floor; if they have not, then advice on these lines may be given. Quinine bisulphate in a dose of 300 mg at bed-time has withstood the test of time as an effective treatment for night cramps, although its mode of action is not fully understood. Some patients are helped by the use of nicotinic acid 50–100 mg at night and this is worth a trial in pregnant patients for whom quinine is contraindicated.

In the management of the restless legs syndrome an important step is to reassure the patient that although the symptoms are difficult to describe the condition is a clearly recognized one. Diazepam or clonazepam (Rivotril)[5] taken at bed-time have been reported to be effective in relieving the symptoms.

References

[1] Hodgkin, K. (1973): *Towards Earlier Diagnosis.* 3rd ed. Edinburgh: Churchill Livingstone

[2] Ekbom, K.A. (1945): Restless legs syndrome. *Acta Medica Scandinavica.* Supplement 158, 1–123

[3] Hussey, H.H. (1976): Restless legs syndrome (Editorial). *Journal of the American Medical Association*, *235*, 2224

[4] Clifford, P.C., Davies, P.W., Hayne, J.A. and Baird, R.N. (1980): Intermittent claudication: Is a supervised exercise class worthwhile? *British Medical Journal*, *1*, 1503

[5] Read, D.J., Feest, T.G. and Nassim, M.A. (1981): Clonazepam: effective treatment for restless legs syndrome in uraemia. *British Medical Journal*, *2*, 885

3.71
The patient complaining of pain in the back

Martin Roland

In community surveys of symptom prevalence approximately one in five adults claim that they have experienced backache in the two weeks prior to interview.[1] Despite the fact that over half of these have taken some sort of medication for their pain, well under 5 per cent actually consult the doctor. Back pain is nevertheless the seventh commonest symptom presenting to the general practitioner who, if he has a registered list of 2,000 patients, will see about 70 new cases of backache each year.[2] Men consult slightly more frequently than women, are more likely to be given a diagnosis of prolapsed intervertebral disc and are much more likely to have prolonged absence from work compared with women. The highest consultation rate is from those in the 45–64 age range — an age group which consults relatively infrequently for most other conditions.[3] Backache is responsible for more certified sickness absence than any other single cause. The lost production from backache has been compared to the output of a town the size of Norwich.[4] People with very heavy manual jobs, drivers and nurses are at particularly high risk of developing back pain. The extensive literature on the relationship between occupation and backache has been reviewed by Anderson.[5]

Presentation

The patient with backache, typically a middle-aged man, usually comes to the surgery a few days after the onset of his pain, though about a quarter of patients have had their pain for over a fortnight before they come to the doctor. Two thirds have been to the doctor on a previous occasion with backache. The pain is much more common in the lumbar than the thoracic spine and often radiates to the buttock, loin or posterior thigh, though it rarely radiates below the knee. Patients often come to the doctor because they have had to stop work as a result of their pain. Others, mindful of the prolonged disability that can result from spinal problems, will be seeking reassurance that there is nothing seriously wrong.

Causes

Most back pain arises from the spine and surrounding tissues. Although there are gynaecological and urological causes for backache, they are uncommonly found in a patient who comes to his general practitioner with a primary complaint of pain in the back.

Pain in the back may arise from ligaments, muscles, nerve roots or dura mater. Injuries to any of these structures may produce pain which radiates into the leg. Pain may also arise in the sacroiliac or apophyseal joints. Disorders of the intervertebral disc probably produce pain by pressing on surrounding pain sensitive structures. The role of the disc in back pain is contentious. While Cyriax[6] claims that most back pain arises from disc disease, the classical syndrome of prolapsed intervertebral disc with root symptoms and neurological signs is rarely seen in general practice.

There is increasing interest in the role of the apophyseal joint in back pain. The apophyseal joint (or facet joint) is a synovial joint, and it is suggested that pain may result from 'nipping' of synovium in the joint. The click heard during manipulation by osteopaths possibly results from temporary gapping of apophyseal joints, though the relationship of this to the relief of pain remains unclear.

Degenerative disease of the spine (usually synonymous with a radiological diagnosis of osteoarthrosis of the spine) becomes increasingly common with advancing age. The relationship between degenerative disease and symptom production is certainly not a simple one for, while degenerative disease is almost universal over the age of 65, patients present to the doctor less frequently with backache in old age than in middle age.

Bone disease, whether from infection, ankylosing spondylitis, spondylolisthesis, tumour or osteomalacia, is a rare cause of backache in general practice, although vertebral collapse from osteoporosis may be recognized in the elderly patient.

Psychological factors are not of great importance in the majority of new presentations of back pain in general practice. While research studies have found an increased incidence of psychological abnormalities in patients seen in hospital with back pain, it seems likely that depression and anxiety in these patients develop as a result of longstanding pain. This generalization will not, of course, hold true for all patients, and most general practitioners know of patients in whom backache has been the presenting symptom of a marital, work or sexual problem.

History and examination

The initial history will normally include enquiry about the onset, duration and nature of symptoms. Brief enquiry about other systems, as appropriate for individual patients, will usually exclude non-mechanical causes for the backache. Pain of sudden onset associated with lifting and twisting may be indicative of a prolapsed intervertebral disc especially if the pain is aggravated by sneezing or coughing. Morning stiffness, especially in a young person, may suggest ankylosing spondylitis or Scheuermann's disease. When a patient presents with pain that is unusual because it is either more severe, protracted or progressive than that seen in most patients, the general practitioner is alerted to the possibility of unusual or serious diagnoses.

The examination of the patient begins as he enters the consulting room with observation of his gait and the way he sits down. The patient with an obvious sciatic scoliosis who prefers to stand presents a characteristic picture.

The patient should be undressed. It is important to realize that doctors, whether general practitioners or specialists, are not able to make a definite diagnosis in most patients with back pain. Even though the general practitioner knows that his examination will be of limited diagnostic value, examination is of considerable therapeutic value for the patient. With the patient facing away from the doctor the site of maximal pain should be identified and the areas to which it is referred. The patient with true sciatica is more likely to have a prolapsed intervertebral disc. The back is then inspected for obvious deformities such as scoliosis or a marked pelvic tilt.

Inspection of movement of the spine will provide the GP with a baseline for future examinations. A secondary scoliosis due to pelvic tilt disappears on forward flexion as does the 'step' which may be felt in the spine of a patient with spondylolisthesis when he is standing upright. A structural scoliosis or a scoliosis due to muscle spasm becomes more obvious on forward flexion. Patients with apophyseal joint disease are said to experience relatively more pain on extension than flexion of the lumbar spine.

Straight leg raising is an important prognostic feature and should be carried out with one hand stabilizing the pelvis on the side of the leg which is being tested. When the leg is raised to the limit of comfort, the foot may be dorsiflexed: this manoeuvre produces pain in the back in patients with nerve root tension. It may be valuable to elicit the reflexes, but muscular power is difficult to test when the patient is in pain. Sensation is probably the least useful neurological sign to elicit except in the rare situation where loss of perineal sensation and bladder or bowel disturbance point to cord or cauda equina compression — a situation which requires emergency referral.

An absence of physical signs on examination of the locomotor system should alert the doctor to the possibility that the pain is gynaecological or urological in origin, and also make him think of a possible underlying psychological problem.

Investigation

X-rays of the spine are of virtually no value to the general practitioner. In the great majority of patients, the site of the pain cannot be identified on a plain X-ray. Plain films are unreliable for detecting prolapsed discs, malignancies, spondylolisthesis or spinal stenosis, all of which require special radiological techniques for their demonstration. Furthermore, many normal people have radiological evidence of degenerative disease in the spine, and the GP may incorrectly attribute his patient's pain to such changes. The plain X-ray is an expensive way of providing misleading information for the doctor and the patient.

In difficult cases an ESR may be helpful; a raised ESR suggests such possibilities as ankylosing spondylitis, infections (tuberculosis of the spine, though rare, is still encountered) or neoplasia. Biochemical tests which may be useful include serum calcium, phosphate and alkaline phosphatase (which may, if abnormal, indicate metabolic bone disease or neoplasia), acid phosphatase (for prostatic carcinoma) and plasma proteins and electrophoresis (for myelomatosis).

Treatment

The patient should be advised to rest. Sitting should be avoided since this produces higher intradiscal pressures than either lying down or standing. When lying down, the patient will be more comfortable if the bed is firm, possibly supported by a board under the mattress, and may find that a pillow under the knees is helpful since this tends to flatten the lumbar spine. Gentle heat from a hot water bottle in the small of the back may be helpful.

Analgesics are usually prescribed. If the patient is resting, aspirin or paracetamol are usually all that is required. Dihydrocodeine may be prescribed for patients in severe pain. An injection of pethidine is very rarely needed. Anti-inflammatory agents and muscle relaxants are probably of little more value than salicylates in non-specific mechanical low back pain.

The GP is sometimes asked by his patient whether he should visit an osteopath. Manipulation has never been demonstrated to be of more than very temporary benefit in controlled clinical trials. If there is severe pain with marked muscle spasm or any evidence of root compression, or if the GP is suspicious of more serious spinal disease, a visit to the osteopath should be discouraged. In other situations, it may be reasonable for the patient to see an osteopath, although repeated visits should not be made unless the benefit of the treatment is very clear.

When giving advice on the prevention of back pain, the GP should tell his patient to avoid stooping down with the legs kept straight; objects should, as far as possible, be lifted with a straight back, bent knees and as little twisting as possible. A number of conventional flexion-extension back exercises impose considerable mechanical strains on the back. Isometric exercises aimed at increasing the strength of abdominal, gluteal and pelvic floor muscles appear to be as likely as conventional exercises to make the patient better, and less likely to make him worse! The patient should be instructed to tense the muscles in these regions in turn for 20–30 seconds at a time, carrying out a series of isometric contractions for 3–5 minutes twice a day. Exercises to strengthen the abdominal muscles are particularly important as these provide a lot of support for the lumbar spine.

Most patients with back pain get better with conservative management within 2–3 weeks. Less than 10 per cent of those presenting with back pain are still unable to work one month after coming to see the doctor. Patients with a short history and normal straight leg raising at presentation are highly unlikely to experience prolonged disability — these two features are the most valuable prognostic indicators.[7]

Referral

General practitioners refer, on average, between 5 and 10 per cent of patients with back pain for a specialist opinion. The referral will usually be made because the pain is either very severe or very protracted. While the GP and the patient often need the reassurance which a referral confers, it should be remembered that the efficacy of most treatments used by rheumatologists and orthopaedic surgeons has yet to be demonstrated in randomized controlled trials.

References

[1] Dunnell, K. and Cartwright, A. (1972): *Medicine Takers, Prescribers and Hoarders.* London: Routledge and Kegan Paul

[2] Morrell, D.C., Gage, H.G. and Robinson, N.A. (1971): Symptoms in general practice. *Journal of the Royal College of General Practitioners*, *21*, 32

[3]Royal College of General Practitioners, Office of Population Censuses and Surveys, Department of Health and Social Security (1986): *Morbidity Statistics from General Practice 1981–82*. HMSO Series MB5 No. 1

[4] Department of Health and Social Security (1979): *Report of Working Group on Back Pain*. HMSO

[5] Anderson, J.A. (1980): Occupational aspects of low back pain. *Clinics in Rheumatic Diseases*, *6*, No. 1, 17–37

[6] Cyriax, J. (1978): *Textbook of Orthopaedic Medicine*. London: Baillière Tindall

[7] Roland, M.O., Morrell, D.C., Morris, R.W. (1983): Can general practitioners predict the outcome of episodes of back pain? *British Medical Journal*, *1*, 523–525

3.72
The febrile patient

Ian Tait

Many patients have short-lived febrile illnesses thought to be of viral origin, in which the practitioner is unable to make any firm diagnosis. In these common situations the doctor holds a watching brief. He uses time as his diagnostic test. If recovery is rapid and complete he is often content to leave the diagnosis unsettled but, if the fever persists, or if the condition of the patient deteriorates, the anxiety of both patient and doctor is quickly aroused. It is with the management of the febrile patient at this stage of the illness, often with a diagnosis of pyrexia of unascertained origin (PUO), with which this chapter is concerned.

Significance of fever

Since the time of Hippocrates fever has been perhaps the commonest passport to the attention of physicians. It is often felt not only to justify but to command his attention. For many patients fever is objective proof that they are ill enough to seek medical advice. Some patients become very alarmed. Others feel that its presence entitles them to make special demands: perhaps for a house visit, or immediate attention. Such demands may have a strident quality which the doctor feels to be unjustified. Special care is then needed to keep a cool diagnostic head. The time for re-education comes later. And it is, of course, true that many patients do need education about the proper significance of fever, and what it is safe to do or not do. It is, for instance, quite reasonable to transport a febrile child in a car, or to have him out of bed in a warm living room. It is not reasonable to take him shopping, or leave him waiting for long periods in a crowded waiting-room.

Doctors are divided in their views on the home use of thermometers. It is reasonable to suggest that individuals should know as much as possible about their illnesses and learn to use that knowledge for the better management of their own medical problems. This means that they should know when they, or those for whom they are responsible, have a fever and what to do about it.

This includes understanding when to seek medical advice or other help.
Although an exaggerated sense of the importance of fever is perhaps the characteristic most often brought to our attention in general practice, there is also a group of patients who seem curiously uninterested or unaware of the presence of fever. These patients present complaining of vague symptoms of lassitude or headache. Many adults, however, take their temperature in response to symptoms of malaise. In the case of children, fever is often perceived by the parents as flushing, sweating, or hotness of the skin. Be all that as it may, taking the temperature, like the examination of the urine, is one of the basic requirements for the proper assessment of any patient with an unexplained illness.

Some causes of unascertained fever (PUO) in general practice

When a fever has continued for more than a week without a diagnosis having been made the general practitioner feels that he cannot any longer remain inactive. It is still quite likely that, despite further investigation, the diagnosis will elude him and the fever disappear spontaneously. But he cannot know this, and a search for treatable causes is demanded of him. The standard textbooks of medicine commonly contain long lists of the causes of pyrexia of unascertained origin and they may indeed sometimes be useful in directing the practitioner's diagnostic thoughts and actions.
There are several conditions that are particularly important in general practice, either because they are relatively common, or because they are easily treated or because they have particularly unfortunate consequences if the diagnosis is missed or delayed. In all these conditions the essential step in the diagnosis is to have thought of the possibility.

Bacterial infections

Urinary tract infection. – At any age this is a common and easily missed cause of fever. It is important both because it is treatable if diagnosed, and of potential danger to the patient if missed. Perhaps it is particularly in young children that this condition commonly presents as a PUO, often with vomiting and irritability, but without any obvious urinary symptoms. The microscopic examination of the urine is an essential diagnostic procedure in the investigation of a PUO and the earlier it is done the better. All practices should have a microscope and all general practitioners should feel confident in the examination of urine. Urine does not travel well and pathology laboratories are not open at weekends. The investigation is best done on the spot by the doctor. The presence of pus cells in a fresh spun specimen establishes the diagnosis which can be confirmed by culture. Its diagnosis is often made more difficult by antibiotic therapy given in the absence of a diagnosis.

Hidden pus. – The three most likely sites are under the diaphragm, in the pelvis, or round the kidney.

Subacute bacterial endocarditis may not be a common disease but it is certainly no less common than it was before the introduction of antibiotics. Increasingly it tends to occur in an older age-group, to attack valves damaged by arteriosclerotic degeneration as well as rheumatic fever, and to be a complication of abdominal or pelvic surgery or instrumentation of the urinary tract, as well as dental work.

Septicaemia is a possibility that should always be in the practitioner's mind; if it is suspected, a blood culture is obligatory.

Pneumonia. – Segmental pneumonia can cause fever with few symptoms or clear diagnostic signs. In the elderly, particularly when they are ill and are lying in bed, pneumonia may be hard to diagnose and the physical signs in the chest difficult to interpret.

Enteric fever (typhoid and paratyphoid) presents with fever in the early stages rather than with any particular localizing symptoms or signs. The diagnosis is best made on a blood culture.

Gall-bladder disease. – Cholecystitis, empyema of the gall-bladder and ascending cholangitis can present as fever without any convincing local symptoms or signs. The patient may be very ill. Blood cultures may be positive.

Diverticular disease. – This is common in the elderly and may cause fever without any clear localizing signs. Abscesses, either paracolic or pelvic, may occur.

Tropical diseases

Perhaps tropical diseases should occupy a special place in our diagnostic thoughts. The ease of modern travel has made tropical diseases a real diagnostic possibility in any case of PUO today. Specific enquiry must be made about recent residence abroad. It is often wise for the general practitioner to refresh his memory and seek advice from a local pathologist over the appropriate investigations to be done if he has evidence to think that his patient might have a tropical disease. The most dangerous condition to leave untreated is *malaria* and every doctor should be prepared to take a thick blood film for examination by the laboratory in patients presenting with high fever in which malaria is a possibility. Some diseases such as *amoebic hepatitis* may present as fever years after the original infection has been contracted.

Virus diseases

There is a group of virus diseases, or diseases of possible viral etiology which may present as a PUO. The commonest are:

Infective hepatitis. – This is a fairly common condition and presents with a fever which may last for four or five days before jaundice becomes clinically evident. Anorexia and nausea are likely to be prominent symptoms. Enlargement of the liver may be noticed before the jaundice appears. Urobilinogen in the urine precedes the appearance of jaundice and of bile in the urine.

Glandular fever can present with fever in the absence of localizing signs and it is worth including a monospot or Paul Bunnell test in the range of tests done to investigate a PUO in general practice. The Paul Bunnell test may be negative in the early stages of the disease and many illnesses that look like glandular fever clinically never produce a positive Paul Bunnell reaction.

Non-infectious diseases

Fever does not, of course, always mean infection and there are some relatively common causes of fever from non-infectious diseases that should be in the doctor's mind. Among these are:

Malignant disease, including leukaemia and Hodgkin's disease.

Auto-immune disorders, particularly perhaps giant cell arteritis or polymyalgia rheumatica. Other collagen disorders such as systemic lupus erythematosus are rare but possible causes. Rheumatoid arthritis causes fever but the local joint signs are likely to make the diagnosis clear.

Venous thrombosis may cause fever without any dramatic local symptoms. Examination of the calves should be a routine in the physical examination of patients with fever, but it should be remembered that thrombosis may affect veins not accessible to external physical examination.

Pulmonary infarction may present as fever.

Myocardial infarction can be silent so far as pain is concerned but still cause a fever.

Dehydration can cause fever. It is particularly important to think of this possibility in the elderly.

Drugs must always be suspected as a possible cause of fever. Even drugs taken for long periods without any ill effect can still cause fever unexpectedly: e.g. sulphonamides, barbiturates and thiouracil. Self-prescribed drugs as well as those given by doctors may be the cause of fever. Careful enquiry must be made about all forms of medication.

Fever of psychological origin

Finally it seems right to mention fever of psychological origin. This is not a comfortable diagnosis but it probably is a real condition. Sometimes it may be necessary to protect a patient who seems otherwise fairly well from an excess of investigations provoked by the persistent presence of fever.

History and examination

Self-limiting febrile illnesses are so common in general practice that once he has excluded an obvious cause the doctor is likely to play for time before he embarks on further investigations. Even his initial history and physical examination are likely to be limited in extent at the time of presentation. The essential question he will ask himself at this stage is: 'Is it safe to wait?' If the patient is very ill or at special risk because of some other factor the answer may be no. But in the great majority of cases it will be perfectly safe to wait.

The 'diagnostic use of time' is an essential problem-solving method for the general practitioner. Certain safeguards, however, are required. First, the patient must understand that the doctor needs to know if the illness changes in a significant way or if his general condition deteriorates unexpectedly. Patients do sometimes conclude that because no treatment has been given the doctor considers the illness insignificant. Developments of importance either for diagnosis or management may then not be communicated to the doctor. The patient should understand what is happening, when the doctor is going to see him again, and under what circumstances he should seek advice before that time. Secondly, the doctor must be available so that it is possible for his patient to find him in case of unexpected or worrying developments, or, if this is impossible, the patient must have clear instructions about whom to contact.

In the modern organization of general practice it often happens that the patient who calls unexpectedly has to be seen by another doctor. This makes it important that the clinical record should make clear the diagnostic and management plans of the original doctor so that any other person who has to take over responsibility for the patient can understand them, and integrate his own actions in line with them. For instance, if the presence of fever and a heart murmur in an elderly patient makes the original doctor think that he should exclude the possibility of bacterial endocarditis, this should be clearly stated in the notes. If not, a second doctor called in unexpectedly is quite likely to prescribe an antibiotic without perhaps considering that a blood culture might be required.

This initial wait-and-see diagnostic period commonly lasts from two to five days. During that time it is useful to have in mind the expected times for the appearance of the rashes of specific fevers. Chickenpox appears on the first day, rubella on the second or third, and measles on the fourth. If by the end of the fifth day no rash has appeared measles can usually be excluded. Most viral illnesses will have run their course by that time. This is the time that both doctors and patients begin to feel that something more must be done. It is often not until then that the doctor feels obliged to treat the situation more seriously and the diagnostic label tends to change from a presumed viral illness to pyrexia of unascertained origin. This is not in fact a common situation in general practice but it is a worrying one for the general practitioner, and an important one for the patient.

In the Morbidity Statistics from General Practice[1] it is this group of patients which is classified under the heading of 'Fever of undetermined cause'. The relevant figures are given in table 1, and

Age	0–4	5–14	15–24	25–44	45–64	65–74	75+
	29	7	2	2	1	1	2

Table I. – Number of episodes of 'pyrexia' (both sexes) in 1,000 patients

give an incidence for all ages of about four cases per thousand patients per year. This means that a doctor with a list of 2,000 patients might expect to be confronted with this problem eight times a year. In two out of three of these times the patient will be a child under five.

We are thus dealing with a situation that is not frequent but when it does occur it challenges the doctor's diagnostic and management skills and exposes him both to the anxiety of the patient and to the potential criticism of his hospital colleagues. In these circumstances the general practitioner needs to have a prepared plan of management in which he feels confident.

The investigation of pyrexia in general practice

The moment at which further investigations are indicated will obviously bear a relation to the severity of the illness. If the general condition of the patient causes concern or seems to be deteriorating unexpectedly, admission to hospital for diagnosis may well be required immediately. If, on the other hand, a decision is made to keep the patient at home, the doctor will need to carry out a basic range of diagnostic procedures. Certainly if the fever continues beyond one week some form of further investigation will be necessary.

It is a great help if the equipment necessary for basic diagnostic investigation is kept ready for use in a convenient form. My personal choice is for a partitioned wooden box, the contents of which are:

Syringes, 20ml, 10ml, and 2ml
Intravenous needles
Iodine in spirit
Spirit swabs and plain swabs
Phlebotomy tourniquet
Laboratory request forms ⎤
Paper and envelopes ⎦ all fixed in the lid
Blood bottles for FBC, ESR, blood sugar
Plain bottles for blood
Blood culture bottles (aerobic and anaerobic)
Swabs and transport media for swabs
Slides for blood smears

The box is kept fully stocked and can be picked up for a home visit with the confident expectation that the diagnostic intention can be turned into effective action. The right moment missed in general practice is all too likely to have gone for ever.

Technique is important in taking a blood culture if false positives are to be avoided. The essential requirements are that all necessary equipment should be prepared before the procedure begins. The skin should be properly sterilized; iodine in spirit is probably best for this purpose, and it should be applied five minutes before the blood is taken. A new sterile needle should be used to inject the blood into the two culture bottles.

To a large extent the order and range of diagnostic tests must be left to the judgment of the individual doctor. The age of the patient may play a large part in this decision. In deciding what investigations to do there is one overriding principle to follow, which is, that, if treatment is to be started which might make it impossible to perform a necessary diagnostic test, that test should be done first. Some obvious examples are blood cultures, throat, urine and sputum cultures, aspiration and culture of joint

effusions.
The investigation programme I most often find myself following is to do a full blood count including a differential white blood count and an examination of a spun deposit of urine as a start. If the condition of the patient causes me concern, or a heart murmur suggests the presence of valvular heart disease, I take a blood culture at the same time. By the time the results of the initial investigations are back the illness is often over, or the diagnosis has become apparent on clinical grounds. If not, further diagnostic efforts will be needed with the conditions listed in this chapter in mind. It will often be at this stage that the general practitioner will feel it right to seek advice from a consultant colleague. If he does so he will feel a great deal more comfortable if he has refrained from using antibiotics without a proper diagnosis, has at least a full blood count result available, has excluded the presence of a renal-tract infection and has perhaps a blood culture safely on the brew in the incubator of the local pathology laboratory.

Management of the febrile patient

The complications of fever likely to be seen in general practice are dehydration and febrile convulsions in childhood, and confusional states in the elderly. Old people also become easily dehydrated when febrile and ill.
Dehydration in children occurs more quickly than in adults and children may fail to drink when ill. Their parents need clear instructions about maintaining an adequate fluid intake. Frequent small drinks are best, and water or simple fruit juices are safest. Isotonic or hypertonic solutions of glucose or electrolytes are dangerous and the doctor should make sure that patients know what this means in language they understand. The urinary output should always be enquired about.
In the elderly, fever, dehydration and confusion are interrelated problems. Confusion results in failure to drink and dehydration increases the confusion. It is just not enough to leave a jug of water beside the bed. At least $1\frac{1}{2}$ litres of urine should be passed daily and this requires a fluid intake of 2 to 3 litres. If doubt exists a regular routine fluid intake should be organized and the intake recorded. In home management the supervision of a district nursing sister is invaluable.
Febrile *convulsions* deserve a special word. The incidence of febrile convulsions in children seems to vary from practice to practice. They occur chiefly between the ages of 1 and 3 years. There is often a family history. These fits are always alarming and parents tend to

invest the event with dire significance, fearing that the child will be a life-long epileptic. These fears should be expressed if present and discussed. If the fit is associated with a temperature over 39.4°C (103°F) in a child under 3 years without a history of birth trauma, or evidence of disease of the central nervous system, then the parents can be honestly reassured. Although there is a greater likelihood of epilepsy developing in an individual who has experienced febrile convulsions the chances are very small indeed.

The most important principle in the management of febrile convulsions is control of the temperature. The parents must be taught to do this with confidence. Over-heating with bed clothes and hot bottles in a febrile illness is always harmful and must be particularly avoided in these cases. Paracetamol in appropriate dosage is indicated and tepid sponging should be advised if the temperature rises above 39.4°C.

If a fit occurs the parent should be advised to remove objects that might hurt the child if he were to strike them, but to use the minimum of force in restraining movements. They should be warned that the child may vomit and so his head should be held to one side and the child nursed head down to prevent any aspiration of vomit. Someone should always stay with the child and this is far more important than running to seek help. Parents can be safely told that these fits are usually brief and children always recover fully.

The single febrile convulsion is not a reason for admission to hospital but, if the fits continue or recur, or if there is any clinical suspicion of meningitis, the child must be in hospital, since a lumbar puncture is the only certain way to exclude meningitis.

If the fit is still in progress when the doctor arrives or he feels the need for some form of active intervention the safest and easiest drug to give is diazepam by intramuscular injection or rectally in a dose of 2.5 to 5 mg.

Reference

[1] Royal College of General Practitioners, Office of Population Censuses and Surveys, Department of Health and Social Security (1986): *Morbidity Statistics from General Practice 1981–82*. HMSO Series MB5 No. 1

Infectious diseases

Disease	*Prodromal stage*	*Duration*	*Incubation*	*Infectivity*
Chickenpox	-	1–2 weeks	2 weeks	1 day before rash appears, till last vesicle has dried
Measles	3–4 days catarrhal symptoms	1–2 weeks	10–14 days	4–6 days before rash appears till 6 days after appearance of rash (or until patient is afebrile – whichever is longer)
Mumps	1 day pain in front of ears	1–2 weeks	2–3 weeks	2 days before swelling appears till swelling subsides
Pertussis	5–7 days catarrhal symptoms and dry cough	1–6 weeks	7–14 days	1 week before 'whoop' or spasmodic coughing appears till 4 weeks later*
Rubella	1 day catarrhal symptoms	3–4 days	2–3 weeks	1 day before rash appears till 2 days after appearance of rash
Scarlatina	1–3 days sore throat	1–2 weeks	1–7 days	3 days before rash appears till desquamation occurs

*The infectivity of pertussis is very variable, and while 4 weeks is a reasonable average guideline, organisms may be recovered after even longer periods.

3.73
The very sick child

Raymond Pietroni and D.W. Holton

In this chapter a very sick child means one in whom there is a real risk of serious complications or death from the illness. With the improvements in the general health and nutrition of the population it is becoming increasingly uncommon in practice to meet the very sick child. Nevertheless, when the general practitioner is faced with such a problem he will need all his reserves of skill and compassion to cope with the situation. Although obviously a proportion will have to be admitted, it is not just a question of sending all such children into hospital. The effects of separating a very sick and frightened child from his parents are now well known and accepted, and parents will increasingly demand that wherever possible their child be kept at home. This will raise the problem of the doctor's own anxiety in this situation and how much uncertainty he is willing to tolerate. It is a sound general rule always to work within the limits of one's knowledge and skills: the same applies to one's anxiety. The general practitioner should never take on a potentially serious situation with which he feels unable to cope because he is uncertain of his own knowledge, skills or feelings.

Presentation

The child may present at home or in the surgery. Because extremely ill children are so uncomplaining the parents may not realize that the child is very sick and the presentation may be such that the doctor himself may not at once be alerted to the severity of the condition. There are, however, certain characteristics of the very sick child. He tends to be apathetic. He is rarely crying, overactive or seeking attention. He is rarely flushed, more often pale. Movement is usually reduced to a minimum as it causes distress. There may be alarming evidence of respiratory distress: consciousness may be disturbed. These signs may be taken in at a glance. It must be remembered that a child's medical condition may alter very rapidly, and general practitioners must be alert to potentially dangerous situations, and act very quickly when necessary.

Causes

The commonest group of causes will be those due to respiratory infections, the agent generally being a virus. In babies this may produce a bronchiolitis usually due to the respiratory syncytial virus which may rapidly lead to respiratory failure. A more common problem is croup, usually due to an acute viral laryngo-tracheo-bronchitis but on occasion associated with infection due to *Haemophilus influenzae*. This organism can also cause acute epiglottitis, a rapidly progressive infection which can cause prostration and collapse within a matter of hours. The possibility of an inhaled foreign body should be borne in mind. Bronchitis is much more common and when associated with wheezing may cause alarm. Asthma is sometimes associated with infection — usually viral, but there are often many other factors. Although very few children die of asthma this is a condition to take seriously. Bacterial infections are less common nowadays but may give rise to serious conditions such as pneumonia and rarely tuberculosis. Children with mucoviscidosis may suffer life-threatening bacterial infections of the lungs due to bronchiectasis. Measles is probably the most common serious infection the general practitioner will meet. The child is often very sick but the prognosis is good. With the advent of immunization, attacks are much less common or severe. Whooping-cough, especially in the very young, may be threatening to life.

A common group of very sick children are those presenting as surgical emergencies of the alimentary tract. Acute appendicitis accounts for 10 per cent of all admissions to surgical wards of children's hospitals. Although uncommon under the age of 5, appendicitis at this age is associated with a high mortality, accounting for 37 per cent of deaths from this condition. Infantile hypertrophic pyloric stenosis and intussusception are rare causes which present in this group. Incarcerated inguinal hernia may easily be overlooked and the later it is detected the higher the morbidity and mortality. Gastroenteritis is still a serious condition, particularly in the very young, and requires prompt action.

The commonest neurological cause of the very sick child is febrile convulsions. In general practice convulsions may rarely be due to meningitis, encephalitis or some intracranial disaster. Bacterial meningitis, though fortunately rare in general practice, has a high mortality and should be diagnosed promptly. Neck stiffness may be present in many infections, particularly of the respiratory tract, but lumbar puncture alone can clarify the diagnosis.

A common cause of death in the 0 to 14 age-group is from accidents, poisoning or violence. Every general practitioner will encounter children in these circumstances who will require careful assessment. Although non-accidental injury is not common in practice, a quoted incidence of 1 case in 5 years in a practice providing care for 2,000 individuals is almost certainly far too low, and the index of suspicion should be high as it has a mortality rate of 10 per cent.

History taking and examination

Very rarely the situation may be so evidently threatening to life (for instance when the child is convulsing, has inhaled a foreign body or has suffered a severe accident) that history and examination will be kept to a minimum and intervention will be immediate. More often the doctor has time to make an accurate assessment of the situation. The history is usually taken from one or both of the parents but if the child is old enough he must be encouraged to give his own account. Apart from the value of this information the child will feel less frightened if he is thus involved. At this time the quality of the information obtained will depend in part on the doctor's earlier relationship with the family. Those previous multiple, often brief encounters, some thought of as being trivial, some not so, will have helped to shape the relationship and in time of crisis this relationship is the main instrument for obtaining an accurate history. Equally, when it comes to the examination, the child will sense whether the doctor is friendly and approachable or whether he is distant and aloof. It is difficult to exaggerate the importance of this relationship and its practical value in eliciting vital physical signs. The crying child is difficult to examine and in the case of a child with abdominal pain, for instance, the doctor may decide on hospital admission reluctantly, simply because he has been unable to examine the abdomen to his own satisfaction. The same child presenting on yet another occasion may associate the doctor's presence with hospital admission and start to cry straight away. And so the unsatisfactory cycle continues.

How should the general practitioner approach the sick child? The child is an individual who deserves courtesy as much as an adult. Permission must be sought before making physical contact, important though this may be. Such permission will be obtained in a variety of non-verbal ways; interest in the child is expressed through questioning about his life at school and at home, and comments about his room and his toys. With the younger child, between the ages of 7 months and 2 years, direct eye-contact should be avoided at first and the doctor should gaze benignly over the baby's shoulder while talking quietly to the mother. During this time he will look directly at the baby for increasing lengths of time until the baby is used to his presence. A small child must be approached on his own level, physically as well as metaphorically, and this may mean kneeling on the floor. The soft repetition of his name will have a soothing effect and facilitate examination. If the child is asleep when the doctor calls he should be wakened by his mother only at the last minute. Much information can be gathered by watching the sleeping child while taking the history from the mother.

Physical handling should be gentle but firm: instruments should be introduced and played with before they are used. Taking the temperature may present problems and it is wise to ask the mother herself to insert the thermometer in a fold of the groin where it must remain for a minimum of three minutes. Oral temperature-taking is unnecessary and difficult in the younger child but in the older one the thermometer can be supported gently by the examiner or the mother. In the infant a rectal temperature may be elicited without causing any distress whatsoever. The examination should be quick but thorough without being exhaustive and exhausting. If it is obvious that the child will have to be admitted to hospital it is kinder not to insist on a detailed examination which may upset him and which will only be repeated in hospital. The doctor's decision is primarily concerned with what action to take rather than the precise diagnosis (although obviously the two often coincide). He can safely limit himself to obtaining sufficient information to indicate the course of action.

The sequence of the examination will vary according to the doctor's training, but many doctors like to examine children from top-to-toe rather than by system. Clothes, and especially the nappy, must be removed, but not all at once as many children quite properly resent being stripped totally naked. At the same time the doctor must remember to look at the whole child rather than just his constituent parts, noting such things as colour, state of activity, disposition of the limbs and general demeanour. He must always ask himself: how ill is this child? Despite the absence of physical signs he must be prepared to act on his overall assessment. Very sick children are often relatively immobile, seem apathetic and protest too little. Often they have an unusual colour and generally they behave unpredictably.

As regards the respiratory system the doctor must naturally listen to the child's breathing and may, of course, have to get quite close to hear a wheeze. In severe respiratory distress auscultation of the chest may produce little in the way of signs. He should look routinely at the alae nasi, the supraclavicular and the suprasternal spaces and the lower rib cage for signs of respiratory distress, distinguishing between inspiratory distress (as caused by croup, epiglottitis or inhaled foreign body) and expiratory distress as in asthma or wheezy bronchitis, although of course they may coexist. The child may be lying still to avoid precipitating a cough which, if heard, may be the only clue to a diagnosis of whooping-cough. Once the doctor has made a provisional diagnosis he can look for specific confirmatory signs which might otherwise be missed, as, for instance, in the case of whooping-cough, small subconjunctival haemorrhages and the torn fraenulum linguae, or, for example, the sparse purpuric spots in early meningococcal septicaemia.

The ear, nose and throat should almost always be examined although this may be left to the last, particularly as examination of the throat is resented by the majority of infants. If epiglottitis is suspected, as when the child's breathing has suddenly become stridulous and he has inspiratory distress, the throat should *not* be examined until immediate tracheostomy is readily available.

In the cardiovascular system particular attention should be paid to the child's colour. If central cyanosis is suspected the nail beds should be examined for the presence of early clubbing which will be most noticeable in the first and second digits of the hands and feet. The warmth of the peripheral limbs will be a guide to the adequacy of peripheral blood flow and the femoral arteries should always be palpated: delay or absence of the pulses may indicate a coarctation of the aorta. The rate and rhythm of the heart beat should be noted and the presence of murmurs recorded. Cardiac murmurs are often heard in association with a fever and tachycardia and may not necessarily indicate a cardiac abnormality. Heart failure in infants is more likely to present as a feeding difficulty, weight gain or enlargement of the liver than in the more traditional way found in adults.

In involvement of the gastro-intestinal system, the tongue and skin should be examined for signs of dehydration. When examining the abdomen a gentle approach is important, and if there is some reluctance on the child's part to allow the examination, his resistance may be overcome by placing his own hand first on his abdomen. The child's attention may also be distracted by asking him to take deep breaths. In the older child localization of abdominal pain is not very accurate and is nearly always related to the main landmark — the umbilicus (which itself should be examined in neonates as being a possible source of sepsis). In boys both testicles are examined and the presence of herniae excluded. An incarcerated inguinal hernia in a baby may be missed if the nappy is not removed. Rectal examination is rarely required especially if the child is going to be admitted to hospital, although it may be indicated as, for instance, when intussusception is suspected.

The neurological system can be more difficult to examine than in the adult. Confusion and disorientation are difficult to assess, particularly if the child has a high fever.

A bulging fontanelle is the best indicator of meningitis in an infant, and in young children the sign of neck stiffness is rarely elicited, even in severe cases. In older children neck stiffness may be elicited by asking them to try to kiss their knees. Headache is a common accompaniment of fever and is not necessarily of any great significance.

Examination of the urine should be routine and may be the only way of detecting nephritis. Pyelonephritis often presents simply as pyrexia, or malaise, but in the older child there may be some loin tenderness and again examination of the urine will reveal the cause.

Management

In the acutely ill child the doctor may have to intervene urgently. This may involve first aid measures such as positioning the unconscious child having fits and clearing the airway. He may have to administer drugs such as hydrocortisone in asthma or anti-convulsants in convulsions. His manner should be confident and quick without increasing the anxiety that is already present. He should 'take charge' of the situation and behave in an authoritative way so as to reassure the parents. When hospital admission is indicated he may have to accompany the patient either by car or in the ambulance. He should be aware of the parents' feelings and always find time when the crisis is over to discuss the situation with them giving them all the information they require. When a child has been admitted to hospital urgently, parents often feel guilty and wonder whether if they had taken earlier action, the crisis would have been avoided. The general practitioner must not rush to reassure these fears until he has explored them. He will remain a link between the hospital and the family and, when possible, should visit the child in the ward.

When the situation is not so urgent and the child is nursed at home, the doctor will have more time but in the long run may find management more demanding. He should provide information and support for the parents and be freely available. He will seek to limit painful procedures and ease them as much as possible. The practice nurse can provide support to parents nursing a very sick child at home.

The general practitioner should facilitate communication with other professionals such as social workers and teachers, and be aware of the overall needs of the child. He will remember the other siblings and gently remind the parents of their needs too.

There can be no more harrowing experience in general practice than to be involved with the management of the child who is about to die. At this time the general practitioner's influence can be of immense importance. He must be aware of the various stages of adaptation to impending bereavement and allow the parents to express their feelings, some of which will be very painful. He will face the child with honesty and courage, genuinely trying to answer his questions with frankness. He may well be surprised at the maturity of the child's approach and his knowledge of what is going on. He must remember that the family will still be his patients after the child has died and that the management of the situation may have far-reaching effects in the future. His only consolation will be that in this time of extreme crisis he is the one professional who is best able to help.

Cot Death

Cot Death or Sudden Infant Death Syndrome is by international agreement understood to mean a death that occurs unexpectedly in a child who was thought to have been previously well. This definition, however, indicates that a post-mortem examination ought to fail to demonstrate an adequate cause of death before the criteria for the diagnosis are fulfilled. The incidence of the condition[1] is between 1 and 3 per 1,000 live births, but no reliable statistics for the United Kingdom are yet available. It is more common in males than females and there appears to be a peak incidence about the age of 8 weeks. It is definitely more prevalent in Scotland than England, but the general practitioner with an average-sized list is likely to see a case only once in every ten years.
The child is generally discovered unexpectedly dead by the parents. Death appears to have occurred peacefully while the child is asleep, often during the night.

Possible aetiological factors

There is still considerable controversy as to whether symptoms in the history or findings on examination of these children prior to death are of significance. The preliminary report[2] of the DHSS multicentre study of post-neonatal mortality[3] indicated that there were several symptoms occurring more commonly in children who died, but most of these would be observed regularly in children presenting to general practitioners, who were not ill enough to merit hospital admission. Fast and noisy breathing, drowsiness and irritability are symptoms which require more detailed assessment, however, and could lead a doctor to consider hospital admission. A recent report from Scotland[4] has produced somewhat different results: almost 40 per cent of their deaths were unexplained; ‘associated findings’ were discovered in another 38 per cent of cases but the authors did not conclude that these were significant pointers to the cause of death. Parents and general practitioners are likely to find some comfort from this report which indicated that there was little evidence to suggest that either group was not reacting appropriately to children’s symptoms of illness.

Prevention

All this may seem to suggest that there is little that the doctor can do to help. Prevention is the principal aim, but general health measures such as better health education, more breast feeding and less smoking by parents, along with better care from general practitioners, have not so far been shown to result in a lower incidence of cot death. Recent research has suggested that overheating of the baby may be a possible factor, and advice should be given to parents to avoid excessive heating of the baby's environment after the neonatal period.

Fortunately the occurrence of cot deaths in siblings still appears to be a relatively rare event. Home apnoea monitors are currently being offered to bereaved families with subsequent children in many areas, and may be welcomed as a supportive measure. As yet, they have not been shown to have significant value as a preventive tool. Immunisation has not been shown to be causally linked with cot death, but there may be an argument for delaying immunisation in subsequent siblings until they are slightly older.

Management

When a family doctor is involved in a case of cot death, he must first of all make certain that there are no suspicious circumstances. He has a duty to report such a death to the Coroner (or Procurator Fiscal in Scotland) and whenever possible a post-mortem should be carried out by a paediatric pathologist. This does not alter the circumstances of the death, but if useful or negative information is uncovered, it may help both parents and doctor.

The principal role, however, must remain the support of the family. Especially if it is a first child, the loss is devastating and the full grief reaction of the parents may take a long period of time. The doctor or health visitor may find that the parents direct a considerable amount of anger towards them, and this must be tolerated and understood. Support from other people, such as friends, priests or ministers may be invaluable. The Foundation for the Study of Infant Deaths (based at 4 Grosvenor Place, London SW1X 7HD) has a useful leaflet to hand to parents, and there may be a self-help group of parents in the area who have found themselves in a similar situation, which could be helpful at this stage. Parents may wish to talk to other medical professionals, including consultant paediatricians. Before embarking on a further pregnancy parents may wish to consult a geneticist, and every opportunity should be offered to help them come to terms with a cot death, and prepare for a further pregnancy, should they reach such a decision.

References

[1] Bain, A.D. and Bartholomew, S.E.M. (1983): A Review of the Sudden Infant Death Syndrome in South-East Scotland. *Scottish Health Bulletin*, *43*, 51.
[2] Stanton, A.N., Downham, M.A.P.S., Oakley, J.R. and Knowelden, J. (1978): Terminal Symptoms in Children Dying Suddenly and Unexpectedly at Home. *British Medical Journal*, *2*, 1249.
[3] Knowelden, J., Keeling, J. and Nicholl, J.P. (1985): *A Multi-Centre Study of Post-Neonatal Mortality*. Department of Health and Social Security.
[4] Arneil, G.C., Gibson, A.A.M., McIntosh, H., Brooke, H., Harvie, A. and Patrick, W.J.A. (1985): National Post-Perinatal Infant Mortality and Cot Death Study, Scotland 1981–82. *Lancet*, *1*, 740.

3.74
The child who fails to thrive

J. H. Walker

The child who fails to thrive

So many children now achieve, and often exceed, the expected milestones of growth and development that the child who fails to thrive may be seen as conspicuously abnormal. The amount of interest which has been focused on infant nutrition has led many parents to have unrealistic expectations of steady growth and regular weight gain. Some become concerned if their child fails to gain a specified number of ounces each week, and many may be equally concerned if, despite regular weight gain, their infant appears to be significantly smaller than his contemporaries. It is therefore important that parents appreciate the variation in growth rate, and the fact that weight at any particular age is related to a variety of factors, of which parental size and birthweight are particularly important.

To allow the growth of infants to be seen in the context of age, birthweight and the population as a whole, weight should always be recorded on percentile charts rather than in absolute figures. By displaying progressive information about growth, the chart may provide the opportunity of detecting any deviation from normal, even before the parents are aware of it, and will certainly allow accurate timing of any deviation which does occur. Growth charts should therefore be instituted for all infants who are under regular health surveillance, and should be used as a prime diagnostic tool in the investigation of the child who is presented because of concern about his growth.

The first step in the investigation is the need to assess whether any failure is real in terms of the expectations for that particular child. Failure to thrive may be due to a variety of causes ranging from feeding problems to rare metabolic disorders. A simple categorization is that of deficiencies of:

1. Intake
2. Absorption
3. Metabolism

although in many situations all three factors may appear to be involved.

Congenital abnormality, particularly congenital heart disease, chronic infection of the renal tract, malabsorption due to coeliac disease or cystic fibrosis, and inborn errors of metabolism all cause failure to thrive. Fortunately in general practice they are rare, and the commonest causes are feeding difficulties and problems of parent/child relationship.

The management of the first consultation should therefore include a detailed history of the pregnancy, the delivery, and in particular the mother's attitude to and expectation of the infant. The type of delivery, whether father was present during labour or delivery, the mother's reaction to the birth, whether she was sedated, whether she and the baby were separated for any reason, or whether the parents were given time with the baby to examine it and to establish a relationship are critical items in the history. In particular, if any abnormality of the baby was present it is important to know what the mother was told, how she was told, and whether, if separation did occur, she was allowed to handle the baby before it was taken to the nursery.

The mother's intentions about infant feeding during the pregnancy should be discussed and the way in which the present feeding pattern was established described. Closer attention to the feeding regime will be needed later. The history may be elicited while the baby is being examined and accurately weighed and measured. A thorough examination should provide some evidence of the child's nutritional state and its relationship with its mother. Weighing and charting will reveal whether the failure to thrive is real or apparent and observation whether the child appears retarded, depressed, anxious or withdrawn and whether the mother handles him with kindness, apprehension or indifference. During the examination particular attention should be paid to the organ systems and the slight possibility of congenital abnormality. Although most infants are thoroughly examined before leaving hospital, the family doctor may occasionally be the first physician to detect a cardiac murmur or signs of other physical disorder.

The urine should be tested for protein, and the examination of the nappy may reveal normal stool or one characteristic of intestinal hurry.

Examination of the child should be accompanied by an assessment of maternal wellbeing. A history of the mother's health during pregnancy, delivery and puerperium may reveal problems which explain her difficulties with the baby. In particular, puerperal depression may have begun a vicious circle of deprivation in which a depressed, exhausted mother finds it impossible to relate to what becomes an unhappy, underfed, underweight baby.

In the majority of consultations, the explanation for the failure to thrive will be found in the areas of feeding or relationship problems.

Feeding

One reaction of parents to the current anxiety about the hazards of obesity in infancy has been a tendency to underfeed. Concern in some mothers about the dangers of hypernatraemia may have led to the offering of dilute feeds, and with some infants mixed feeding may be unnecessarily delayed. An assessment as to whether inadequate intake really is the cause of failure to thrive can therefore only be made by accurate history-taking and by observing an actual feed.

The ability of the family doctor or the health visitor to visit at the appropriate time of day is paramount. In babies who are bottle fed, the complete feed from mixing to winding should be observed. Particular attention should be paid to the measuring of powder and water, the type of bottle, the size of teat and hole, and the mother's technique of feeding and winding. The atmosphere of the home, practical aspects of hygiene, and the role of other family members can all be assessed.

Observation of a breast-fed baby who is failing to thrive is equally important. One of the major problems of breast feeding is the mother's inability to see actually how much milk the baby takes. Any breast-fed baby who is failing to thrive must be weighed before and after feeds if an assessment of quantity is to be made. It is not safe to assume that all is well because the breast is not completely empty at the end of the feed and the babe appears to be content. Many underfed infants appear tranquil before they become lethargic and it is important both to assess the amount the babe takes at each feed by test feeding and to test the residue available in the breast by expression.

The symptoms of feeding disorders cover the whole field of self-expression in infancy—crying, vomiting, development of diarrhoea, constipation, colic and wind. Underfeeding is most likely in babies who fail to thrive. Their hunger may be expressed by crying before a feed, which is then taken ravenously. Even though the quantity may be inadequate, the baby will sleep for an hour or two, but then waken and cry again. Crying may lead to air-swallowing which in turn will produce flatulence, vomiting and colic. Frequently small green 'starvation' stools may be seen, but the situation should correct if the right volume of milk is offered. Normally 2½ oz per lb of body weight (150 ml per kg) is required. In the child who has been underfed, or has particular metabolic needs, such as the premature, 3½ oz per lb (200 ml per kg) may be necessary.

Breast-fed babies who are not receiving the appropriate quantity may need complementary bottle feeds. An inadequate flow may be the result of tension between mother and child, and often the relief of anxiety produced by complementary feeds will allow more milk to be produced, with the resolution of the problem.

Perpetual crying or the evening crying of 'three-month colic' may have become a habit which requires sedation. Occasionally patterns of behaviour may have become so entrenched that the baby needs to be sedated, using a simple sedative such as paediatric choloral elixir BPC. Occasionally the mother and baby may need to be admitted to hospital to allow the situation to be resolved.

For both bottle- and breast-fed babies the observation of a feed will provide the most effective method of diagnosing defects in feeding technique and of assessing the relationship between mother and child. The importance of this relationship has been highlighted by recent studies which have shown that once simple feeding problems have been eliminated psychosocial problems are the most common and important causes of failure to thrive. A system of comprehensive maternal and child care based on general practice is therefore the most likely to provide opportunities for early diagnosis, treatment and anticipatory prevention.

The mother/child relationship

Emotional deprivation as a cause of failure to thrive might be anticipated by a knowledge of the mother, her family background, marital relationships, attitude to the pregnancy, delivery, and early bonding experience with the child. Kempe[1] has shown how the early moments and hours of mother/child interaction relate to subsequent child abuse. Failure to thrive due to emotional causes can be regarded as one variation of this syndrome. Any abnormalities in the pregnancy or the child should raise suspicions. Prematurity is recognized as a significant risk factor, not only because of the special metabolic and dietary needs of the premature infant, who requires a higher-than-average intake per pound of body weight, but because prematurity may have categorized the baby as 'different'. In his book *The Abused Child*,[2] Martin lists some of the factors which influence the quality of bonding between parent and child. In the parent these include:

Expectation of the child
Desire for the child
Capacity to give
Ego-strength to adapt to stress
Ability to accept imperfection
Realistic fantasies of the child

The factors in the child:

Absence of defects

The ability to match the parents' expectations
Good health
Loving behaviour, including smiling, cuddling and thriving

Disturbance of any of these factors may lead to relationship difficulties. Knowledge of the parent, gained through antenatal care, and of the child, through early routine health surveillance, is particularly valuable. The likelihood that the baby will not have been born under general-practitioner care underlines the importance of information from the hospital. A history of early separation because of infant or maternal distress, or of disappointment with the infant, its sex, appearance, size or weight, are particularly important. Patterns of parental visiting have also been shown to be predictive of relationship problems, failure to thrive, and child abuse. Babies in special-care baby units who are visited less than three times during their stay have a 23 per cent probability of being abused, whereas those visited more than three times only a 2 per cent probability. Although this information is unlikely to be immediately available to the family doctor, it may be sufficiently important to seek.

The management of failure to thrive due to psychological factors may be complex. At the simplest level, the recognition by the mother that she is having difficulty in relating to her baby is essential, and the reassurance that not all babies are equally lovable and manageable may help. The diagnostic home visit often provides the setting for this type of therapy and the provision of empathetic support and supervision of the feeding regime may be all that is required. The child who fails to thrive, and is in real danger of physical abuse, however, represents the other extreme of the syndrome, and will require referral and admission. As the effects of deprivation become increasingly understood, the importance of early referral for specialist help cannot be emphasized too strongly.

Rare disorders

Other reasons for paediatric referral will include suspicion of one of the rarer causes of inadequate growth. Malabsorption syndromes are extremely rare, but cystic fibrosis and coeliac disease may be responsible for the malabsorption of fat and the presence of steatorrhoea. Cystic fibrosis can be an early cause of failure to thrive, but coeliac disease will only develop after the institution of mixed feeding and the introduction of gluten to the diet. Superficial examination of the stool is unlikely to help, and stool-fat estimation will be required. A sweat test will be necessary for the diagnosis of cystic fibrosis. A family history is not always present, and although the incidence of approximately 0.4 per 1,000 births makes each of these conditions extremely rare, they should be borne in mind.

The disorders of carbohydrate metabolism are even rarer. Some, such as galactosaemia, will normally present dramatically during the neonatal period; continuous vomiting, persistent diarrhoea, lassitude, fits, and jaundice, will have led to the diagnosis being made in hospital before discharge. Despite careful neonatal examination, however, some abnormalities, particularly congenital heart disease, may have been missed, and it is for this reason that careful physical examination following accurate history-taking are so important in family practice. Chronic urinary infections, associated with congenital abnormalities of the renal tract, and other infections, are important but rare causes. Cretinism, growth-hormone deficiency, chromosomal abnormalities, birth trauma and idiopathic hypercalcaemia are even rarer causes which the paediatrician may consider.

Older children

When an older child is presented because of failure to thrive, it is essential to assess whether this is of recent origin or is the continuation of an earlier pattern of abnormal growth. The growth chart is therefore again the most effective preliminary diagnostic aid, and if the child's practice record does not contain details of height and weight, these should be sought from health visitor, child health clinic, or School Health Service.

Many of the items in the differential diagnosis of failure to thrive in the younger child are equally appropriate when considering the problem in the older. A full history and physical examination must therefore again be the basis of investigation. The evidence of slow growth during the earlier years, and a knowledge of the size of the parents and the growth of siblings may suggest that the child is simply going to be genetically of short stature. Alternatively, a satisfactory early growth pattern which subsequently becomes abnormal is a cause for concern. Particular care in history-taking and physical examination should therefore be taken in eliciting any suggestion of previously undetected physical abnormalities.

In common with the younger child who fails to thrive, the older may be suffering from malabsorption syndrome, congenital heart disease, chronic respiratory disease, or abnormality or chronic infection of the renal tract, hepatic disease, anaemia, or a rare chromosomal or metabolic disorder. Malignant disease, tuberculosis, diabetes, rheumatoid arthritis or chronic liver disease may present as failure to thrive, and it is necessary to exclude organic disease before considering the more common emotional causes.

Physical examination should therefore be followed by haemoglobin, white-cell count and ESR determination. Tuberculosis can be eliminated by Haef or Mantoux testing, some abnormalities of the urinary tract by urinalysis and culture, and malabsorption by the estimation of faecal fat.

As in infancy and early childhood, however, psychosocial causes, particularly frank or occult emotional deprivation, will be found to be the most common. Although the family doctor should be in a position from which emotional problems can be readily recognized these are often disguised behind a façade of minor physical illness. A failure to thrive associated with frequent school absences, apparently due to repeated upper respiratory tract infections, will suggest the need for further social investigation. In many cases, the schoolteacher or school nurse may be able to provide valuable information, and it will often be found that the child has been referred to an educational psychologist because of declining school performance or frank emotional disturbance. Many children whose failure to thrive is found to be due to emotional deprivation put on weight and grow normally when separated from their parents by admission to residential school or foster home.

The usefulness of percentile charts as diagnostic aids in assessing failure to thrive must be emphasized. Four examples are shown here:

In Figure I the chart shows the pattern of growth of a boy whose mild asthma was accentuated by his home environment. Admitted to a residential school, a normal growth rate during term time was interrupted by return home during the holidays. A completely normal pattern was finally established when he was taken into care and permanently separated from his parents.

In Figure II the growth pattern of a premature infant is illustrated. This shows the corrective effect of a high calorific intake in raising the weight from below the tenth centile to the 75th centile in the baby's first 9 months.

Figure III shows the pattern of failure to thrive becoming apparent after the introduction of mixed feeding, pointing to a diagnosis of coeliac disease, and the subsequent restoration of weight gain on a gluten free diet.

In Figure IV the effect is shown of the mother's puerperal depression on her infant's development in the early months and the restoration of a normal growth pattern parallel with the mother's recovery.

It is unfortunate that while many physical causes of failure to thrive in the older child respond to specific therapy, the treatment of those whose problems are rooted in psychosocial disorder are much more difficult.

Investigation and management

Problems of failure to thrive initially fall into two categories: those where the child is presented by parents who have recognized the problem, and those where the failure is discovered by other means — the health visitor, clinic, or as a result of consultation for some other reason. It is suggested that the investigation begins with a full family, obstetric and neonatal history, followed by a competent physical examination during which close observation can be made of the relationship between mother and child. When this reveals no abnormality, it is important that arrangements are made to observe one or more feeds. This can be arranged at home and provides further opportunity for the assessment of the attitude of the mother and other members of the family. The weighing before and after feeds of breast-fed infants and a study of the mixing and offering of a bottle will usually reveal correctable factors. Unless a profound relationship problem is detected, it is likely that this degree of interest and support and the correction of minor management irregularities will produce the desired improvement within a period of one or two weeks. It is essential that a developmental assessment of the child should be made and that growth and development charts should be instituted so that response to therapy and possible relapse is detected early. Lack of response or the persistence of important symptoms should lead to paediatric referral for exclusion of the rarer causes, or to provide the opportunity of in-patient care in which closer observation and more intensive support can be provided.

Failure to thrive in the older child must be investigated using the same basic methods, but in the knowledge that a more extensive range of diagnoses must be considered. If physical causes have been eliminated by normal examination and investigation, helpful information about the child's social and emotional development may be obtained from school teachers, nurses and psychologists, who together with social workers may play an important part in management.

References

[1] Helfer, R.E. and Kempe, C.H. (1968): *The Battered Child.* University of Chicago Press
[2] Martin, H.P. (ed.) (1976). *The Abused Child.* Cambridge, Mass.: Ballinger

BOYS 9 - 18 NUDE WEIGHT

Name .... Birth Date .... Reg. No. ....

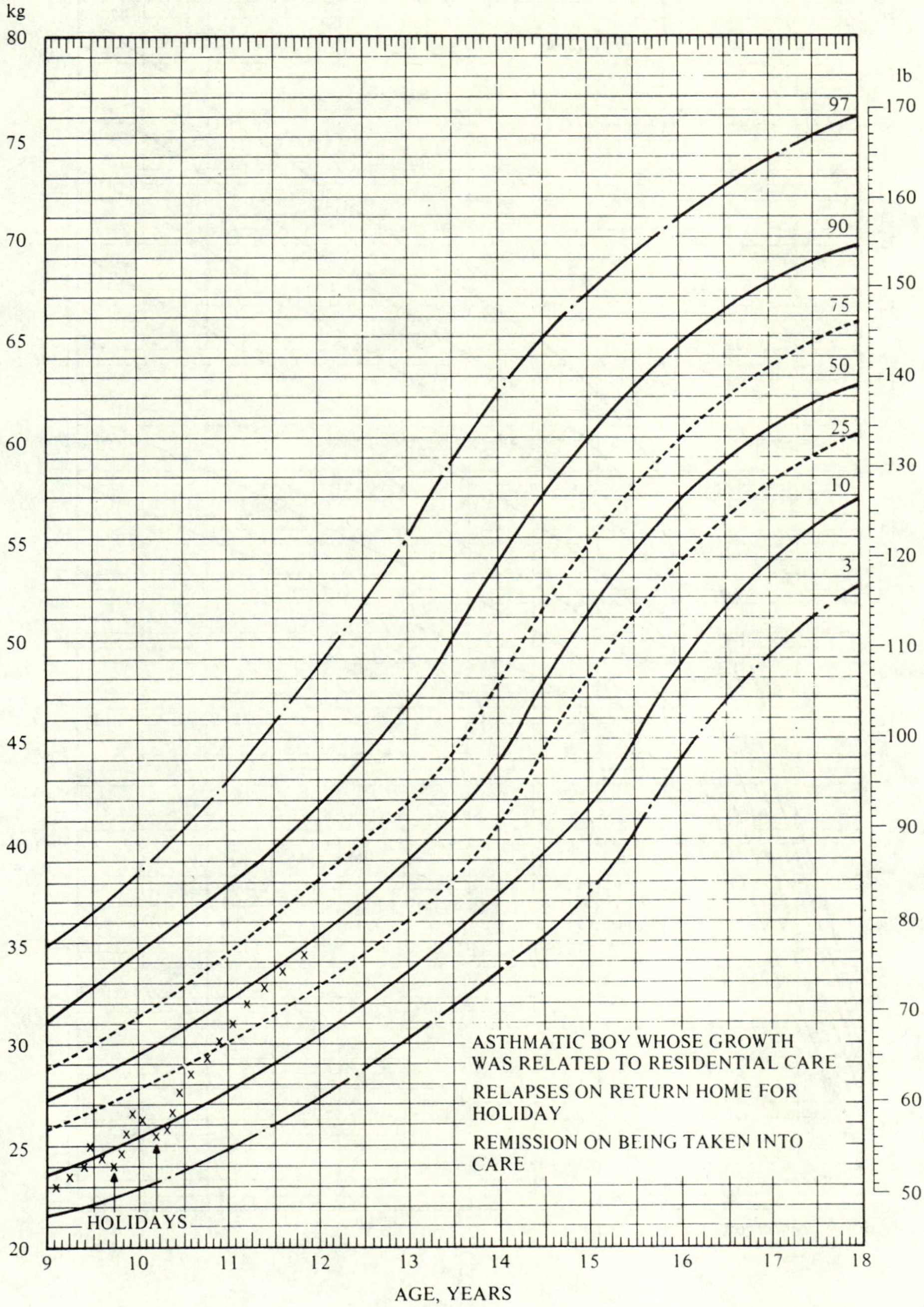

FIGURE I

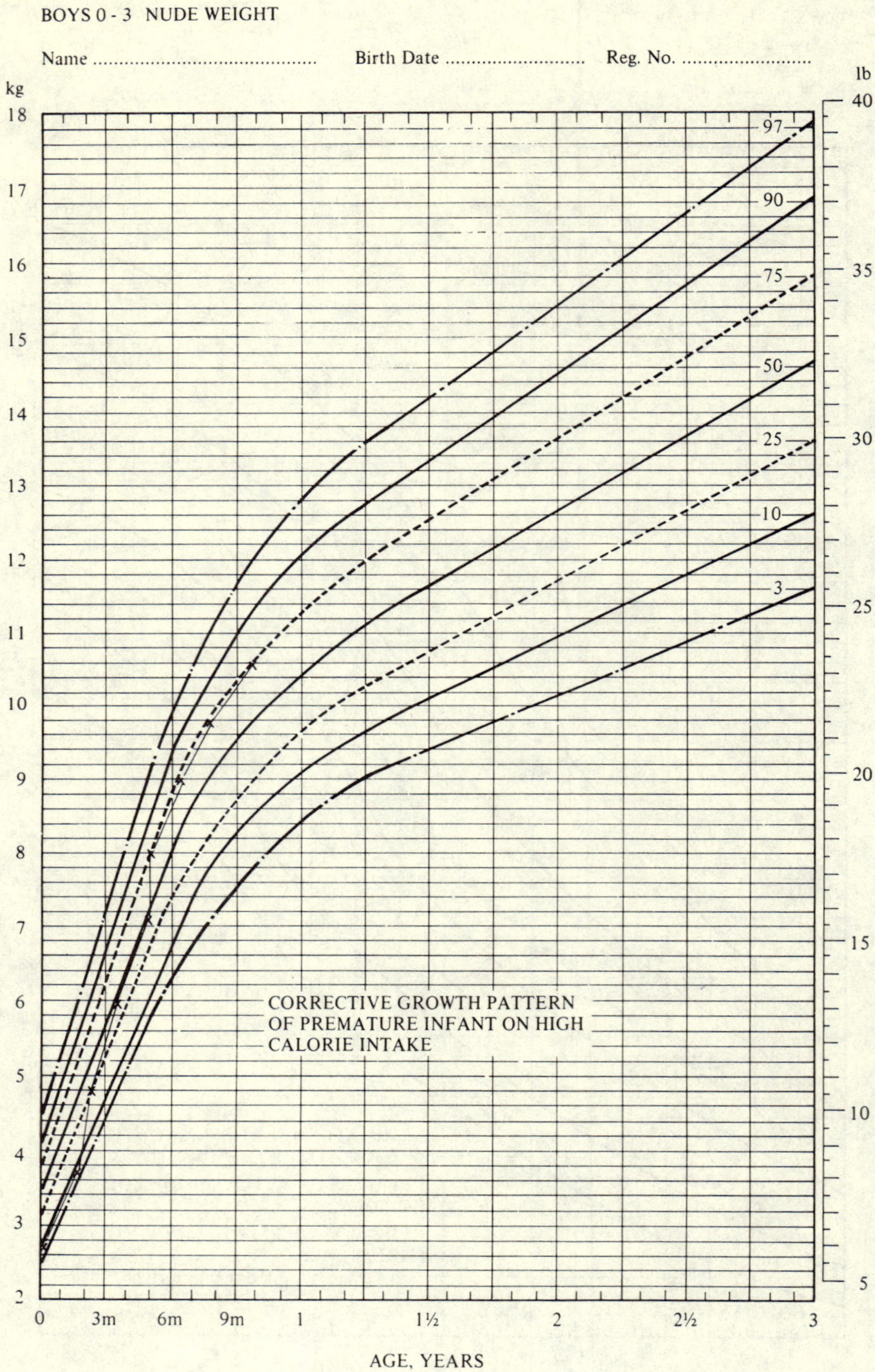
BOYS 0 - 3 NUDE WEIGHT
Name ....
Birth Date ....
Reg. No. ....
kg
lb
97
90
75
50
25
10
3
CORRECTIVE GROWTH PATTERN
OF PREMATURE INFANT ON HIGH
CALORIE INTAKE
0
3m
6m
9m
1
1½
2
2½
3
AGE, YEARS

FIGURE II

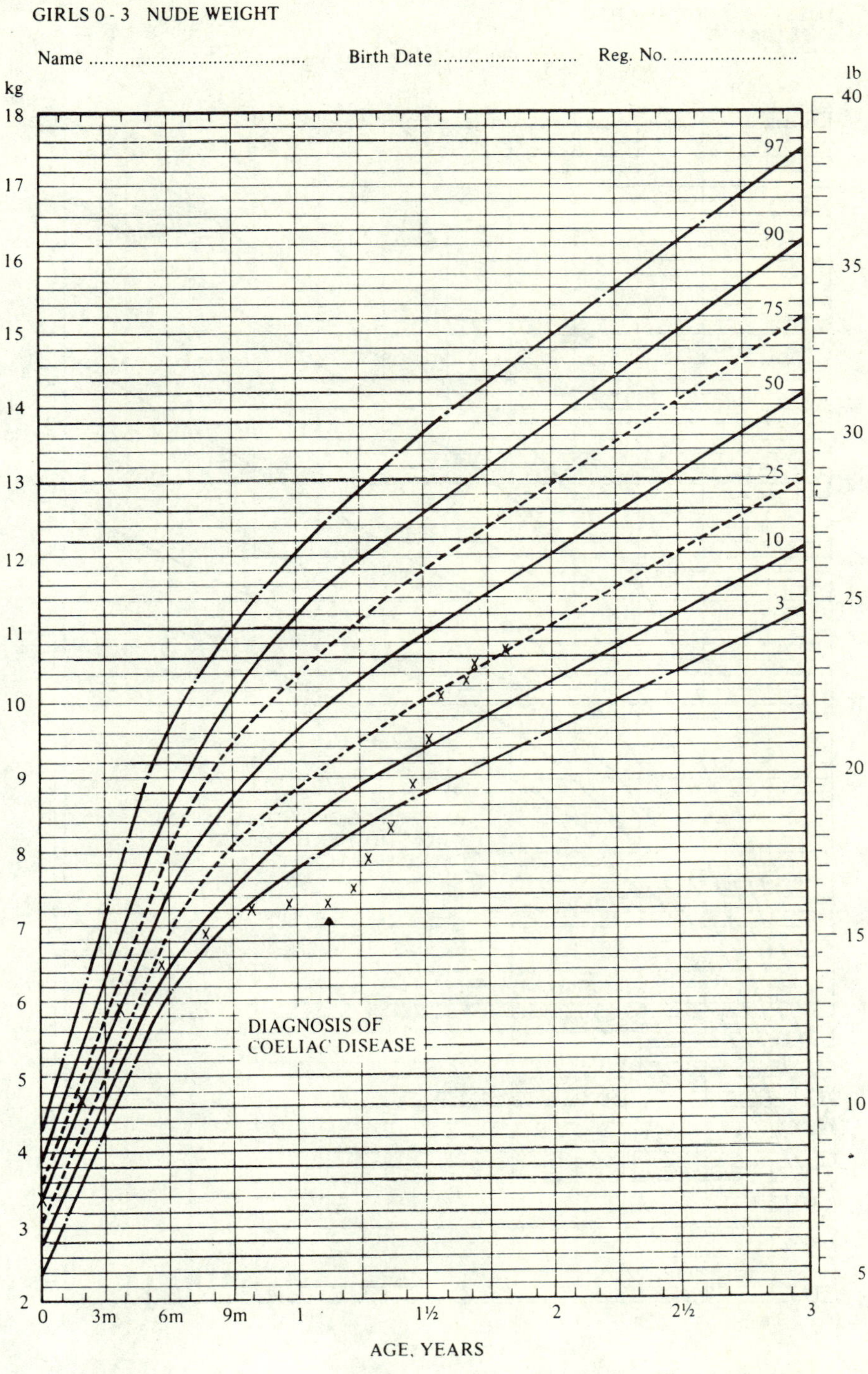
GIRLS 0 - 3 NUDE WEIGHT
Name .... Birth Date .... Reg. No. ....
kg
lb
18
17
16
15
14
13
12
11
10
9
8
7
6
5
4
3
2
40
35
30
25
20
15
10
5
97
90
75
50
25
10
3
DIAGNOSIS OF
COELIAC DISEASE
0
3m
6m
9m
1
1½
2
2½
3
AGE, YEARS

FIGURE III

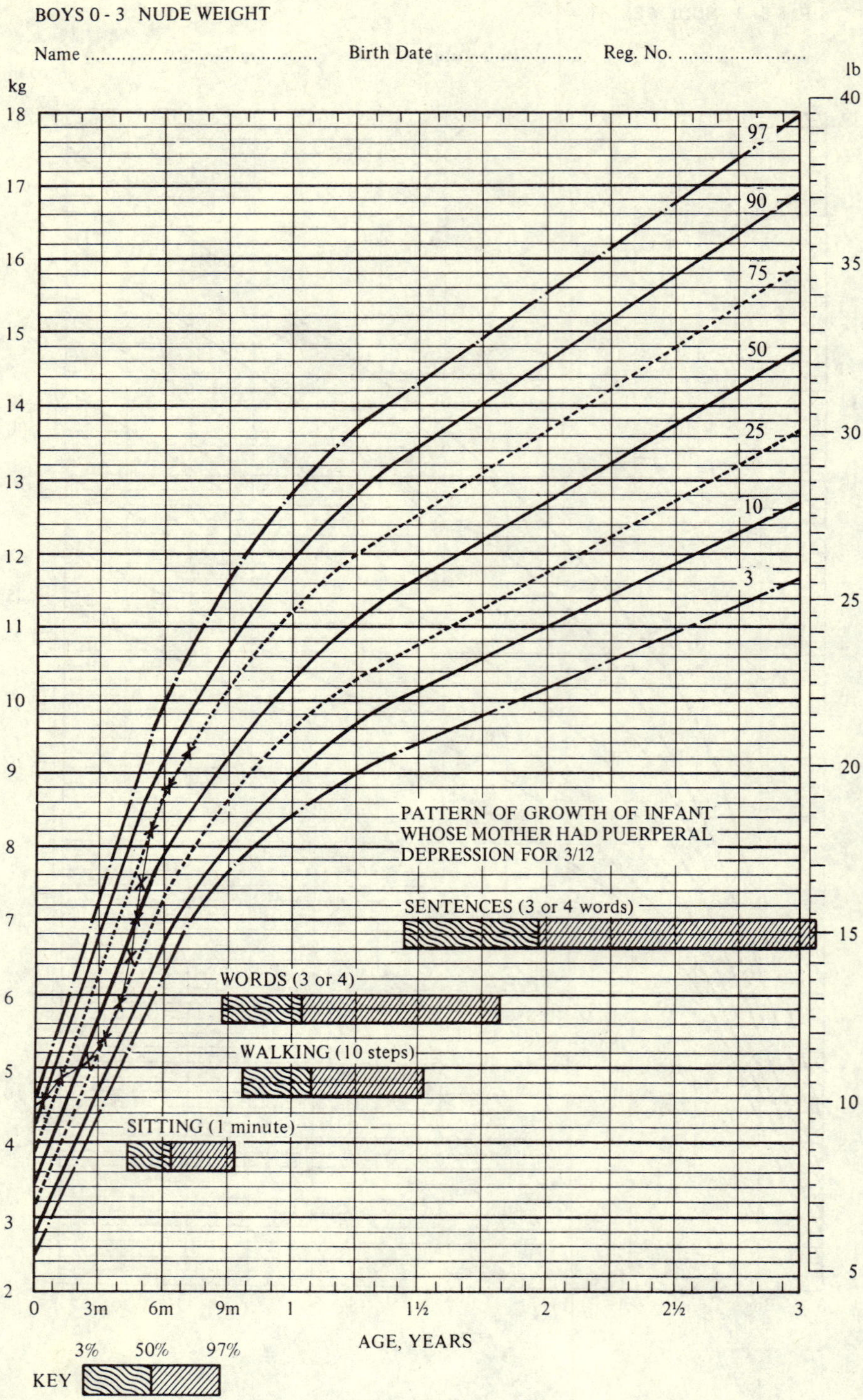

BOYS 0 - 3 NUDE WEIGHT
Name .... Birth Date .... Reg. No. ....
kg
lb
97
90
75
50
25
10
3
PATTERN OF GROWTH OF INFANT
WHOSE MOTHER HAD PUERPERAL
DEPRESSION FOR 3/12
SENTENCES (3 or 4 words)
WORDS (3 or 4)
WALKING (10 steps)
SITTING (1 minute)
0
3m
6m
9m
1
1½
2
2½
3
AGE, YEARS
3%
50%
97%
KEY

FIGURE IV

3.75 The poisoned patient

M.E. Preston-Whyte

In 1971,[1] 50,000 adults in the United Kingdom were admitted to hospital because of poisoning, representing 10 per cent to 25 per cent of all acute medical emergencies. The vast proportion, 85 per cent, of these cases were due to self-poisoning or 'parasuicide' in which there is no real wish for self-destruction; genuine attempted suicide represented 10 per cent of cases with accidental poisoning forming the remainder. The annual mortality from poisoning is 7,000 (approximately equal to that due to road deaths).

Whilst deliberate self-poisoning is a disease of adults, accidental poisoning is an increasingly common problem of children under the age of 5. Approximately 40,000 children are poisoned annually, 20,000 of whom are admitted to hospital. Each year, 200 children under the age of 15 die from poisoning.[2]

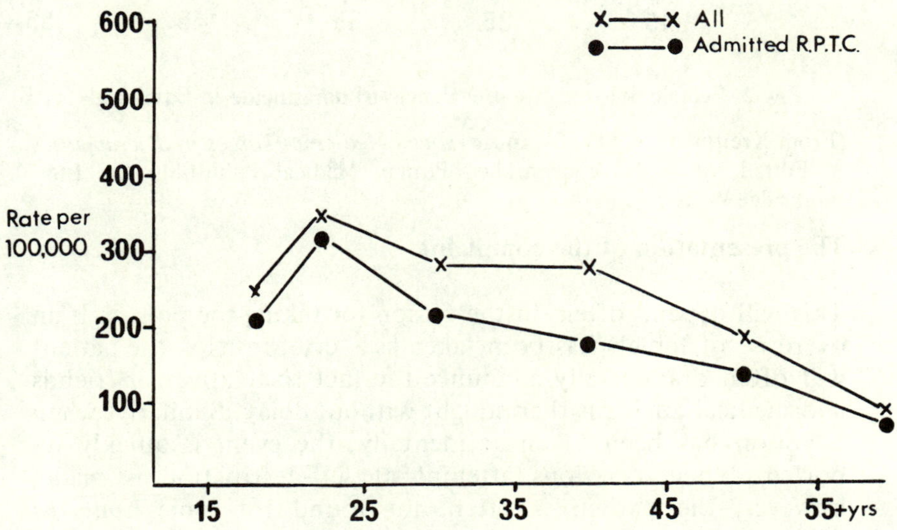

Fig. 1. Male persons: age prevalences of parasuicide in Edinburgh

(From Kreitman, N. (1975): in *Advanced Medicine: Topics in Therapeutics 1.* Edited by A.M. Breckenridge. Pitman Medical Publishing Co. Ltd., Tunbridge Wells.)

Figures from the Regional Poisoning Treatment Centre in Edinburgh demonstrate that the incidence of cases of poisoning occurring in the community closely resembles the pattern of hospital admissions. The accompanying graphs (figures 1 and 2) show that deliberate self-poisoning occurs more often in the 18–25 age group and that women are more likely than men to take an overdose.

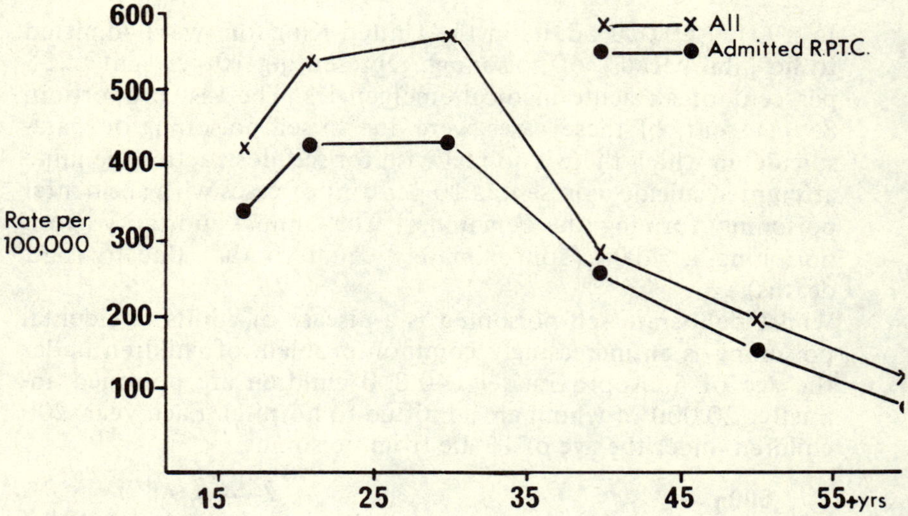

Fig. 2. Female persons: age prevalences of parasuicide in Edinburgh

(From Kreitman, N. (1975): in *Advanced Medicine: Topics in Therapeutics 1*. Edited by A.M. Breckenridge. Pitman Medical Publishing Co. Ltd., Tunbridge Wells.)

The presentation of the complaint

This will depend often on the reason for taking the poison. If an overdose of tablets has been taken as a 'cry for help', the patient will often dramatically announce the fact to relatives or friends and medical advice is then sought without delay. Similarly, when a poison has been taken accidentally, the event is quickly reported. When a serious attempt at self-destruction is made, however, the patient is often not found for some hours as deliberate measures for preventing discovery are usually taken (booking into a hotel, or parking a car in a remote spot) and may as a result be deeply unconscious. Occasionally, the patient who may not intend to kill himself misjudges the dose of tablets or takes them with alcohol and may be found dead or comatose the following morning.

Recognition of the patient who will make a successful suicide attempt is important. These are predominantly the elderly and more often those living in remote rural communities, usually suffering from chronic physical disease. Members of the medical profession, particularly women, have a higher suicide rate than other professions. When a depressed patient is seen by his general practitioner, he should be asked directly about any suicidal thoughts. There is a high incidence of patients having seen a doctor two to four days prior to their admission suffering from self-poisoning.

It should be noted also that there is no correlation between the dose of drug taken, and the patient's mental state and the risk of a subsequent attempt. Patients are not usually pharmacologists and cannot predict the physical sequelae of the act with any accuracy.

It has been shown that the parasuicide rate is higher among unemployed persons, and that there is a marked increase in rate for Social Class V and where overcrowding occurs (this relates particularly to women).

Causes

Figures obtained from the Edinburgh Poisons Unit show that the following drugs are involved in more than 90 per cent of admissions: barbiturates, methaqualone (Mandrax), benzodiazepines, tricyclic antidepressants, phenothiazines, salicylates, and paracetamol.

In 1967, barbiturates accounted for 50 per cent of drug overdoses; in 1973 this figure had fallen to 20 per cent. Their place has been taken by the benzodiazepines and tricyclic antidepressants; whilst the former are less dangerous drugs, the tricyclics have been shown to be highly toxic in overdose. The increased prescribing of these drugs to those patients who are depressed and anxious will inevitably increase the risk of self-poisoning. The reader is referred to Chapters 3.2 and 3.3 for discussion of appropriate management of these patients.

Although these drugs are most commonly involved in deliberate overdose by adults, children are often the victims, attracted to brightly coloured tablets while visiting 'Granny' who dislikes the child-proof containers because of the difficulty she has in opening them. Poisoning with these drugs present the following clinical features:

Barbiturates are unpredictably absorbed but drowsiness and coma develop quickly. The duration and depth of cerebral depression vary greatly with the drug, the dose, and the tolerance of the patient. The severity of the poisoning is greater with a large dose of a short- or medium-acting barbiturate than with long-acting phenobarbitones.

Benzodiazepines seldom cause more than a prolonged but reversible period of unconsciousness unless the patient suffers from chronic respiratory disease.

Tricyclic antidepressants cause coma of varying degree; dilated pupils, intestinal ileus, and urinary retention occur due to their anticholinergic effects. More dangerously, hyperreflexia with convulsions and, in a late stage, cardiac arrhythmias occur. Such arrhythmias should only be treated at home if electrocardiographic control is available. Intravenous lignocaine is the drug of choice for ventricular tachycardias but propranol is needed if a supraventricular tachycardia is diagnosed. However mild the overdosage, these patients should be referred for further treatment in hospital and intramuscular valium 10 mg may be needed to sedate them for the ambulance journey.

Phenothiazines commonly cause hypotension, hypothermia, or sinus tachycardia but there is less disturbance of consciousness and respiratory depression than with the barbiturates. Symptoms of muscle spasm and tremor are common and convulsions may occur in severe cases.

Salicylates cause hyperpnoea, tinnitus, and sweating. Coma is uncommon except in children. There are complicated metabolic disturbances and patients are often more ill than is at first apparent. Gastric emptying is delayed and secretion of salicylates back into the stomach from the blood-stream occurs.

Paracetamol seldom causes coma but severe liver damage, which may be fatal, may occur after several days. This is one of the few situations where delay of a few hours in initiating treatment in a conscious patient may mean the difference between life and death. As it is becoming an increasing problem in parasuicide, doctors should be aware of paracetamol's danger and emptying the stomach of its contents has the highest priority. Measurement of plasma paracetamol levels gives a guide to prognosis but offers no direct help with the management which is essentially supportive.

The following substances are far less common causes of poisoning but are important in that they represent the 2 per cent of poisons where a specific antidote exists:

Poison	*Antidote*
Iron salts	Desferrioxamine
Opiates	Nalorphine/naloxon

Poison	*Antidote*
Heavy metals	Dimercaprol
Cyanide	Cobalt edetate
Organophosphorous compounds	Atropine and pralidoxine
Carbon monoxide	Oxygen

More recently, intensive research has suggested that paracetamol and paraquat may eventually be treated by specific antidotes.

The general practitioner will rarely have to deal with poisoning which would necessitate him including the specific antidotes among his armamentarium of emergency drugs unless he is practising in an area remote from a centre where such treatment could be undertaken.

A recent article[3] which investigated the size of the problem of poisoning with household products concluded that the age-group predominantly involved was 1 to 5 years old, that the intrinsic toxicity of most household cleaning products on sale in Britain is not high, and that the accidental ingestion of amounts commonly taken by children hardly ever endangers life.

Out of doors, children are at risk from eating berries (e.g. deadly nightshade which causes atropine poisoning), or seeds (e.g. laburnum), or drinking horticultural chemicals left in old lemonade bottles, of which paraquat is the most common and lethal.

Carbon monoxide as a cause of poisoning has declined rapidly as a result of the introduction of natural or methane gas instead of coal gas.

History

The information that the doctor needs to obtain when poisoning is suspected should be restricted to the following questions, remembering that the informant may be distraught and unable to give accurate answers:

1. What has been taken, how much and when?
2. Has the patient vomited subsequently?
3. Is the patient rousable or not?

What has been taken? The type of drug taken should alert the doctor to the need for urgent treatment when:

1. The poison has delayed effects on specific organs, e.g. paracetamol on the liver, which can be fatal.
2. Its delayed metabolic effects are serious, e.g. aspirin.
3. Its effect is to depress respiration and circulation, e.g. barbiturates, morphine.

4. Serious arrhythmias and convulsions may occur, e.g. tricyclic antidepressants.
5. More than one drug has been taken, the action of the one potentiating the other, e.g. barbiturates and alcohol.
6. A caustic or similar substance has been ingested, causing local damage.
7. A specific antidote exists (see below).

How much? As a general rule, the greater the quantity of a drug taken, the greater are its harmful effects. Patients may, however, deliberately over- or under-estimate the amount taken. No decisions on management of the patient should depend on the answer to this question alone.

When? The length of time that has elapsed since the poison was taken will determine to some extent the patient's management as well as corroborate the details of the history so far obtained. One would regard with suspicion the story of a patient having swallowed a handful of barbiturates but being fully conscious some hours later.

Has the patient vomited? The conscious patient who has vomited may prove a less urgent problem than the patient who has not. But absorption of the drug may have already occurred if the stomach had been empty when the drug was taken and vomiting may only yield 30 per cent of the drug ingested.
The unconscious patient who has vomited may require extremely urgent medical attention. Aspiration of stomach contents as a result of vomiting may cause mechanical obstruction to respiration as well as generalized bronchospasm (Mendelson's syndrome) and later pneumonia.

Is the patient rousable or not? The unconscious patient requires immediate assessment – often this is the only history that is available. The conscious patient on the other hand may be brought to the surgery if transport is available.

Examination

The examination of the conscious patient may be limited to pulse rate and possibly temperature (to provide a base-line reading when salicylates have been ingested). The unconscious patient should be more carefully assessed as follows:

Depth of coma. The lightly comatose patient will have the eyelid reflex still present, the pupil will react to light and there will be withdrawal response to mildly painful stimuli. At this stage, the pharyngeal reflex will be preserved and the larynx will thus be

protected if spontaneous regurgitation or vomiting occurs.
As coma deepens, these reflexes disappear and when the patient presents with absent corneal reflex, an inactive pupil, and is unresponsive to marked painful stimulation, e.g. supra-orbital pressure, his condition is critical.

Depth and rate of respiration. Respiration becomes progressively slower and more shallow as coma deepens with increasing hypoxaemia. Conversely, salicylates result in hyperpnoea as a result of metabolic acidosis.

Pulse rate, regularity, and blood pressure. The depressant effect of the drug on the heart and circulation adversely affects the perfusion of the tissues and shock occurs as indicated by a feeble pulse and falling blood pressure.

Temperature. Patients who have been unconscious for some time, particularly in cold weather, are often hypothermic. Salicylate poisoning, however, causes pyrexia.

If at this point, examination reveals a deeply unconscious patient showing signs of shock, immediate transfer to hospital is indicated. The lightly comatose patient may be examined more thoroughly, the doctor's interest centring on other signs of attempted suicide, e.g. cut wrists, or physical signs of associated disease which may be contributing to or may be the cause of the patient's condition, e.g. hypoglycaemic coma or cerebrovascular accident.

Management

At home or surgery

The first decision to be made as a result of the information received is whether the doctor should attend the patient himself or immediately refer the patient to hospital. If it appears that the poison involved is one where any delay in treatment may be critical, e.g. paracetamol, or where the patient is described as deeply unconscious, then it may be more appropriate for the doctor to order an ambulance and to ring the local Casualty or Poisons Unit to inform them of the patient's expected arrival.
Brief, clear instructions should be given to the caller on the care of the unconscious patient (see Chapter 3.6) while the ambulance is awaited. These same instructions could form the basis of a typewritten card for the receptionist's use when the doctor is not available; included should be advice on what action the receptionist

must take: namely, to tell the caller that she will order an ambulance to transfer a patient, if unconscious, to hospital, or that the conscious patient can be taken directly to the nearest Casualty Department together with such evidence of what poison has been taken as is available.

If the practitioner decides that he should see the patient himself then he should do so at once. If the patient is conscious, the details of the history should be confirmed and checked against the available evidence. He must then decide whether an attempt should be made to empty the stomach by induced vomiting. Normally gastric emptying is complete after four hours but gastric stasis due to the drug (e.g. tricyclics, iron, salicylates, and phenothiazines) fear or nausea may result in delay considerably longer than usual and emptying of the stomach may still be of benefit twelve hours later. The amount of drug recovered is rarely more than 30 per cent but the advantage of emesis is that it can be done on first seeing the patient whereas gastric aspiration and lavage should be done in hospital.

If it is decided that emesis should be tried, then the safest, most effective method is 5–20 ml Syrup of Ipecacuanha followed by a glass of water (for children Paediatric Emetic Draught B.P.C. should be used, 10 ml from 6 to 18 months and 15 ml if older). This usually results in vomiting occurring within twenty minutes. The dose can be safely repeated if vomiting does not occur.

Apomorphine is no longer recommended[4] as it can cause coma, especially if given to a patient whose central nervous system is already depressed. The traditional salt-and-water emetic may precipitate acute heart failure in the elderly and is also contra-indicated. Mechanical methods, e.g. tickling the back of the throat, are rarely effective. Corrosive poisons, e.g. bleach, lysol, are an absolute contra-indication to emesis as vomiting may result in perforation of a viscus, and petroleum products may be aspirated into the lungs where they cause more damage than in the stomach.

If emesis is successful in the conscious patient (it should never be induced in the unconscious patient) the next decision is whether the patient should be observed at home or referred to hospital for further treatment. The patient who can be observed at home is the one who has taken a known small dose of a drug, e.g. benzodiazepine, some hours previously and who is still conscious or easily rousable from sleep. If the patient is unconscious (the exception is the example just given), referral to hospital is always indicated, the general practitioner supervising the position of the patient in order to maintain a clear airway during the journey. There is no place for the systemic administration of analeptics (respiratory stimulants) or vasoconstrictor drugs, and positive-pressure ventilation with an Ambou bag will result in overdistension of the stomach with regurgitation of its contents.

At hospital

The detailed management of the patient in hospital does not concern the general practitioner but the information he can supply may be invaluable in deciding treatment. A directive from the Central Health Services Council in 1962 suggested the setting up of special Poisons Treatment Centres and Poisons Information Services to aid the emergency treatment of cases of acute poisoning.
In the U.K. a 24-hour Poisons Information Service is available at the following numbers:

Belfast	0232 40503
Cardiff	0222 33101
Edinburgh	031-229 2477
Leeds	0532 32799
London	01-407 7600
Manchester	061-740 2254
Newcastle	0632 25131

If the patient is unconscious, gastric aspiration and lavage is usually performed if the drug has been taken less than four hours previously (the exceptions are those drugs which may remain in the stomach for twelve hours or longer). This procedure should only be carried out after a cuffed endotracheal tube has been passed to protect the airway. Removal of the poison should not take precedence over other more urgent resuscitative measures. Few specific antidotes are available and supportive treatment based on the following non-specific measures form the basis of treatment:

1. Maintenance of an adequate airway with endotracheal intubation and assisted ventilation.
2. Treatment of circulatory failure and hypothermia.
3. Correction of acid-base and electrolyte abnormalities.
4. Unabsorbed drug removed by gastric aspiration and thorough lavage.
5. Identification of drug taken and estimation of plasma levels to indicate amount ingested. (See following list.)

Drugs for which positive identification is particularly helpful in deciding therapy

Phenobarbitone	Methanol
Barbitone	Iron
Meprobamate	Chlordiazepoxide
Salicylates	Tricyclic antidepressants
Paracetamol	Organophosphorous compounds

Forced diuresis and peritoneal or haemodialysis are of little value in the majority of cases. With such measures as the above, the overall mortality of cases of poisoning admitted to hospital has been reduced to less than 1 per cent.

The aftercare of the poisoned patient

As has been shown, the vast majority of cases of poisoning are due to deliberate overdose, usually of a non-lethal quantity of a drug. As the patient is seldom in hospital for more than twenty-four hours, the aftercare of this patient is particularly relevant to his general practitioner. All Poison Units and most Casualty Departments at the larger general hospitals arrange for the patient to be seen by a psychiatrist. Brandon[5] in 1970, suggested that it was vital to interview the patient in addition to nearest relatives before important factors became obscured and the event rationalized. The psychiatrist's assessment of the precipitating factors and the need for further treatment will determine whether the patient requires immediate admission to a psychiatric hospital (25–40 per cent of parasuicides) or whether the patient can be discharged home either for follow-up by a social worker or to continue follow-up with the psychiatric clinic as out-patient or as an attender at a day centre. Some patients may be more appropriately discharged to the care of their general practitioner who should be familiar with their family circumstances and therefore better able to intervene when interpersonal relationships have broken down. He may find that involving his practice team, particularly if this includes a psychiatric nurse, will help in a situation where a supportive role may be needed for some time.

The problem of repetition of the act must always be remembered. Approximately 40 per cent of episodes of self-poisoning admitted to hospital are not the first-ever episodes and the rapid increase in parasuicide noted in recent years may reflect an increased liability to repetition rather than an increasing number of individuals becoming parasuicides for the first time. Therapeutic endeavour may have to be switched from the possibilities of preventing first attempts and concentrating on the question of effective secondary prevention. It has been shown that inflicting unpleasant procedures, e.g. unnecessary stomach wash-outs, does not lead to any reduction in subsequent episodes.

When a case of accidental poisoning involves a child, again admission to hospital is rarely longer than 24 to 48 hours. The general practitioner should be alerted by the event to possible problems within the family for these cases often occur in homes where parental care is poor or where the mother is depressed and apathetic. The health visitor may be the most appropriate person to make a follow-up visit to offer advice on the prevention of similar accidents in the future. She could also play a major preventive role by stressing safety in the home with posters and film shows for mothers attending clinics, such as the infant welfare clinic (cartoon films can be obtained by written application to the local Health Education Council).

The pharmaceutical industry is producing more drugs in individually-packed foil sheets which should decrease the risk of accidental poisoning. Recent legislation has been directed towards limiting the sale of drugs 'over the counter', which may help to deter the parasuicide but will do little to reduce the risk of a serious suicide attempt.

References

[1] Goulding, R. (1971): Self-poisoning. *British Journal of Hospital Medicine*, *5*, 249

[2] Jackson, R.H., Walker, J.H. and Wynne, N.A. (1968): Circumstances of accidental poisoning in childhood. *British Medicdal Journal*, *4*, 245

[3] Goulding, R., Ashforth, G.K. and Jenkins, H. (1978): Household products and poisoning. *British Medical Journal*, *1*, 286

[4] Lawrence, D.R. (1973): *Clinical Pharmacology*. 4th ed. Edinburgh: Churchill Livingstone

[5] Brandons, S. (1970): Crisis theory and possibilities of therapeutic intervention. *British Journal of Psychiatry*, *117*, 627

3.76
The injured patient

David Morrell

The Third National Morbidity Study shows a consultation rate for accidents, poisoning and violence of 182 per 1,000 patients at risk.[1] The highest consultation rates for these causes are found in males aged 15 to 44 years and females aged 75 years and over. In a study of new symptoms presented in general practice Morrell and colleagues[2] found that complaints of trauma to various parts of the body acounted for 4.8 per cent of symptoms. Many of the complaints presented did not however mention trauma and patients simply complained of pain. In a further report[3] we demonstrated that 43 per cent of patients presenting with pain in the back and 11 per cent of patients presenting with pain in the chest or abdominal pain were diagnosed as suffering from strains or sprains. It is apparent from these studies that injury of one sort or another is responsible for many of the new symptoms presented to the general practitioner.

The extent to which the general practitioner is concerned with the management of injury is influenced by his place of practice. The Second National Morbidity Study revealed that consultation rates for accidents, poisoning and violence were 1.9 per 100 patients at risk in rural areas compared with 1.4 in urban areas. This may reflect the availability of accident departments to patients living in urban areas, while the general practitioner may be the first doctor consulted in rural areas. The place in which the doctor practises does however affect the types of injury with which he will be presented. In farming districts he must expect injuries varying from major tractor accidents to simple lacerations. Some doctors practise in close proximity to trunk roads and must develop special skills in the management of road accidents. Others must develop particular skills in the management of mining accidents or mountain rescue. This chapter is not concerned with these rather special situations which are well described in a book edited by Easton[4] to which general practitioners concerned with such work contribute.

Presentation

The important factors determining when a patient experiencing injury will consult are the anxiety produced by the accident and the disability engendered by the injury. The general practitioner is commonly consulted by a patient with an apparently trivial injury. It is important in such cases that his diagnosis should include some explanation of the excessive anxiety provoked. In the case of a child this may be the first indication of child abuse. Injury in a young wife may be the first sign of marital disharmony and represent a cry for help. Individuals involved in competitive sport frequently react excessively to minor injury for they fear that this might threaten their sporting career. Sometimes an apparently inappropriate response to minor injury may be provoked by over-critical spouses, parents-in-law or neighbours. An inexplicable injury or repeated injury may be the first indication of an alcohol problem. A proper understanding of the factors which may provoke the request for care in response to minor injury is a prerequisite for proper management.

Injuries to certain parts of the body tend to produce more anxiety than injuries to other parts. Head injury evokes fears of brain damage; facial injuries fears of permanent disfigurement; and abdominal injuries fears of 'internal damage'. Quite minor injuries during pregnancy cause fears concerning the wellbeing of the unborn child.

In all cases the doctor should take a careful history of the cause and circumstances of the injury and should attempt to identify the major reason for the patient's anxiety. There is a temptation in these cases to proceed at once to examination of the injured part, but with the exception of the rare serious injuries, the history is usually the more important.

It is not possible in a book of this type to consider all the possible injuries which a general practitioner may be called upon to manage. Some problems which are commonly presented will be described and some general principles of management outlined. Further information about injuries to specific joints will be found in Chapters 3.64 to 3.69 and injuries to the eye in Chapter 3.18.

Contusions

These may be defined as tissue damage resulting from trauma which does not cause laceration of the skin.

Presentation

The patient who presents to the general practitioner with a contusion usually consults in order to receive relief from pain, or reassurance that there is no bony injury, or a certificate for sickness benefit. The doctor should however always bear in mind that the complaint may reflect some underlying problem such as child or wife abuse or a desire to adopt the sick role for reasons unassociated with the injury.

History and examination

In history-taking the most important factors to record are the cause of the injury, i.e. the forces likely to have been applied and the patient's immediate response to injury. In a fall, the age and weight of the patient may be important in assessing the probability of bony damage. If the patient is able immediately to resume the activity in which he was engaged bone damage is unlikely, even though some hours later he may be severely disabled by pain and swelling. The circumstances of the injury are important to ascertain and in the case of an industrial injury or road traffic accident where legal action may be forthcoming, particular care should be exercised in recording all the facts.

Diagnosis

The classical signs of a fractured bone are pain, swelling, deformity and impairment of function. In the presence of a fracture these usually follow immediately on the injury, although there are some exceptions such as a fractured scaphoid bone. Injuries which do not cause a fracture may some hours later produce all these signs due to haematoma formation. In the presence of a fracture however there is usually localized tenderness at the site of the fracture. The haematoma or bruising occurring in a contusion in the absence of a fracture more often causes generalized tenderness. Where the contusion is produced by abnormal stresses on joints such as the ankle or knee localized tenderness may be elicited over a torn ligament and pain produced by tension of this ligament. The most common site where doubt exists is injury to the ankle. Pressure applied directly to the medial or lateral malleolus will produce acute pain in the presence of a fracture, whereas ligamentous tears will be indicated by tenderness to pressure applied below the malleolus on the medial or lateral ligaments. Rib injuries are another common source of anxiety in general practice and again direct pressure over a rib will usually indicate a fracture rather than bruising. Where abdominal injuries occur it is always important to bear in mind the possibility of damage to the spleen or kidneys. The patient should be examined to determine whether there are any signs of shock such as a raised pulse rate or fall in blood pressure;

there should be an examination for abdominal tenderness and urinalysis should be carried out.

Management

Fractures. If the patient has an obvious fracture with deformity of one of the long bones this should be splinted as it lies using either a malleable wire or inflatable splint or if one is not available a plaster of Paris backslab. The type of equipment carried by the general practitioner will be influenced by his place of work, the types of injuries he commonly encounters and the distance he works from the nearest hospital. To transport a patient with a displaced fracture without support over long distances causes unnecessary suffering and possibly further shock, and some form of splinting in the most comfortable position should always be carried out. The patient and relatives should be told not to give anything by mouth as this will delay reduction of the fracture under anaesthetic. In the United Kingdom patients will rarely be travelling such long distances that they will require powerful analgesia, but if this is required the patient should be labelled with the time and dose of the drug administered.

In the case of undisplaced fractures adequate support may be provided by a crepe bandage or elastoplast strapping. Not uncommonly the general practitioner is called upon to see a patient where there may be bony damage but where there is no evidence of bone displacement. In these cases support and analgesia should be provided and the patient should be x-rayed at his own and the hospital's convenience. Sending such a patient to hospital for x-ray out of hours usually leads to a long wait in the accident department when he would be much better resting following injury in his own home. By the following day the need for an x-ray may seem much less immediate and if it is required may be dealt with much more expeditiously.

Any suspicion of injury involving the neck or spine must be treated with extreme caution. Such patients should be admitted to hospital without further examination which may in itself lead to irreversible damage to the spinal cord.

Sometimes the general practitioner will be called upon to supervise the transport of patients suffering from spinal injury. Some general principles should be observed:

1. Do not attempt to move the patient until adequate help is available.
2. In transferring the patient to a stretcher endeavour to keep the spine supported throughout its length. This may be achieved by inserting a blanket beneath the patient and lifting with the help of six to eight helpers, ensuring that the spine is kept at all times horizontal.

3. If injury to the cervical spine is suspected, the patient should be fitted before moving with a supporting collar which may be very simply made from a rolled-up newspaper in a head-scarf or sling.
4. If the patient must be extracted from a damaged vehicle or from under a collapsed building, for instance, support for the spine can be assured by the use of a blanket held by four to six helpers. It is important in extracting the patient that the spine should never be twisted, flexed or extended in this process.

Simple contusions. If seen at once the disability produced by a contusion can be relieved by measures designed to reduce haematoma formation. The part affected should be cooled by bandages soaked in water or icepacks. Firm pressure should be applied and the injured part elevated. In muscle injuries spasm may cause severe pain and this may be relieved by splinting the joint above and below the injury using either light aluminium splints or a plaster backslab. Severe contusions of large muscle masses, e.g. the quadriceps, may lead to the loss of large quantities of blood into the muscle and signs of shock.

In most minor contusions bleeding will have ceased within 24 hours and gentle support followed by graded exercises will lead to a gradual resumption of activities. In severe muscle injuries, however, a much longer period of rest may be required.

Many of the contusions seen in general practice result from sports injuries and the patient should be advised to graduate his rehabilitation slowly before exposing the injured part to the stresses demanded by active sport. Following joint injuries the use of supporting elastic bandages is popular among sportsmen but the stability of the joint is dependent on the rehabilitation of surrounding muscles which may waste rapidly following injury and require several weeks to return to normal. A piece of elastic is little substitute for this and may give rise to false confidence.

Relief of pain. Contusions may be very painful and disturb sleep. Adequate analgesics should be prescribed, and in the presence of severe pain the short-term use of such drugs as pethidine or methadone should be considered.

Head injury

Presentation

The general practitioner is rarely presented with a patient suffering from severe head injury, such as those following road accidents or falls from a height, or those occurring in industry. These patients are most frequently taken directly to accident or emergency departments. The general practitioner is most commonly asked to express an opinion about a child who has fallen from a swing or a chair, or an adult who has fallen downstairs or struck his head on a shelf or door.

History and examination

In cases of minor head injury, the patient and doctor are anxious to exclude the possibility of any intracranial damage. The history in these cases is all important. The exact nature of the injury should be determined and the patient's memory of the event should be elicited. A period of amnesia preceding the injury suggests at least some degree of concussion. Loss of consciousness following the injury is similarly significant and its duration should be recorded. Injury to the temporal region is more likely to cause intracranial haemorrhage from the middle meningeal artery than trauma to the frontal or occipital regions. A history of vomiting following the injury is important to elicit. Headache is common following head injury and, in the absence of any loss of consciousness or impaired memory for the event, is not necessarily significant. Changes over time are really the most important facts to be determined from the history. Any impairment of consciousness or memory or concentration after a period of lucid behaviour is serious.

In minor head injuries examination is usually much less rewarding than history-taking. In major head injuries where the doctor is presented with an unconscious patient there should be an immediate examination to ensure that the patient has a clear airway. Further examination should determine the respiration and pulse rate and the characteristics of the pupils and their reaction to light. The patient who is still unconscious by the time the general practitioner reaches him will almost always require immediate admission to hospital and little is gained by a more detailed examination before arranging this. It is however of value to record the level of consciousness before referral to hospital so that any deterioration with the passage of time may be noted. This should be recorded in functional terms such as the patient's response to the examiner's voice or instructions, and response to tactile or painful stimuli. The patient who, shortly after an accident, can respond to instruction and 30 minutes later, on admission to hospital, fails to respond to painful stimuli such as pressure on the achilles tendon or eyeballs is clearly in need of urgent surgery. Conversely any return to consciousness is an important prognostic indicator.

Examination of the patient who has lost consciousness only transitorily, or not at all, and is later seen by the general practitioner is usually unhelpful. A superficial examination of the skull for any evidence of fracture, particularly in the temporal region, is important. The state of the pulse, pupils, respiration and blood pressure should be recorded as they form a base line for subsequent observation. A brief examination for any localizing neurological signs, including a test for muscle power and reflexes, will usually conclude the examination.

Management

The unconscious patient should be admitted at once to hospital after an adequate airway has been ensured and the patient has been placed in the semi-prone position to protect against inhaled vomitus should vomiting occur. If the patient is deeply unconscious, insertion of an airway, if this is available, is desirable. A note should accompany the patient describing the level of consciousness and giving any other relevant information.

With less severe injuries the doctor should, in the absence of any localizing signs or signs of deteriorating consciousness, arrange for the patient to be nursed at home. Very frequently the anxiety aroused by the injury is unjustified and in these cases the doctor should attempt to reassure the patient or parent. Occasionally, the general practitioner is faced with a patient who has received a severe blow on the head but shows no signs of impaired consciousness. In this situation it may be important to keep the patient under careful observation while at the same time avoiding excessive anxiety. To achieve this satisfactorily demands careful evaluation of the resources available. Ideally, the patient, while being encouraged to rest, should not be allowed to fall into a deep sleep for several hours after the injury. The parent or other attendant should, therefore, be encouraged to rouse the patient at two-hourly intervals and establish that there has been no change in consciousness. For the sensible parent this is sometimes possible, but when in doubt hospital admission is preferable. In some cases a home visit by the doctor or practice nurse three to four hours after the accident is reassuring to the patient and doctor alike. It may be helpful to provide the patient's relations with written instructions, such as those set out in an appendix to this chapter.

Many patients experience headache following a head injury. This should be treated as required by analgesics, and in the case of more serious injuries the patient must be advised that this may continue for several weeks. After a severe head injury return to work may be delayed for several weeks or months. In addition to headache, the patient may experience difficulty in concentrating, impaired memory and depression. It is important in these cases for the doctor to protect his patient from the demands of his occupation, until he is really fit to respond to them. This will often be influenced as much by the particular occupation of the patient as by the specific symptoms experienced.

Lacerations

Presentation

Most lacerations seen in general practice are caused by blows, or falls on sharp objects, or in manipulating knives or other sharp instruments. They usually bleed freely and may cause undue concern. If a patient seeks advice on the telephone following a laceration, he should always be carefully instructed to apply pressure to the bleeding part and if possible to elevate it. In many cases no further treatment is required.

History and examination

The history should attempt to define the cause of the injury, and if possible the depth of the injury. This is particularly important in perforating or stabbing injuries such as may be caused by garden implements or screwdrivers, or falls on sharp points such as garden stakes or sharp toys. It is important to know if the injury has taken place through clothes which may clean the implement before it enters the skin, but may also result in a particle of clothing being incorporated in the wound. In lacerations caused by glass, it is useful to know whether the glass has shattered, allowing particles to enter the wound. The doctor should try to find out if the patient or parent is particularly anxious about the injury. This anxiety may arise from fear, for instance, of tetanus, following an injury in the garden, or rabies following a dog bite, or from fear of retaliation from a self-righteous spouse or parent.
Most lacerations seen in general practice are superficial, and after stopping the bleeding require only simple inspection and dressing. The doctor should however be very circumspect in examining lacerations of the hands and feet and those around joints. In the case of penetrating wounds, a small laceration at the point of entry may belie injuries of deep structures. In these cases the doctor should carefully examine the patient for any impairment of function, bearing in mind especially injuries to tendons and nerves.

Management

Where lacerations are superficial, treatment consists simply of bringing the skin edges together to facilitate healing. Most superficial lacerations have bled freely and infection is rare. Very often simple butterfly sutures, or the application of micropore tape, together with splinting of the injured part will lead to satisfactory healing. If difficulty is experienced in getting sutures to adhere to the skin, the application of Tinct. Benz. Co. to the skin on each side of the wound may solve this problem. If the edges cannot be apposed in this way, a local anaesthetic should be injected and the wound sutured. In scalp injuries it is often difficult to maintain good apposition, and sutures may be required. If the laceration is jagged the skin edges should be trimmed under local anaesthesia before suturing. In superficial lacerations of the face, particularly those which run counter to the normal skin creases, specialist assistance may lead to a more satisfactory cosmetic result.

Deeper lacerations may need to be explored under local anaesthesia to remove foreign material. This will depend on the nature of the injury elicited in the history. If the general practitioner is in any doubt about the possible involvement of deep structures such as tendons or nerves he should seek specialist assistance at once, and this should apply to all but the most superficial lacerations of the palmar surface of the hand and wrist.

Some lacerations result in the loss of skin and must be allowed to granulate. The management of these will depend to a large extent on the site of the injury. Scarring of the knees and elbows from such injuries is common in most adults in the population and is of little consequence. Conversely, lesions of the face or hands may cause serious disability and may require early intervention by the plastic surgeon.

Perforating injuries often cause the general practitioner anxiety. In these cases good records displaying the immunization status of the patient can be reassuring. If tetanus toxoid is to be administered the following guidelines may be useful.

The administration of tetanus toxoid:

Patient known to have had a tetanus booster or complete course within the last five years (unless wound regarded as carrying a very high risk of tetanus, when this interval may be reduced to one year)	No toxoid required

Patient known to have had a course of tetanus toxoid and/or booster, but with the last dose more than five years ago	Tetanus toxoid one dose
Patient has not had previous tetanus toxoid, or tetanus immunization status unknown	Full course of tetanus toxoid (0.5 ml of toxoid subcutaneously, followed by a further 0.5 ml six weeks later, with a third dose six months after that)

Perforating injuries and major lacerations also tend to turn septic and an initial injection of one million units of Triplopen should be followed by oral therapy (a seven day course of erythromycin or flucloxacillin).

In patients who are not known to have been actively immunized against tetanus and who have serious wounds (with significant devitalization or clinical evidence of sepsis or puncture-type wounds or direct contact with soil) the additional injection of human tetanus immunoglobulin (in another limb from that used for the toxoid) should be administered.

Abrasions

Abrasions are caused when the skin is traumatized by a rough surface insufficient to cause a laceration. In general practice they are most commonly seen after falls on a rough surface.

History and examination

It is important to determine the cause of the abrasion and the likelihood of foreign material being forced into the skin. An abrasion caused by a fall on gravel for instance is likely to cause more problems than a fall on a wooden or plastic surface. Examination must determine the extent to which foreign matter has contaminated the skin. Abrasions due to a fall on tarmac may cause subsequent tattooing of the scar if this is not thoroughly cleaned.

Management

Abrasions should be cleaned thoroughly with an antiseptic soap such as Cetavlon 5 per cent. If a great deal of foreign matter has entered the abrasion it should be scrubbed after injection of a local anaesthetic. It should then be sprayed with an antibiotic spray such as 'Polybactrin' and left exposed to form a scab. Severe abrasions on the face may require plastic surgery, but this is unusual.

Burns

Presentation

Most burns seen in general practice are superficial, and the cause of the burn, which may be interpreted as reflecting parental or personal neglect, may be an important factor in leading to a consultation.

History and examination

It is important to determine the cause of the burn. First degree burns caused by steam and boiling water are probably those most commonly seen in general practice. Superficial burns cause blistering and on examination the floor of the blister is seen to be red and very tender. Burns resulting from flames and electrical burns may be deeper. Deeper burns produce a white, yellow or brown ulcer which is often insensitive. It is important to determine the degree of burning. First degree burns will heal with little scarring, but second degree burns may result in extensive scar formation which in certain sites, such as the hands or face or over joints, can cause severe disability.

Management

In superficial scalds and burns considerable pain relief may be obtained by applying 1 per cent hydrocortisone cream. Blisters should be left intact and covered by a dry dressing. More severe burns of limited extent may be treated by the general practitioner by exposure so that a scab forms and healing occurs by granulation. Burns of any serious extent, or those affecting the flexor surface of joints, the hands or face should be referred to a specialist as they may require skin grafting. Burns are always painful and adequate analgesia should be provided.

References

[1] Royal College of General Practitioners, Office of Population Censuses and Surveys, Department of Health and Social Security (1986): *Morbidity Statistics from General Practice 1981–82*. HMSO Series MB5 No. 1

[2] Morrell, D.C., Gage, H.G. and Robinson, N.A. (1971): Symptoms in General Practice. *Journal of the Royal College of General Practitioners*, *21*, 32

[3] Morrell, D.C., Gage, H.G. and Robinson, N.A. (1971): Symptom Interpretation in General Practice. *Journal of the Royal College of General Practitioners*, *22*, 297

[4] *Rescue and Emergency Care*, ed. Easton, K. (1977): London: Heinemann Medical Books Ltd.

Appendix

Instructions to patient after a head injury

The doctor should be contacted if the patient complains of:
(a) increasingly severe headache, or
(b) continuous vomiting, or
(c) double vision, or
(d) if the patient becomes unconscious, or
(e) if the patient becomes unnaturally drowsy.

To check on the last point, the patient should be wakened every two hours during the night in the 24 hours following the injury.

3.77 The patient who consults for contraception

Mairi G. B. Scott and Marshall Marinker

Presentation

The development of sophisticated biological techniques has today made it possible for every woman to control her own fertility with relative safety and with little disturbance of physical sexual function. While this has been the most important development in the social history of man since the introduction of agriculture, there have been profound psychological consequences. Human sexuality and fertility are fundamental in the human experience. They were the object of taboo, ritual and superstition long before the birth of the great world religions and remain a major subject of moral dictat in contemporary religious thinking. They provide the mainspring of psychoanalysis, which is certainly one of the most powerful expressions of Western man's psychology, whatever its limitations as a form of therapy. Because of this, the availability, use, effectiveness and consequences of contraceptive techniques present major problems and challenges for society and for contemporary medicine.

For the most part it is women who consult doctors about birth control. Increasingly the request is straightforward. Often the woman has already made up her mind what sort of method she wishes to try, or is already using a method successfully but wishes to change to an alternative method which may interfere less with sexual intercourse, or which she knows to have a lower failure rate. In the UK it is not uncommon today for adolescent girls to request oral contraception at the time of their first sexual relationships. Sometimes they make such requests in anticipation of their first sexual encounters and here the request for contraceptive advice may mask another sort of request. Such a young woman may in fact be asking the doctor for permission to have sexual intercourse. She may see the prescription for the Pill as resolving a situation about which she has not yet been able to make up her mind. Quite apart from her own feelings, and the fears and desires that she is experiencing, there will be pressures on her to conform to the group. Often these group pressures will be in conflict. It may be part of the customs of her family or her church to reject intercourse before marriage. On the other hand, the customs of her peer group, at school, club or work, may be very different. It is part of the doctor's job to explore these pressures and to relate them to what it is that the patient wants and needs. Here the doctor's clinical skills are deployed on the frontier between his own system of beliefs and that of his patient. Sometimes the patient may look to the doctor to protect her from a sexual encounter for which she is still unprepared and sometimes she looks to the doctor for the permission that is denied her elsewhere. Some doctors feel that they have a duty to impose their own morality on the patient; others feel that their task is to help the patient to identify and understand her own morality and to live safely with it. There are no easy nostrums.

General practitioners are aware, however, how recent and uncertain is the contemporary habit of openness and frankness about sexual matters. Many men and women continue to find it painful to encounter such openness, still less to be honest about their sexual experiences and needs. For this reason the request for help with contraception is often covert. The request to go on the Pill may lie undetected in the patient's complaint about backache, menstrual difficulties, sleeplessness, depression and so on. It is a self-evident truth that the doctor who advises his patient about contraception cannot do so without in some way considering the patient's sexuality and relationships, and the effect of his intervention on the patient's sexual life. It may seem daunting to suggest that whenever a young woman asks to go on the Pill, the doctor will be involved in taking a full sexual history, in sex education and psychotherapy. In fact he is involved in all three, and more besides. Because the general-practice consultation integrates the physical, psychological and social aspects of the patient's problem, sex education and counselling will be integrated in the routine of family planning, and because they will be tailored to the needs of the individual patient, may be as brief as they are effective. Advice and help with contraceptive technique must be an essential component of any sexual counselling. By the same token sexual counselling is an essential component of all effective contraceptive advice.

The most vulnerable group of patients needing contraceptive advice are those who do not seek advice. Many general practitioners are invited to give talks to schools and young people's clubs on the availability and techniques of contraception. Increasingly, practices display posters in their waiting-rooms stating that the doctor is willing to talk about this topic and advise. The patient who has a termination of pregnancy will certainly expect to discuss contraception, but inquiry about the woman's wishes and beliefs concerning contraception should be made in the course of all maternity care, and specifically discussed at the last postnatal consultation. Similar opportunities present when young people are examined prior to employment, or university, or even in the course of other routine consultations.

The individual's sexuality is a private affair. It may be determined by strong religious belief, strong family custom or unspoken fears or shameful fantasy. Because of this, the offer to discuss contraception with a patient who does not ask for help, requires tact in approach and the closest attention to the way in which the patient responds. In the postnatal consultation, the question, 'What did you do about birth control in the past?', may be a gentler opening than 'What are you going to do about birth control now?'. The answer to the first question will involve the patient in talking about her experiences and beliefs in a way which may not come easily in response to the second. In the case of a consultation with a young person, the doctor may simply say 'I don't want to pry, but I like my young patients to know that if they want to discuss contraception now or at some time in the future, I would be happy to do so.' The aim of contraceptive advice is to help the patient to live his or her own life without the pain and burden of unwanted pregnancy, or the misery of a sexual experience damaged by the fear of unwanted pregnancy. The aim, however, must never be to impose on the patient the doctor's own model of sexuality or birth control. An evangelistic fervour for contraception on the part of the general practitioner is as destructive as ignorance, indifference and hostility.

Choices

Coitus interruptus, the withdrawal of the penis from the vagina before ejaculation, with ejaculation being completed on the woman's abdomen, is a widespread method. It is fraught with hazards both physical and psychological: seminal leakage may occur before withdrawal, the man may fail to withdraw before full ejaculation, the sex act is fraught with apprehension and the woman is usually denied an orgasm. Nonetheless, although doctors have long given the method a bad name, many couples seem to use it successfully, and to be content with their sexual lives. As with any medical intervention, the doctor must be quite sure that he has something better to offer the patient before he dismantles what may be a highly satisfactory adaptation to the needs and customs of his patient.

The choices available to the patient are:

1. The rhythm method or 'safe period'
2. Mechanical occlusion: sheath or vaginal diaphragm or cervical

cap, usually with chemical spermicides
3. Oral contraception
4. Intrauterine contraceptive device (IUCD).

Permanent contraception by means of male or female sterilization will be considered later.

The decision to choose a particular form of contraception is a complex one. The first component of choice is patient acceptability. For example a woman who simply says 'I would not feel a proper woman if I took hormone pills', is making a relevant statement about her own sexuality, and should never be persuaded to take oral contraception. By the same token fears about the permanent presence of a foreign body in the uterus, particularly if it is associated with fears of a deformed baby resulting from an unplanned pregnancy, are themselves a contraindication to the use of an IUCD. The couple may express a wish to use the sheath because both wish the man to be 'in charge' of the situation, and to take the responsibility. When the use of occlusive diaphragms and caps with spermicides was virtually the only form of contraception offered by doctors, the patient's interaction with her device was often seen as illuminating her sexuality. The woman who could not bear to touch her vagina, or check that the cap was in place, often indicated in this way a rejection of her own sexual feelings, a fear about her own vagina or her partner's penis.

The second component of contraceptive choice concerns the effectiveness of the method in preventing pregnancies. Surveys of contraceptive methods are reported in terms of the number of unwanted pregnancies that occur per 100 woman-years. A woman-year refers to the continuous use of the method for 12 months. As with most surveys of this kind, the crude rates hide large individual variations. A method which is highly acceptable to a patient will be conscientiously used with good results; most failures with modern methods are related to mistakes and omissions by the patient. A method like the Pill, which has a very low reported failure rate, may carry a much higher risk of failure for a particular couple if the woman feels less feminine because she is taking these substances.

The third component of choice concerns the unwanted effects of these methods on general health. Some contraceptive methods, particularly the Pill and to a lesser extent the IUCD, have unwanted effects on general health which may constitute absolute contraindications to their use. The Pill, however, may confer health benefits, and these must also be taken into account.

Methods

The rhythm method or 'safe period'

Where mechanical or chemical methods of contraception are unacceptable, fertility can be reduced by relative sexual abstinence. The rhythm or 'safe period' method applies precise biological information to sexual abstinence so that intercourse may be avoided specifically at those times when conception is most likely to take place. This method is of particular importance to practising Roman Catholics since it was considered permissible in the Papal Encyclical of 1968.

Ovulation takes place on or about the fourteenth day before the onset of the next menstrual period. The ovum is capable of fertilization for up to 48 hours after ovulation, and sperm may remain active for up to three days after entry into the vagina. Given that ovulation may occur one to two days earlier or later than the fourteenth day, a woman with a 28-day cycle would be considered fertile from the ninth to the eighteenth day of that cycle. With a shorter cycle, or prolonged menstruation, the number of days when sexual intercourse is relatively safe, is reduced. If menstruation is irregular, some authorities advise that a record be kept of each cycle length for up to one year. Nineteen days is then deducted from the number of days of the shortest cycle; this marks the beginning of the 'unsafe period'. Ten days is deducted from the number of days of the longest cycle, and this gives the last day of the 'unsafe period'.

An important refinement of the rhythm method is based on the keeping of a temperature chart. Ovulation accompanied by a rise in progesterone causes a rise in body temperature of about 0.5°C. Once the temperature has been maintained at this higher level for three days, it is assumed that ovulation has taken place and intercourse is unlikely to result in pregnancy. The observation that the character of the mucus in the vagina changes from thick and sticky immediately following menstruation to clear and slippery just before the time of ovulation is used as an extra safeguard in detecting ovulation.

Clearly such a method requires careful advice, accurate temperature measurement by the patient, a certain measure of intelligence and a lot of motivation. Marshall[1] gives precise and excellent instructions for the patient on the use of the combined mucothermal method. The patient must first be taught how to use a special ovulation thermometer. Following instruction in the use of the thermometer, her ability to read variations in temperature should be tested. The thermometer is then kept by the bedside and preferably the rectal temperature is measured first thing in the morning before rising or taking a warm or cold drink. The temperature should then be recorded on a special chart. The patient is also taught how to notice and record the characteristics of the vaginal mucus which is also recorded on the chart. The booklet, which is written in a question and answer form, deals with all the major problems likely to be encountered by a patient attempting to use this method of family planning. It is often claimed that intercurrent fevers caused by colds, sore throats and so on, may render this method of family planning extremely difficult. However, this rarely causes any problems as the temperature rise caused by the intercurrent infection is usually considerable and can be seen to be different from that due simply to ovulation.

Using the calendar method only, the failure rate varies in different series from 14 to 40 pregnancies per 100 woman-years. Results from studies in western Europe, using only the post-ovulatory phase as determined by the temperature chart, reveal a failure rate of 0.8–1.4 per 100 woman-years. Using the combined calendar and temperature method the effectiveness varied in the studies between 3.2 and 8.0 pregnancies per 100 woman-years.[2] Results depend on the intelligence, motivation and quality of instruction of those employing this method more than any other.

Occlusive methods and spermicides

Although they are frequently used in this way, most manufacturers discourage the use of spermicidal preparations without occlusive methods. Delfen, either as a cream with applicator or as a vaginal foam, has been advocated as a sole method for nulliparous women who have not had a previous cervical dilatation. Most commonly, spermicides and occlusive methods are used in combination: it is the mechanical occlusion which provides the major effect, the spermicide affording an additional margin of safety.

The condom, or sheath, is perhaps still the commonest method of contraception. Because the use of the condom is likely to reduce the risk of infection with HIV, this method will remain the method of choice for those who continue to have casual intercourse. Combined packs containing both sheath and some form of chemical spermicide are now marketed.

The vaginal diaphragm is a thin rubber dome within a thickened rim which contains either a coil or a flat spring. Sizes vary from 50 to 100 mm. The sprung rim extends from the posterior fornix to the symphysis pubis. Spermicidal cream squeezed from a tube on both sides of the rubber dome, provides both a spermicide and a vaginal lubricant.

The cervical cap is a thicker rubber dome some 20–30 mm in diameter and fits over the cervix, keeping its position by suction. Spermicidal cream is squeezed into the cup before fitting.

The vault cap has a rubber dome, and a thickened rim which is not reinforced with a spring. Spermicidal cream is used in the same way, and the cap keeps in place over the vault by suction. The diameter varies from approximately 50 to 75 mm. The 'vimule' is simply an elongated vault cap, which is used when the cervix is particularly long.

It is important to stress that the proper fitting of such occlusive caps, and the proper instruction and monitoring of patients in their use, require training. The Family Planning Association and other bodies make such training available for doctors, and no practitioner should undertake the provision of these methods unless properly accredited.

The vaginal diaphragm cannot be used unless the pelvic musculature is intact. Lax vaginal walls, or some degree of prolapse, is a contraindication to its use. When the musculature is poor the cervical cap may be used, provided there is a good cervix. If the cervix is small and flat, the vault cap should be used, and if the cervix is very elongated, the 'vimule'.

Failure rates as low as four pregnancies per 100 woman-years have been reported with the condom.[3] Failure rates for combined vaginal occlusive methods with spermicides are reported averaging some 12 pregnancies per 100 woman-years.[1]

Health hazards are few with these methods. Rarely, there is a skin sensitivity either to rubber or to one of the spermicidal preparations. On the positive side, there is some evidence that the use of the diaphragm offers some protection from the risk of preinvasive carcinoma of the cervix. Wearing a condom reduces the chance that the man will acquire gonorrhoea from his partner,[4] or will infect her. It also reduces the transmission of HIV.

Oral contraceptives

The pill has proved to be the most effective form of contraception and because it involves no physical interference with intercourse and imposes no sanctions on when intercourse may take place it has proved to be acceptable to many women. At least 50 million women in the world now use the Pill and in Britain the number is 2.5 million. Because of the growing evidence of contraindications to taking the Pill, and the many side effects, manufacturers have produced a wide range of oral contraceptives, each designed to reduce either risks or side effects. There are three sorts of combined preparations: single level, biphasic and triphasic. There is also a progestogen-only pill. The combined pill is normally taken for twenty-one days followed by seven tablet-free days, when a withdrawal bleed takes place. There is evidence of much confusion among patients, and a consequent lack of compliance. A recent study in two general practices[5] has shown that 27% of the women receiving prescriptions for contraceptives fail to take their pill reliably. It was thought that the confusion arose with the starting day of the course and with the tablet-free week. Some manufacturers have now produced an every day (ED) package which, by inserting seven placebo tablets, allows the patient to take continuous medication. The failure rate for all combined contraceptives is 0.5 pregnancies per 100 woman-years.

The progestogen-only pill, sometimes called the mini-pill, is taken continuously and, unlike the combined pill, can be used during lactation. It has an increased incidence of amenorrhoea and irregular periods. The failure rate is estimated at 2–2.5 pregnancies per 100 woman-years — approximately the same as that for the IUCD.

The major adverse effects which are now well established refer to the cardio-vascular system: deep venous thrombosis and pulmonary embolism; hypertension and stroke, and acute myocardial infarction.[6] Vessey[4] estimated that 100,000 pill users when compared with 100,000 women using either the diaphragm or IUCD would experience an excess of about 35 hospital admissions for stroke, 70 for venous thrombosis and embolism and 10 for acute myocardial infarction. The possibility of these events occurring increases when other risk factors are present: smoking, increased age, obesity, diabetes mellitus and hypertension. These figures refer to the combined pill and those with over 50 micrograms or more of oestrogen.

There is increasing evidence to show that the Pill also affects lipid metabolism. Progestogens are known to alter cholesterol metabolism and alter the plasma levels of high- and low-density lipoproteins. As there is a strong association between lowered HDL-C and raised LDL-C levels and arterial disease this is causing some concern.[7] Some of the triphasic formulations may have the opposite effect and increase HDL-C.[8]

Risks are reduced with lower dosage so that it is now current practice to prescribe 30-microgramme pills. The use of biphasic or triphasic pills allows the dose to be lowered more in the early part of the cycle while still inhibiting ovulation in the later part of the cycle and also minimising breakthrough bleeding. These pills are effective, but are critically dependent on good compliance in order that the correct strength of medication is taken at the correct time.

Minor side-effects are also extensively reported. These include nausea and vomiting, although this may be short lived. Breakthrough bleeding may occur when the dose is too low. There may be weight gain, leg cramps, exacerbation of migraine, persistent amenorrhoea or depression. On the positive side women on the pill achieve a regular cycle, a decrease in blood loss, less dysmenorrhoea and premenstrual symptoms and an improvement in acne. It seems unlikely that the pill is associated with an increase in risk from either breast cancer or carcinoma of the cervix;[7] however there is substantial evidence that oral contraceptives reduce the risk from ovarian and endometrial carcinoma to about half that of non-users.[9,10,11]

Oral contraception is contraindicated in any woman suffering from a hormone-dependent carcinoma. A history of liver dysfunction is also a contraindication. Care must be taken with concomitant medication: drugs such as anticonvulsants, barbiturates, chloramphenicol, chlordiazepoxide, chlorpromazine, meprobamate, rifampicin and sulphamethoxypyridazine can affect the rate of hepatocellular metabolism. Patients on these drugs should be advised to take a higher dose of oral contraceptive therapy.

Antibiotics such as ampicillin can alter the absorption of the oral contraceptive from the bowel. If patients on the Pill require a course of broad spectrum antibiotics it is recommended by the manufacturers that they should use barrier methods of contraception in conjunction with the oral contraceptive.

High blood pressure and diabetes mellitus are now thought to be contraindications to the use of oral contraceptives. It would seem reasonable to allow women who have no risk factors to remain on the combined pill up to the age of 45 years.

Women who smoke or who have other risk factors should be advised to stop the combined oral contraceptive pill at the age of 35 years. Although the progestogen-only pill has not been linked to thromboembolic disease, it would seem prudent to avoid these preparations also in high-risk groups.

Women who wear contact lenses may be warned that in a small minority of cases changes in the curvature of the eye, local oedema or changes in viscosity, may render the wearing of these lenses unbearable.

Following confinement, if a woman is not breast feeding, oral contraception may be initiated at the six-week post natal examination, or sooner. There is no need to await the reappearance of menstruation. When breast feeding is continuing, the use of the progestogen-only pill is an acceptable method of contraception for the patient who is reluctant to use occlusive methods, and who wishes to avoid the risk of inhibiting lactation.

Oral contraception should be withdrawn if the patient gives a history of calf pain, unexplained chest pain, severe headache or transient paralysis. Whenever possible oral contraception should be withdrawn at least three months before planned surgery.

Injectable contraceptives

These products date back to the early 1960s. The two best-known progestogens used are depot medroxyprogesterone acetate (DMPA) and norethisterone oenathate (NET EN).

DMPA is currently available for long-term use in more than 80 countries and in 1984 it was finally approved for use in the UK for selected women after full counselling. Only about 1 per cent of women practising birth control in the UK currently use this method. It is available in aqueous microcrystalline suspension and is normally given in a dose of 150 mg every twelve weeks.

The overall failure rate of these two products is 0–1 pregnancies per 100 woman-years. The failure rate is marginally higher in women who are underweight. The major advantage of this method is that compliance is assured on the basis of each injection.

There are, however, a number of disadvantages. The injected drugs cannot be withdrawn if side-effects occur. There may also be a wide variety of disturbances of menstruation both between patients and in the same woman over a period of time. There may also be delays in the return of fertility, there may be weight gain, galactorrhoea, mild androgenic effects such as acne and the other minor side-effects already described with hormone contraceptives.

There appears to be no effect on blood coagulation, on carbohydrate metabolism or on liver function. Similarly, there appear to be no data to link their use with cancer of the breast, endometrium or cervix, nor has any link been established with raised blood pressure, myocardial infarction or stroke.

Overall it would seem that injectable progestogens provide a very effective and safe contraceptive method. The only significant disadvantage is that of irregular bleeding. However, in the United States the FDA has so far refused to grant DMPA a licence, and this may limit the widespread use of these products in developed countries.

Post-coital contraception

This method of contraception has been used for thousands of years. Vigorous douching and the insertion of chemical agents into the vagina were widely advocated, as was physical exertion such as sneezing and jumping about!

The currently accepted methods are less spectacular. If the patient presents within seventy-two hours of unprotected intercourse she can immediately be given two tablets each containing 250 micrograms of levonorgestrel with 50 micrograms of ethinyloestradiol (Eugynon 50 or Ovran), followed by two more tablets twelve hours later. Other dose regimes have been tried but as the side-effect of nausea is common the lowest dose possible seems to be desirable. The failure rate of this method varies enormously depending on the likely fertility at the time of intercourse.

If the patient presents more than 72 hours after intercourse but before five days from the most probable date of ovulation, a copper-bearing intrauterine device can be inserted. This method works by preventing implantation and the failure rate is very low indeed (2 per 100 woman-years). It is important to bear in mind that some patients may find totally unacceptable any method of contraception which acts after fertilization as it may be seen as no different from induced abortion. Lastly, post-coital UCD is an unsuitable method for a woman who has had a previous ectopic pregnancy.

Intrauterine contraceptive devices

A variety of intrauterine devices are available. For older women and those who cannot or choose not to take the contraceptive pill, the IUCD offers a useful and effective form of contraception. It is estimated that 60 million IUCDs are in use worldwide and about 4 per cent of women in Britain are using them. The failure rate is 0.3–6 per 100 woman-years. This decreases with the length of time the device is *in situ*. The failure rate also depends on the skill of the person who inserts the device. At present there are three marketed varieties of IUCD: inert, copper-bearing and hormone releasing.

The main mode of action is by blocking implantation. The copper and inert devices lead to elevated levels of prostaglandins and the copper enhances the foreign body reaction causing a variety of changes in the endometrium. The progestogen-releasing IUCDs alter endometrial cells and also reduce sperm penetrability.

Side effects of bleeding and pain are related to the size of the surface area of the inert device. Smaller devices, however, are associated with larger failure rates. The use of copper devices has increased in recent years, in preference to inert devices. The extra contraceptive action of the copper permits smaller devices to be used effectively. Copper devices currently available are: Multiload; Ortho Gyn T; Novagard and Nova T.

The IUCD has a number of major disadvantages. There is an increased risk of extrauterine pregnancy or risk of miscarriage if the device fails and the patient becomes pregnant. The device may cause pelvic infection and resulting infertility. There is an increase in menstrual blood loss with consequent cramps and iron deficiency anaemia which is worse with malposition of the device. Also the threads can be lost making removal difficult. During insertion there is a small risk of perforation of the uterus, although this is minimized with adequate training.

Contraindications to the use of IUCDs include a history of previous ectopic pregnancy, past history of tubal surgery, distorted uterine cavity or one sounding to less than 5.5 cm depth, and known true allergy to a constituent. Less clear-cut contraindications are nulliparity, previous pelvic infection, fibroids, endometriosis and suspected subfertility.

Inert IUCDs can be left *in situ* for as long as necessary. Replacement is only indicated when the woman wishes a pregnancy, or in the presence of side-effects. The device should be removed one year after menopause. The copper devices have an officially approved duration of three years except Novagard which has a silver cored copper wire and can be left for five years.

The standard copper wire devices begin to lose copper at an accelerated rate from about twenty-seven months onwards. After four years, 28 per cent of removed IUCDs show fragmentation of the wire. This does not happen with the silver cored wire.

It would appear that some 15 per cent of women who choose an IUCD change their method within the first year.

History, examination and follow-up

As already noted, consultations about contraception are anything but 'routine'. They provide opportunity to establish or further a therapeutic relationship with the patient. All the elements of clinical problem-solving (Chapter 1.2) and counselling (Chapter 3.2) must be brought into play. The opportunity exists to detect early signs of disease, early signs of emotional disturbance, and to monitor the development of unwanted consequences of the help being given.

No matter which method is contemplated, mechanical occlusion, the Pill or an IUCD, the history should include a search for all those conditions which might be contraindications to any of the three methods. Since a high proportion of women change their method over the course of time, a comprehensive data base is essential. The physical examination should always include an examination of the breasts and urine and a recording of the blood pressure.

An examination of the pelvis or, on the rare occasions when the patient is a man, of the penis, is important for a number of reasons. Perhaps the least important is the search for disease and deformity. So far as the Pill is concerned, there are few contraindications apart from carcinoma that would be found on pelvic examination. The presence of vaginal candidiasis is an indication for treatment, not the withholding of the Pill. An estimate of uterine size, position and mobility, as well as the state of the cervix is essential prior to the fitting of an IUCD. The state of the pelvic musculature and the state of the cervix are similarly important in the placing of a diaphragm or cap.

Of no less importance is the patient's physical and emotional response to the examination itself. Women may show a timidity and fear about this examination; they may exhibit adductor spasm or vaginismus, or an anaesthetic indifference to the procedure. Each reaction gives a clue to the possibility of a problem in the patient's sexual life and gives an opportunity to broach the subject, however delicately. Readers would do well to read the literature on this aspect of contraceptive care.[12,13,14]

It is important not to confuse the relationship between the taking of a smear for cervical cytology, and contraceptive care. There is no proof of increased risk of carcinoma of the cervix from taking oral contraceptives. Accordingly after one or two negative reports, cervical cytology need be repeated only every three years, whatever the frequency of Pill 'check-ups'.

Follow-up and monitoring depend on the method used.

Women using the diaphragm or cap, after the initial period of patient training, should be seen at three months, six months after this, and then every year. This presupposes that they can be adequately trained to detect any damage to their device, particularly the vaginal diaphragm. Individual women who are highly motivated and intelligent may need to be seen less often than yearly, once a satisfactory fit and regime have been achieved. Women are always instructed to insert the diaphragm or cap before the consultation, so that the doctor can check correct position and fit.

Patients taking the Pill should initially be seen three months after the first prescription. Instructions will have been given to the patient to return if untoward symptoms are experienced.

When the patient commences tablets on the fifth day of the period, she should be warned that adequate contraceptive cover cannot always be guaranteed during the first cycle, and that some other method of contraception, for example the sheath, should be used additionally during this time. This is not necessary if the woman starts taking tablets on the first day of her next period. Once the Pill regime has been established, there is probably no need to see the patient more often than once a year, when, in addition to checking for any symptoms that may be developing, the blood pressure should be checked and the urine tested for sugar. It is always important to take the opportunity to palpate the breasts, but in the absence of menstrual or vaginal symptoms, it is probably not necessary to repeat the pelvic examination more often than once in every three years, when a cervical smear should be taken.

The IUCD is normally inserted three or four days after the onset of menstruation. There is some evidence that failure rates are higher in the first two or three months following insertion, although few doctors recommend additional use of the sheath during this time. The patient should be taught to check the presence in the vagina of the nylon thread which is attached to the IUCD, and may be warned that some irregular bleeding may take place. Many women experience some lower abdominal cramp and backache during the first day or two after insertion, but these should be controlled by simple analgesics. The patient should be seen six weeks after the first insertion, and annually thereafter, when a pelvic examination should always be carried out.

Sterilization

Sterilization, whether by vasectomy or by ligation of the Fallopian tubes, should always be regarded as a final and irreversible procedure. Because the operation on the man is much simpler, cheaper and less hazardous than interruption of the Fallopian tubes, vasectomy is being increasingly sought by couples who feel that under no circumstances will they want a subsequent pregnancy. The difficulty of making such a judgment constitutes one contraindication to the method. There are few physical consequences, but the procedure carries with it potential psychological hazards. It is difficult to predict what part a man's fertility plays in the way in which he sees his own sexuality. There is no physical reason why a loss of fertility should affect potency, or libido, but it may. Because of the rich investment of anxiety in human sexuality, referred to earlier in this chapter, and because of the close association between sexuality and fertility, there is a minority of men in whom the operation may be psychologically damaging. It is therefore of paramount importance when considering sterilization either of the man or the woman, that the patient's consent is both informed and freely given and that the partner's consent should be considered too.

The doctor

This chapter has made much of the patient's needs, feelings and beliefs. Some practitioners, because of their own moral or religious persuasion, are unhappy about the use and consequences of contraceptive techniques. Just as the doctor has no right to impose his own religious or political beliefs on his patient, so the patient has no right to demand a service from his doctor which his doctor's conscience forbids. Perhaps the majority of patients are aware of their own doctors' beliefs and practices. But patients may well be helped if doctors with conscientious objections display a notice in his waiting-rooms, for example, 'Your doctor is willing to discuss family planning with you, but does not prescribe the Pill or other contraceptive devices. Should you require this sort of help the address and times of Family Planning Clinics in the neighbourhood is appended.'

Finally, the general practitioner should be neither surprised nor dismayed that some of his younger patients seek advice on contraception from Family Planning Clinics and similar organizations. The limitations, crises of confidentiality and conflict of interest implicit in the notion of family doctoring, often make it easier for a young person to approach a strange doctor who will know in advance the nature of the problem that the patient is bringing.

References

[1] Marshall, J. (1977): *Family Planning by the Mucothermic Method*. Portsmouth: Eyre & Spottiswoode.

[2] *Biology of Fertility Control by Periodic Abstinence* (1967): Report of a W.H.O. Scientific Group. W.H.O. Technical Report Series Number 360.

[3] Peel, J. (1972): The Hull Family Survey II. *Journal of Biosocial Science*, *4*, 333.

[4] Vessey, M.P. (1978): Contraceptive methods: risks and benefits. *British Medical Journal*, *2*, 721.

[5] Finlay, I.G., Scott, M.G.B. (1986): Patterns of contraceptive pill-taking in an inner city practice. *British Medical Journal*, *293*, 601–602.

[6] Royal College of General Practitioners (1974): *Oral Contraception and Health*. Tunbridge Wells: Pitman Medical.

[7] Kay, C.R. (1984): The Royal College of General Practitioners' oral contraception study. *Obstet. Gynaecol*: *11*, 759.

[8] Bergink, E.W., Borglin, N.E., Klottrup, P. and Liukko, P. (1982): Effects of desogestrel and levonorgestrel in low-dose oestrogen oral contraceptives on serum lipoproteins. *Contraception*, *25*: 477.

[9] The Centers for Disease Control Cancer and Steroid Hormone Study (1983): Long term oral contraceptive use and the risk of breast cancer. *Journal of the American Medical Association*, *249*: 1591.

[10] The Centers for Disease Control Cancer and Steroid Hormone Study (1983): Oral contraceptive use and the risk of ovarian cancer. *Journal of the American Medical Association*, *249*: 1596.

[11] The Centers for Disease Control Cancer and Steroid Hormone Study (1983): Oral contraceptive use and the risk of endometrial cancer. *Journal of the American Medical Association*, *249*: 1600.

[12] Tunnadine, L.P. (1970): *Contraception and Sexual Life*. London: Tavistock Publications.

[13] Friedman, L.J. (1962): *Virgin Wives*. London: Tavistock Publications.

[14] Courtenay, M. (1969): *Sexual Discord in Marriage*. London: Tavistock Publications.

3.78 The patient who seeks help about hereditary diseases

Pauline and Brian McAvoy

At the beginning of the twentieth century hereditary diseases were relatively unimportant causes of ill health. Since then, however, there have been major advances in environmental conditions, nutrition, control of infectious diseases and therapeutics, resulting in a dramatic reduction in infant deaths. Consequently genetic diseases have assumed a greater importance in present day mortality and morbidity statistics.

Accurate figures for the overall incidence of genetic diseases are difficult to obtain. However, it has been calculated that about one in 20 paediatric admissions and one in ten childhood deaths in hospital can be attributed entirely to genetic disorders.[1] Clearly, hereditary diseases make a major contribution towards present day morbidity and mortality, particularly in children.

Types of hereditary diseases

Hereditary diseases can be divided into three main groups:

1. Chromosome disorders.
2. Single gene (unifactorial) disorders.
3. Polygenic (multifactorial) disorders.

1. *Chromosome disorders*

Here there is a demonstrable abnormality in number or structure of the chromosomes. These disorders can be classified according to whether the autosomal or sex chromosomes are affected (Table I). Recent studies have shown that approximately one in 200 newborn infants has a significant chromosomal aberration.[2]

In general, chromosome disorders occur sporadically, and thus the risk of recurrence in other family members is low. With the exception of Turner's syndrome, the older the mother the greater the risk of her child having a disorder of chromosome numbers.

By far the commonest autosomal chromosome defect is Down's syndrome which affects one in 700 live births. Ninety-five per cent of cases have an extra chromosome 21 — trisomy, the frequency of this increasing markedly when mothers are over the age of 35. Four per cent have a translocation chromosome and this is associated with a considerably higher risk of recurrence within the family. One per cent are mosaics who possess both normal and trisomic cell lines.

1. *Chromosome disorders*
   - (a) Autosomes
     - (i) Down's syndrome (trisomy 21)
     - (ii) Edward's syndrome (trisomy 18)
     - (iii) Patau's syndrome (trisomy 13)
     - (iv) Cri du chat syndrome (deletion of short arm of chromosome 5)
   - (b) Sex chromosomes
     - (i) Turner's syndrome (XO)
     - (ii) Klinefelter's syndrome (XXY and variants)
     - (iii) XYY male
     - (iv) Triple X female (XXX)
2. *Single gene (unifactorial) disorders*
   - (a) Autosomal dominant
     - (i) Achondroplasia
     - (ii) Huntington's chorea
     - (iii) Marfan's syndrome
     - (iv) Osteogenesis imperfecta
     - (v) Polycystic kidney disease
     - (vi) Polyposis coli
   - (b) Autosomal recessive
     - (i) Albinism
     - (ii) Cystic fibrosis
     - (iii) Friedreich's ataxia
     - (iv) Hurler's syndrome
     - (v) Phenylketonuria
     - (vi) Sickle-cell anaemia
   - (c) X-linked recessive
     - (i) Duchenne muscular dystrophy
     - (ii) Haemophilia
     - (iii) G-6PD deficiency
     - (iv) Partial colour blindness
   - (d) X-linked dominant
     - (i) Vitamin D-resistant rickets
3. *Polygenic (multifactorial) disorders*
   - (i) Atopy
   - (ii) Cancer
   - (iii) Cleft lip ± palate
   - (iv) Congenital dislocation of the hip
   - (v) Diabetes mellitus
   - (vi) Epilepsy
   - (vii) Hypertension
   - (viii) Ischaemic heart disease
   - (ix) Schizophrenia
   - (x) Spina bifida

Table I. Types of hereditary diseases

The next most common chromosome disorders after mongolism are trisomy 13 (Patau's syndrome) and trisomy 18 (Edward's syndrome), which affect approximately one in 14,000 live births. Structural abnormalities of autosomal chromosomes affect one in 500 live births, but rarely cause significant clinical abnormalities. One in 500 live births involves a sex chromosome abnormality, the majority of which affect number rather than structure. The commonest of these disorders are the triple X syndrome (one in 800 live born females), the XYY syndrome (one in 800 live born males), Klinefelter's syndrome (XXY, one in 900 live born males) and Turner's syndrome (XO, one in 2,500 live born females).

2. *Single gene (unifactorial) disorders*

Since these disorders are due to a single mutant gene, the laws of Mendelian inheritance can be used to predict the likelihood of recurrence in a family.

Unifactorial disorders include autosomal and X linked traits, and can be dominant or recessive (Table I).

Autosomal dominant traits are expressed when only one mutant gene is present. Therefore they are transmitted directly from affected parent to affected child, the ratio of normal to affected offspring being one to one with no sex differences. In practice, however, genetic counselling for autosomal dominant traits is complicated by the varying severity of the clinical condition in individuals (variable expressivity). An affected individual may show only minimal manifestations of the full syndrome but 100 per cent of his offspring are at risk of inheriting the trait, and for each the risk is 1 in 2. Consequently, before giving genetic counselling it is vitally important to examine carefully the parents of affected individuals.

Autosomal recessive traits are expressed when a mutant gene is present in a double dose. They are not transmitted directly from generation to generation but occur when two healthy parents who carry the single gene (heterozygotes) produce a child who possesses both genes (homozygote). Males and females are affected equally and the chances of their future offspring being similarly affected are one in four.

Due to common ancestry, autosomal recessive disorders occur more frequently in the children of consanguineous marriages. In first cousin marriages, the risk of development of such a disorder is twice that of the normal population.

X linked recessive disorders affect only men but are passed on by healthy female carriers. Half the male offspring of such a woman will be affected, and half her female offspring will be carriers like herself.

Much rarer are X linked dominant disorders. Here both males and females can be affected, heterozygous females usually less severely than males. All the sons of an affected male are normal, whereas all the daughters are affected. Half of the sons and half of the daughters of an affected female will inherit the disorder themselves.

3. Polygenic (multifactorial) disorders

Both genetic and environmental factors are thought to play a part in the aetiology of these disorders which include many of the common diseases and congenital malformations (Table I). The polygenic nature of these disorders makes it impossible to apply Mendelian principles to predict the pattern of inheritance. Instead empiric risks of recurrence derived from large family studies must be used. In general, this figure is in the region of 2 to 5 per cent.

In practice it is with this last group of genetic disorders that the family doctor will find himself most involved, since chromosome and single gene disorders are relatively rare, and are generally diagnosed at birth in hospital. Consequently, individual multifactorial disorders will be discussed in detail later in this chapter.

How the problems of hereditary diseases present in practice

In practice most general practitioners will encounter problems of hereditary diseases in relation to certain events in the life of an individual or a family; these may be considered under the following headings:

1. Premarriage.
2. Miscarriages and stillbirths.
3. Birth of an abnormal child.
4. Recognition of a disease in an individual or another family member.

1. *Premarriage*

In the United Kingdom first cousins are permitted to marry, and a general practitioner may be consulted regarding the advisability of this. It is important to establish whether there is any family history of an autosomal recessive disorder since, for a child to be affected, both parents must be carriers of the abnormal gene. Normally this would be a rare occurrence but consanguineous individuals are at risk of having inherited the gene from a common ancestor. In short, in first cousin marriages, the risk of the development of an autosomal recessive disorder is twice that of the normal population. If there is no such family history, the couple can be reassured that there is only a small increase in the risk of their producing a child with a congenital malformation or mental retardation.

An individual with an established disease may consult his general practitioner before marriage about the risk of having an affected child. If the disease is one with a clearly recognized genetic basis, advice from a geneticist is probably indicated. Fortunately, such conditions are rare, and it is much more likely that the individual will be suffering from a disease which either has no genetic basis or belongs to the group of multifactorial disorders, e.g. diabetes mellitus or epilepsy. In such cases, if the necessary information is not to hand, a telephone conversation with the local geneticist may be all that is required.

2. Miscarriages and stillbirths

Spontaneous abortion is estimated to occur in 12 to 15 per cent of all pregnancies.[3]

Many women ask why the miscarriage occurred and if there was anything wrong with the baby. It is rarely possible to give an answer for an individual miscarriage, but various studies have shown that 50 per cent of spontaneous abortions have a gross chromosomal abnormality. The earlier the abortion, the greater the incidence of chromosome abnormalities. The knowledge that this was 'nature's way of correcting a mistake' can be very reassuring and allay fears that the miscarriage resulted from a perceived personal misdemeanour, e.g. over exertion or sexual intercourse.

A couple who have had recurrent miscarriages may ask if this has been due to some genetic defect in themselves. Surprisingly, in only a very few cases, probably less than 3 per cent, is there evidence of a gross transmissible chromosomal defect.[4]

Chromosome abnormalities are found in about eight per 1,000 stillbirths and abóut six per 1,000 neonatal deaths.[5] Since both these events usually occur in hospital, discovery of such a disorder generally results in direct referral for genetic counselling.

3. *The birth of an abnormal child*

This event will often give rise to the question 'Will it happen again?' Referral to a geneticist may have been initiated by the attending paediatrician or obstetrician, particularly if the child has a clearly recognizable genetic disorder or multiple congenital abnormalities. However, many congenital anomalies have a multifactorial basis, and in this situation figures are available for the empirical risk of recurrence. In general terms, for the common congenital defects there is a 2 to 5 per cent risk of recurrence when both parents are normal and have had one affected child. More precise figures are available for specific conditions (Table II).

Congenital anomaly	Frequency per 1,000 total births	Percentage risk of recurrence in future child
Spina bifida	2.5	4—5
Anencephaly	2.0	4—5
Congenital heart disease	6.0	2—4
Pyloric stenosis — male index	5.0	2
— female index	1.0	10
Cleft lip ± cleft palate	1.0	4
Club foot	1.0	3
Congenital dislocation of hip (late diagnosis)	1.0	4

Table II. Empiric risks of recurrence for some common congenital anomalies

4. *Recognition of disease in an individual or another family member*

It is well recognized among the medical profession and the lay population that many common diseases have a familial tendency. The main difficulty posed by the so-called multifactorial conditions is that the risk of recurrence within the family cannot be predicted as readily as with the single gene disorders. Instead, statistical risks based on large family studies must be given.

When such a condition arises or is recognized within a family, the general practitioner may be approached by the affected individual or a relative wanting to know if the condition can be 'passed on' or if he or she is likely to develop it.

Numerous conditions have a familial tendency, but here we will mention only those which the general practitioner most frequently encounters, or which, because of their prognosis, can cause particular concern to the individual.

Atopy. The incidence in the general population is 10 per cent. If one member of the family is atopic the risk of recurrence is in the order of 20 to 30 per cent.

Cancer. Certain types of cancer have an increased incidence in families, e.g. breast and stomach. The occurrence of different types of cancer within a family does not significantly increase the individual's risk of developing the disease. However, if only one type of cancer, e.g. breast or stomach, appears in the family the individual is at greater risk than the general population; studies have shown this risk to be in the order of five to 15 times that in the population as a whole. Knowledge of this may encourage women to be more conscientious with regard to periodic breast examination, and prompt seeking of medical advice.

Cancer accounts for one in five deaths in this country. This is an important figure to bear in mind when advising individuals who are concerned about the number of relatives who have died of cancer.

Coronary artery disease. There is a well recognized increased familial tendency to coronary artery disease, but the respective contributions of genetic and environmental factors are disputed. Cigarette smoking, blood pressure and serum cholesterol levels are powerful predictors of coronary artery disease and tend to be familial, but whether they outweigh a genetic predisposition is uncertain.
First degree relatives of an affected individual are six times more likely to develop coronary artery disease than the average population.
Most varieties of hypercholesterolaemia are polygenic but about one in 500 of the population has a familial hypercholesterolaemia which is inherited as an autosomal dominant. Coronary artery disease affects 40 per cent of these males and 20 per cent of these females before the age of 40, almost a quarter of the males dying from this before they reach 50.[6]

Diabetes mellitus. Diabetes mellitus affects 1 per cent of the population. The younger the individual is when he or she develops diabetes the greater is the risk of close relatives becoming affected. As with the general population such risk increases with the age of the individual relative. A table of probable ranges of empiric risks in relatives which makes it possible to advise an individual has been compiled by Darlow.[7] For example, a 45-year-old individual, one of whose parents developed diabetes when aged 30, has a 2 to 3 per cent chance of being affected (population risk equals 0.5 to 0.9 per cent). If both parents were affected at the same age, this risk increases two to four fold.

Epilepsy. 0.5 per cent of the population suffers from idiopathic epilepsy. With one affected parent the risk of epilepsy developing in offspring is 5 per cent. If both parents are affected this risk increases to 10 per cent.

Hypertension. It is well recognized that blood pressure tends to be higher in first degree relatives of hypertensive patients than in the general population. However, as with coronary artery disease and migraine it is difficult to assess the respective contributions of genetic and environmental factors to the increased familial tendency.

Migraine. 5 to 10 per cent of the population are affected by migraine at some time in their lives, with a 60 to 70 per cent predominance in females. The well-recognized familial tendency results again from shared genetic and environmental factors within families. Risks to first degree relatives are probably of the order of 10 per cent.

Multiple sclerosis. Although this condition affects only about one in 1,200 of the population, it can be a devastating disease. Studies have shown a ten to 30 fold increased risk in a family which already has one affected member. The recurrence risk in first degree relatives is 1 per cent.

Rheumatoid arthritis. This affects 3 per cent of women and 1 per cent of men. The risk of recurrence in first degree relatives is increased one and a half to five fold, the higher figure applying if the affected family member is male.

Mental illness
(a) *Schizophrenia.* 1 per cent of the population suffers from schizophrenia and it is generally agreed that there is a genetic component in its aetiology. If one parent is affected the risk of recurrence in offspring is 10 per cent. If both parents are affected this risk increases to 40 per cent.
(b) *Affective psychosis.* The risk of recurrence of manic-depressive psychosis in first degree relatives is 10 per cent or more. With depression alone the risks are less, probably somewhere in the region of 5 per cent.

Screening

Screening techniques for genetic disorders are now being used in the following areas:
1. Prenatal diagnosis.
2. Neonatal diagnosis.
3. Carrier detection.

1. Prenatal diagnosis

There is no point in undertaking prenatal diagnosis unless the parents are already prepared to consider the possibility of termination. Four groups of disorders can be detected at a sufficiently early stage of pregnancy to allow termination if the parents so wish:
(a) Chromosome disorders.
(b) Open neural-tube defects.
(c) Certain inborn errors of metabolism.
(d) X linked recessive disorders.

(a) *Chromosome disorders*. The commonest condition in this group is Down's syndrome (trisomy 21), which affects one in 700 live births. However, the frequency of mongolism is closely related to maternal age, e.g. one in 2,300 under the age of 20 and one in 40 over the age of 45.
Amniocentesis makes foetal chromosome analysis possible, and many centres now offer this service to mothers aged over 38 and to those who have previously had an affected child. This procedure is generally performed around 16 weeks' gestation, and in skilled hands carries an increased risk of foetal loss of only 1 per cent.
Other chromosomal disorders detectable by amniocentesis include Patau's syndrome (trisomy 13), Edward's syndrome (trisomy 18), Klinefelter's syndrome (XXY) and triple X syndrome.

(b) *Open neural-tube defects*. Spina bifida occurs in 2.5 per 1,000 total births and anencephaly in 2 per 1,000.
The measurement of maternal serum alpha feto protein at 16 to 17 weeks' gestation is now widely used as a screening procedure for open neural-tube defects. It is estimated that this procedure will detect 80 to 90 per cent of affected foetuses. Mothers whose raised serum alpha feto protein levels are confirmed on repeating the test are offered amniocentesis and termination of the pregnancy if the diagnosis is confirmed. Care must be taken in the interpretation of serum alpha feto protein levels, as the results can be misleading in twin pregnancies, missed and threatened abortion and patients with 'wrong dates'.

(c) *Certain inborn errors of metabolism*. There are over 60 metabolic diseases inherited as autosomal recessives which are detectable by biochemical testing following amniocentesis, e.g. the thalassaemias, sickle-cell anaemia, Gaucher's disease, Hurler's syndrome and Tay-Sachs' disease. Unfortunately, no reliable prenatal tests are yet available for the more common autosomal recessive conditions, e.g. cystic fibrosis and phenylketonuria.

(d) *X linked recessive disorders*. Duchenne muscular dystrophy and haemophilia are the two commonest conditions in this group. Foetal sex determination following amniocentesis offers the carrier mother the opportunity of aborting a male foetus whose chances of being affected are 50 per cent. Recent work shows it is now possible to differentiate affected males from unaffected males.

2. *Neonatal diagnosis*

Detection of certain inherited disorders in the neonatal period allows intervention and can prevent development of particular sequelae. In general, such testing is useful for certain autosomal recessive metabolic disorders, for example phenylketonuria, galactosaemia, amino-aciduria.

The Guthrie test for the detection of phenylketonuria (one in 10,000 live births) is now performed in all neonates between the fifth and fourteenth day of life. A modification of this test can be used to detect several other inborn errors of metabolism.

Certain centres are screening for cystic fibrosis (one in 1,800 live births) by biochemical testing of meconium or faeces in neonates, but although early diagnosis and treatment may improve the life expectancy, more specific tests are needed before mass neonatal screening can be recommended.

Other centres are measuring serum T4 levels on heel stab samples from neonates as a screening procedure for hypothyroidism (one in 3,000 to 4,000 live births).

3. *Carrier detection*

Recent advances have made it possible to detect healthy carriers for several X linked and autosomal recessive disorders, e.g. Duchenne and Becker muscular dystrophy, haemophilia, glucose-6-phosphate dehydrogenase deficiency, ocular albinism, sickle-cell anaemia and Tay-Sachs' disease. Unfortunately, in some of these conditions not all carriers can be detected by the presently available tests. For example, only two-thirds of the carriers of Duchenne muscular dystrophy have an elevated serum creatine kinase. However, combining the biochemical information with the pedigree studies can enable the geneticist to provide a more accurate estimate of the likelihood of an individual being a carrier.

Genetic counselling

The main aim of genetic counselling is to enable couples to make an informed decision on whether or not they should have a child. However, quoting genetic risk figures alone is not sufficient. It is important to take time to discuss prognosis and availability of treatment as it has been shown that parents are often influenced as much by the 'burden' of a disease as they are by the chances of recurrence.[1]

Skinner[8] has suggested that ideally counselling should involve consideration of at least the following points:

(a) Confirmation of the diagnosis.

(b) Discussion of diagnosis and prognosis, including what treatment, if any, is available.
(c) Explanation of recurrence risks in terms understandable to the particular couple.
(d) Discussion of available courses of action — contraception, prenatal diagnosis, termination of pregnancy, adoption.
(e) Helping to dispel feelings of guilt which parents often experience after the birth of a child with a genetic disorder.

Role of the general practitioner

In many straightforward situations, e.g. congenital malformations, in which the diagnosis is clear, many multifactorial disorders and clearly defined unifactorial disorders, the general practitioner is ideally suited to provide genetic counselling. His knowledge of the social, psychological and educational background of families can enable him to tailor the information given him to the individuals concerned. However, specialist advice is often essential. This need not always involve a formal referral of couples to a genetic clinic since the relevant information may be readily obtained by the general practitioner telephoning or writing to the geneticist.

Every Region now has at least one Genetic Centre which usually runs clinics in several towns. Seventy to 80 per cent of the population live within ten miles of such a clinic. The general practitioner also has a role in reinforcing the information given to patients by the geneticist, and, when necessary, clarifying this.

It is difficult to assess the value and effectiveness of genetic counselling but a prospective study (by Emery)[9] of 200 couples with significant genetic problems has shown that the proportion deterred from having children increased with time and over one third of those deterred had been sterilized within two years of counselling.

Conclusion

Genetic factors are an increasingly important cause of present day morbidity and mortality. It is therefore important that the general practitioner has a clear understanding of basic genetic concepts, the scope and methods of screening and his role in genetic counselling. Because he is in the ideal position to develop an extensive understanding of patients' social, psychological, educational and family backgrounds the general practitioner can play a key role in this rapidly expanding field.

References

[1] Emery, A.E.H. (1974): Genetic counselling — or what can we tell parents? *The Practitioner*, *213*, 641

[2] Neilsen, J. (1976): Chromosome examination of newborn children: purpose and ethical aspects. *Humangenetik*, *26*, 215

[3] Bobrow, M. (1978): Chromosomal abnormalities. *Medicine*, Series 3, *2*, 73

[4] Ferguson-Smith, M.A. (1979): Notes on chromosomal abnormalities in obstetrics. *Practical Obstetric Problems*, 6th ed., p. 111. London: Lloyd-Luke

[5] Carter, C.O., Ash, P. and Vennart, J. (1977): The incidence of hereditary disease in man. *Lancet*, *i*, 849

[6] Thompson, G. (1978): Plasma lipoproteins and their disorders. *Medicine*, Series 3, *11*, 562

[7] Darlow, J.M., Smith, C. and Duncan, L.J.P. (1973): A statistical and genetical study of diabetes. *Ann. Hum. Genet.*, *37*, 157

[8] Skinner, R. (1980) Tracing the pedigree pattern of genetic diseases. *Medical News*, *13*, 30

[9] Emery, A.E.H., Raeburn, J.A., Skinner, R., Holloway, S. and Lewis, P. (1979): Prospective study of genetic counselling. *British Medical Journal*, *1*, 1253

3.79
The patient who is worried about sexually transmitted diseases including AIDS

F. M. Hull

The history of sexually transmitted disease in man has been the subject of much speculation and controversy. Perhaps societies reveal themselves to historians, in this matter, much as patients reveal themselves to doctors. There is shame, guilt, blame and denial. Opinion is divided as to whether bony lesions discovered in the remains of early inhabitants of Europe and Africa are those of syphilis, which would suggest that the diseases were endemic in those continents from a very early stage. Other historians have suggested that the disease was imported to Europe by Columbus's sailors returning from the New World.

Wherever it came from there was a European pandemic at the end of the fifteenth century, the spread of disease impelled by the ubiquitous wars of the age. To a greater or lesser extent this pandemic continued throughout the rest of European history. In Peter Schaeffer's play *Amadeus*, one of the characters says '[Mozart] died of syphilis like the rest of us'.

The pattern of STD changed with the discovery of penicillin: the incidence of syphilis declined, except among homosexuals. The invention of the oral contraceptive, on the other hand, increased the incidence of STD. The 'pill' not only removed the thin barrier (first of sheep gut, later of latex) between penis and vagina which had afforded major protection against STD, but it also freed women from the fear of pregnancy. Social scientists have speculated that this may have been partly responsible for the change to what has sometimes been called 'the permissive society'. How far protection against unwanted pregnancy, and the promise of penicillin were responsible for a change in sexual mores, remain matters for speculation. Doctors, no less than patients and societies, can easily become trapped by shame, guilt, blame and denial when they come to deal with this particular category of man's afflictions.

The incidence and clinical picture in sexually transmitted diseases may also have changed because of changing attitudes to forms of sexual behaviour, long practised, but now openly discussed in publications, about a wide variety of genital, oral and anal methods of achieving sexual gratification with either sex. The incidence of sexually transmitted diseases has increased among male homosexuals, but has actually decreased among female homosexuals.[1]

Despite this increase in the incidence of STD, they are, with the exception of monilial and trichomonal vaginitis, relatively rarely presented to the general practitioner. It seems likely that where facilities are accessible, many patients who suspect that they are suffering from these diseases go directly to 'special clinics'. For the general practitioner diagnostic probabilities should therefore be influenced by the age and sexual mores of the community in which he practises. In a recently reported controlled trial and review of the literature[2] it has, for instance, been demonstrated that chlamydia trachomatis is an uncommon cause of dysuria in women in a London general practice, but is a relatively common cause of this symptom presented in special clinics and in a practice of doctors providing care for students in a North American university campus. Lack of adequate research in general practice, combined with the fact that in morbidity studies, STD may be coded under a variety of non-specific rubrics, makes the epidemiology of these diseases in primary care very uncertain.

Coincidentally new diseases have been recognized as being sexually transmitted. With new manifestations of old diseases and many new diseases as well it is hardly surprising that patients often become worried about sexually transmitted disease. Table I clearly shows how STD has increased and that the increase is largely due to infections other than the notifiable trio of syphilis, chancroid and gonorrhoea.

Year	*Syphilis*	*Chancroid*	*Gonorrhoea*	*Others**	*Total* (100%)
1925	26.6%	1.5%	42.7%	38.9%	71,000
1945	12.4%	0.5%	24.6%	62.5%	134,000
1965	2.6%	0.4%	23.1%	74.3%	159,000
1979	1.0%	0.01%	13.1%	85.9%	427,000

* Includes those with no demonstrable infection

Table I. — Reports from venereal disease clinics in England and Wales

Causes

Patients who are worried about STD vary from those whose cause of concern is little more than a guilty conscience to those with florid symptoms. The principal causes of STD are listed in Table II together with details of causative organisms and a guide to frequency of presentation in general practice.

Agent	*Organism*	*Disease*	*Incidence in general practice*
Viruses	Papilloma virus	Condylomata acuminata	
	Pox virus	Molluscum contagiosum	Increasingly common
	Herpes virus	Herpes genitalis	
	(Hepatitis B virus)	(Hepatitis)	
Spirochaetes	*Treponema pallidum*	Syphilis	Rare
Bacteria	*Gonococcus*	Gonorrhoea	Common
	Ducrey's bacillus	Chancroid	Very rare
	Donovania granulomatis	Granuloma inguinale	Exceedingly rare
	Mycoplasma hominis *Haemophilus* (now *Gardnerella*) *vaginalis* *Chlamydia trachomatis*	Non-specific urethritis or vaginitis	Common
	Shigellae salmonellae	Gastrointestinal infection	Unknown
Protozoal	*Trichomonas vaginalis*	Vaginitis and, rarely, male infections	Unknown
	Amoembae *Giardia lamblia*	Gastrointestinal infection	Unknown
Fungi	*Candida albicans*	Thrush	Very common
Parasitic	*Acarus scabie*	Scabies	Common
	Phthirus pubis	Pubic lice (crabs)	

(Organism and disease in brackets occurs particularly in homosexuals)

Table II. — Causative agents

Even in today's society STD causes an emotional reaction in the patient: anger, despair, shame or embarrassment, and it is therefore important to consider the patient's worry about the disease. As in many other aspects of medicine the incidence of anxiety about STD is greater than the incidence of the diseases themselves. There is no category of diseases where it is more important that the nature of the patient's beliefs should be extensively and sensitively explored. Unless this is done reassurance will be uncertain when the disease is not present; compliance (and help with tracing contacts) will be uncertain when the disease is confirmed.

Opportunistic health education is vital. A young person who has plucked up courage to consult his doctor and meets anything less than sympathy and reassurance that all STD is treatable, may fail to consult again when serious disease is contracted later.

There is growing evidence to suggest that the likelihood of developing carcinoma of the cervix may also be linked to sexual behaviour. There is a known higher incidence among patients of low social class, and in urban areas compared with rural ones. The incidence is higher among blacks and Puerto Ricans, and lower among Jews. High parity, early age of first sexual intercourse and a large number of sexual partners are all associated with increased incidence. Because of this the development of cervical carcinoma has been linked to circumcision, smegma, sexually transmitted diseases and semen. Though the trends of (standard cohort) mortality from cervical cancer and of new cases of gonorrhoea over 50 years[3] show remarkable similarity, there is some evidence that the most likely infective aetiological factor is the herpes genitalis virus, which is associated with tumour formation elsewhere in the body. At first, circumcision was thought to account for the low Jewish incidence, but the hygiene dictated by religious practice is now thought to be a more likely factor. Smegma is no longer thought to be carcinogenic to the cervix, but the possibility that protein breakdown products from sperm may induce malignant change in cervical cells at a particular stage of cell division may explain the relationship between some patterns of intercourse and the disease. Perhaps cervical cancer too will one day come to be viewed largely as a sexually transmitted disease.

Presentation

STD may be totally asymptomatic, or may present with life threatening symptoms. Perhaps the commonest presentation is of anxiety about STD in the embarrassed youngster worried about the consequences of early sexual contact. Here the task is to investigate seriously the possibility of STD, but also to encourage the confidence of the young person that he will be accepted and cared for, not rejected and punished.

The simplest way of considering the presentation of the many diseases grouped under the rubric STD is to consider them by causative agent. This is shown in Table II. Each disease may produce early, intermediate or late symptoms which may vary with the sexual roles of the patient: male, female or homosexual of either sex.

Presentation of virus STD

Anogenital warts (condylomata acuminata) are increasingly common, they are of long incubation (up to three months) and, on moist areas of vulva, glans or anal margin, produce cauliflower like lesions, though on drier areas they may be more keratotic. In moist areas secondary infection is common, especially when hygiene is poor. These lesions may be confused with syphilitic warts (see below).

The pox virus which produces the characteristic pearly lesion of *molluscum contagiosum* may be transmitted sexually and causes considerable worry when discovered on the skin of the genitals. Fortunately the condition is harmless.

Herpes genitalis, caused by herpes virus II (HV1, which causes the typical cold sore, is usually isolated from lesions above the waist) is a disease currently causing much concern. This is partly due to its association with cervical carcinoma and partly due to the fact that this STD, like syphilis, poses a threat to the developing foetus. The disease may be spread by genital, oro-genital or ano-genital contact. It presents early (within four or five days of contact) with painful vesicles around the anus or genitals. The vesicles may coalesce and become secondarily infected leading to severe vulvitis or balanitis with considerable systemic upset. Recurrence is common, but is usually associated with less generalized illness.

Infective hepatitis, due to hepatitis B virus, is increasingly seen in homosexuals who may also be drug addicts.

Spirochaetal STD: syphilis

Syphilis classically presents with early, intermediate and late (primary, secondary and tertiary) stages. Tertiary syphilis is outside the scope of this chapter. In primary syphilis the typical chancre, or sore, appears in about two to four weeks from exposure: in the male the lesion is often on the penis, but in women it may affect the internal genitalia and so be unnoticed. Oral or anal chancres also occur and the latter are becoming increasingly common because of a marked increase in the incidence of syphilis among homosexuals.

The intermediate symptoms of syphilis are variable and usually appear from six to 24 months after exposure. Commonly there is a generalized rash often associated with multiple genital or mouth lesions.

Bacterial STD

Gonorrhoea is increasingly common: although Table I shows a fall in the proportion of gonorrhoea among causes of STD presenting to special clinics, this is because of a rise in other causes of STD rather than a reduction in incidence of gonorrhoea. Between 1950 and 1976 the number of known cases of gonorrhoea in the UK rose from about 22,000 to 70,000 per annum.

The early symptoms are more marked in males than females. In men there is profuse urethral discharge associated with severe dysuria usually within a day or two of exposure, but sometimes delayed for as long as two weeks. In the female there may be vaginal discharge or dysuria, but frequently women may be asymptomatic. Increasing oro-genital sexual practice has placed the gonococcus in the differential diagnosis of pharyngitis. Gonococcal proctitis may occur in either sex and may be asymptomatic. Especially in men, it may give rise to rectal pain and tenesmus. It should be noted that as many as 10 per cent of men with urethral gonorrhoea have no symptoms at all: the disease only comes to light through contact tracing. These unusual presentations of STD, and the possibility of STD when the patient presents with common symptoms, emphasizes the need to make a diagnosis in the context of the whole clinical and social picture. Later symptoms in the male are dysuria, caused by urethral stricture, and, in women, symptoms relating to ascending genital infection especially salpingitis.

Chancroid and *lymphogranuloma inguinale* are tropical STDs which are rare in general practice. Both produce large tender lymph nodes.

Non-specific urethritis. A series of bacteria are grouped together as causes of non-specific STD which are common causes of non-specific urethritis (NSU) in males and vaginitis in women. Such organisms include *Gardnerella* (formerly *Haemophilus*) *vaginalis*, *Chlamydia trachomatis* and *Mycoplasma hominis*. In males these organisms cause urethritis, usually occurring several days to weeks after exposure, which is associated with a thin glairy discharge. This is quite distinct from the thick yellow pus of gonorrhoea and is usually accompanied by far less dysuria. Untreated the discharge may become chronic, but sometimes disappears spontaneously. In some cases urethral stricture may develop.

In females non-specific infection may be a cause of vaginal discharge or pelvic inflammatory disease which is difficult to identify. In a series of 166 women with cases of pelvic inflammatory disease investigated in Aarhus, Denmark, 55 per cent were caused by *Mycoplasma hominis*, 37 per cent were caused by *Chlamydia trachomatis* and 5 per cent were caused by *Neisseria gonorrhoea*.[4] In Britain it is recognized that *Chlamydia* is the commonest cause of non-specific genital infection.[5]

Other bacterial STD include enteric diseases, shigellosis, salmonellosis and Campylobacter infection due to oro-anal contact among homosexuals.[1]

Reiter's disease. The syndrome comprising purulent urethritis, inflammation of synovial membranes and conjunctivitis called *Reiter's disease* is of unknown aetiology though it has been associated with several infections including gonorrhoea and dysentery; currently it is thought that *Chlamydia* may be the responsible organism. The disease is frequently missed since the triad of urethritis, arthritis and conjunctivitis do not always co-exist.

Protozoal STD

Here the common disease is *trichomoniasis*, whose spread is not only related to sexual activity. In the male this is usually asymptomatic though it may produce balanitis or urethritis. In females there is a typical greenish, frothy discharge (see Chapter 3.59). As with enteric bacterial disease there has been a considerable increase in gut protozoal infections due to giardiasis and amoebiasis in those practising oro-anal sexual contact.[1]

Fungal STD

Thrush, caused by *Candida albicans*, is one of the commonest minor gynaecological conditions seen in general practice (see Chapter 3.59). Candida is often present in asymptomatic women and a sudden change from symbiosis to overt infection may be precipitated by a number of causes including diabetes, drugs and sexual activity. In men Candida rarely causes symptoms though it may give rise (especially in diabetics) to balanitis (see Chapter 3.52). Proctitis caused by Candida may occur in both sexes but is especially common in homosexual males.

Parasitic STD

Close physical contact encourages the spread of many contagious diseases, among which *scabies* (due to *Acarus scabiei*) and *pubic lice*, or crabs, are particularly regarded as STD. Both present with pruritus and a skin rash; with scabies this is generalized and with pubic lice is usually limited to the area covered by pubic hair.

It is important that the presence of any one possible STD should alert the physician's mind to the possibility of all others.

History

History taking is crucial and should be undertaken with due regard to the patient's emotional reaction. Sympathy is vital in order not to alienate the patient since follow-up and contact tracing may be very important.

Because of the varying presentation of the many diseases within the group of STD, many symptoms may be offered. However, the *worry* that the fear of STD generates will often be predominant.

The social standing of the patient is no guide. Precise details of the duration and severity of presenting symptoms must be taken together with the date of exposure if it is known. General questions about the sexual contact should be put at this stage in order to establish whether the contact was casual or with an established partner, within or without marriage and whether it is known if the partner has symptoms. Though later it may be necessary to know the identity of the partner at this stage preserving anonymity is likely to give the patient confidence. Exploring the sexual practice of the individual can be undertaken by questions relating to the frequency of sexual contact, whether sexual contact always leads to intercourse, whether contraception was used and if so what method. Was sexual contact always genital, if not what other contact may there be, such as oro-genital, oro-anal, ano-genital? It is important to ask about the patient's general health to discover any constitutional symptoms which may have been caused by STD or could indicate generalized disease (e.g. diabetes) which may influence the patient's symptoms.

The possibility of pregnancy should be considered and an assessment made of the patient's psychological attitude towards the symptoms. Because there is an association between drugs (including alcohol) and STD the opportunity should be taken to enquire about the possibility of such concurrent problems.

Examination

The patient should be undressed from the waist downwards, further stripping may be needed later, but initially total nudity may only increase what may already be severe embarrassment. The exposed skin should be carefully examined for evidence of the rash of secondary syphilis or of scabies or pediculosis. The conjunctiva should be examined for jaundice or for inflammation which may suggest Reiter's syndrome. The mouth should be carefully examined for evidence of herpes, candida, secondary syphilis or pharyngitis. The presence or absence of swellings, sores or ulcers on the external genitalia should be noted. In men the meatus should be examined for discharge. In women the vulva must be carefully inspected before speculum examination of the vagina and cervix followed by a bimanual pelvic examination to test for pain on moving the cervix, and for adnexal swelling or tenderness which might indicate pelvic inflammatory disease.

The physical signs of the common gynaecological STD are described in Chapter 3.59. Finally, when indicated, rectal examination with proctoscopy should be undertaken in both sexes noting the presence of warts, ulcers, inflammation or discharge.

Investigation

Once any STD is suspected the doctor must be alert to the possibility of any other STD which may co-exist. Investigation depends on virology, cervical cytology, serology, bacteriology and microscopy.

Viral disease

Condylomata acuminata and molluscum contagiosum are diagnosed clinically; the former may be confused with condylomata lata of secondary syphilis, but serology, which should always be undertaken, will reveal this. Herpes simplex virus may be recognizable from standard cervical smears. Serological diagnosis of Herpes simplex II is possible, but there may be confusion because of false positive tests caused by Herpes simplex I. The specimen should be taken from the cervix or from external genital vesicles on cotton wool swabs and sent to the laboratory in Stuart's medium as soon as possible.

Syphilis

When there is clinical evidence of primary syphilis patients should be referred for investigation which involves isolation of the treponemes and dark-ground microscopy. Serological tests for syphilis do not become positive until four to six weeks after the appearance of the primary lesion. There are now many tests available and accurate diagnosis depends on close collaboration between clinician and serologist who needs an accurate history (with each specimen) which should include the clinical state of the patient, the date of exposure if known and whether screening, diagnostic or prognostic tests are required.
Tests are broadly of two sorts: non-specific tests used for screening and those that test for specific anti-treponema antibody. There are now so many tests that reference to a venereological textbook is necessary for details. Table III may help the confused clinician through the welter of abbreviations which exist, and to understand which tests are used as screening and which are specific.

Bacterial disease

The diagnosis of gonorrhoea depends on the isolation of the organism, *Neisseria gonorrhoeae*. Swabs should be taken from the urethra, the pharynx and the rectum in both sexes and from the cervical canal in women (it is important to note that a high vaginal swab is useless since gonorrhoea does not infect the vaginal epithelium). Dry swabs should only be used when they can be

Abbreviation	*Full name*	*Antibody*	*Antigen*	*Principle*
ART (Sc)	Automated Reagin Test	Non-specific (anti-lipoidal)	Cardiolipin coated particles	Flocculation
CWR (Sc)	Cardiolipin Wasserman Reaction	Non-specific (anti-lipoidal)	Cardiolipin	Complement fixation
ELISA (Sp)	Enzyme linked immunosorbent assay	Specific for pathogenic treponemes	Disrupted *T. pallidum*	As column 2
FTA (abs) (Sp)	Absorbed fluorescent treponemal antibody test	Specific for pathogenic treponemes	Dead *T. pallidum*	Immuno-fluoresence
RPCFT (Sp)	Reiter protein complement fixation test	All treponemes	Extract of non-pathogenic treponemes	Complement fixation
RPR (Sc)	Rapid plasma Reagin test	Non-specific (anti-lipoidal)	Cardiolipin coated particles	Flocculation
TPHA (Sp)	*Treponema pallidum* haemagglutination assay	Specific for pathogenic treponemes	Disrupted *T. pallidum* coated in red cells	Haemagglutination
TPI (Sp)	*Treponema pallidum* immobilization test	Specific for pathogenic treponemes	Live *T. pallidum*	Immobilization
VDRL (Sc)	Venereal disease research laboratory test	Non-specific (anti-lipoidal)	Cardiolipin coated particles	Flocculation

Sc = Screening. Sp = Specific

Table III. — Serological tests for syphilis

delivered to the laboratory within half an hour. Otherwise swabs should be transported in Stuart's medium or Transgrow which will allow a delay of up to four days. The organism can be identified in smears of urethral pus quite simply and the author became adept at examining such smears, stained with methylene blue, at sea while serving in the Royal Navy.

The group of organisms including *Gardnerella*, *Chlamydia* and *Mycoplasma* are extremely difficult to culture. Careful investigation of cervicitis may often fail to incriminate possible causative organisms such as *Chlamydia*. Pelvic inflammatory disease caused by *Chlamydia* or *Mycoplasma* and vaginitis caused by *Gardnerella* may also be very difficult to prove. Similarly Reiter's disease is impossible to prove by investigation since there are no specific tests for it. Rare cases of shigellosis or salmonellosis transferred sexually will require faecal culture.

Protozoal disease

The commonest protozoal disease is trichomoniasis which may be diagnosed from cervical smears or from high vaginal swabs. Occasionally the organism may be isolated from male urethral discharge particularly if taken early in the morning before micturition. Rare sexually transmitted protozoal gut infection due to amoebae or *Giardia lamblia* requires stool examination.

Other STD

Candida may be identified from cervical smears and high vaginal swabs or, in the male, from subpreputial swabs by microscopy and culture. Pubic lice can be identified by naked eye or low microscopy which is also used to identify acari extracted from skin burrows.

Management

The guiding principle in the management of sexually transmitted disease is the eradication of disease in all the sexual partners. With promiscuous individuals where there may be many partners of either or both sexes, this presents a major exercise in epidemiological investigation. The eradication of gonorrhoea from a man's urethra is relatively simple, but if this is done without also treating the asymptomatic gonorrhoea of his partners the opportunity to prevent considerable morbidity and even mortality has been missed. It follows that such cases, though quite treatable in general practice, should be referred to the local special clinic where organization exists for contact tracing. However, this places the general practitioner in a dilemma for if he were to refer every case of candidiasis or trichomoniasis to the special clinic he would rapidly overload the clinic and alienate his patients. These two common diseases are often sexually transmitted, but may also be spread in other ways and it is important to recognize that the proven presence of either of these diseases may be an indication of more serious, but covert, STD. It follows that the most important aspect of management is a high index of suspicion and full investigation of *any* case of STD. Once full investigation has been made the general practitioner must make a careful and considered decision as to whether or not the patient should be referred to a special clinic. In making such a decision he will have to review the effect that this is likely to have on the sexual partners within or without marriage and to be prepared for detailed and tactful explanation of his referral.

The management of STD thus falls into two groups: those who require reference to a venereologist for treatment and contact tracing immediately because there is strong ground for a presumptive diagnosis of syphilis and/or gonorrhoea, and those who can safely be treated by the general practitioner after adequate laboratory investigation to exclude syphilis and gonorrhoea. Unfortunately, as in all medicine, there is a grey area between these clear extremes occupied by non-specific urethritis in males and vaginitis.

Candidiasis and trichomoniasis respond to nystatin or drugs of the imidazole group or to metronidazole respectively (see *British National Formulary* or *Treatment* Chapter (B)6.2).[6] Patients are increasingly informed about STD; the advice to husband via his wife that he must undergo treatment because of his wife's vaginal candida or trichomoniasis may cause quite unjustified suspicions and so it is important that full tactful explanation is given to both patients.

Non-specific genital infection is a difficult matter since no obvious cause can be found for the persistence of vaginal discharge or urethral discharge. In addition to the possible causes listed above a common cause of such complaints is abnormal awareness either of normal vaginal discharge or of penile moisture which in some patients can become an obsession. In the presence of persistent observable penile or vaginal discharge with no positive laboratory findings the general practitioner has to decide whether to start treatment empirically. In some cases he, or the patient, may be unhappy to do this without appropriate consultant opinion. In non-specific vaginal discharge (which may be due to vaginitis or cervicitis) metronidazole will eradicate *Gardnerella*, tetracycline is useful in mycoplasma infection and *Chlamydia* will respond to tetracycline or erythromycin. In males non-specific urethritis will often respond to tetracycline.

Finally, problems may occur where a patient refuses the doctor's recommendation of referral to a special clinic. Here the overriding consideration must be that of confidentiality, but although the patient's wishes must be respected, every effort should be made by the doctor to ensure the proper tracing and treatment of contacts.

References

[1] Williams, D.C. (1981): Hepatitis and other sexually transmitted diseases in gay men and lesbians. *Sexually Transmitted Diseases*, *8*, 330–332

[2] Burney, P., Marson, W., Evans, M. and Forsey, T. (1983): *Chlamydia trachomatis* and lower urinary tract symptoms among women in one general practice. *British Medical Journal*, *286*, 1550–52

[3] Beral, V. (1974): Cancer of the cervix: a sexually transmitted infection? *Lancet*, *1*, 1037

[4] Moller, B.R., Mardh, P., Ahrons, S. and Nussler, E. (1981): Infection with *Chlamydia trachomatis*, *Mycoplasma hominis* and *Neisseria gonorrhoea* in patients with pelvic inflammatory disease. *Sexually Transmitted Diseases*, *8*, 198–202

[5] Anonymous (1983): Sexually transmitted disease surveillance (1981). *British Medical Journal*, *286*, 1500–1

[6] Hull, F.M. (1978): Vaginal discharge, in *Treatment*, Chapter (B)6.2. London: Kluwer Medical

Further reading

Barlow, D. (1979): *Sexually Transmitted Disease*. Oxford: University Press

Felman, Y.M. (1980): Homosexual hazards. *Practitioner*, *224*, 1151–1156

Murray, D.P.J. (1980): Asymptomatic gonorrhoea in the male. *Practitioner*, *224*, 1141–1144

Schofield, C.B.S. (1979): *Sexually Transmitted Disease*. Edinburgh and London: Churchill Livingstone

Willcox, R.R. and Willcox, J.R. (1982): *Venereological Medicine*. London: Grant McIntyre

Appendix
Acquired Immune Deficiency Syndrome (AIDS)

Marshall Marinker

In 1981, a number of reports of *Pneumocystis carinii* pneumonia and Kaposi's sarcoma in homosexual men, were reported in the USA. These patients were subsequently found to have a severely impaired cellular immune response, and to succumb to the unchecked development of malignancies and so-called opportunist infections. Since then the disease has assumed epidemic proportions in the USA, where the number of reported cases has doubled each month, and in parts of West Africa. The disease is now achieving epidemic proportions in some parts of the UK population. It remains to be seen whether or not government, the public and the health care professions can learn sufficient from the American experience to modify what could be a devastating effect on our society. The facts suggest that the general practitioner, the primary health care team and the community services will be the key elements in the medical profession's response to this urgent challenge.

The disease is caused by a retrovirus, a group previously thought to have a very low infectivity. This human immunosuppression virus (HIV) has already become widely established among homosexual men, intravenous drug misusers, and haemophiliac patients previously treated with unscreened blood products. Infection appears to be blood borne, and the virus is excreted both in the semen and the saliva. Although homosexual men are at greatest risk, the disease has been shown to spread as a result of heterosexual intercourse with an infected partner of either sex.

The disease appears to be invariably fatal, death ensuing from opportunistic infections and neoplasia, which result from a breakdown of the immune defences. The progress of the disease is variable, the course seems to be about two years, and some 25–50 per cent of those affected develop dementia.

Presentation

The commonest presentation of the disease is a persistent generalized lymphadenopathy (PGL). This lymphadenopathy is thought to be a reaction to the HIV, and it is sometimes preceded by an acute phase marked by fever, muscular pains and headaches, not unlike influenza.

These clinical findings are not uncommon in a variety of infections, and the approach of the general practitioner will be modified by what he knows of the 'at risk' status of the patient. It will also be modified by the patient's own anxieties. At the time of writing there is a widespread health education campaign, designed to raise the awareness of the public about the nature and danger of the disease, and about prevention. The general practitioner is therefore now able to assume that the majority of adult patients are aware of the dangers, and might expect that the doctor's line of enquiry will include questions relevant to the disease.

A minority of patients with generalized lymophadenopathy go on to develop what has been described as the AIDS-related complex (ARC). Here there are symptoms and signs of infections such as fever, night-sweat, loss of weight and oral candidiasis. Not all patients who develop ARC will necessarily have suffered from PGL, and not all patients who progress to AIDS will necessarily have manifested ARC. Because of public awareness, the general practitioner will now increasingly be faced with questions which arise not from a clinical manifestation of the syndrome, but from anxiety, social pressures and the wish to avoid infection, or to avoid the possibility of spreading the disease.

History and examination

The most important task of the history is to elicit the likelihood of risk. The following are the major risk categories: male homosexuals; heterosexuals who believe that they may have had intercourse with an infected person, or with someone in a high risk group; intravenous drug misusers; and persons with a promiscuous sexual lifestyle. Most haemophiliac patients who have been treated in the past with pooled blood products are by now most likely to have been screened for HIV, but this needs to be checked. Despite the public anxiety about AIDS, and the likely effects of explicit health education programmes, it is more than likely that patients will continue to be sensitive about questions concerning their sexual preferences and lifestyle. This is scarcely surprising because of the intensely personal nature of sexual life, and because judgements about sexual preferences, practices and lifestyles, are not only clinical but also moral. The doctor who holds strong views about these matters (however deeply held the moral or religious convictions from which they stem) will be disabled from helping his patient, and is likely to fail in his attempt to prevent the spread of the disease, if he allows himself to express these views in critical or condemnatory terms.

Because of the protean nature of the disease and its presentation, the general practitioner cannot rely on the hypothetico-deductive line of clinical reasoning, which is described in Chapter 1.2, Clinical Problem Solving in General Practice. If the disease is suspected, the general practitioner must carry out a systematic and full history and examination. In particular he should look for a history of feverish illnesses, the appearance of firm swellings in the neck, axillae and groin, loss of energy, marked weight loss, rashes, recurrent or persistent diarrhoea, soreness in the mouth, dysphagia and dyspnoea. Similarly, a full examination should be carried out, with special attention being paid to lymph nodes, the buccal mucosa and the entire skin area, which should be searched for the signs of Kaposi's sarcoma.

Investigations

A positive HIV antibody is strongly indicative. It should be recalled that there is often a three-month lag between infection and the appearance of detectable antibodies, although this is unlikely to be an important factor in the investigation of a patient who presents with either symptoms or signs of the disease. Further investigation includes a full blood count with a differential white count and platelets. A swab from the buccal mucosa should be taken to look for candidiasis.

Management

It would be rash to assume any significant biomedical breakthrough in the management of this syndrome within the next few years. Management of the patient with the established syndrome is similar to that of patients with other diseases who are dying. The problems of terminal care for these patients, however, are likely to be particularly taxing. Most people dying from AIDS will be in a younger age group than those dying of the other major causes of adult mortality. All the other emotional and economic problems associated with death in youth may be exacerbated by personal and family rejection. It is in this context that the reader is referred to Chapter 4.8, Terminal Care and Bereavement.

To date there have been some 600 cases reported in the United Kingdom, and although epidemiological predictions are difficult to make, it has been suggested that by 1992, 145,000 will have contracted the disease in this country. In 1984 there were 59,000 acute medical beds, so there is a distinct possibility that by the early 1990's the number of people dying from AIDS will have swamped the acute hospital services in this country. Diagnosis and management of these cases will rapidly exhaust the resources of genito-urinary clinics and infectious disease units. Increasingly, the diagnosis and management of AIDS patients will become the responsibility of the primary health care team.

The major management tasks in general practice will be concerned with health education and counselling. The problems are not only interpersonal, but demand answers to difficult ethical questions. The following seem to be the most important.

How should the general practitioner respond to the patient who requests to be tested for HIV? It might seem sensible and humane to acquiesce. But should the patient first be asked if he/she understands the consequences of a positive finding? If he/she proves to be HIV positive, this will have the most devastating effect, personally, socially, sexually and financially. Two years ago one in ten HIV positive persons were reputed to develop the full syndrome. Currently the figure is three in ten. The developing epidemiology looks alarming. When a patient makes a request for a test, it is important to ensure that he/she understands the consequences.

A different dilemma is posed by the patient presenting with vague malaise and some lymphadenopathy. The general practitioner in the past has had no difficulty in explaining that he wishes to carry out a blood test to exclude infectious mononucleosis. He would almost certainly make no reference to the fact that he was also looking at other blood components, which would help to exclude the unlikely diagnosis of leukemia. This reticence, in order to avoid anxiety at the margins of possibility, poses few ethical problems. But what of the need now to look for HIV? The issue may be very similar to that posed in the case of the patient asking to be screened.

If the general practitioner cannot test for HIV without explaining the purpose and possible consequences of this search, there is a danger that the doctor may avoid the investigation, delay diagnosis and fail to limit spread. If he does not inform the patient about the true nature of his investigation, is he not guilty of an assault? These problems have been with us for a long time, but AIDS, because of its devastating consequences, illuminates them in a new and urgent way.

AIDS sharpens the debate about confidentiality. Those members of the primary health care team who may be put at risk from taking blood or dressing wounds may have the right to know which patients are HIV positive. If that is the view taken, it may be very difficult to contain that confidentiality within the team. If the records are flagged, the information could soon spread beyond the confines of the practice. If confidence in the doctor's confidentiality is damaged, patients may remain secretive and valuable opportunities to limit the spread of the disease will be lost.

What is the position of the general practitioner whose HIV positive patient refuses to disclose the information to a sexual partner? Imagine the dilemma of such a general practitioner, if the unsuspecting wife of a HIV positive individual announces that she intends to become pregnant. The ethic of confidentiality may here be overtaken by a precedent ethic to avoid the harm which one individual may do to another.

Perhaps the most important task for the general practitioner is to contribute to the health education of his patients. Here again, the doctor will be confronting some of the most personally sensitive and morally difficult aspects of human experience. Promiscuity is a major risk factor. The biological advantages now of keeping to one sexual partner may be stressed. If the lifestyle of the individual is such that an exclusive sexual relationship is not possible, advice must be given about which sexual practices are safer, and which more dangerous. The use of condoms is strongly recommended. Avoidance of oral and anal sex with new or casual partners is equally important. Open-mouthed kissing appears not in itself to be particularly hazardous with such partners. It is important to remember that the duty of the doctor is not to choose the sexual preferences, sexual practices or lifestyle of the patient: it is to explain the consequences of these, and then to give the best advice available.

At the other end of the scale, many patients are unnecessarily anxious about the infectivity of HIV. They are concerned that infection may arise from communal activities such as swimming, contact sports and parties, or may take place through close contact at work. In this context, it is important to stress that the transfer of infection is limited to direct contact with blood and body fluids and is unlikely to occur casually. People in certain occupations are clearly at special risk, such as the medical care professions, police and ambulance drivers, but they will normally have received personal guidance in the light of the particular hazards to which they are exposed. It is important that reassurance to those not at risk should be widely disseminated, lest fear of infection leads to suspicion where this is not justified, and intolerance.

There is an increasingly strong argument for providing clean needles (on an exchange basis) to patients who are intravenous drug misusers, but here again there is a division of opinion in the profession.

Much of this section has been written in the form of questions, rather than in the form of hard and convinced advice. The writer takes a libertarian view of such matters as sexual preference, sexual practices and lifestyle. Those who take a different view must interpret this chapter in the light of their own beliefs. As with so many other aspects of the practice of medicine (for example, termination of pregnancy, terminal care, *in-vitro* fertilization) differences between doctors about what they believe and what they regard as permissible or tolerable will be no different from those which divide society at large. What should unite us is the desire to remain sensitive to the differences, and to respond as sympathetically as we can to what it is that the patient believes and can tolerate.

3.80
The patient who does not complain

Ann-Louise Kinmonth and J.J.C. Cormack

The National Health Service is geared more towards salvage than towards pre-empting established disease. Thus the consultation in general practice is more likely to be taken up with the palliation of the presenting symptom than with a consideration of the possible risk factors for ill health associated with it or with the person presenting. It is much easier to give advice to a patient suffering from a specific complaint than to burden someone who feels relatively well with the knowledge that they are at uncertain individual risk of an unpleasant disorder in the future. Yet, those working in primary medical care are being exhorted to change their approach, and to take on the responsibility of diagnosing presymptomatic disease among their patients so that they can invest in their health for the future.

This approach to disease depends on the ability to identify factors which consistently predict future ill health and whose modification is not only possible by methods acceptable to the patient but will result in less ill health.

However, many of the known risk factors for disease are genetic and so at present are relatively immutable; where they are open to modification, this usually requires a change in lifestyle which may be hard for the individual to achieve; finally, even where risk factors can be modified, situations in which their reversal has been shown to reduce untimely death or morbidity are few. A good example of success is smoking which is a major risk factor for coronary heart disease. Doctors have in the main been able to give up smoking, and thereby reduced their expected death rate from coronary heart disease by 50 per cent within 5 years[1]: thus they may also have provided their profession with the necessary motivation to be effective in helping their patients to stop smoking.[2]

Similarly there is good evidence that reducing severely or moderately raised blood pressure lessens significantly the risk of stroke in men under 70 years old.[3]

However modification of other strong risk factors for coronary heart disease (blood pressure, moderately elevated blood lipids, or hyperglycaemia) has not been shown conclusively to reduce risk of death from myocardial ischaemia. Nor is there any evidence that large scale, 'multiphasic' screening delays among the screened group.[4]

Controlled clinical trials able to show up differences in outcome due to modification of such risk factors require large numbers of patients to follow sometimes difficult protocols for many years and are expensive and difficult to mount. It is thus perhaps not surprising that good evidence of the benefits accruing from control of asymptomatic increases of blood pressure or blood glucose has been slow in coming.

The sections that follow discuss the management of some of those biological variables that have no clear cut-off points for normal and abnormal with the aim of providing those facts at present available to help the general practitioner in decision making about further investigation and treatment of individual patients.

High blood pressure

The detection and treatment of raised blood pressure presents one of the greatest clinical challenges facing general practitioners in the last quarter of the twentieth century. Tudor Hart[5] writes:

> 'The arrival of effective drugs in the 1950s and of tolerable drugs in the late 1960s, with good evidence of the effectiveness of reducing pressure in preventing stroke, renal damage, retinal damage and heart failure, imposes a duty on doctors to make this treatment available to those who need it.'

In the National Morbidity Survey[6] essential hypertension (benign or unspecified hypertension with or without heart and/or renal disease) showed an episode rate of 41.4 and a consultation rate of 135.2 per 1,000 population per annum. These figures should however be interpreted with caution as no criterion was given for the blood-pressure levels which constituted the basis for the diagnosis of 'hypertension'. Sinclair[7] has suggested that it may well be that for every patient with hypertension attending a general practitioner or a hospital clinic, there are two or three others of the general population unaware that their blood pressure is raised, and that there may be as many as a million undiagnosed cases in the United Kingdom. The logistic and economic dilemmas which these figures pose must be faced.

The case yield under the age of 30 is too small to justify active case finding on present evidence, and finding asymptomatic hypertension over 70 probably does not appreciably influence outcome. As the proportion of the registered population of all ages who consult at least once during the year is 67 per cent[6], over a period of 5 years it should be possible to ensure that the blood pressures of about 90 per cent of the population are measured and recorded during that time.

There is, as yet, no universally agreed definition of 'hypertension'. It is, however, generally accepted that high blood pressure is not a disease but a risk factor — the higher the level of pressure (particularly diastolic pressure) the greater the risk of cerebrovascular accidents, coronary heart disease, left ventricular failure and renal failure. Using the fifth phase (disappearance of sounds) as the diastolic measurement point mild hypertension may be defined at levels between 95–104 mmHg, moderate hypertension at 105–120 mmHg and severe hypertension levels above 120 mmHg[8].

The results of the Medical Research Council's trial on the treatment of mild to moderate hypertension and the European Working Party's study of hypertension in the elderly have not provided unequivocal answers to the questions 'whom to treat' or 'when to treat'. Evidence of benefit was most striking in males over the age of 45 with diastolic pressures exceeding 100 mmHg. One striking finding in the MRC study was that the adverse effects of cigarette smoking were greater than any benefit conferred by drugs. There is at least some evidence that good control of hypertension at all levels and in both sexes is justified by reduction in morbidity and that even a lesser level of control is of considerable benefit.

Any policy of selective screening must depend heavily on adequate record systems so that the age and sex of patients selected for screening can be clearly identified; their blood-pressure readings should also be readily accessible and the screening criteria adopted adhered to.

Causes of high blood pressure

While there are many hypotheses about possible factors contributing to the development of hypertension (e.g., age, heredity, diet, anxiety, weight), there are relatively few identifiable reversible primary causes. These include

1. Coarctation of the aorta
2. Primary aldosteronism
3. Phaeochromocytoma
4. Renal disease:
   — Congenital kidney deformities (including polycystic kidneys)
   — Chronic pyelonephritis
   — Gout nephropathy
   — Hypercalcaemia
   — Renal artery stenosis.

Coarctation should be suspected if there are absent femoral pulses or femoral pulsations delayed in comparison with radial pulsations, a systolic murmur over the sternum and back and notching of the ribs on the chest X-ray.

Primary aldosteronism (Conn's syndrome) may be suspected if the serum potassium is low and also if there is T-wave depression on the electrocardiogram.

Phaeochromocytoma may be suspected if there is no response, or an anomalous response, to treatment, and such suspicions should call for a twenty-four-hour urine collection to estimate vanillylmandelic acid (VMA).

Renal disease may be suspected from the history (symptoms of renal colic, recurrent urinary infections or a family history of polycystic kidneys, which are inherited as a simple dominant), or from a finding of bacteriuria or uraemia or raised serum uric acid (gout nephropathy). In such cases an intravenous pyelogram should be arranged.

The diagnostic/management pathway following the initial history and examination will therefore be:

1. Absent or delayed femoral pulses:? coarctation: refer to specialist
2. Lowered serum potassium:? primary aldosteronism: refer to specialist
3. Failure to respond to treatment:? phaeochromocytoma: twenty-four-hour urine for VMA — if raised refer to specialist
4. Raised serum uric acid:? a possible contraindication to the prescription of thiazides
5. Raised blood urea:? congenital renal lesion: intravenous pyelogram
6. History of recurrent urinary infections or finding of bacteriuria:? chronic pyelonephritis: intravenous pyelogram
7. Raised serum calcium:? hypercalcaemic stones: intravenous pyelogram
8. History of renal or ureteric colic:? hypercalcaemic stones: intravenous pyelogram

If renal lesions are confirmed by intravenous pyelography, or if there is doubt about the findings or their management, further referral is indicated.

History and examination. — Once the base-line for diagnosing hypertension is identified the patient's entry into the investigation and treatment group (as opposed to simply a surveillance group) should be based on at least three separate resting readings of the blood pressure.

The history which is taken is not, of course, a history of the condition itself (it is after all simply an incidental finding), but of possible associated events and background. A minimal check-list would include:

— Family history of hypertension, cardio- or cerebro-vascular disease or renal disease
— Facial or other paresis and/or dysphasia (however transient)
— Breathlessness

— Anginal pain
— Symptoms of renal disease
— Current drug therapy (especially oral contraceptive pills, or antidepressants)
— Smoking habits.

Physical examination. — After checking the blood pressure this should include:
— Auscultation of the heart (for triple rhythm and murmurs)
— Auscultation of the lung bases
— Palpation of kidneys
— Auscultation of abdomen (for bruits)
— Femoral pulses
— Weight and height
— Ophthalmoscopy.

Base-line investigation. —
— Urine for protein, sugar and culture
— Electrocardiography for LV strain and as a base-line and/or X-ray chest for heart size
— Blood: — Plasma electrolytes
— Urea and/or creatinine
— Uric acid
— Calcium.

Management of high blood pressure

Once the rare cases of hypertension secondary to remediable conditions are excluded, the management of the majority of identified hypertensives may be provided by the general practitioner.
There is no evidence that hypertension first identified over the age of 70 (unless there are acute symptoms such as left ventricular failure) should be actively treated. The patient whose vascular tree has withstood raised arterial pressure to this age is likely to have adjusted to the situation to a degree where treatment (which to be effective has to be prolonged and carefully monitored and may have its own hazards) could be seen as meddlesome interference rather than genuine therapeutic endeavour.
For the rest there are three principal lines of management:

1. The control of obesity
2. Advice on smoking, alcohol and salt
3. Drug therapy

Obesity. — There is little doubt that there is an association between obesity and hypertension. The effectiveness of treatment of obesity is disappointing. Nevertheless, the attempt should be made to encourage patients to achieve and sustain a realistic target weight by dietary advice, exhortation, encouragement and willingness to follow-up. Drugs have little, if any, place in the management of obesity but the establishment of a good doctor–patient relationship can in certain cases lead to real progress (see Chapter 3.41).

Smoking. — There does not appear to be any direct relationship between smoking and the development of high blood pressure, but as one of the outcomes of high blood pressure is ischaemic heart disease the proven connection between cigarette smoking and coronary artery disease makes advice and encouragement to patients to stop smoking an important aspect of management.

Alcohol. — There is some evidence that a high alcohol intake contributes to an increase in arterial pressure and the finding of asymptomatic hypertension may be a suitable occasion to counsel a patient about excessive alcohol intake.

Salt. — Debate continues about the contribution of salt in the diet to the pathogenesis of hypertension, but it is reasonable to advise patients in whom a diagnosis of hypertension is established that they should avoid particularly salty foods and should not add salt at table.

Drugs

The aim of drug treatment must be to lower the blood pressure without unacceptable side-effects. A target figure of 140/90 would be reasonable but in individual cases higher levels may be quite acceptable bearing in mind the fact that for moderate or severe hypertension any degree of control is better than no control.

Beta-blockers. — The treatment of hypertension with drugs is a constantly changing picture. At the present time the use of beta-adrenoceptor blocking drugs seems to offer the greatest prospect of success, particularly in patients under the age of 55. Although there are many beta-blocking drugs now available and they are probably equally effective in lowering blood pressure there is some evidence that less adverse effects (fatigue, cold extremities, cardiac failure, bronchospasm) are experienced with cardioselective beta-blockers than with other drugs in this group, and that water-soluble beta-blockers are less likely to cross the blood brain barrier and cause depression and sleep disturbances than lipid soluble drugs.

Compliance is particularly important when very long-term (possibly lifelong) treatment is used to reduce an asymptomatic risk. Once daily dosage of drugs with proven 24 hour action is probably the best method to secure compliance. Atenolol (Tenormin) —

which is water soluble, and sustained release metoprolol (Betaloc SA) — which is lipid soluble, meet these criteria.
Atenolol should be started at a dose of 50 mg per day and sustained release metoprolol at 200 mg daily: if after a month target reduction of pressure is not achieved these doses can be increased to 100 mg or 400 mg respectively.

Thiazide diuretics. — These diuretics can be used alone or in combination with other drugs in the treatment of hypertension. Their hypotensive effect is independent of their diuretic effect and is probably due to action on peripheral vascular resistance. All thiazides are equipotent and the cheapest currently available is bendrofluazide, which should be given in a dose of 5 mg per day. The dose range is narrow as there is no further hypotensive response to doses greater than 5 mg daily. The side-effects which must be monitored are potassium depletion (though potassium supplements are only rarely required), and the possible precipitation of diabetes mellitus or hyperuricaemia.

Combined drugs. — If the blood pressure cannot be adequately controlled with either a beta blocker or a thiazide diuretic the next step should be to try a combined preparation. For the sake of compliance these are best prescribed in single daily dose formulations; the recommended preparations are atenolol/chlorthalidone (Tenoret 50, Tenoretic), metoprolol/hydrochlorothiazide (Co-Betaloc SA) or acebutolol/hydrochlorothiazide (Secadrex).

Third-line drugs. — If control is not achieved with a combined beta blocker/thiazide preparation the practitioner may well wish to refer the patient for specialist advice. Many doctors, however, would be prepared to prescribe a 'third-line' drug at this stage and the most appropriate, currently, are the calcium channel antagonist nifedipine (Adalat Retard) 20–40 mg twice a day, or the angiotensin converting enzyme inhibitor captopril (Captopen, Acepril) 12.5–25 mg twice daily. Captopril should be used with caution as the first dose may induce marked hypotension within three hours and therefore the patient should be warned and the doctor readily available during this time. The other ACE inhibitor, enalapril, has probably not yet been sufficiently fully evaluated to justify its use without specialist advice.

Vasodilator and other drugs. — If nifedipine or captopril are contraindicated as third-line drugs a vasodilator such as hydralazine (Apresoline) may be used: the initial dose is 25 mg twice a day increasing to a maximum dose of 100 mg twice a day. Adrenergic blocking drugs (such as bethanidine, debrisoquine or guanethidine) and methyldopa, all used quite extensively in the past for the treatment of hypertension are no longer recommended for routine use because of their high incidence of undesirable side-effects.

Follow-up

Once the diagnosis of hypertension is established and treatment started the patient has to be made aware that he is at the start of a process which will generally be life-long. The implications of this to a relatively young patient must be explained and explored and repeatedly reinforced. Not only must the blood pressure itself be monitored, but the patient must be constantly encouraged to maintain treatment in the absence of symptoms. To maintain supervision and follow-up, efficient organization and clear records are essential. This is a situation where the use of flow sheets in recording would undoubtedly assist, and some practitioners and some practices are already devising their own examples. It is to be hoped that they will publish and share their experiences. Some further suggestions on follow-up are contained in Chapter 4.9.

Decisions have to be made about the rational sharing of care where specialists are involved. All too often, patients are referred for initial assessment and then followed-up in a sometimes arbitrary fashion by constantly changing junior hospital staff, with the general practitioner relegated to the role of signing prescriptions. This is a situation which calls for local initiative and discussion, if continuity of care is not to degenerate into a circus of clinic attendances with unclear objectives.

The problems do not end — indeed they only begin — with the definition of high blood pressure and the identification of patients who suffer (or more accurately will suffer) from it. There is not yet any consensus to guide us on treatment and follow-up — only the responsibility and challenge which are inescapably posed by the possession of a sphygmomanometer.

The paralysis and incontinence of our hemiplegic patients, the relentless downhill progress of those with failing kidneys, the painful and dyspnoeic misery of those with heart failure and severe ischaemic heart disease, and not least the suffering of their caring relatives must all prompt us to use the instruments of secondary prevention we do have to edge back the tide of cerebro- and cardio-vascular damage which threatens an unacceptably large segment of an unsuspecting population.

Hyperglycaemia

It is now recognized that the clinical state of diabetes mellitus represents one end of a spectrum of glucose tolerance. Blood glucose in young people is usually maintained between 4 and 6 mmol/l irrespective of feasting or fasting. In the diabetic state, this tight control is lost and in the majority of patients presenting with characteristic symptoms of hyperglycaemia the diagnosis can be simply established by a single random plasma glucose level which will be greater than 11 mmol/l.

It is estimated that at least 1 per cent of patients on any doctor's list may fall into this category but the overall prevalence increases with age and half the people with diabetes are older than 60 years. A general practitioner caring for a population including 500 young people (0–16 yrs) is unlikely to make the diagnosis of insulin dependent diabetes (IDD) in this age group more than once in 20 years. In contrast more than one patient with non insulin dependent diabetes (NIDD) would be expected to present each year.

Each list of 2,000 patients will contain at least 20 people with frank diabetes. Among these, about 30 per cent will be treated with insulin and 70 per cent will be managed on diet or tablets. The natural history of diabetes in the generation living over the last 50 years has been characterized for insulin dependent and non insulin-dependent patients (Tables Ia and Ib). The younger the age of onset the greater the reduction in life expectancy, and in the past no more than 50 per cent of juvenile onset patients could expect to live beyond the age of 50 years. Excess early deaths among IDD patients are mainly due to renal failure, while myocardial infarction and cerebrovascular accidents kill both groups earlier and at least twice as often as the rest of the population. Morbidity is also serious. Diabetes is the most common cause of blindness in the middle-aged, while uraemia and gangrene contribute to a burden of disability which doubles the hospitalization rate compared with an age-matched general population.[9] Among both IDD and NIDD groups, the risk of early morbidity and mortality is strongly associated with the duration of hyperglycaemia. Epidemiological studies also suggest that the risk of premature large vessel pathology (macroangiopathy) is directly related to rises in blood glucose concentration, however small. The risk of small vessel disease (microangiopathy) may be related in a similar way to postprandial blood glucose levels above 11 mmol/l. Blood glucose concentration, like blood pressure, is a continuously distributed variable in Caucasian populations. Thus for every established diabetic patient there is probably at least one other undiagnosed patient, whose lesser degree of glucose intolerance has not brought him or her to diagnosis but who is at increased risk of arterial disease and of worsening clinical diabetes.

To accommodate better understanding of the risks associated with hyperglycaemia, new diagnostic criteria have been recently defined based on a 75 g glucose tolerance test. The current criteria for the diabetic and glucose intolerant states are shown in table II. There are, however, a few occasions when the general practitioner will need to perform a glucose tolerance test. They include cases where diabetes is suspected but fasting and postprandial blood glucose levels are not diagnostic and in cases where it is necessary to establish the renal threshold for glucose.

Why bother?

Effective treatment for diabetic complications, especially retinopathy, is now available and clinical trials using the new methods of monitoring blood glucose control are providing increasing evidence that tight metabolic control can reduce the incidence and severity of tissue damage, especially of the kidney. In addition, close attention to blood pressure, smoking, infection and foot care may delay the progression of tissue damage.[10] The tools are thus available to improve significantly the prognosis of the next generation of patients with diabetes.

Presentation

The alert general practitioner will not miss the diagnosis in those patients with characteristic symptoms of polyuria, polydipsia and weight loss. However only half the patients will present in this way (Table III) and only a small minority with florid ketoacidosis.

How far should the doctor look for diabetes among the rest of his or her patients? Studies on the value of unselected screening suggest that this is not a cost effective plan. However, it is known that the majority of undiagnosed patients will be found among patients with the specific risk factors shown in Table I.

Diabetes mellitus is a great mimic and should be considered, especially among the at risk groups such as older patients presenting with recurrent infections especially of the genitals or urinary tract or with non-specific tiredness or malaise. Screening of all stressed, fat, elderly patients might be worthwhile. Among children and young people, suspicion should be raised by weight loss and chronic malaise as well as the more easily recognized thirst and polyuria.

Glycosuria

About 2 per cent of ordinary people (more in pregnancy) with glycosuria do not have hyperglycaemia. On the other hand, 26 per cent of people with a degree of glucose intolerance may not have glycosuria. Testing the urine, especially after meals, remains a useful diagnostic tool. However, it is a coarse one, and may delay diagnosis among asymptomatic patients, especially older patients with renal impairment in whom the renal threshold for glucose is raised. A fasting or one hour post breakfast capillary blood glucose level is the best tool widely available for early diagnosis at present. Glucose intolerance increases with age, and it may be wise to rely on fasting rather than postprandial hyperglycaemia before diagnosing 'diabetes' in patients over the age of 60 years (table II). It should also be remembered that laboratories can make mistakes, and a single

	I *Insulin dependent diabetes (IDD)*	II *Non insulin dependent diabetes (NIDD)*
1. Risk factors:		
Family history:	+	++
Genetic lesion	Histocompatibility (HCA) specificities	?
	Islet cell antibodies	—
Age	Throughout life with peak at 12–14 yrs	the majority > 50 years
Other	—	Obesity Physical inactivity
		Gestational diabetes Delivery of baby ≥ 4.5kg (10lb)
2. Presentation:	Usually acute over days and weeks	Often over months or years
	Usually symptomatic; polyuria; polydipsia, weight loss	Often asymptomatic or with Infection – especially genitourinary Pruritus vulvae Tissue damage
3. Major causes of death	Renal failure Coronary heart disease	Coronary heart disease Stroke

Table Ia. — Characteristics of the major subtypes of diabetes mellitus

1. Microvascular, e.g. renal glomerulopathy, retinopathy.
2. Macrovascular, e.g. coronary heart disease, peripheral vascular disease.
3. Neuropathy (sensory, motor and autonomic; gastrointestinal and vascular).
4. Lens opacification.
5. Collagen change.

Table Ib. — Types of diabetic tissue damage

Blood Glucose	*Diabetes*	*Impaired glucose tolerance (IGT)*	*Normal*
Fasting (mmol/l)	≥8	<8	<6
Two hours after a 75 g glucose load (mmol/l)	≥11	8–11	<7

(NB: Values are for venous plasma; for venous whole blood subtract 1; for capillary blood subtract 1 from the fasting values, add 1 to the two hour values.)

Table II. — W.H.O. criteria for diagnosis of diabetes mellitus[9]

	Insulin dependent patients %	Non insulin dependent patients %
Hyperglycaemic ketoacidosis	30	0
Polyuria; polydipsia; weight loss	60	30
Infections + pruritis vulvae especially vaginitis, balanitis, UTI, skin infection	5	25
Tissue damage especially cataracts, neuropathy	0	5
Incidental to hospital admission, investigation or screening	5	40
	100	100

Table III. — Common presentations of diabetes mellitus (based on an audit of 390 patients from 8 practices)

abnormal blood glucose level in an asymptomatic patient requires confirmation.

Causes

It is now well recognized that the syndrome of diabetes includes a number of clinically and genetically distinct disorders resulting from absolute or relative insulin deficiency. The usual characteristics of the two major sub groups are shown in Table I.

There is a strong genetic predisposition to diabetes, especially among non insulin dependent patients. In insulin dependent patients the genetic mechanisms appear to be associated with changes in the immune defences of individuals. Specific circulating and cellular antibodies are found in patients developing insulin dependent diabetes, and it is thought that viral infection may trigger a pathological-immune reaction which leads to islet cell destruction and diabetes.

History and examination

Where any degree of hyperglycaemia has been confirmed, a careful history and examination is necessary to define the current status and future risks for that individual; the acutely ill, ketotic, insulin dependent patient will need rapid admission for intensive care. The following remarks apply to all patients at diagnosis and subsequent review.

1. Family history and patients' beliefs. Many patients will have had experience of diabetes through a friend or relative. Discussion of this allows the doctor to explore the fears the patient may entertain about the effects of 'sugar' on him or herself; these often include fear of hypoglycaemia, inevitable blindness, gangrene or 'rotting kidneys'. In addition patients are afraid of the impact diabetes will have on their lives; especially their present employment prospects, and chances of marrying and having children. They fear the disciplines of management; 'the diet' and 'the needle'. It is a challenging task to help each patient separate real from imagined risks and to enable him or her to understand that complications are not inevitable and can be minimized by good management.

2. Existing tissue damage. Non insulin dependent patients may have a long history of hyperglycaemia before diagnosis. It is particularly important to establish the presence of:

(a) *Ischaemic heart disease* increasing the risk of myocardial infarction (a history of angina; an abnormal ECG).
(b) *Peripheral vascular disease* increasing the risk of gangrene and foot ulcers (rest pain; absent pulses; poor capillary return).
(c) *Neuropathy* increasing the risk of foot damage (paraesthesia; absent ankle jerks and sensory loss), of urinary stasis (leading to infection) and of impotence.
(d) *Cataracts and retinopathy* both of which can be treated. Virtually all patients with long duration of disease have detectable background retinopathy which does not affect vision. Vision is threatened by proliferation of new vessels and macular exudates which can be detected by fundoscopy through dilated pupils. It is also threatened, especially in non insulin dependent patients by macular oedema which can be detected by loss of visual acuity. Both can be effectively treated by early photocoagulation using laser-therapy.
(e) *Nephropathy* Persistent clinical proteinuria (>30 mg/dl by Albustix) reflects established renal disease; exclude infection and treat hypertension.

3. Exacerbating factors

(a) A high calorie diet low in dietary fibre and high in sugar and fat.
(b) Drugs which alter glucose tolerance.

Thiazide diuretics, Corticosteroids, Oral contraceptives } decrease glucose tolerance.

Alcohol may exacerbate reactive hypoglycaemia and delay recovery from it. It is also high in calories (7.5 Cal/g).

Beta blockers may block warning symptoms of hypoglycaemia.

(c) Obesity.
(d) Other risk factors for organ damage:

Hypertension
Smoking
Urinary tract infection
Hyperlipidaemia.

Management

The aims of management are:

1. Prevention or treatment of acute complications associated with extremes of blood glucose (mainly in insulin dependent patients).
2. Prevention or treatment of the chronic complications of hyperglycaemia.

Treatment

1. Diet. The majority of new cases of maturity onset diabetes are manageable by diet alone. The aims in this group are:

1. To avoid obesity by caloric control based on avoidance of energy dense sugar and fat (e.g. sweet fizzy drinks, table sugar, confectionery, fried food, crisps, fatty meats and cheese).
2. To improve glucose tolerance by eating a liberal carbohydrate diet based on unrefined foods high in fibre, especially legumes (e.g. dried beans, peas, sweetcorn, jacket potatoes, Weetabix, wholemeal bread).

If tablets are required as an adjunct, meals should not be missed since hypoglycaemia can occur. If patients are insulin dependent the basic dietary advice is the same but it becomes even more important to eat the right amount of carbohydrate at the right time, and exchange lists of carbohydrate foods are usually used.

Changing dietary habits is difficult; attempts should be based on a history of what the person usually eats, and dietetic follow up is essential to solve problems and reiterate advice. A dietitian's help is therefore invaluable and direct referral should be made whenever possible. Useful patient manuals on dietary advice, alcohol use, and recipes are available from the British Diabetic Association (Chapter 4.9).

2. Tablets. Where diet fails, but ketosis is absent, a sulphonylurea (e.g., tolbutamide, chlorpropamide) should be tried. Sulphonylureas stimulate the appetite, and in obese patients the biguanide, metformin may be preferred instead (though it frequently causes diarrhoea and may precipitate lactic acidosis).

Chlorpropamide is long acting and may cause hypoglycaemia especially in the elderly and patients with renal disease. It can also be associated with an unpleasant flush, tachycardia and sweating after alcohol. Tolbutamide which is shorter acting or Glibenclamide are our drugs of choice for the majority of elderly non insulin dependent patients.

3. Insulin. Ketotic hyperglycaemia requires treatment with insulin. Therapy is usually initiated in hospital, but fine tuning can only be effectively carried out at home.

Insulin concentration is now standardized at 100 units/ml and each doctor should be familiar with the types in common use in his or her

area. Commonly a fast acting 'clear' insulin is combined with a medium acting 'cloudy' insulin and given twice daily (table IV). Beef, pork, and human insulins are available. Pork and human insulin are less antigenic than beef and are preferred for new patients. Well controlled patients should not have their insulin type changed on theoretical grounds of type or purity.
Patients should if possible learn how to alter their dose in the light of home blood glucose results but should be warned never to omit their dose completely, especially in the morning.

Monitoring blood glucose

1. Symptoms. Symptoms of high blood glucose, especially nocturia, are a useful alert to patients that all is not well and mild symptoms of hypoglycaemia are supportive evidence of good control. The asymptomatic patient may, however, be at risk from hyper- or hypoglycaemia and so must rely on biochemical tests for monitoring control.

Type	*Species*	*Highly purified examples*
Rapid action: (approx 6hr)		
Regular, soluble, crystalline	Beef	Insulin injection BP
Neutral	Beef Pork Human	Quicksol/Neusulin Velosulin/Actrapid Humulin/Human Actrapid
Intermediate action: (approx 20 hr)		
Insulin zinc suspension (amorphous; semilente)	Pork	Semitard
Insulin zinc suspension (crystalline plus amorphous; lente)	Beef Pork Human	Tempulin Monotard Human Monotard
Isophane (protamine)	Beef Pork Human	Hypurin/Monophane Insulatard Human Protaphane
Long action: (approx 30 hr)		
Insulin zinc suspension (crystalline; ultralente)	Beef	Tempulin Ultratard
Protamine zinc insulin	Beef	Hypurin

Table IV. — Insulins

2. Urine tests. Where the renal threshold is known, semiquantitative tests for glycosuria using e.g. Clinitest tablets or Diastix (Ames) can provide a guide to the pattern of hyperglycaemia through the day. However, their most useful role may be in conjunction with Ketostix (Ames) in confirming states of acute insulin deficiency. Aglycosuria is not necessarily synonymous with good control.

3. Blood glucose. Capillary blood glucose levels can be measured by each patient using indicator sticks. An autolet (Owen Mumford) can reduce the pain of blood-letting and the use of a reflectance meter is an added refinement. The measurement of blood glucose by patients themselves at different times through the day is a great advance in maintaining satisfactory control and should be used if possible by all insulin dependent patients and by non insulin dependent patients at least occasionally before breakfast (fasting). It is the only way that asymptomatic patients can establish the presence of low or high blood glucose in time to do something about it.

4. Glycosylated haemoglobin. Glucose in the blood glycosylates haemoglobin in direct proportion to the degree of hyperglycaemia. The proportion of glycosylated haemoglobin at any time depends on both the average blood glucose concentration and the red cell life span. Measurement of glycosylated haemoglobin can thus give a useful indication as to whether control has been poor (or too tight) over the previous 6–8 weeks. Patients can thus be identified for closer attention when control is poor.

At one extreme, the life of the recently diagnosed patient depends on regular injections of insulin, a regular pattern of meals and a suitably adjusted lifestyle including a method for monitoring the diabetes. At the other extreme weight reduction by caloric restriction may correct the metabolic disturbance completely. Every case will require an individual management plan, but success will depend on regular follow up and patient support and education.

Follow up. — Diabetic patients who stay in regular contact with professional advice live longer than defaulters[11] and motivation by a concerned professional can achieve significant improvements in blood glucose control.[12]

Systematic follow up is therefore essential, but who should be responsible? Hospital diabetic clinics are overstretched despite seeing only 50 per cent of the diabetic population in many areas[10] and up to 25 per cent of patients may be receiving no follow up at all. How can we most effectively spread the load so that all patients at least are reviewed annually? Patients fall into several 'care groups' and the responsibility for follow up of each group must be decided at a local level. In general this might be:

General practitioner:

1. Adult patients without complications treated with diet, tablets or insulin.
2. The very old and frail.
3. More complicated cases who persistently default from specialist care.
4. Shared care of other cases.

Specialist in diabetes:

1. Children and adolescents, and child-bearing women.
2. A proportion of insulin dependent adults.
3. Complicated cases of all kinds.

Effective follow up requires a recall register and systematic surveillance. It can be made easier if someone in each practice takes a specific administrative or clinical interest in diabetic care, be it doctor, nurse or receptionist. One such solution is the 'mini-clinic' in which a designated general practitioner takes the major responsibility for diabetic follow up, with the help of the treatment room nurse. In the Wolverhampton area the default rate is lower from these mini-clinics than from the hospital clinic and regular mini-clinic attenders show as good blood glucose control as hospital attenders.[13] In other areas shared care schemes operate where the hospital takes responsibility for regular review and the general practitioner for intervening follow up.[10]
It is notable that among patients accustomed to attending a hospital, discharge to general practitioner care without ensuring a system for regular recall has resulted in generally poor surveillance, and morbidity and even mortality over 5 years have tended to be higher than among continuing attenders at hospital.[14]

Other resources. — Effective management of diabetic patients requires access to dietitian, ophthalmologist and chiropodist, as well as the availability of indicator sticks for home blood glucose measurement and laboratory access for measurement of glycosylated haemoglobin. Local solutions for these needs are required before general practitioners will feel professionally justified in following up many patients with diabetes entirely themselves. Solutions will be best found where specialists and general practitioners are united in their efforts to provide care for the 2 per cent of the population at risk from hyperglycaemia.

Aims of follow up

1. Motivation and education. Successful management of diabetes depends in large part on patients understanding and carrying out their own treatment and monitoring of control. Education to do this is time consuming, and diabetic liaison sisters and treatment room sisters with an interest may do much to help. The British Diabetic Association (Chapter 4.9) welcomes new members and provides a wealth of advice and support through branch meetings, summer camps and publications.

2. Control of glucose. Ideally we should aim at:
(a) absence of symptoms of high or low blood glucose;

(b) near normal blood glucose;

—aglycosuria at all times (except where the renal threshold is low)

—fasting blood glucose 4–6 mmol/l; 1 hour post prandial blood glucose <10 mmol/l

—near normal glycosylated haemoglobin. (Local laboratories vary in their normal range; often about 3–6 per cent.)

Non insulin dependent patients can be managed on the basis of occasional normal fasting blood glucose levels alone. Patients on insulin should keep a written record of blood glucose tests through the day and bring them to consultations where their discussion can fulfil a powerful educational role.

3. Control of weight. Especially in non insulin dependent patients. This requires weight charts, dietetic assistance, and continuing motivation (e.g. weight watchers etc.).

4. Monitoring other risk factors. Especially smoking, blood pressure and infection.

5. To monitor and manage microangiopathy, macroangiopathy and neuropathy especially:

(a) *Vision* Examination of lens and retina through dilated pupils annually; examination of visual acuity using a Snellen Chart and pinhole annually at least.

(b) *Renal* Urine for protein at every visit.

(c) *Feet* Neuropathy, macroangiopathy, and microangiopathy can all jeopardize the feet by ulcers, infection and gangrene. Self-care (hygiene, inspection and well-fitting shoes) supervised by nurse, doctor and chiropodist can help prevent this, and the feet should be examined at least twice a year.

6. Treatment. Discussion and modification of diet, tablet, or insulin therapy. This should include the technique of insulin injection and examination of injection sites for lumps or hollows.

7. Monitoring. Discussion of monitoring techniques and supply of equipment.

8. Social and emotional support. The general practitioner is used to managing many of the kinds of social problems that can accompany diabetes and its treatment throughout life; the parents who feel bereaved of their 'normal' child because he now has diabetes; the adolescent who experiments by omitting her insulin, the young man or woman afraid of impotence or of having an abnormal child. However the practising doctor may feel less sure of his or her role with the apparently unconcerned patient; there may be a fine balance between ensuring that patients understand the risks of diabetes to their health and saving them from undue anxiety.

Most patients with diabetes will benefit from specialist advice and resources at some time of their lives, but general practitioners have a major continuing responsibility through medical advice and counselling to help their patients avoid the complications of diabetes. When this fails, and myocardial infarction, blindness or gangrene supervene the responsibility continues, with other members of the health care team and social services, to minimize the impact of the condition on the lives of individual patients.

Anaemia

Anaemia is a sign, defined as a level of haemoglobin below an arbitrary limit, and is not in itself a disease. In the Third National Morbidity Survey 5.3 episodes of iron deficiency anaemia were diagnosed per annum per 1,000 patients (although the haemoglobin level on which the diagnosis of anaemia was made was not defined). There was a marked sex variation: 1.7 episodes for men and 8.7 for women. For pernicious anaemia the figures were 0.8 for men and 1.7 for women, with a mean of 1.2, and for other anaemias 0.4 for men, and 0.9 for women with a mean of 0.7. Fry[15] quotes even higher figures showing a prevalence of anaemia (Hb less than 12G/100 ml) of 26.2 per cent for women and 4.1 per cent for adult males. In women the highest prevalence rate was noted between the ages of 30 and 50 and in men the peak of prevalence was found in the elderly. These last figures are based on a single practice survey taking a 1 in 8 sample of all adults aged over 15, while the National Morbidity Survey deals with anaemia diagnosed on clinical suspicion, or as an incidental finding.
Elwood and his colleagues, in a classic paper[16] based on a study of a random sample of 880 women, showed that haemoglobin levels between 10.0 G and 12.0 G/100 ml are not harmful in themselves and do not cause symptoms. Thus while iron deficiency (which is by far the commonest cause of anaemia as currently defined) is widespread, it probably does not in itself cause any interference with function unless the haemoglobin falls much below 8.0 G/100 ml. Mass screening for anaemia therefore cannot be expected to have a great effect in terms of reducing morbidity or improving well-being, or in reducing mortality from serious disease (Moore[17]).
There are, however, certain groups who should be regarded as particularly vulnerable to anaemia and for whom a case can be made out for selective case-finding. These are:

1. Those especially liable to dietary iron deficiency or deficiency of other substances essential for haemopoiesis:
   Dysmature or low birth weight infants (under the age of 6 months)

The elderly (over the age of 70)
Immigrants in poor social circumstances
Alcoholics
Patients who have had a gastrectomy.

2. Those with evidence of blood loss or found to have occult blood loss:
   Patients with persistent: — menorrhagia (and patients fitted with an intra-uterine device)
   — epistaxes
   — haematemeses or melenae
   — haemorrhoids

   Patients with gastro-intestinal lesions: — hiatus hernia
   — peptic ulcer
   — colitis
   — diverticular disease

   Patients on long term salicylates, indomethacin, anticoagulants or anticonvulsants.
3. Pregnant women
4. Patients liable to hereditary haemoglobinopathies:
   — Negro patients liable to sickle cell disease
   — Patients of Mediterranean origin liable to thalassaemia.

History and examination. The discovery of a low haemoglobin is in itself a pointer to the taking of a fuller history which in turn will indicate the appropriate examination and investigation pathway. By far the most important group of anaemias numerically are those due to iron deficiency with a *hypochromic* picture. Here the history and examination must be directed to a search for sources of:

(a) Blood loss, overt or occult, from the gastro-intestinal tract or female genital tract
(b) Nutritional deficiency (especially in the elderly and the poor)
(c) Malabsorption (particularly gluten enteropathy).

Failure to find such causes and/or failure to respond to treatment, will lead to a search for a further explanation such as uraemia, rheumatoid arthritis or malignant disease.

A *normochromic* anaemia may be associated with scurvy (especially in immigrants) or myxoedema (especially in the elderly), although both of these conditions may also show a macrocytic picture.

The commonest *macrocytic* anaemias are those due to vitamin B_{12} and folate deficiencies. A serum B_{12} and folate estimation may be all that is required to establish the diagnosis and initiate treatment (especially in frail elderly patients in whom extensive investigation is not indicated).

Fuller investigation of macrocytic anaemia in younger patients by bone-marrow studies enables a further division to be made into

megaloblastic macrocytic anaemias, which in addition to B_{12} and folate deficiency may be caused by the megaloblastic anaemias of infancy or of pregnancy, and the megaloblastic anaemia associated with the administration of anticonvulsants, especially phenytoin. *Normoblastic* macrocytic anaemia may be due to:
— Haemolysis
— Aplastic anaemia
— Leukaemia
— Hepatic cirrhosis
— Myxoedema.

Management. The management of patients with anaemia naturally depends upon its causes. The vast majority are iron deficient and respond to oral iron (such as ferrous sulphate tablet, B.P., 200 mg twice or thrice daily with or after food). Overt bleeding will probably require definitive treatment, although patients with menorrhagia may respond simply to oral iron and their menorrhagia may diminish as their iron stores increase, without the need for hormonal or surgical intervention. Occult bleeding should lead to a search for its cause, but in some cases, such as hiatus hernia, haemorrhoids or bleeding due to salicylate ingestion and even many cases of peptic ulcer, symptomatic treatment will often suffice.

Failure to respond to treatment or suggestive symptoms will lead to fuller investigation, especially of the lower bowel for diverticular disease or malignant lesions.

The nutritional anaemias will also respond to therapy simply monitored in general practice (with iron, B_{12}, folic acid or ascorbic acid, as appropriate) and the health visitor will often help with the necessary dietary advice.

It should be reiterated that anaemia is not a diagnosis, but simply a pointer to the further diagnostic pathway which should lead to the unravelling of the primary cause. While population screening is not justified, the general practitioner's alertness in relation to vulnerable groups should help to ensure early intervention when it is indicated but protect from over-zealous investigation when simpler procedures are appropriate.

More detailed discussion of the anaemias is to be found in Chapter 3.34.

Albuminuria

Apart from contamination (e.g. in women who are menstruating or who have vaginal discharges), the commonest causes of albuminuria as an incidental finding are early manifestations of pre-eclamptic toxaemia in pregnancy and infection or inflammation of the urinary tract.

Albuminuria can also occur after exercise or prolonged standing (orthostatic albuminuria), and in severe cardiac failure.
An incidental finding of albuminuria should lead to an examination of an early morning specimen of urine passed soon after rising. If the finding is confirmed on an early morning specimen a mid-stream specimen should be sent to the laboratory for culture (or a dip-slide taken).
Further examination of the patient may help to indicate the câuse of the albuminuria:
—Ankles, fingers and sacrum for the presence of oedema (found in cardiac failure, the nephrotic syndrome and in some cases of pre-eclampsia).
—Estimation of the blood pressure (for hypertension).
If pre-eclampsia, urinary tract infection, cardiac failure or hypertension do not appear to be underlying factors, the patient with persistent albuminuria should be referred to a physician or nephrologist for further assessment.

High ESR

The erythrocyte sedimentation rate (ESR) is a non-specific test normally used to confirm the presence or monitor the progress of organic disease. When an unexpectedly raised ESR is found as an incidental finding further history, examination and investigations should be directed towards seeking further evidence of:
—Acute or chronic infection (including unsuspected pulmonary TB)
—Inflammatory or collagen disease, especially rheumatoid arthritis
—Neoplasia
—Anaemia
—Multiple myelomatosis.
It is important to stress that a raised ESR does not necessarily indicate disease (especially in the elderly, or in pregnancy) and also that a normal ESR does not exclude organic disease.
If an unexpectedly high ESR is found the estimation should be repeated, along with a full blood count to include haemoglobin and white cell count.
If the figure is still raised above local laboratory normal values and there is no obvious sign of acute infection, it is reasonable to arrange a chest X-ray, to check further for signs of either breast or prostatic carcinoma and to look further for the possibility of previously unsuspected joint disease.
If the value is very high myelomatosis may be suspected and in this case blood should be sent to the laboratory for protein and electrophoresis along with 10 ml of urine to test for the presence of Bence Jones proteins.

References

[1] Doll, R. and Peto, R. (1976): Mortality in relation to smoking: twenty years' observations on male British doctors. *British Medical Journal, ii,* 1525

[2] Russell, M.A.H., Wilson, C., Taylor, C. and Baker, C.D. (1979): Effect of general practitioners' advice against smoking. *British Medical Journal, ii,* 231

[3] Veterans Administration Study (1972): Effects of treatment on morbidity in hypertension. *Circulation,* 45, 991

[4] Fowler, G. (1983): *Screening in Preventive Medicine in General Practice.* Eds. Muir Gray and G.H. Fowler. Oxford: O.U.P.

[5] Hart, J.T. (1975): The management of high blood pressure in general practice. *Journal of the Royal College of General Practitioners, 25,* 160

[6] Royal College of General Practitioners, Office of Population Censuses and Surveys, Department of Health and Social Security (1986): *Morbidity Statistics from General Practice 1981–82.* HMSO Series MB5 No. 1

[7] Sinclair, R.G. (1975): In *Screening in General Practice* Ed. C.R. Hart, p 193. Edinburgh: Churchill Livingstone

[8] Lothian Hypertension Group (1984): Guidelines in the management of hypertension in general practice — detection and assessment of hypertension. *Journal of the Royal College of General Practitioners, 34,* 405 and 460

[9] W.H.O., (1980): WHO Expert Committee on Diabetes Mellitus. *Technical Report Series 646, Geneva*

[10] Home, P. and Walford, S. (1984): Diabetes care: whose responsibility? *British Medical Journal, ii,* 713

[11] Deckert, T., Poulsen, J. and Larsen, M. (1978): Prognosis of diabetics with diabetes onset before the age of 31. I & II. *Diabetologia, 14,* 363

[12] Worth, R., Home, P.D., Johnston, D.G., Anderson, J., Ashworth, L., Burrin, J.M., Appleton, D., Binder, C. and Alberti, K.G.M.M. (1982): Intensive attention improves glycaemic control in insulin dependent diabetes. *British Medical Journal, 2,* 1233

[13] Singh, B.M., Holland, M.R. and Thorn, P.A. (1984): Metabolic control of diabetes in general practice clinics: comparison with a hospital clinic. *British Medical Journal, 2,* 726

[14] Hayes, T.M. and Harries, J. (1984): Randomised controlled trial of routine hospital clinics versus routine general practice care for type II diabetics. *British Medical Journal, 2,* 728

[15] Fry, J. (1966): *Profiles of Disease.* Edinburgh: E & S Livingstone

[16] Elwood, P.C., Waters, W.E., Greene, W.J.W., Sweetnam, P. and Wood, M.M. (1969): Symptoms and circulating haemoglobin level. *Journal of Chronic Diseases, 21,* 615

[17] Moore, R.M.A. (1975): In *Screening in General Practice.* Edinburgh: Churchill Livingstone

4
Continuing Care

4.1 The nature of continuing care

Marshall Marinker

The members of a profession and the people whom they serve tend to share ideals, models of professional behaviour. The nature of these models is, in part, a legacy from the history of the profession in a particular society. In part it is a reflection of these memories and beliefs in the mass media. These images are in turn modified by individual experience – the experience of the professionals in their work, and the experience of the persons whom they serve. These models and ideals, which owe much to myth, beliefs and aspirations, have an important effect in shaping professional services. They become incorporated into both the professional ethos and the character and standards of the service which a society expects.

The public and professional image of the district general hospital is rooted not only in the development of biotechnology applied to medicine, but in its reflection in articles and documentaries in the mass media – in books of fiction, films and television serials. The medicine practised may be described as crisis medicine and a high degree of technology is in evidence. The treatment of the patient is humane but anxiety levels are high, technical competence is the most valued characteristic, there is evident critical peer group review, and so on. This popular view of hospital medicine affects not only the expectations of patients, but also the expectations of doctors. Hospital medicine which concerns itself with quite a different sort of care, for example of the elderly infirm or of the mental defective, is known to be professionally less attractive. Indeed among the attempts to make these branches of hospital medicine more attractive are moves to introduce high technology: for example in the name of research, into human development in these fields.

The reason for this preamble in a chapter on the nature of continuing care is that the same forces are at work in shaping general practice. The nature of continuing care is in part rooted in the reality of our social history, but it is also rooted in what we, both patients and doctors, want to believe and in the way in which our image is both reflected and created by the media. Ivan Illich[1] makes the point that our definitions of health are simply a reflection of our cultural values. Indeed, he says that health is a synonym for culture. By the same token medical care intimately reflects what we value in our culture. General practitioners wish to become like the image which they themselves have had an important part in creating.

Perhaps the archetype of this image is the old family doctor. He has been in the same practice for most of his professional lifetime; the people whom he serves have mostly been born, grown up and worked, and will eventually retire and die in his neighbourhood. He delivers the babies of women who were themselves delivered by him. He provides primary and personal care, but above all he provides continuing care. He is totally accessible to his patients, his knowledge of their lives is encyclopaedic and enriched by his knowledge of the families or the individuals. He provides continuing medical care and is himself the embodiment of the continuity of his community. The enormous success of the television series Dr Finlay's Casebook had much to do with the way in which this fictional general practice set in rural Scotland in the 1920s approximated to some sort of cultural archetype with instant appeal for contemporary patients and their doctors. What of the present-day reality?

Continuity and accessibility

There is a remarkable paucity of information concerning the length of time that doctors spend in a particular practice. Traditionally, the career of the general practitioner has been a geographically static one. The doctor entered practice as a young man, either as an assistant or a junior partner, or he established a new practice and for many years thereafter was described as 'building' his practice. By this was meant the establishment of professional relationships with patients, so that he got to know an increasing number of them and they came to look upon him as their own doctor – the first person to whom they would turn with a medical problem. In the United Kingdom it has been the exception rather than the rule for the established general practitioner to move from one locality to another. There are probably many reasons for this relative absence of mobility: first, the emotional investment which the general practitioner makes in his practice; second, the fact that under the National Health Service he cannot sell the goodwill of his practice, and so for most established principals a move from one practice to another is unlikely to bring financial benefit, and is more likely to involve at least a temporary loss of income. Lastly and perhaps most important, the doctor becomes aware that his own diagnostic skills are linked to the vast store of implicit information that he has about those for whom he provides continuing care.

By the same token we know relatively little about the movement of patients between doctors, although potentially much of this information is recorded in the files of Family Practitioner Committees. The estimated annual turnover of 10 per cent of patients[2] conceals considerable differences between the relatively unchanging practice populations of rural areas or the residential neighbourhoods of market towns on the one hand, and practices in metropolitan conurbations on the other. Even if we take the 10 per cent figure as representing the mean of a so-called average practice, this in no way implies that the total practice population changes once in every ten years. Almost certainly this 10 per cent represents a more geographically mobile sub-stratum of the total population, who therefore in themselves present a particular problem in providing and achieving continuity of medical care.

Cartwright,[3] in her study of patients and their doctors, found that two-thirds of the adults whom she interviewed had had the same doctor for at least five years. Half of them had had the same doctor for at least ten years, and just over a third for at least fifteen. She found that 78 per cent of those adults who had been with the same practitioner for fifteen years or more believed that their doctor would know their name if they were to meet in the street. Asked if they thought they might be able to get hold of their general practitioner, or someone acting for him, if they needed him on a Sunday afternoon, or in the middle of the night, 84 per cent of those interviewed thought that they would be able to do so. Cartwright concludes that continuity of care, taken as having the same doctor over several years, is very much a reality in the National Health Service. Her researches, however, also throw light on the personal nature of this continuing care. She took four characteristics of the so-called 'personal doctor', and found the following:

1. Of those interviewed, 66 per cent thought that their doctor would know them by name if he met them in the street.
2. 44 per cent regarded their relationship with him as friendly, rather than business like.
3. 28 per cent thought that they might discuss a personal problem which was not a strictly medical one with him.
4. 75 per cent thought that he was good about explaining things to them fully.

Although only 11 per cent of the patients interviewed had a general practitioner who fulfilled all four of these criteria of personal doctoring, 88 per cent of them had a doctor who met

one or more of the criteria.
Two other findings in Cartwright's study have a bearing on continuity. The first is her measure of the geographical proximity of the doctor's surgery to the patient's home. Four-fifths of the patients said that it took them less than a quarter of an hour to get to their doctor's surgery and just over half of them normally walked all the way. The second concerns the role of the general practitioner as a family doctor. In her sample, Cartwright found that 72 per cent of the people who lived in households with relatives had the same doctor as all their relatives in the household, while 85 per cent of patients had a family doctor in that at least one other relative had the same general practitioner.

How often do doctors and patients meet?

There have been several studies which measure the frequency of contact between patients and their doctors. Reports from a number of practices suggest that the number of consultations per person per year is steadily falling. Some 25 years ago figures of four consultations a year for male patients and five for female patients were the norm. Average rates found in 1981–82 Study of Morbidity in England and Wales[4] were 2.7 for males and 4.0 for females. Much more dramatic has been the decline in home visiting. From a comparison of figures from a number of practices a mean trend reduction of 60 per cent is calculated for the years 1949–1971.
The Third National Morbidity Survey suggested that in the year 1981–82, 65 per cent of male persons on the general practitioner's list and 77 per cent of female persons consulted. These figures do not vary much with age or sex, except for children of both sexes under the age of 5: over 98 per cent of these children attend at least once a year. The Second National Morbidity Survey shows that these average figures conceal a number of interesting variations. For both sexes the decade between the ages of 5 and 15 is characterized by a relatively low annual consultation rate, less than 2. In the three decades which follow between 15 and 45 years, this consulting rate remains approximately the same for males, but more than doubles for females. For both sexes after the age of 75 years the rates are at their highest: 4.5 per annum. In the same study some 23 per cent of males and 32 per cent of females consulted the doctor four times or more during the year. Around 13 per cent of males and 20 per cent of females consulted six times or more.
In two studies,[5,6] despite the commonly held belief that there is a tendency for members of the same family to consult frequently, no significant correlation was found between parents and

children, or between spouses, or between siblings in their rates of consultation.

Marsh[7] records that in his own practice, where as a result of management decisions the consultation rate was reduced to 2.3 per patient per annum, the rate of contacts with families was quite high. He recorded contacts with at least 82 per cent of households where two individuals were registered with the practice. Where three or four individuals were registered, 95 to 96 per cent of households were contacted. In those households with five or more persons registered with the doctor, there was contact with 100 per cent in the course of one year.

Studies in the United Kingdom show that consultation rates differ between one region and another. Consultation rates in Scotland are two or three times higher than those in England, and within England there is a high to low gradient of consultation between areas in the north and south. A number of studies[8, 9, 10] show higher than average consulting rates in mining areas: these rates can only in part be explained by such features as morbidity or sickness certification of miners, since similarly high rates are found for women and children in mining areas. Consulting rates have also been shown to vary with the type of area: residential, urban, rural and so on.[8]

What becomes clear from an examination of the evidence about consulting rates is that each particular part of the country, perhaps each individual general practice, develops an idiosyncratic frequency and rhythm of doctor/patient communication, which in part reflect the general culture in which we live, are modified by local circumstances like tradition, industry, patterns of morbidity and so on, and are finally mediated by the personality of the doctor providing care, and by his practice organization. For example, it has been found that older and more experienced doctors tend to have lower consulting rates than younger ones.[8, 11] Consultation rates seem to vary inversely with list size[12] and fall when an effective appointment system is introduced.

The pattern of primary, personal and continuing care which was built into the structure of the National Health Service may have been based on a mythology about general practice in the past, but it appears to be a present reality. The advent of group practice seems to have done little to erode the one-to-one nature of the doctor/patient relationship, but the considerable growth of the primary health care team may be a threat to continuity of care by a personal doctor: when care of the individual is split between doctor, community nurse, health visitor and social worker, there is a danger that a dilution of responsibility will take place which Balint[13] described as a 'collusion of anonymity'.

Further, the introduction and growth of deputizing services in general practice, such that night and weekend calls are dealt with by doctors other than those in the group or partnership, have seemed to pose a further threat to continuity of care. A study of one such deputizing service[14] showed that calls handled by the deputizing services represented approximately 1 per cent of all the subscribers' consultations, 5 per cent of all their home visits and half of those calls received between midnight and 07.00 hours. The author of the study concluded that at this level of activity the concept of personal doctoring was not threatened.

So much for the data concerning the patterns of doctor/patient contact. What does continuity of care mean, other than that patients see their doctors on average about three times a year? In what way is continuity of care different from episodic care? The nature of continuing care is related to the natural history of man and the natural history of unhealth.

The natural history of man

From the general practitioner's point of view the care of the unborn baby poses particular problems. The physical health of the mother, her state of nutrition, control of disease processes such as diabetes mellitus or high blood pressure, drugs both prescribed and unprescribed which the mother takes, and the cigarettes which she may smoke can all affect the integrity of the developing foetus. It is at this stage of life that the general practitioner will need to be particularly sensitive to the emotional environment into which the child will be born. Is the child wanted? By both parents? What does the mother feel about the baby inside her, and about the coming labour? Such considerations are an essential part of the care which the general practitioner must provide for the pregnant mother, and the importance of these aspects of general practice care is in no way diminished by the fact that increasingly the confinement will take place in a hospital obstetric unit under the care of a specialist obstetrician.

The infant is vulnerable to all sorts of physical and emotional hazards. The role of the general practitioner in monitoring the development of the growing infant, the provision of immunization against infectious diseases, and in observing the changing patterns of emotions and communications within the family are dealt with in chapter 4.2. The attention which the doctor gives to the care of a particular baby will in part be influenced by his perception of the levels of risks involved.

More than anything else, the health of infants may be predicted by the social circumstances of the parents. Social class remains the most sensitive predictor of perinatal mortality. The infant born out of wedlock to a 16- or 17-year-old girl from social class 5, living in an overcrowded household, is more likely to have an undeclared congenital abnormality, or to succumb to an infection, than a child of similar age and weight who has been born into a middle-class marriage. In making a decision about how and where to manage a respiratory illness in an individual infant, the general practitioner must not only weigh the evidence from clinical findings, but also from the social circumstances which may predict the outcome of the illness much more powerfully than the clinical findings.

During the first five years of life the general practitioner will have monitored the development of the infant, ensured adequate immunization against infectious diseases (and here again he will need to ensure that children from socially vulnerable families are not omitted from these programmes), and for the most part he will be dealing with minor upper respiratory episodes of illness experienced by the 'catarrhal child'. Here the problems are not only those of the sensible management of minor self-limiting illnesses, but also the importance of early intervention in the more serious illnesses of childhood, a task made particularly difficult by the notorious suddenness with which a clinical picture can change in the course of a child's illness. The sudden onset of massive respiratory failure in a toddler who, only a few hours before, seemed to have mild coryza is among the unavoidable accidents of even the most careful health care. The presentation by the parents of a sick child, and the way in which the doctor responds to this, lay down the future pattern of health and health care for the growing individual. The frequency and the urgency with which a child is presented to the doctor may be factors not only of the child's inherent morbidity, but of a parent's anxiety about the health of the child, or about the mother's uncertainty about her own competence or even 'goodness' as a mother.

With the onset of puberty and the subsequent adolescence of the individual, the major problems, by and large, are not those of physical morbidity but of psychological and social adjustment to the adult world. The young person is now encountering his or her own sexuality, is negotiating new relationships with peers and with parents and, particularly later in adolescence, is often in healthy rebellion against the status quo of which the general practitioner may be seen as an arch proponent. As chapter 4.3, on adolescence, discusses, there is a particular problem for the general practitioner who may be seen by the adolescent patient as an extension of unwanted parental authority.

For the young adult physical health will be at its peak. The young men will be infrequent attenders except when minor and recurrent infections or injury force them to seek certification of incapacity for work, and young women will seek advice about birth control, sexual adjustment, pregnancy and the care of their babies. The unskilled worker will be at the height of his earning power, and will quickly assume the independence of what Maslow calls self-actualization. At the other extreme the professional men or women may still be postgraduate students, or at best will be novices, and relatively low paid ones, in a long professional life. For them total independence and self-actualization may be delayed by one or two decades. Depending on the social class and culture of the individual, there will be different patterns of family support from the grandparent generation, and so different emphases on the need for health care.

Some of the chronic diseases, for example those conditioned by congenital defects, or diabetes mellitus, epilepsy, peptic ulceration, asthma and so on, will already have made their appearance in the life of the young adult. By middle age physical health is beginning to deteriorate, even though psychological maturity and social power may be at their maximum. The young adult who was a heavy cigarette smoker from youth is now producing a great deal of sputum, and is becoming short of breath even on mild exertion. It is now that he can no longer be described as suffering from a smoker's cough, but as a chronic bronchitic. The house-owner has been examined for further life insurance, and is found to have a raised blood pressure which may require life-long treatment. The risks from cancer and coronary thrombosis are at their height.

For all except the unskilled labourer, middle age marks the peak of social status. In work, a plateau of promotion has been reached, the family will be at its geographically most stable and involvement in the social life of the neighbourhood will be at its greatest. By that very same token, life's disappointments may be at their keenest. The fact that many of the goals which the individual has set himself cannot be achieved becomes self-evident. The physical and emotional changes of the menopause, the climacteric which may well have an emotional reality, even if it does not have a proven physical one, are underscored by the natural diminution in physical standards, the break up of the original nucleur family as children grow up, leave home and get married themselves, and the increasing loss by death of parents or older siblings. Many of these losses, both actual losses and imagined ones whose reality for the individual is indisputable, may be expressed to the doctor in the form of a so-called depressive illness. Much more than the exhibition of psychotropic drugs will be required in helping the individual to accommodate to fundamental changes in life style, life expectations and life supports.

In old age the individual may face an increasing physical disability, a slow deterioration of the senses which keep him or her in touch with the environment, a social isolation all the more barren because it may be hidden within the constructs of what appears to be an intact family, and the emotional isolation which comes from lack of social contact, and from an increasing loss by death of others in the same age-group: spouses, siblings and friends. In our own contemporary culture, which is youth oriented and relatively materialistic, the elderly are peculiarly vulnerable. The advent of the printing press and literacy in western society has robbed the old of their traditional wisdom: they are no longer the memory bank from which the culture renews itself. The increasing sense of privacy in family life and the growing social and geographical mobility of the modern family in our society tend increasingly to leave old people bereft of the physical, emotional and social supports which make life bearable. Through its institutions a welfare state attempts to make good some of these losses, and the general practitioner has an important role both in identifying need and mobilizing resources.

Like birth, death may be wanted or unwanted, unexpected or planned, damagingly premature or damagingly delayed. The physical event itself may be painful or easy and the emotional and social setting in which it occurs, supportive or non-existent. When death occurs in the family, it is followed, as a birth is followed, by a period of readjustment. The coming to terms with a loss may be as emotionally demanding and sometimes as stormy as the coming to terms with the arrival of a first child.

This brief description of the human life span is, of course, much more a caricature than an account. Each individual and each family will depart in many important ways from the characteristics and events which have been described, much as the individual experience of a disease will depart in many ways from the classical descriptions of the textbook. But medical care takes place against some such shifting patterns of physical endowment, emotional experience and social support as that set down in this chapter. At every stage of human life the individual is vulnerable in a particular way, and the general practitioner must be sensitive to the particular vulnerabilities of each individual. A perspective based on the facts of human development is at least as important to the general practitioner, as a perspective based on the facts of human pathology.

The natural history of unhealth

It is impossible to describe a disease without reference to changes over time. Even throughout the classical period of medicine, from the days of Hippocrates to the sixteenth century when medical theory was concerned with the constitution of the individual rather than with disease entities, doctors recognized the importance of prognosis. With the advent of Sydenham in the sixteenth century the description of diseases in terms of the march of events opened up the way, for example, to differentiate rashes and fevers into the discrete entities of measles, scarlatina and so on. Because of the infinitely slower tempo of the chronic diseases, the later description of these depended not on a chronicle of events over time, but on the findings of the pathologist. Even now the natural history of many chronic diseases and conditions has yet to be described, although much good work has already emerged from research in general practice. For example, Fry's study of catarrhal children[15] helps us to understand the natural course of events, what sort of outcomes to expect, and how to judge the results of our own interventions.

Preventive medicine in general practice has had a variable success. Immunization against infectious diseases has certainly transformed the picture of child health, although the most vulnerable children are the most likely not to be presented for immunization. Health education, despite the impressive rhetoric of those who advocate it, has yielded poor results. The majority of infants continue to be fed on cow's milk, despite the clear advantages of breast feeding, although there is some current evidence of a reversal of this trend. Mothers continue to produce obese infants, teenagers begin the crippling habit of cigarette smoking, unwanted infants are conceived, venereal diseases, chronic bronchitis and lung cancer, coronary thrombosis, obesity and road traffic accidents remain major health hazards, although in theory much could be done to reduce these risks for the individual. Nonetheless, despite these gloomy facts, much may be accomplished by the general practitioner which may be of great value despite the difficulty of quantifying the results.

If the model of health education is simply the transmission of an authoritative message from doctor to patient, assessed in terms of the number of messages remembered, the number understood and the compliance of resulting behaviour, little can be expected. What is required is not the transmission of messages but changes in the beliefs of the patient.[16] It is not enough for doctor and patient to share the knowledge that heavy cigarette smoking is associated with heart and lung disease. The doctor must also understand the role of cigarette smoking in the life of his patient, the cultural values of the group within which the patient lives, the meanings that he ascribes, for example, to the symptoms of chronic bronchitis. For the doctor, chronic bronchitis means the slow progression from morning cough and sputum to increasing shortness of breath, exacerbations of acute infection, the short-term success of therapy, the days off work which lengthen into weeks and then into months as the years go by, early retirement, the strain on family finance and family relationships, the gradual impoverishment of life and the insidious onset of heart failure. For many patients this picture represents the norm of life experienced in the neighbourhood and the family, and the price of deviating from the normative behaviour of heavy cigarette smoking, or the deprivation of what cigarette smoking gives and represents, may be too high a price to pay. Unless the general practitioner is prepared to understand his patient's values, and to try to change the patient's beliefs about life styles and life chances, so-called health education will result in nothing but the clash of mutual disappointments. More than this, a didactic and insensitive approach to health education which becomes doctor-oriented propaganda may so damage the doctor/patient relationship, that neither doctor nor patient can make effective use of the relationship then or later.

Early diagnosis demands a knowledge of the natural history of diseases: the management of recurrent sore throat, or frozen shoulder, or bereavement is rooted in the doctor's knowledge of what to expect, and his vigilance when the natural history of the patient's disease deviates markedly from what is to be expected: when he suspects that the sore throat may be infectious mononucleosis, the frozen shoulder the site of a secondary carcinoma, the bereavement a deepening or suicidal depression. Not only is prognosis important, but a knowledge of how the patient endured previous episodes of unhealth can be helpful. Not only the patient's drug idiosyncrasies, but also the ability to tolerate feeling ill, the amount of present or future oriented anxiety which illness brings, what frightens the patient, how much anxiety he is able to tolerate, how compliant he is likely to be in taking tablets, or staying in bed – all have much to add to the doctor's individual management. Much of this information may be recorded in the previous notes (see chapter 1.4), but much often remains implicit in the doctor's knowledge of his patient, so that the doctor who knows his patient well is able to respond to the patient's problem in such a way as to meet the peculiar characteristics of the individual's strengths, weaknesses, anxieties and patterns of behaviour.

In Chapter 1.1, on Health and Unhealth, I suggested that disease processes alone account only for a part of the morbidity with which the general practitioner is asked to deal. More therefore than a knowledge of the natural history of disease processes, is required. Thus, it is an accepted part of the corpus of medical knowledge that epilepsy is more common in children who have experienced febrile fits, but this is not very useful knowledge, because there is no known way of preventing the onset of epilepsy, and the fact is only available to us with hindsight. There are other, much less well documented observations about the natural history of unhealth which may be more useful, even though they have not been adequately described or quantified. The way in which individuals within a family tend to occupy the sick role can sometimes help to elucidate the most puzzling of consultations. The young girl who presents with painful periods and eventually has one or two admissions to hospital for a dilatation and curettage, who presents with mysterious abdominal pain and eventually has a relatively normal looking appendix removed, may well go on to present with infertility or dyspareunia in her twenties or thirties, when it may be possible to uncover the deep uncertainty that she feels about her body and about her role as a woman. The schoolboy who is identified by his mother as 'frail' and is often absent because of recurrent upper respiratory-tract infections, becomes the young man who settles for a lifetime of unemployment with a chronic back condition for which there is never convincing physical evidence.

A common criticism of medicine in the United Kingdom is that we have a disease service rather than a health service. Implied in this criticism is the recommendation that good primary medical care is anticipatory care, and that we should be involved in much presymptomatic diagnosis. Resources for presymptomatic diagnosis are, of course, strictly limited, but it would be wrong to imagine that the arguments against prescriptive screening in general practice are concerned only with the finite nature of resources (see Chapter 1.6).

It is common knowledge that a large proportion of patients with high blood pressure and diabetes mellitus are undetected until late in the natural history of the diseases, when symptoms are becoming evident. A number of criteria by which the appropriateness of presymptomatic screening may be judged has been developed.[17] These are that the clinical problem must be important in terms of frequency and seriousness; that the diagnostic criteria for the condition are not equivocal; that there must be an acceptable and successful treatment and that screening is acceptable in terms of the discomfort which it may cause the individual and the public expenditure which it may entail for society. When these criteria are applied to the major conditions normally considered as possible subjects for screening in general practice – diabetes mellitus, cancer of the cervix, iron-deficiency anaemia, or bacteriuria of pregnancy – no clear-cut case emerges. In considering the challenge presented by moderate to severe hypertension, where the health sequelae are known to be serious and the advantages of treatment have been proven, the arguments for case finding are thought to be superior to those of screening.[18, 19] In considering the pattern of contacts between doctors and patients in his own practice, Tudor Hart concluded that every patient in his practice who had a raised blood pressure would be seen at least once in the course of five years. Consequently over a five-year period, a policy of case finding would result in a complete index or list of patients with the condition, who might then be offered treatment.

Continuing care which is also anticipatory requires choices to be made in the allocation of scarce resources. For example, as yet there is no convincing argument in favour of developmental assessment of infants in general practice. In terms of yield, a search among the elderly members of a practice will undoubtedly reveal much in the way of locomotor and sensory losses; what has still to be proven is that identifying these disabilities will result in interventions which improve the health of the individual old person, when this is measured not by morbidity labels alone, or volume of treatment given, but in terms of physical and social function.

The doctor/patient relationship

Balint[13] describes the doctor/patient relationship as a mutual investment company. Into each consultation the doctor and the patient bring the investment that they have made in the relationship with one another. The way in which the patient presents the complaint, the sort of questions that the doctor can ask, and the sort of answers which may be expected, the areas of life which will be dealt with and those which will be alluded to but not explored, the decisions that the doctor makes about a physical examination, and the way in which he will conduct it, the decision to refer, and to whom to refer, and so much more will depend on a whole series of negotiated agreements between doctor and patient which can never have been chronicled in the medical record. Before the advent of the National Health Service when a doctor moved his practice he would sell its good will to the incoming doctor. What was sold was the habit of the patient to consult at a particular place. What can never be sold, what can never be transferred from one doctor to another, is the stock of the mutual investment company.

The characteristics of the doctor/patient relationship, the skill in using it both for diagnosis and treatment are outside the scope of this chapter. The reader is referred to the relevant literature. Just as, outside the consulting-room, each relationship develops within its own time span, and according to its own inherent tempo, so does the doctor/patient relationship. The ease and intimacy which may develop quickly with one patient, may take years to develop with another. Sometimes the patient may test the ability to trust a doctor through a number of episodes of illness before real trust will be given. Much depends also on the personality of the doctor, on his ability to understand himself and not to fall into the trap of allowing each consultation merely to rehearse the ways in which he deals with his own feelings of anger, sadness, anxiety or need to be loved. It is for this reason that skill in the handling of the doctor/patient relationship cannot come from reading alone, but from the careful monitoring of real life experience.[13]

Family doctoring

Because of the relatively long period of association between individual doctors and their patients, and because of the fact that most families tend to register with the same doctor, or practice, the general practitioner is often described as a family doctor, and tries in all conscience to behave in accordance with this public image which he and his patients have created. Among those who seek to create a theory of general practice, the perspectives of family medicine have proved most attractive.[20] These perspectives are reinforced for general practitioners by the proponents of family psychiatry.[21] There are, however, many pitfalls, both for the general practitioner and the patient, in the ideologies of so-called family medicine.[22] There are problems of confidentiality. Much information about family life and the behaviour of individual members of the family may be given to the doctor, but the only information which the doctor is able to use with a particular patient, is information which is common ground between them. A young man may present with depression. The general practitioner may know from his wife that their sexual life is unhappy, but the information is of little use to him unless the patient himself can talk about it. Instinctively, the doctor might be motivated to explore this area of the patient's life, but may be inhibited from doing so because he wishes to avoid the danger of breaking the confidence of his patient's wife: for example, that she has become emotionally involved with another man.

The family perspective involves the general practitioner in the question of conflict of interest. An elderly incontinent patient may want to go on living at home for as long as possible. The general practitioner may believe that this would be in the old person's best interests, but her daughter, on whom she relies for a certain amount of help, has had recurrent bouts of depression, and now feels that she cannot cope. The rebellious adolescent may want to open up about all sorts of anxieties, but may see the so-called family doctor, precisely because he has been such a good friend to the family, as an agent of the parents. Lastly, there is a danger that, by focusing on the family relationships rather than on the needs of the unique individual, that continuing care may no longer be also personal care.

A patient is not a person who has a disease, or the precursor of a disease. A patient is simply someone who consults the doctor. The individuals on the general practitioner's list are not patients at risk, they are persons at risk. It is a dangerous assumption to make that, because the doctor or a member of the family believes that a particular medical problem involves other members of the family, these individuals can unilaterally be accorded the status of patient. They cannot. To summon the husband of a frigid wife, or the mother of a depressed adolescent, is bad general practice, in the name of good family medicine. This can only result in a professional invasion of privacy, a confusion about the goals of medical practice and a loss of integrity in the doctor/patient relationship.

Conclusion

In a strict and literal sense continuing care is an illusion. Totally continuing care, in this sense, would be claustrophobic and controlling: it would confine rather than support the individual. The care of the general practitioner is intermittent, and sometimes the gaps between consultations may be months or years. The practitioner seen by the individual patient as 'his own' may not always be available when he is wanted. Sudden illness may occur when the patient is away from home, or in the middle of the night when a particular practitioner is not on call. On the other hand, because each doctor will be involved with a number of members of the same family, and because one or other member of the family may be consulting at any particular period, there often grows up a network of intimate familiarity between the general practitioner and his patients, which could not be gauged from an examination of the medical record alone.

In the chapters which follow the nature of continuing care is looked at in relationship to the stages of human development. As life progresses, the physical, emotional and social experiences of the individual undergo many changes, and the family itself develops from courtship to retirement. The doctor who is called upon to intervene, often in the most intimate way, in these life events, does not do so only from the static position of a professional role, a status ascribed by society. He is himself a participant in the development of the doctor/patient relationship, and each relationship will bear the stamp not only of the patient's personality and the patient's location in his family and society, but also of the doctor's personality, of the stage of his own human development and his professional development. The skills of continuing care no less than the skills of personal care demand of the doctor an awareness of his own human predicament, and his own professional values.

Previous Chapters (1.4, 1.5) have put forward the case for reforming the record keeping systems of general practice in order to provide effective personal and continuing care. The medical record itself must become a sensitive tool for diagnosis and management. A demographic profile of the practice population in the shape of a card index age/sex register will sooner or later come to be seen as essential in the provision of anticipatory care. By the same token disease indices for conditions like hypertension, diabetes mellitus and so on may become common place. It would be foolish to underestimate the magnitude of work involved in such reforms, work both by general practitioners and by their clerical staff. The wish to carry out these reforms will only follow on their proven utility in improving the health of the people for whom general practitioners care. Much research in the field remains to be done. The motivation to reform will come from the general practitioners' desire to provide that personal and continuing care which is still best expressed, not in the results of empirical research, but in our myths, our traditions and our professional rhetoric.

References

[1] Illich, Ivan (1974): *Medical Nemesis.* London: Boyar

[2] Royal College of General Practitioners (1973): *Present State and Future Needs*, 3rd ed. Reports from General Practice No. 16

[3] Cartwright, A. (1967): *Patients and their Doctors.* London: Routledge & Kegan Paul

[4] Royal College of General Practitioners, Office of Population Censuses and Surveys, Department of Health and Social Security (1986): *Morbidity Statistics from General Practice 1981–82*. HMSO Series MB5 No. 1

[5] Marinker, M. (1969): Unpublished data

[6] Courtenay, M.J.S., Curwen, M.P. Daw, D., Robinson, J. and Stern, M. J.: (1974) Frequent Attendance in a Family Practice. *Journal of the Royal College of General Practitioners, 24*, 251.
[7] Marsh, G.N.: Data from M.D. thesis
[8] Williams, W.O. (1970): A Study of General Practitioner's Work Load in South Wales 1965–1966. *Journal of the Royal College of General Practitioners, 19*, Supp. 1
[9] Ryder, J.G., Waters, W.H.R., Charnock, R.B. and Lunn, J.E. (1969): A Study of Work Load in a Mining Area Practice. *Journal of the Royal College of General Practitioners, 17*, 361
[10] Art, J.T. (1971): The Health of Coal Mining Communities. *Journal of the Royal College of General Practitioners, 21*, 517
[11] Morrell, D.C., Gage, H.G. and Robinson, N.R. (1970): Patterns of Demand in General Practice. *Journal of the Royal College of General Practitioners, 19*, 331
[12] Wright, P.J. (1968): General Practice in South West England. *Journal of the Royal College of General Practitioners.* Report from General Practice No. 8
[13] Balint, M. (1964): *The Doctor, His Patient and the Illness.* London: Pitman
[14] Williams, B.T., Dickson, R.A. and Knowelden, J. (1973): BMA Deputising Service in Sheffield, 1970. *British Medical Journal, 1*, 593
[15] Fry, J. (1961): *The Catarrhal Child.* London: Butterworth
[16] Bennett, A.E. (1976): *Communication Between Doctors and Patients.* Nuffield Provincial Hospitals Trust, Oxford University Press
[17] Wilson, J.M.G. and Junger, G. (1968): *Principles and Practice of Screening for Disease.* HMSO
[18] Adler, M.W. (1976): Detection of Blood Pressure in General Practice – Screening or Case Finding. *Journal of the Royal College of General Practitioners, 26*, 171
[19] Hart, J.T. (1975): The Management of High Blood Pressure in General Practice. *Journal of the Royal College of General Practitioners, 25*, 160
[20] Williams, J.I. and Leaman, T.L. (1973): *In Family Practice.* London: W.B. Saunders
[21] Howells, J.G. (1970): Family Psychiatry and Family Practice. *The Practitioner, 205*, 280
[22] Marinker, M. (1976): The Family in Medicine. *Proceedings of the Royal Society of Medicine, 69*, 115

4.2 Infancy and childhood

David Morrell and Margaret Pollak

More lives are lost during the fifteen months spanning the last three months of pregnancy and the first year of life than in the succeeding twenty-five years. The dangers in late pregnancy are mainly those associated with a failure of foetal growth. In labour death is most commonly due to complications affecting the blood supply to the brain and to severe congenital malformations. In the peri-natal period the precise cause of death is often obscure, but is often associated with low-birth-weight babies. In the first year of life death is most commonly due to respiratory infections and unexplained sudden death (cot deaths): these tend to occur in 'disadvantaged' children such as those of low birth weight. All these problems are more frequent in socially deprived families. Accidental injury is the most common cause of death between 1 and 15 years and shows a social class gradient.

These facts provide a clue to the way in which health care for children should be organized. It must be based on a system which offers continuity from the ante-natal period onwards, and in which the providers of care possess information which will help them to identify the most vulnerable children and make special provision for them.

Organization of care

The organization of the National Health Service, which makes the general practitioner the normal portal of entry to the Service and in which patients normally register and remain with the same general practitioner over a period of years, provides a continuing relationship between patients and general practitioners. Many studies have shown that women in the reproductive age-group and children under the age of 5 years consult the doctor on average about five times each year. This means that a mother of a young family will have plenty of opportunities to get to know her doctor, and he in turn may gather a great deal of information about the young family registered with him. Home visiting, although less common than in the past, still accounts for about one-fifth of the consultations carried out by general practitioners and provides special opportunities for the doctor to learn about the patients' homes and family relationships. A single home visit well used will tell the doctor a great deal about the physical cleanliness of the home, the way food is stored and prepared, over-crowding, the role of the television set and of toys in the life of the family, and in the evening or at a weekend it may tell much about the relative roles of mother and father in the family.

This frequent contact and developing personal relationship forms the ideal setting for the continuity of medical care so desirable for the children. The families for whom an individual doctor is responsible may be identified by keeping an age/sex register, and this makes it possible for the doctor to relate the care he is providing to the population for whom he is responsible. He may then investigate situations where the demand for his services seems either excessive or unusually low, and provide comprehensive programmes of preventive care and surveillance for these families.

To achieve this ideal requires regular information about the care being provided, which means an efficient record system; it also requires an efficient organization to follow up those who fail to avail themselves of the services available. This organization and the provision of preventive and educational services for young families are time consuming, and indeed expensive, and in the past impossible to achieve in many cases. To fill the gaps the local health authorities were given certain statutory responsibilities for the care of children under the age of five. Developments in general practice in the last three decades have led to the concept of the primary health care team consisting of general practitioner, nurse and health visitor and this has greatly altered the situation. At the present time over 75 per cent of the health visitors employed in this country are attached to specific general practices. In this situation some have taken over the administrative arrangements which ensure comprehensive care for the children in the practice under the age of five. The doctor's role remains important, but he is freed from the difficult and time-consuming work of ensuring that all children receive care, that adequate health education and surveillance are provided and that those at special risk are identified. There is, however, some way to go before every general practitioner works alongside a health visitor. In rural communities this may be difficult to achieve for geographical reasons, but in many ways it is less crucial because the rural general practitioner tends to be in much closer day-to-day touch with the patients in his practice than the doctor working in the urban setting. In the big city centres, however, there are still single-handed general practitioners who do not have attached health visitors and in whose practices there is great social and medical need.

It is sometimes difficult to define where the continuing care of young families starts. All births are notified to the health authority and this leads to a visit by the health visitor to the new-born infant within fourteen days of birth. Statutorily, the new-born infant therefore enters the medical care system at this time, but clinically it is much more appropriate for the child to enter the system at the time of conception. This implies that the general practitioner and health visitor should be involved in the care of the infant in the ante-natal period and demands a major commitment of the general practitioner to ante-natal care. In the 1950s general practitioners played a large part in obstetric care and home delivery was then common. Since that time there has been a shift towards institutional obstetric care. At its worst this may mean that the mother on reporting her pregnancy to her general practitioner is referred to hospital and not seen by him again until she has had her baby. During pregnancy she is seen by an ever-changing series of junior hospital doctors. It has been appreciated that this form of care is extremely unsatisfactory, and to counteract it the general practitioner in many cases provides the bulk of ante-natal care in his surgery, the hospital specialist seeing the patient perhaps three or four times during the course of the ante-natal period and delivering the patient in the hospital specialized unit.

In the last five years there has been an increasing realization of the important part which the general practitioner has to play in ante-natal care, and in some of the most enlightened areas the obstetrician has now come out of the hospital and works alongside the general practitioner in his surgery. In such a setting the patient is delivered in the specialist unit but receives all her ante-natal care in the familiar surroundings of her own practice; the first person she may see in the ante-natal clinic is the health visitor who will in due time help her to adapt to her new role of motherhood. This is clearly not possible in every single-handed practice, but it does establish an ideal which may be achieved in many group practices and health centres. It offers continuity of care at a time when it is possible to establish the most important relationship between general practitioner and patient. This is the time to identify the special problems which may occur in the first year of life of the new baby, in terms not only of medical but also of social morbidity.

Objectives of continuing care of children

Given the opportunities of providing continuity of care from the ante-natal period onwards, through infancy and childhood, the general practitioner's role may be considered under the following headings:

- Health education
- Immunization against infection
- Early detection of illness or disability
- Continuing care of children suffering from important disabilities
- Episodic care in response to patient demand.

Health education

The ante-natal period provides an ideal time for health education. There is regular contact with the doctor and health visitor and towards the end of pregnancy the expectant mother will usually have given up work and have time to prepare for the new baby. In many hospitals classes are run to teach mothers techniques to enjoy their experience. In some of these time is also given to instruction about infant feeding and child rearing.

Practices vary in the way they organize their ante-natal care, but many run ante-natal clinics separate from the normal consulting sessions. These have the advantage that they can often be more carefully planned and more leisurely than the normal consulting hours, and those members of staff particularly concerned in obstetric and paediatric care can all be available. Some practices run special classes for expectant mothers, but there is a lot to be said for building education into the routine attendance of each mother. The expectant mother may, for instance, be given an opportunity to talk to the health visitor at each attendance, and the health visitor may initiate this contact where she feels there is particular need. Classes, however, are often attended by those who least need them, while the poorly educated, socially deprived and poorly organized are less likely to attend, and if they do attend are less likely to be able to learn. A more personal approach allows the health visitor to identify the individual's particular problems and communicate in a way which that individual can understand.

The relative contribution of health visitor, midwife and doctor varies in different settings, but it is important that they should have a common policy and not give conflicting advice. This is much easier to achieve in a practice setting than in hospital and is a major argument for the preparation for childbirth to take place in general practice.

The individual mother's needs vary depending particularly on whether she is primigravid or has other children at home. In the former situation education focuses on infant feeding and the general care of the newborn. In the latter it is important to help the family to welcome the new baby without jealousy. Attention must be given in particular to the existing siblings.

Education in the ante-natal period will continue naturally into the post-natal period, early infancy and childhood. At first it will focus on such problems as feeding, sleep patterns, care of the skin. Later, the mother will need to learn what to expect in terms of the child's development and ways in which she can facilitate toilet training, walking, talking and playing and later still discipline. Some special problems, such as accident prevention in the home and the management of the common illnesses of childhood, must also enter the educational programme. Most of this can be built into the normal consultations with the health visitor and doctor and should be seen as a continuing responsibility by both.

Feeding. – There are numerous books on infant feeding, and only general principles will be considered here. Perhaps the most important is that the practice should have an agreed policy. Nothing is more confusing to a young mother than a multiplicity of pieces of conflicting advice. At the same time it is important to be able to tailor advice to the individual. To achieve this it is necessary to understand the special problems and pressures under which the individual is living. The acceptability, for instance, of advice to breast feed will be influenced by the mother's attitude to her own breasts, her husband's attitude, the opinion of mother and mother-in-law, the type of housing and privacy available to the mother and her need to return to work.

In recent years the advantages of breast feeding have been clearly demonstrated, and may be summarized:

1. Breast milk is correctly constituted in its nutritional elements. The baby is less likely to become obese, is less subject to the dangers of electrolyte imbalance which may occur through improperly prepared artificial feeds or at times of illness or climatic extremes.
2. It is sterile and delivered at the right temperature. There is also sound evidence that the breast-fed baby is more resistant to infection and less susceptible to atopic problems.
3. It is easily accessible and cheap.
4. It brings mother and child into a close relationship and there is evidence that this conveys significant psychological advantages (bonding).

These very real advantages are, however, unlikely to convince a mother who, for cultural or personal reasons, finds the whole exercise repugnant, or who has to return to work six weeks after delivery. It is also important in discussing this subject with expectant mothers to stress that like all skills it takes a little time to acquire and she must be prepared to encounter and overcome early difficulties.

Discussion of feeding should start at the first antenatal visit when the doctor will normally examine the breasts and nipples. There are few contraindications to breast feeding and also few pointers as to whether it will be successfully established. The size of the breasts is no guide to success or failure, but a badly inverted nipple may cause problems unless it can be drawn out in pregnancy. Sore and cracked nipples are a common cause of failure and their preparation by regular rough towelling and expression of colostrum in later pregnancy may be helpful. Following delivery breast feeding will normally be established in hospital. A crucial time for ensuring success is when the mother returns home. She is likely to become more active. The baby is likely to react to a change in surroundings, and this is a time when a mother can lose her confidence and decide that it is easier to measure out the feeds and see that they are consumed than trust to her own body. This is therefore a time for close supervision and support from the health visitor and general practitioner.

If artificial feeding is selected by the mother it is important that she should not be made to feel a failure. She should be advised that low solute milks have considerable advantages. Their protein content is more closely similar to breast milk and they contain less sodium and phosphorus than the old full cream milks. It is most important that mothers feeding their babies with dried milks should be supervised in the preparation of the feed. There is a tendency to use heaped rather than level measures of milk and this can lead to overfeeding and electrolyte disturbance. The old formula of 2½ ounces per pound body weight still holds good, but may be translated into 150 millilitres per kilogram body weight. Babies, however, like adults, vary in their food requirements and generally make their feelings known. If a baby is being correctly fed the fact that he is restless or apparently dissatisfied should never be an excuse for changing from one artificial preparation to another. The baby may be having too little or too much, or the hole in the teat may be too small or too big, but the formulation of the milk is rarely to blame.

Accident prevention.– Accidents are the most common cause of death in children aged 6 months to 15 years and the home is more dangerous than the roads; burns are the most common cause of serious injuries. This is therefore an important subject for health education. The hazards to which a child is exposed can best be judged by a home visit. This is undertaken by a health visitor shortly after birth, but the doctor should be equally aware of this common cause of morbidity when he visits young families in his practice.

The unguarded fire is perhaps the most common hazard encountered in the home. Others include the saucepan handles extending outwards from the cooker which may be grabbed by the curious child. Detergents, disinfectants and drugs which are stored at floor level or within easy reach of the exploring child are a common cause of disaster. Some toys are potentially lethal as is the long flex to the iron or television set. Recently the dangers of some imported medicines, e.g. 'Asian Tonic', have been demonstrated. The doctor who is consciously looking for these hazards will encounter them all too often in his home visits. A personal word of advice will do far more good than posters and television programmes.

Minor illness in infancy and childhood. — The infant and young child suffer many minor illnesses as they build up their resistance to common infections. Mothers are often concerned as to when it is appropriate to consult the doctor and when they should be capable of coping with the problem on their own. While the doctor should always be prepared to advise a mother about her child's illness if it is causing anxiety, there are many common problems which can be managed at home if the mother is taught how to manage them. Respiratory and gastrointestinal infections are by far the most common cause of illness in childhood. In the first year of life they may be life-threatening, but in later childhood they are common and usually self-limiting and mothers should be taught about the significance of common symptoms.

The catarrhal period of development has been well described by Fry[1] and mothers should be helped to understand this difficult phase of child development. The symptoms of diarrhoea and vomiting occur in the same age-group as the catarrhal syndrome[2] and clearly the gastrointestinal tract responds in the same way as the respiratory tract to new infectious challenges. Mothers may be helped to respond to these problems by advance warning and specific advice. Appropriate positioning of a child with coryza at night with no pillow and the foot of the cot raised will often ameliorate a troublesome night cough. Maintaining a warm moist atmosphere in the bedroom will help the child with a dry cough. Immediate restriction of food but not fluid in a child suffering from vomiting or diarrhoea will usually bring such episodes to a halt within twenty-four hours, and before any serious complications have occurred. The correct management of minor trauma in the home can prevent secondary infection.

Mothers are usually eager to receive advice on these common problems. If they do not receive it from the doctor or health visitor they will seek it elsewhere, and not uncommonly this leads to unnecessary anxiety and alarm for the patient and out-of-hours calls for the doctor. The positive approach to the education of parents in managing the common illnesses of childhood, including the value or otherwise of prescribed medication, should form part of the continuing care of children and clear guidance should be given as to when and how to seek medical aid.

Immunization

Immunization against infectious diseases has been one of the main reasons for the fall in morbidity and mortality from these diseases in the last fifty years. Despite this there are many children who are incompletely protected against these diseases. This represents a major challenge to the general practitioner. If he maintains an age/sex register and good records he should be able constantly to monitor the immunization status of the children in his practice. If a health visitor is attached she will normally undertake this task and will follow up those who fail to attend for immunization.

In some practices immunization is undertaken in the context of the normal surgery consultation, but many general practitioners set aside time for a special clinic for under-five-year-olds at which developmental tests and immunization are carried out. This certainly facilitates the supervision of children in this particular respect.

The recommended schedules for immunizations are constantly under review. It is generally agreed that the immune response is improved if immunization is given after the age of six months. At the same time it is equally clear that the dangers of whooping cough are greatest in the first six months of life. Most authorities now recommend that immunization against pertussis, diphtheria, tetanus and polio should be commenced at the age of three months. A second dose is given six to eight weeks later and a third dose after a further five to six months. Immunization against measles is recommended about the age of one year. Vaccination against smallpox is not recommended routinely. Before school entry a booster injection against diphtheria, tetanus and polio is usually given. B.C.G. is administered at the age of 10 to 12 years for Mantoux negative children, and rubella vaccine is given to girls at the age of 11 to 12 years.

Immunization against whooping cough and measles may very rarely be followed by neurological complications. The risk of severe and permanent disability from these procedures has been estimated in a recent study as 1 in 300,000.[2] The risks of morbidity and mortality from whooping cough and measles in an unimmunized population are estimated to be far greater. There is some evidence that the risks to children with a past or family history of convulsions in first degree relatives or neurological damage in infancy is greater than to those without such a history and for this reason such children should not be immunized against pertussis and should be given immunoglobulin with their measles immunization.

Early detection of illness

By virtue of the fact that he has a defined population for whom he is responsible, and that he has a continuing relationship with them, the general practitioner is well placed to identify those families in his practice who are particularly vulnerable to illness. He may in addition provide continuing developmental assessment for all the children in his practice. Resources in general practice, however, are always limited and the object of identifying vulnerable families is to ensure that they in particular receive adequate supervision.

Identifying vulnerable children. — Children may be particularly vulnerable to physical illness as a result of antenatal or perinatal complications. A small-for-dates infant is the classic example and requires close follow up in the first year of life. Less common examples are infants who have suffered respiratory problems in the first hours of life, infants delivered after an antepartum haemorrhage, or infants subjected to traumatic deliveries. The general practitioner involved in the antenatal and early postnatal care of these children will be aware of their special needs.

There are, however, many other factors best known to the general practitioner which influence the likely progress of the newborn through infancy and childhood. These are not simply gross deficiencies in housing or resources. Pollak[3] has shown that children may live side by side in neighbouring houses in the same street but their developmental levels will differ if the content of their lives is different. The factors which influence the development of children are complex. Bowlby[4] stressed the need for a warm, intimate and continuing relationship for a child to achieve mature emotional development. Pringle[5] has described how the emotional climate of the home depends on the success of the parents' marriage, and that temperamental, intellectual or sexual incompatibility may lead to a tense atmosphere which almost inevitably affects the child's adjustment to life.

There is abundant evidence that the battered child is likely to be born of parents who have been treated similarly themselves, who have been subjected to constant parental criticism and deprived of good mothering. As parents themselves they often have unrealistically high expectations of their baby, are frequently socially isolated and fail to find in each other the fulfilment of their personal needs.[6] It has been shown that there is a higher incidence of behaviour disorders in the children of parents who suffer from chronic psychoneurosis, but that this is not true of parents suffering from psychoses.[7] These and other studies will guide the general practitioner in drawing up a list (Table I) of the children in his practice who are particularly vulnerable to physical, emotional and intellectual problems in the early years of childhood.

The baby

Antenatal
Multiple pregnancy, antepartum haemorrhage, toxaemia of pregnancy, rhesus incompatibility

Intranatal
Prematurity, small-for-dates baby, complicated delivery

The family

Problem families, broken homes, one parent families, marital disharmony, low social class

Parents

Psychoneurosis, chronic physical illness, alcoholism, working mothers with inadequate child minding

The home

Overcrowding, multiple occupancy, homelessness, a history of accidents in the home

Siblings

Truancy, children kept at home without adequate reason, poor readers or children with learning problems, children attending special schools

Table I. – Salient factors leading to physical and other problems in early childhood

It is not difficult for the doctor or the health visitor to apply these criteria to every child born into the practice. The information required to make a decision should be known to the doctor and should be noted in his records; in this way he can identify those children at particular risk and make special provision for them.

Developmental examination. — During the last two decades there have been a number of reports including recommendations about primary care for children and the objective of these has been to set goals and establish uniform standards for paediatric services in the United Kingdom.[8,9,10] Among these reports the subject of a routine examination of the pre-school child has loomed large. A few definitions about examining young children are probably in order. Screening is the practice where a health professional initiates contact with an apparently healthy child and applies a test in order to detect deviations from normality. In the case of children its purpose is the detection of mental and physical handicaps, defects of hearing and vision, behaviour disorder and neurological disability.

Surveillance refers to an ongoing process which includes a number of preventive and anticipatory measures going beyond the mere quest for disease. This is part and parcel of the day-to-day contact that general practitioners have with children during surgery consultations and home visits.

Assessment refers to a more specialized examination carried out because of suspected abnormality or the presence of risk factors and is usually performed by those with additional skills in the examination of children. Although the term is sometimes used synonymously with screening it is probably more appropriate to use it when referring to more extensive examination procedures. The following section is principally concerned with the subject of screening.

While it is necessary to submit any screening test to the criteria for all screening procedures,[11] developmental screening covers a wide variety of tests of motor, visual, hearing and emotional development and too strict an interpretation of Wilson's criteria may not be possible when many of the tests still used in screening have not yet been fully validated. The situation in paediatric screening is different in that normal development is often dependent on the appropriate maturation of interdependent skills: thus hearing defects will affect speech, squint may affect binocular vision and vision and hearing will affect intellectual development. In addition, social behaviour may have permanent affects on emotional and intellectual development and learning skills.

A wide variety of screening tests for physical, emotional and intellectual impairment have been developed. Some may easily be learned and applied by the general practitioner and health visitor. Others are more sophisticated or time consuming and require special skills and the general practitioners' role may simply be to be alert and refer doubtful cases to the paediatrician.

The logistics of organizing screening clinics within a practice with the aim of achieving acceptable attendance rates are not to be underestimated. In most practices such clinics are a combined operation between general practitioner and health visitor. In some partnership practices one doctor develops special skills and undertakes all the developmental work. Where general practitioners have accepted responsibilities for comprehensive child care including screening, there has been no evidence of interference with the all purpose concept of the general practitioner. Most general practitioners still look to the health visitor to take the initiative in preventive paediatrics. Relationships with health visitors have been greatly helped by health visitor attachments to general practice. The contention that health visitors are less effective than doctors in detecting early signs of abnormality in children may only be true for a limited range of conditions and for the majority of developmental problems the health visitor may be in the best position, both by training and inclination, to note the potential abnormalities. Some doctors combine immunization with well baby care; others prefer to separate them. There has been little evaluation of different ways of delivering this type of care. Whatever the method, it is important that there should be a clearly defined practice policy and Curtis Jenkins' guidelines for the practice teams' activities are worthy of recognition.[12]

1. The commitment to the philosophy of prevention should be shared by all members of the primary care team.
2. Effective organization is the key priority to ensure that no child is 'lost' and that all are seen at regular agreed intervals.
3. It is essential to free developmental clinics for screening from the inappropriate task of treating sick children and it is advisable to separate the 'sick' from the 'well' during such a clinic.
4. Continuous monitoring of: the team's effectiveness, immunization rates, non-attendance rates and disorder rates. Regular spot checks of the team's target population register against the practice age-sex register to ensure that no child is lost.
5. All members of the practice staff including receptionists need to know what goes on in the child prevention programme and why.

The intervals at which children should be assessed are subject to constant review, but as a minimum examinations at 6 weeks, 7 months and then 3 times before the age of 5 years at roughly equal intervals come within most recommended schemes. There is some evidence that the Identification of abnormalities tends to increase with advancing age and this indicates the importance of reviewing children at about 3 and 4½ years of age. It is important that the developmental clinic should not degenerate into a situation in which a series of tests is carried out but little time is allowed to observe the mother/child relationship. A few minutes spent talking to the mother and watching the child playing with toys and communicating with the mother and doctor can be more revealing than a wide variety of tests. At the end of such an unstructured interview the doctor may be tolerably certain whether the child's locomotor development, social skills, hearing and vision are likely to be within normal limits. In addition, the doctor will try to relate this observation to his/her knowledge of the family situation acquired in the ante-natal period and during the continuing relationship with the patient and he will assess the security of the mother in handling her infant.

Several books have been published such as that by Egan and his colleagues describing tests which may be applied at various stages in development.[13] Others (e.g. Illingworth — *The Normal Child*[14]) discuss in some detail the common problems encountered by mothers such as sleep problems, feeding difficulties, temper tantrums, toilet training and discipline. Barber *et al.* have produced a chart in which the child's development can be plotted allowing visual comparison within the normal range of the child's previous development[15] and a developmental chart available from the Health Departments is reproduced in the Appendix to this chapter.

It is not difficult for the general practitioner to attain skill in detecting *physical abnormalities* in the first 5 years of life and by careful review he should be able to identify those children who are failing to reach their milestones. Some of the abnormalities in vision, hearing and intellectual achievement are more complex and will require either additional training to acquire skills in examination or advice from a specialist. Certain physical disabilities, such as evidence of congenital dislocation of the hip or squint demand immediate referral to a specialist. Others may simply increase the general practitioner's suspicion that development is retarded and that further review will be called for. If there has been no improvement at follow-up the child should then be referred for a specialist opinion. Observations concerning hearing and vision are crucial in the early period of life because any impairment may well be remediable and will affect the development of vocabulary and fine social skills unless dealt with at as early a stage as possible. Such children should always be referred for further investigation. Delays in the development of vocabulary may be evidence of hearing defects or more complex problems of mental retardation or lack of stimulation in the family.

It is worth bearing in mind that a child with one handicap is more likely to suffer from another than a normal child. The discovery or suspicion of a handicap should therefore lead to a careful search for others, or referral to a specialist.

There is now a clear policy within general practice in favour of greater integration of the preventive and therapeutic services. There is increasing emphasis in child health on comprehensive care and this will need to go hand-in-hand with careful audit, both at national and local level. Wilmot *et al.*[16] give an example of how goals can be set and outcome measured in an individual practice and the establishment of computer recall systems both at practice and at district level will help in the administration and review of any screening programme.

With greater awareness on the part of doctors of the role played, not only by parents, but by teachers, child minders and nursery staff in health promotion, their relations with these groups will come increasingly to resemble a partnership. Indeed the time may come when the parents and nursery staff receive training in certain of the more straightforward screening tasks themselves.

Pre-school developmental screening is part of the broader issue of child surveillance. Whatever system of screening emerges it will need to exploit the potential of the primary health care team and will have to be flexible enough to allow variations in the system to be based on local needs of children and their families.

Continuing care of disadvantaged children

The vast majority of children grow up normally and their progress is only interrupted by the recurrent infections of childhood. The majority of these are respiratory infections which tend to reach their peak in the age-group 3 to 7 years. Some children seem to be particularly vulnerable to infections of the throat, others to otitis media and yet others to bronchitis. This is all part of the process of acquiring immunity to infection. Some of these infections may lead to disability and the doctor providing continuing care will attempt to identify any complications, such as hearing loss following acute otitis media.

On school entry the child often experiences an increase in the number of infections and there may occasionally at the same time be behavioural problems as the child adapts to a new way of life. From the age of about 7 onwards, however, illness becomes less common and the general practitioner often sees little of his young patients from the age of 7 until they begin to approach puberty. A few children, however, suffer chronic or recurrent physical disorders in childhood and need special supervision from the general practitioner. These must be viewed in the context of the whole family and indeed identifying the implications of such illness for the child and the rest of the family and his future schooling is an important function which the general practitioner is uniquely placed to carry out.

Descriptions of the management of the acute episodes of disabling conditions of childhood, such as eczema, enuresis, asthma and epilepsy, will be found in the relevant chapters in Part 3 of this book. The long-term management, particularly where continuing therapy is concerned, presents special problems. The general practitioner will be keen to ensure that the epileptic or asthmatic child regularly receives suppressive drugs such as phenobarbitone or sodium cromoglycate. This demands a high degree of compliance from parent and child and at the same time it is important that these children should not be seen by their siblings or peers as sick. It is often difficult for the parents of children with chronic disability to avoid becoming over-protective, but this is of great importance both for the child and the siblings. Children who are disabled should be encouraged to live to the limit which their disability allows. It would be foolhardy to allow the epileptic child to ride a bicycle or swim unsupervised but he should be encouraged to play other games like football, cricket or tennis and to take a full part in such school activities as summer camps. It is often difficult for the parent of an asthmatic child to allow unrestricted physical activity, even when the illness is well controlled with sodium cromoglycate which may indeed make it possible for the child for the first time to take a part in physically demanding activity.

The general practitioner has an important role to play in counselling the parents of physically disabled children, and, even more important, the children themselves as they approach puberty.

There are other children who while physically healthy are at a disadvantage as a result of emotional or intellectual impairment. The prisons and the schools for the maladjusted in this country are inhabited largely by people who were deprived of a secure loving relationship in childhood. There are those who are frankly rejected and they occur in every social class, although the way they present to the doctor varies in different social classes. Where there is money available they may be handed over to the 'au pair', despatched to boarding school or bribed to keep out of the way. Where there is chronic unemployment, poverty, alcoholism or mental illness the parents may simply lack the resources to provide the love which a child needs and love which they themselves have never experienced. In some cases severe marital disharmony leads to a constant insecure and stressful situation. The children of such homes tend at first to present behaviour disorders. Later it becomes clear that they have never learned to control their anger or hatred or to show concern for others and this leads to violence and vandalism.

The general practitioner is in a position to realize, and will indeed often know, that particular children in his practice are at risk in these situations. It is often easy to make an accurate diagnosis and prognosis. It is much more difficult to intervene. If he is to do so successfully he must seek the possible source of strength or security in the situation and not be put off by the apparent hopelessness and inevitability of the outcome. He may find unexpected resources in a hopeless hen-pecked husband or in an unhappy battered wife, or in an older sibling or a grandparent. He may then with the help of a social worker or health visitor be able to build on this source of strength.

Sometimes he will encounter situations where the disturbed behaviour of the child is exacerbating an already disturbed marital situation. The classical example is a child who will not sleep until he gets between his parents in bed. This effectively puts an end to the sexual life of the parents. The doctor's intervention in prescribing a sedative for the child may reduce the emotional tension in the home and cut across a vicious circle. In some cases, however, this sort of situation is the result of parental collusion and the child's behaviour may bring about a covertly wanted situation for the parents. Occasionally appropriate treatment of the over-stressed mother or alcoholic father may bring about the desirable result. Rarely there will be no resources in the home and the general practitioner will feel constrained to recommend that the child be taken into care which may in time lead to fostering or adoption. It used to be said that a bad mother is better than no mother. This is no longer tenable and the provision of a loving adoptive parent may be the solution to some of these problems.

Another group of children whom the general practitioner will encounter are those who fail to develop intellectually because they are not exposed to the necessary stimuli in early life. The toddler should be constantly enjoying new experiences and challenges, while insufficient sensory stimulation can lead to retardation. Pollak[3] demonstrated this in her study of three-year-olds in London. Probably the most important factor in intellectual growth is the child's speech environment. Unfortunately this is most likely to be impoverished among those who are culturally most likely to be retarded. By developing an awareness of those who are most vulnerable the general practitioner and his health visitor should be able to intervene by parental advice and in some cases early admission to nursery schools.

Finally, there is a small group of children who are mentally retarded. This may present as part of a more complex picture in which there are associated abnormalities which may be congenital or acquired. Mental retardation is not a diagnosis which a general practitioner will normally make. He may suspect this when he finds that a child with normal vision and hearing is slow to speak and shows poor social adaptation or locomotor skills. He will then normally refer the child to a specialist. For a variety of reasons it is not uncommon for intellectually normal children to be retarded in their development and there are numerous examples in history, such as Newton, Darwin and John Hunter, all regarded in childhood as slow learners, or even fools. In cases of slow development the general practitioner's role will be to try to identify the cause. In others, however, there will be real impairment of intelligence. In some of these children it will have been suspected at birth, such as mongols; in many it will come as an apparent surprise. It is important, however, to realize that the parent is often not as surprised as the doctor and that for some time they may have suspected that their child was abnormal. The doctor may be tempted to prevaricate but he should be wary of depriving a parent of the opportunity of discussing a problem which has for a long time been worrying them.

The parent of a mentally retarded child will often react to this finding with hostility and guilt feelings. The practitioner has a vital part to play in dealing with these. He may, for instance, have a clue as to their cause. The child in question may not have been planned and he may suspect that it was rejected in early pregnancy. There may be some 'skeleton' in the family cupboard, such as a mentally or physically disabled relative and the parent concerned may feel a special responsibility for the child's disability. There may be factors in the antenatal or intranatal period which the parent construes as responsible for the present predicament, such as taking drugs, smoking, induction of labour or a difficult delivery. All of these the general practitioner should explore in the hope that he can resolve some of the feelings of guilt and hostility and help the parents to accept their problem and the challenge which it offers to them. Unfortunately, the families affected are often those who have the least economic and emotional resources to respond to this challenge. Parents will also have other anxieties concerning the work a disabled child will impose on the family. What will the neighbours think? Where will he go to school? All these problems should be discussed by the doctor, the health visitor or a social worker. The ultimate placement of the child will often depend on specialists in educational psychology or child psychiatrists, but in the intervening years it is the general practitioner and his team who must provide support in coping with the problems of feeding, sphincter control and the impact of a mentally retarded child on the developing family.

Integration of episodic and continuing care

There is a risk in separating the continuing care of childhood, as reflected in the educational and preventive work in the antenatal clinic and the developmental examinations in the first five years of life, from the episodic care demanded by parents when their children fall foul of some new virus, bacterium or traumatic challenge. This is an over-simplification of the situation. Every contact between doctor and child should be seen as an opportunity to increase the doctor's knowledge of the child and the family and to form a relationship. It is this relationship which will determine whether or not the worried mother will present her anxieties or her child to the doctor. It will determine whether or not the doctor can carry out a satisfactory examination of the child's abdomen when he develops appendicitis or his ear when he develops otitis media. It will help the parent who makes inappropriate demands on the doctor accept the doctor's criticism and hopefully his constructive advice. It is this relationship which will allow the parent faced with serious or, in rare cases, fatal disease turn to her general practitioner with confidence and receive from him the support that she requires.

References

[1] Fry, J. (1961): *The Catarrhal Child.* London: Butterworths

[2] Morrell, D.C., Gage, H.G. and Robinson, N.A. (1971): Symptoms in General Practice. *Journal of the Royal College of General Practitioners, 21*, 32

[3] Pollak, M. (1971): *Today's Three Year Olds in London.* London: William Heinemann Medical Books

[4] Bowlby, J. (1951): *Maternal Care and Mental Health.* World Health Organization. HMSO

[5] Pringle, M.J. (1977): Parental Deprivation in Under Fives. *Proceedings of the Royal Society of Medicine, 70*, 24

[6] Jobling, N. (1976): *The Abused Child.* London: National Children's Bureau

[7] Rutter, N. (1966): *Children of Sick Parents.* Institute of Psychology, Maudsley Monographs. London: Oxford University Press

[8] Scottish Home & Health Department (1973) *Towards an Integrated Child Health Service*, Edinburgh: HMSO

[9] Report of the Committee on Child Health Services (1976) *Fit for the Future.* London: HMSO

[10] Royal College of General Practitioners (1982) *Healthier Children — Thinking Prevention.* London: RCGP

[11] Wilson, J.M.G., (1966): *Some Principles of Early Diagnosis and Detection in Surveillance and Early Diagnosis in General Practice.* London: Office of Health Economics

[12] Curtis-Jenkins, G. (1982) The First Five Years of Life *British Medical Journal 285*, 1175–1176

[13] Egan, D.C., Illingworth, R.S. and Mackeith, R.C. (1971): *Developmental Screening 0–5 years.* Ipswich: Lavenham Press Ltd

[14] Illingworth, R.S. (1975): *The Normal Child.* 6th ed. Edinburgh: Churchill Livingstone

[15] Barber, J.H., Boothman, R. and Paget-Stanfield, J. (1976): A Visual Chart for Pre-School Developmental Screening. *Health Bulletin, 34*, 80–91

[16] Wilmot, J.F., Hancock, S. and Ullyet, P. (1984): Paediatric Surveillance: Performance Review and The Primary Care Team. *Journal of the Royal College of General Practitioners, 34*, 152–154

Appendix 4.2-(1)

PAEDIATRIC DEVELOPMENT SHEET

SIGNIFICANT FAMILY HISTORY:

♂ ♀

Sibling name & year of birth ☐ ☐ ☐ ☐

PRENATAL HISTORY:

AT RISK FACTORS such as: Diabetes Toxaemia Jaundice

CONFINEMENT:

BREAST FEEDING Nil ☐ 2/12 ☐ 2–4/12 ☐ 4/12+ ☐

Solids Started

NEONATAL EXAMINATION

Weight Kg

Skin...

Spine...

Hips...

Feet...

Digits...

Skull...

Palate...

Ears...

C/V/S (Femoral pulses).........................

Eyes...

Tongue...

Chest...

Abdo. & Genitalia.............................

Hernia...

Moro Reflex...................................

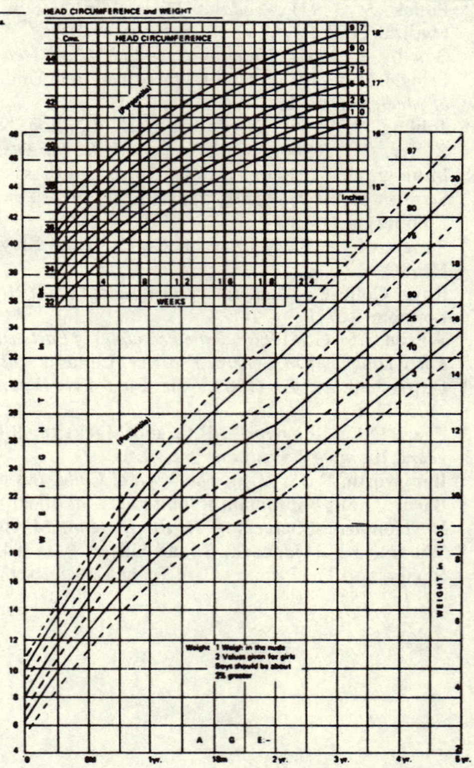

Form GPIII K

The development charts on this and the following two pages are based on the work of the Research Unit of the Royal College of General Practitioners and modified by the Joint Working Party of the Department of Health & Social Security on A4 Records to whom we express our gratitude. *Eds.*

DEVELOPMENT CHART

Appendix 4.2-(1) contd.

1. Mark "X" for items which child performs.
2. Mark "O" for items which child could not perform.
3. It is suggested that test ages marked ☐ are carried out by the doctor.
4. Record mother's observations and reactions under "Observations".

	TEST Actual Age	6/52	3/12	6/12	9/12	12/12	18/12	2 yrs	4 yrs	Observations	Immunisations
6 weeks	Lifted prone, momentarily holds head in line with body										
	Pull to sit. Head lag partly controlled										
	Hands closed									PKU	
	Grasp reflex +									Hips	
	Smiles									Physical Examination	
	Follows objects side to midline										
3 months	Lifted prone, holds head up										
	Lying prone, lifts head 45–90°										
	Pull to sit – only slight head lag										
	Holds rattle momentarily										
	Supine, watches own hands										
	Follows objects from side to side									Hips	
	Squeals of pleasure										
6 months	Lying prone, back is extended and weight on hands (not arms)										
	Rolls prone to supine										
	Sits up with hands forward for support										
	Weight bearing on legs										
	Transfers cube from one hand to another										
	Reaches out for objects										
	Alert: responds to examiner and mother										
	Smiles and laughs										
	Syllables ba, da, ka										
9 months	Sits steadily										
	Stands up, holding on										
	Creeps on hands and knees										
	Crude thumb-finger grasp										
	Waves "bye-bye"										
	Knows own name										
	Hearing responses at 46cm (18") (Lt. and Rt.) such as rattle, cup and spoon									Hips Squint Examination of Testicles Physical Examination	

DEVELOPMENT CHART

Appendix 4.2-(1) contd.

1. Mark "X" for items which child performs.
2. Mark "O" for items which child could not perform.
3. It is suggested that test ages marked ☐ are carried out by the doctor.
4. Record mother's observations and reactions under "Observations".

	TEST Actual Age	6/52	3/12	6/12	9/12	12/12	18/12	2 yrs	4 yrs	Observations	Immunisations
12 months	Pivots stably while sitting										
	Walks – one hand held										
	Fine pincer grasp – finger/thumb										
	Plays "Peep-bo"										
	Responds to simple commands										
	Uses 2-3 words with meaning										
18 months	Throws ball without falling										
	Walks upstairs, one hand held										
	Builds 3-4 cubes										
	Feeds without rotating spoon										
	Dry by night mostly										
	Understands simple orders										
	Several intelligible words										
2 years	Kicks ball without overbalancing										
	Walks backwards in imitation										
	Unscrews lids, turns door knobs										
	Builds 6-8 cubes										
	Can put on shoes and socks										
	Asks for food, drink, toilet										
	Joins 2 or 3 words in sentences										
	Hearing responses at 122 cm (4 feet) (Lt. and Rt.)									Hips Squint Physical Examination	
4 years	Hops on one foot									Physical Examination and Pre-school Assessment	
	Can button clothes fully										
	Attends to own toilet needs										
	Imaginative play										
	Tells stories										
	Counts up to ten										
	Questioning at its height										
	Hearing responses at 122 cm (4 feet) (Lt. and Rt.)										

(553) 402292 100M 8/76 HN&M 278

4.3 Adolescence

Pauline Watson

Adolescence may be defined as that period in a person's life which extends from the onset of the physical changes of puberty until the achievement of adulthood and independence. It is a period of rapid change and great turmoil, as the adolescent endeavours to come to terms with himself, his limitations and his potential, and with the world outside himself. Everyone has a picture of the adolescent at this stage: a pimply youth, a podgy girl, easily embarrassed and often awkward, sometimes rude or withdrawn, self-absorbed and often sullen, generally wasting his own time, and difficult to respond to. Keats described it brilliantly: 'The imagination of a boy is healthy' he wrote in the preface to *Endymion*, 'and the mature imagination of a man is healthy; but there is a space of life between, in which the soul is in a ferment, the character undecided, the way of life uncertain, the ambition thick-sighted . . .'

The general practitioner needs to be aware of these uncertainties and upheavals which occur at adolescence, and of the various means which the adolescent uses to survive the physical and psychological stress. It is often difficult to provide satisfactory continuity of care because adolescents can become resentful and reluctant patients. As children they were brought by parents, but subsequently they come less often and the practitioner may find when he treats patients in this age group that it is not always an advantage to be a 'family doctor'. The adolescent may be willing to talk frankly about his problems only if he feels sure that his doctor will not discuss them with his parents. This is particularly true if he has had a difficult relationship with his parents, or if he has been behaving in a way of which he knows they would disapprove. In older adolescents the rights to confidentiality are those of an adult, but for those under 16 the doctor has to decide whether or not to share the problem with the parents, in the knowledge that if he does so he may well damage the relationship between himself and his patient. At this age, however, he may feel that to involve the parents is in the best long-term interests of the patient.

Many adolescents are unsure about what is normal and what is abnormal in their physical development, and are often too afraid or embarrassed to seek help. There is a wide variation in the normal physical and psychological development at this stage, and the doctor must be able to reassure the adolescent when development or signs of stress are within the normal range. He also needs to be able to see the danger signs of more serious problems which may require treatment. This is difficult, because in a consultation an adolescent will often be silent and withdrawn, and may have trouble in articulating his fears or even in understanding them himself. The first meeting with the doctor will often be an occasion on which the doctor is tested as to whether or not he is 'safe' and can be trusted; he will not be accorded a 'divine right' to help merely because of his title or qualifications.

The onset of the physical changes of puberty in girls precedes that of boys by about two years, but there is a wide variation in the time of onset and in the rate at which the changes occur. The onset is marked by a sudden spurt in growth, and an associated increase in strength. In girls this usually occurs between 10 and 11 years, and in boys between 12 and 13 years. As a result girls are often taller than boys at this age, although eventually they are overtaken. This is the last period in which girls can compete with boys on physical terms, and it may therefore be a time during which a boy may be anxious about his growth because he does not seem to be keeping up with his sisters or peers. An early onset of the physical changes of puberty and an advanced rate of growth are thought to be associated with good intellectual achievement. Early adolescents are often gawky and clumsy, and seem to have little control over their lengthening limbs, but there is an improvement in co-ordination which develops from the onset of puberty, and movement becomes gradually more controlled and elegant. Puberty may be delayed by poor nutrition over a long period, or postponed by major illness. Childhood diabetes mellitus may cause a delay in the onset of puberty or result in depression of the growth rate before and during adolescence, so that the diabetic may fail to reach his expected height.

Sexual maturation

Sexual maturation in girls begins with breast development and is followed by the growth of pubic hair and then axillary hair. This is succeeded by the onset of menstruation. The onset of breast development is variable, and it is not uncommon for a child of 9 or 10 to be brought to the doctor with a small tender swelling of one breast, which is merely a manifestation of precocious breast development. The onset of menstruation or the development of secondary sex characteristics before the age of 10 years is said to be abnormal, but in the majority hormonal studies are within the normal range. Tanner[1] quotes data showing the average age of menarche in 1950–60 in girls in schools in the south of England as approximately 13.2 years. His figures also show that the age at menarche has been reduced over the past century by about four months per decade.

It is common for periods to be irregular in adolescence. They may also be scanty, or heavy and prolonged. Dysmenorrhoea is a frequent complaint, and the pain may be severe and accompanied by vomiting and fainting. Usually as menstruation becomes established and more regular these disturbances become less severe. Normal activities should be encouraged, and mild analgesics may be given if necessary; but if dysmenorrhoea is severe and disabling it can be controlled by suppressing ovulation by cyclical hormone therapy. Menorrhagia in adolescence improves spontaneously in most cases. A dilatation and curettage can be physically and psychologically harmful, and is unnecessary provided pelvic examination is normal. In persistent cases, a bleeding tendency from any cause should be excluded, and severe and persistent bleeding may require cyclical hormone treatment for its control.

A girl's attitude to her periods and to the discomfort which she experiences will be greatly affected by what she has been led to expect by her mother, and by her mother's attitude to her own menstruation and her own sexuality. If a girl has not had menstruation explained to her, she will be very frightened if she wakes up one morning to find a patch of blood on the sheet. She may fear that she is seriously ill, and be afraid to confide in anyone. If a mother has complained of pain and of feeling ill every month, it is likely that the girl will fit in with this pattern and feel ill as well. There are many myths associated with menstruation which may worry an adolescent girl who has some abnormality in the menstrual pattern: she may have been told that if her period is late, or she has missed a period, the blood will 'go to her head'; she may fear that to bath, wash her hair, eat ice-cream, or swim during menstruation will be harmful.

During adolescence, the regularity of periods may be easily upset by emotional disturbance. For instance, if a girl leaves home to go to college, or if a close relative dies, or if an important relationship with a boy-friend comes to an end, she may miss several periods and become worried about the possibility of being pregnant. This may worry her even if she has not had sexual intercourse. Anorexia nervosa most commonly presents in adolescence (see Chapter 3.42), and amenorrhoea may be the presenting symptom.

A girl's complaints about irregular or painful periods may well be a manifestation of a deeper unease about her femininity. This difficulty in coming to terms with herself as a woman is often associated with a mother who has given the impression that sex is dirty or sinful, or who has punished or disapproved of her as a child for touching her vulva or vagina. When she becomes an adolescent she may be unable to accept her vagina as a normal part of her body; she may be unable to touch herself, and be afraid to attempt to use tampons during menstruation. It may be helpful if the doctor 'gives permission' for her to touch herself, and shows her how to examine her own vagina; with simple explanation, and by allowing her to discuss what she feels on examination, she may be helped to dispel any frightening fantasies she may have about her body, and reduce her anxiety about sexual intercourse in the future.

Hormonal imbalance can result in premenstrual tension or premenstrual depression, in adolescence as at any other time: an adolescent may be more easily upset and irritable before and during periods, and it is well established that academic performance in examinations is poorer at this time. There is also an increase in the incidence of minor delinquency. [2, 3, 4]

Sexual maturation in boys begins with an increase in the size of the penis, testes and scrotum, followed by the growth of pubic and axillary hair. Later there is an appearance of the beard and bodily hair on the limbs and trunk, and a change in the voice, which occurs gradually over a period of months. Adolescents tend to be preoccupied with these changes: there is endless comparison between themselves and their peers, and as the time of onset and rate of development are variable, this results in a great deal of anxiety. They may have fears that they are not developing normally, or that they will never become mature. This concern will occasionally present to the doctor as a worry about one particular aspect of development, or a seemingly trivial physical discomfort; boys may complain of a lack of height, of being too fat, of not being strong enough, of acne, or of excessive axillary sweating. They may present with painful swelling of one or both breasts, which gives rise to a great deal of anxiety about normal male sexual development; this clears spontaneously in a variable length of time. In the same way girls may complain of being too tall, too fat, having unusual facial features or breasts which are too large or too small, acne, or greasy hair. The symptom of which the adolescent complains may appear to be within the normal range, but the view of his or her body will be coloured by attitudes which have been formed in childhood. If there are feelings of inadequacy, the body may well be regarded as inadequate, in spite of reassurance.

Problems of adolescence

Acne is a common problem in adolescence. When it is severe or prolonged it can result in considerable disfigurement, but even in a mild form it can be distressing. At a time when an adolescent is anxious to be particularly attractive to the opposite sex, and when he feels insecure about the changes occurring in his body, acne may disrupt his social life, make him feel ugly, and result in depression (see Chapter 3.38).

Adolescent girls sometimes present with abdominal pain which is of psychological rather than physical origin, but it is important to exclude any organic cause of the pain. In such cases physical examination, and particularly vaginal examination, should be undertaken circumspectly: the majority of adolescents have no qualms about a physical examination (and may see it as a sign of the doctor's interest), but some may feel threatened. It may even be seen as a physical assault, or a seduction; and many young adolescents may be embarrassed by an examination when they are barely accustomed to their newly acquired sexually mature bodies. This situation can usually be resolved by the way in which the doctor approaches his patient.

Anxiety about bodily function and development may present as a physical symptom in this way, but it may also manifest itself as depression or in a falling-off of performance at school. Early or delayed development in any marked degree can result in psychological problems. Early maturation, for instance, may mean that the social expectations of the adolescent are too high: he looks like an adult and is expected to behave like one, when in fact he is emotionally immature. On the other hand, if puberty is delayed he may become embarrassed and shy because he is small and undeveloped in comparison with his contemporaries, and he may resent being treated as a child.

Physical illness in adolescence

Illnesses diagnosed in childhood or adolescence, such as diabetes mellitus, epilepsy, eczema or asthma, which require the co-operation of the patient in keeping the disease under control, present problems in adolescence and require special care in their management. For instance, a diabetic child who has been careful and co-operative in testing his urine regularly and recording the results may appear to lose interest in doing the tests, or cheat in his recording of them. Whereas previously he has kept faithfully to his diet, he may now eat sweets or drink sugary drinks, so that his diabetes gets out of control. He may also resent having to attend the clinic. Even if an adolescent is co-operative, he may find it more difficult than before to control his diabetes, because of the rapid physical and psychological changes that are taking place.

Adolescents with such diseases resent the limitations imposed upon them by the illness, for this is a time when they would like to conform in every way to the behaviour patterns of their friends. A diabetic must always make sure that he can get his insulin injections at the appropriate time, and so he must plan his day in advance; his peers may be experimenting with food or alcohol, and may be staying away from home for long periods without warning or forethought. While the others are carefree, the diabetic has to keep to his diet and give himself the injections, and the epileptic must remember to take his treatment. This emphasizes the difference between himself and his peers at the time when he is most anxious to appear the same. He will require a considerable amount of support and patient explanation if he is to learn to accept his condition, and co-operate with the doctor in controlling it.

Anorexia nervosa. — Anorexia nervosa has its highest incidence in adolescent girls. It involves a persistent refusal of food, resulting in loss of weight and emaciation, and in secondary amenorrhoea. Often the adolescent does not consider that she needs treatment, and she is brought by her mother.

Authorities differ in their views on the cause, course, and treatment of anorexia nervosa.[5] For instance Bruch describes the control of eating in anorexia nervosa as an effort of self-assertion in patients with 'a paralysing sense of ineffectiveness',[6] while Crisp relates its onset to a sexual experience causing alarm in patients with poor premorbid sexual adjustment.[7] Crisp describes a high incidence of higher birth weight and early menarche in such girls, and postulates that the onset of early puberty in a girl who is ill-prepared leads to guilt, fear, and disgust about sex, so that she resorts to severe restriction of food in an effort to return to a pre-pubertal physical state. The current emphasis on the desirability of being slim, with pressure from the media, is also likely to be of significance.

The adolescent often has a distorted perception of her body image, and will continue to regard herself as fat, however much weight she loses. She has a horror of fatness above all things, and associates it with ugliness, though she is also preoccupied with food for much of the day and she will often spend long periods of time gazing at food in shop windows. Eating is associated with feelings of revulsion, and is followed by a sense of guilt, especially if a period without much food is followed by a bout of overeating. She may resort to bingeing, with vomiting and purging in order to maintain weight loss. Anorexia nervosa is frequently associated with depression, anxiety, phobic, or obsessional symptoms.

Such adolescents present against a background of marked family tension, and treatment is difficult. Early mild cases may improve spontaneously with sympathetic discussion of the fears of the patient and her family. Snaith describes areas to be explored with such patients: these involve her fears surrounding eating and loss of control, exploration of family relationships, sexual fears, and other stresses. Her co-operation should be sought in fixing a realistic target weight and diet, and in agreeing to regular consultations with weighing. He suggests that psychiatric referral should be made in the following instances:

1. a weight which is 15 per cent below matched population mean weight;
2. general family friction;
3. severe vomiting and purging, making hypokalaemia a danger;
4. persisting evidence of associated psychiatric disorders, especially depression;
5. at the patient's request.

Glandular fever. — Infectious mononucleosis has its highest incidence in teenagers (Stokoe[8]). The symptoms, sore throat, lymphadenopathy, and pyrexia, however, are anything but distinctive, and may be due to other causes (e.g. streptococcal tonsillitis). Thus, Stokoe found that it is not possible on clinical grounds to identify Paul-Bunnell-positive cases of glandular fever. On the other hand, it is important to consider infectious mononucleosis in a teenager who presents with a sore throat which does not respond to treatment, and the diagnosis should be confirmed, though no specific treatment can be given. It pursues a protracted course, and an accurate prognosis can only be given when the doctor is sure of the diagnosis: a positive Paul Bunnell is pathognomonic of the disease but in its absence the practitioner must decide on other grounds whether or not the patient is likely to have glandular fever. In Stokoe's series, the following features were more commonly found in sero-positive than in sero-negative cases: many atypical monocytes, palatal petechiae, hepatomegaly, splenomegaly, and abnormal liver function tests. The presence of these features would therefore tend to confirm the diagnosis even in sero-negative cases.

If a patient is thought to have glandular fever, he will need a much longer period of rest than is necessary with simple tonsillitis. On advising when a patient should return to school or work the doctor should remember that patients with glandular fever often have prolonged malaise with tiredness and anorexia lasting for several weeks. This may be due in some cases to associated hepatitis or myocarditis: Dunnet[9] found that a large majority of his series of patients with glandular fever had abnormal liver function tests. The maximum level of enzyme activity showing hepatocellular damage occurred between the second and fourth week of the disease and returned to normal in the majority within six weeks. Dunnet also found ECG changes indicating non-specific myocarditis in 16 per cent of his patients, and the possibility of myocarditis should be considered in patients presenting with a tachycardia disproportionate to their fever.

Psychological aspects

In examining problems which are likely to occur in adolescence, it is important to observe the psychological tasks which are understood to be normally performed at this stage. In our modern society, the time-scale over which they arise has inevitably changed. An adolescent is now physically and sexually mature long before he is economically independent; his education may be prolonged, sometimes into his twenties, and over this period he will still be dependent on his parents, and as a result they may continue to exert their authority over him as if he were a child. In primitive societies, when an adolescent moves from one phase to another, the moment is usually marked by a definite ritual, or *rite de passage*, which leaves him in no doubt about his status and what is expected of him. In modern sophisticated society, the moments of transition are blurred, and an adolescent may feel isolated and confused because he is unsure of the role which is expected, and he has to struggle to achieve each new status.

Since social changes and expectations are changing so rapidly, the behavioural standards of two generations may be widely different, and an adolescent who identifies closely with his peer group will probably find that he is in conflict with parents or teachers. This 'generation gap' is probably greater at the present time than it was previously because of the opportunities for higher education which exist, irrespective of financial background; while the influence of television and the other mass media makes it less likely that adolescents will accept the values and standards of their parents without question.

Adolescence is a vitally important period in an individual's life, not only because failure to pass satisfactorily through each stage of psychological development will undoubtedly prejudice his mental health in the future, but also because serious disturbance at this time may affect important decisions which have to be taken. It is during adolescence that a career is chosen, and sometimes a marriage partner; and if these choices (or some academic performance) are affected by a temporary inability to cope with stress, his whole life may be the worse for it. It is important therefore to be able to assess what is a normal reaction to stress in adolescence, and what is a sign of more serious disturbance. In order to be able to do this it is necessary to have a model of what is regarded as within the normal range of psychological development.

As Laufer[10] pointed out, all adolescents are subjected to stress from the environment, but it is the reaction to the stress which is important, and not the stress itself. Laufer describes three main areas of tension: 1. in the relationship with parents; 2. in the relationship with peers; 3. in the adolescent's view of himself as a physically mature person.

An adolescent will be subject to stress in his relationship with his parents as he strives to become independent from them. For most adolescents this process is far from smooth, and it is a cause of many of the emotional upsets which occur at this time. The child who previously idolized his parents becomes an adolescent who is critical of them and provocative in his behaviour. The parents need to modify their attitude, by allowing him more freedom to become independent, but at the same time they must exercise a certain amount of control over his conduct. It is often difficult to maintain a steady balance between these two, and as a result there is often a great deal of tension between parents and adolescent children. The toleration and understanding of the parents are stretched to the limit, while the adolescent is easily upset and unpredictable in his behaviour. At one moment he will be very grown-up and independent, and then under stress he will become childlike again and require the protection and support of his parents, as if alarmed by his daring. If the relationship again becomes too like that of his childhood, he will retreat from it and become inaccessible and awkward once more (Henry[11]).

The process of becoming independent is difficult enough when parents are able to be understanding and helpful, but their behaviour may be affected because they are jealous of their children's opportunities, or because they relive some conflict which was unresolved in their own adolescence. As a result they may be unreasonable in their demands, or afraid to allow the adolescent enough freedom in which to grow up. Although the adolescent may not be economically independent, he will wish to make his own decisions about his clothes, his friends, his religion, his political opinions, and about how he spends his time. As he becomes more independent, he should be able to uphold his own opinion or way of behaving and justify it, even at the risk of parental disapproval. Parents, for their part, have to walk a kind of tight-rope between too much and too little restraint; and for the adolescent too little restraint may imply a lack of concern.

Until now the adolescent has relied on his parents to impose standards of right and wrong upon him. At adolescence he is concerned with working out his own standards, and these must be consistent with his own image of himself. This is not to say that he necessarily flouts the parental code of conduct, but he will adhere to a way of behaving only if it is of his own choosing. Late adolescence is concerned with consolidating these aspects of his character: at this stage the adolescent is preoccupied with matters of conscience, and he becomes idealistic in religion or politics. He will feel extremely guilty if he fails to live up to his ideal of himself. An older adolescent will often be uncompromising in his views, and regard himself as almost omniscient on various issues of morality; it is only later that he will dare to allow himself to question these issues or doubt his original point of view.

The relationship of an adolescent to his peer group is another potential source of stress. As a child becomes adolescent the importance of the peer group is greatly increased. His life tends to become dominated by its activities and opinions; it gives him an opportunity of close relationships outside the family when the tensions within the family make it difficult for him to confide in his parents. As opposed to the expectations of his parents, the expectations of his peers are not those of childhood, and in this way the adolescent's friends help him to become more mature. Within a small group of friends, the adolescent can learn a great deal about personal relationships. He is able to discuss his fears and anxieties with others at the same stage of development, who have similar problems, without feeling threatened. He feels emotionally secure in the group, and gets a certain prestige from belonging to it. It may also be a useful way of assuaging his guilt, by blaming his unacceptable behaviour on the whole group or its leader. The group is, in a way, a rehearsal for adult life: its members learn to be loyal and committed to the group, and sanctions can be imposed if behaviour is unacceptable. The group also provides competition and motivation for achievement in work or recreational activities. Identification with a peer group can lead to tension between an adolescent and his parents if the parents consider the dress, language, or behaviour of the group is not to their liking. But if the adolescent is not accepted by his peers, a great deal of distress and unhappiness will result.

The third main area of stress is in the adolescent's image of himself. If he is unable to see himself as growing into a sexually mature adult, and if he cannot accept the sexual changes which are occurring in his body, anxiety will result, in a way which has already been described.

Sexual development

Alongside his transition from dependence to independence, an adolescent passes through a transitional stage in his sexual development, at the end of which he should be able to have an adult heterosexual relationship involving tender love and sexual intercourse. There has been no qualitative change in his sexual feelings from the age of 5 or 6, when he enters the latency period of childhood, until the beginning of adolescence. At this time there is a marked increase in his sexual feelings. In boys particularly, excitement at this age may be a sign of general tension, and they may have erections or emissions when they feel any strong emotion, such as fear or anger. It is only when they are more mature that they respond specifically to heterosexual stimuli (Blos[12]).

It is well known that at different stages in their development adolescents spontaneously group themselves in different ways. Their friendships fall into certain patterns. In early adolescence they tend to form groups of the same sex which have little contact with groups of the opposite sex. Later they tend to form an idealized relationship with an older member of the same sex. This gives way to a phase when again they form groups of the same sex, but the members of one group have short-lived and sometimes simultaneous relationships with several members of a group of the opposite sex. These are often based on similar interests, and do not usually involve sexual intercourse. Late adolescents pair off in more permanent heterosexual relationships.

When considering problems of a psychological nature in adolescents it is interesting and helpful to examine the theories which explain these groups and relationships in psychoanalytical, sociological and anthropological terms. The psychoanalyst would say that there is a resurgence of 'pregenital' instinctual drives in boys at puberty, and a resurgence of their Oedipal conflict.

In these terms, the process of adolescence is concerned with the relinquishing of incestuous parental love-objects, and their replacement by mature heterosexual love-objects. If there is a failure to pass from one phase to another, i.e. if a fixation at one level occurs, the individual will not achieve sexual maturity.

The choice of friends and spontaneous formation of groups in different stages of adolescence can also be viewed in sociological or anthropological terms. In these terms, the pattern which is adopted will be modified by social pressures, and will vary between different races and cultures. The psychological task of the adolescent in becoming independent from the parents is universal, but the means by which it is achieved will vary in different societies.

Hadfield[13] has described the process of psychological development at this stage as the growth of the ability to love, in all senses of the word. From the friendship of early adolescence, to personal affection for a friend of the same sex, to sexual curiosity and the desire to attract, and finally to complete love for one person of the opposite sex. This mature love is at first romantic and idealized, and then leads to a strong desire for sexual intercourse and a permanent relationship. As Meyerson[14] has written:

> This is the rapprochement: the meeting of the two persons to experience deep reciprocal involvement that can surpass past fixations in ways that are loving, conciliatory and emotionally fulfilling rather than pain-inflicting and continuously littered with the debris of unforgotten emotional shrapnel.

The doctor can use any model to describe the psychosexual development of the adolescent as a means of understanding what can be regarded as within the natural limits of feelings and behaviour. A promiscuous 13-year-old, for instance, will not be thought of as over-sexed, but as behaving in a way which is inappropriate to her age and as searching for love and affection rather than sexual satisfaction. She may well be completely anaesthetic when sexual intercourse occurs. Similarly homosexual relationships in adolescence may be worrying for parents, but can be seen as normal and transient unless there has been some disturbance in childhood sexual development which has resulted in fixation at this level. An ambivalent relationship with the parents may be viewed as a manifestation of Oedipal conflicts, and hence elucidate otherwise inexplicable behaviour.

Masturbation. — Adolescents are often worried by their need to masturbate. They may be perturbed by a sudden unexpected nocturnal emission, or be afraid that they may have in some way damaged themselves by producing an emission by masturbation. They have difficulty in talking to a doctor about such anxieties, and typically present with some other complaint or symptom.

Masturbation is a normal part of adolescence, and is part of the general increase of sexual feelings which occurs. It is a means of regulating sexual tension, and in masturbating an adolescent can come to terms with the sexual functions of his body in the comparative safety of his fantasies. Masturbation is a part of the normal psychosexual development of adolescence, and is part of the process by which the sex drive is channelled from the auto-erotic to more mature objects. Accordingly, the fantasies associated with masturbation will change at different stages of adolescence, from narcissistic fantasies to fantasies involving the opposite sex.

An adolescent may worry that masturbation will result in physical injury, or it may represent a loss of control over himself which he fears will lead to madness if it persists unchecked. These fears are reinforced by the many myths which have been handed down from generation to generation and which may even be told by parents in an effort to discourage their children from masturbation: these include suggestions that it will lead to infertility or insanity. An adolescent may find it helpful merely to be reassured that there is no substance to such stories, and that he is in no way abnormal because he has nocturnal emissions or masturbates frequently.

Although masturbation is normal in adolescence, excessive and compulsive masturbation can occur, usually as a result of deprivation of love or feelings of inferiority. The adolescent seeks reassurance in masturbation. If masturbation is orgastic and satisfying it may lead to a failure to progress to a more mature phase and normal heterosexuality. Compulsive masturbation may result in a preoccupation with the body, and the strong associated guilt feelings can interfere with a normal development.

Other adolescents cannot allow themselves to masturbate at all. For them, masturbation is associated with infantile sex drives which have been repressed to such an extent that masturbation is not permitted. Such individuals cannot cope with the increase in their sexual drives at adolescence, and normal psychosexual development cannot occur, so that a boy who denies having masturbated is a cause for concern. In girls, on the other hand, such a denial is not necessarily pathological. Many deny any history of masturbation, or at least are unwilling to talk about it; and in girls sexual feelings may be demonstrated as a more general concern with physical appearance, rather than genital stimulation as in boys.

Psychiatric illness

Adolescents can present with emotional, behavioural, or psychotic disorders. The traditional psychiatric view is that great upheaval and disturbance, with turmoil and alienation, are to be expected, and that psychiatric problems of this period of life have variable symptoms which are transient and benign. Rutter[15] has questioned this view, based on his epidemiological study of 14–15 year olds in the Isle of Wight (and his reviews of other studies).

The evidence points to the view that in early adolescence symptoms are no more variable than at other times, that prognosis is not different from similar disorders in earlier childhood, and that prognosis depends mainly on diagnosis, i.e. psychosis has the worst, neurosis the best, and behaviour disorders an intermediate outcome.

Parent–child alienation is not common except in children with psychiatric problems, but 'inner turmoil' with feelings of misery, self-deprecation, and ideas of reference are quite common in 14 year olds and often unnoticed by adults. Psychiatric disorder is probably only a little commoner than in middle childhood, but the pattern changes in that there is more depression and more school refusal.

Rutter concludes that adolescent turmoil does in fact exist but that its importance may have been over-estimated in the past. He also emphasizes that it is unwise to assume that adolescents will 'grow out' of their problems.

All adolescents are subject to stress and react with anxiety or disappointment: to assess whether or not an adolescent is psychologically healthy it is necessary to build up a picture of his relationships with his parents and friends. It is also necessary to discover whether or not his job, or his academic work, is beyond his powers; and to find out what kind of image he has of himself, and how he views his future. The presentation of psychiatric illness in adolescence may be atypical, and it may be overlooked if the signs are not appreciated. A dramatic, florid anxiety state, for instance, which is frightening for the adolescent and his friends and family, may settle down quickly with simple reassurance, whereas schizophrenia may develop slowly and insidiously, with a gradual falling-off in academic or job achievement, while the withdrawal from social life may escape notice.

Periods of anxiety or depression occurring in adolescence in response to various pressures, such as failed examinations, broken relationships, or some inner conflict, may settle spontaneously. They may, however, become incapacitating and require active treatment.

Henry[11] describes what he believes to be the commonest psychological disorder of late adolescence: a sudden state of anxiety and distress provoked by the appearance of some conflict in the adolescent's life, which focuses on some personality problem that is the result of an earlier unresolved conflict. He cites the following as common causes of such a breakdown: dependence–independence conflicts, inability to cope with anger (one's own or other people's), fears of failure in the adult role (socially or sexually), and difficulty in making adult relationships.

Depression in adolescents may present as failure to keep up with school work, as school phobia, or as a physical symptom such as headache, abdominal pain, or tiredness. On examination, however, a history can often be obtained of weeping, suicidal thoughts, thoughts of running away, loss of a sense of pleasure, sleep disturbance, or poor appetite.

Depression can result in suicide attempts in adolescence (as at any other time) and, although suicide gestures are common, especially in adolescent girls, it is always necessary to treat them seriously. They are always a manifestation of serious distress. Ridicule or a failure to provide necessary help may provoke further and successful suicidal attempts. Adolescents are alarmed by thoughts of suicide, and will have difficulty in talking about them to other people. It is therefore necessary to ask specifically about them if there is thought to be a risk.

The risk is particularly high in a depressed adolescent who is isolated or who has a previous history of suicidal attempts, especially if the life situation provoking the previous attempts has not changed. Often the behaviour is an attempt at communication, and treatment therefore involves establishing more appropriate and less dangerous ways of communicating between the adolescent and the doctor, and between the adolescent and his family. In addition other sources of stress should be explored.

In the case of most emotional disturbances during adolescence, the role of the doctor may be simply to allow the patient to share some of his anxieties. The adolescent will need to build up a trusting relationship with the doctor and this may take time — not necessarily long interviews, but a succession of short consultations during which the adolescent tests the doctor to see how far he can be trusted. All that may be required is that the young patient should be reassured that his feelings and behaviour are not clinically abnormal or morally bad.

But this sort of reassurance will not help the patient unless the doctor who reassures has earned his confidence. Often these testing consultations can be trying ones. The adolescent patient may re-enact his domestic rebellions in the consulting room and he may do this again and again before he accepts that he himself is accepted.

Cases not responding to support and reassurance may need psychiatric referral, possibly for individual psychotherapy or (if there is significant family psychopathology) for family therapy. Psychotropic drugs alone for anxiety or depression in adolescence are unlikely to be successful and may well be inappropriate.

Schizophrenia and affective disorders increase in incidence after puberty and may be difficult to distinguish from the shyness, vagueness, and introspection of normal adolescents. The diagnosis may only become clear after a period of time with careful observation, but it is important to bear it in mind.

Conduct disorders in adolescence vary from difficult, anti-authoritarian behaviour to delinquent acts which lead to involvement with the courts. Mild cases may settle spontaneously if they are treated with understanding but firm control. When, however, the behaviour reflects a disturbance in family relationships, family therapy or social work involvement may be necessary.

Early emotional deprivation leading to later severe conduct disorders in an adolescent with poor impulse control, little ability to form close relationships, and little sense of guilt, is likely to need prolonged treatment in a residential setting. Even here, treatment is likely to be difficult, and may be unsuccessful.

Changing social attitudes

In recent years there has been a change in the attitudes of society towards young people. They are criticized by the mass media for their sexual promiscuity, irresponsibility, long hair and 'way-out' clothes. These criticisms have not been confirmed by research into the sexual behaviour of adolescents. Schofield[16] found that in the age group 15–19 over two-thirds of boys and three-quarters of girls had not had sexual intercourse. Perhaps the most important change in recent years is the change in the attitude of young people towards sexual behaviour, rather than any change in practice; and while the majority behave according to the moral code of their parents, they do not condemn those of their peers who behave differently. In sexually experienced girls Schofield found that most of them had had sexual intercourse within a secure setting — usually with a steady boy-friend or fiancé. Boys, on the other hand, were more likely to have had sexual intercourse casually. More boys than girls had had intercourse, and this disparity is accounted for by the existence of a small percentage of very promiscuous girls. Although reports of teenage sexual behaviour in newspapers and magazines may be based more on fantasy than fact, they are not without effect on the adolescents themselves and may influence their behaviour. Schofield found that non-experienced boys were usually under the impression that their peers had more experience than was the case; they were therefore under pressure to experiment sexually or feel left out. Similarly girls who believe that their friends have sexual intercourse with their boy friends may feel afraid that they will be thought prudish and that their boy friends will leave them if they do not follow suit. A girl, however, may also feel (having been told by her mother that 'boys do not marry the girls they sleep with') that to have sexual intercourse would mean that she was 'easy' or promiscuous, and prevent a stable relationship from developing. The resulting conflict can cause a great deal of anxiety.

Conventional education from teachers or parents may be of little value for adolescents. Most of their information, accurate and inaccurate, is derived from their friends. As they are often in the process of rebelling aginst their parents, they may class their doctor and their parents together, and so find it impossible to ask for the doctor's advice and help. This is particularly true if the doctor looks after the whole family. In a group practice it is sometimes helpful if the adolescent is treated by one partner and the parents by another. Alternatively the adolescent may prefer to get help from a quite separate agency like the Family Planning Association or a Student Health Service.

The resistance by teenagers to instruction from those who are regarded as authoritarian may partly explain the increasing rates of premarital pregnancy and venereal disease in young people, despite efforts to spread information about contraception and the presenting signs and symptoms of gonorrhoea.

Venereal disease

In recent years the incidence of venereal disease in young people has shown a considerable increase and the doctor dealing with adolescents should have a high index of suspicion when there is a possibility of infection. The problem of diagnosis is made more difficult by the adolescent's vague knowledge about the ways in which venereal diseases present. It is complicated by the fear, common in adolescents, that any symptom (or even no symptom) occurring after sexual activity must mean that he has become infected by venereal disease. Moreover, the presenting symptoms are not always classical, and may draw attention to other systems, while gonorrhoea and non-specific urethritis can be symptomless in girls.

Symptomless girls do not come for treatment, and thus form a reservoir of infection which leads to increasing spread of the disease. In addition, there will be disastrous results if a urethritis due to the gonococcus is treated as a urinary-tract infection. The presence of dysuria should therefore raise the question of venereal infection in a girl at risk, particularly if no growth is obtained from a midstream specimen of urine. Similarly, a girl treated blindly for a vaginal discharge, which is assumed to be monilial because she takes the oral contraceptive pill, may well have gonorrhoea. It is important therefore to consider the possibility of venereal disease if a girl presents with dysuria, vaginal discharge, perineal or anal warts, or abdominal pain (Chapters 3.51, 3.59 and 3.77).

If there is a likelihood of venereal disease the diagnosis is best confirmed in a venereal disease clinic. Such a referral may demand a great deal of tact. If the adolescent denies that there has been genital contact but the doctor feels that the symptoms suggest infection, to persist with the referral implies that the patient is lying, but not referring risks the possibility of missing the infection. Results from swabs sent off in transport media alone are not so reliable as fluorescent smears and cultures taken by a venereologist.

Some adolescents will understand the complications of venereal disease and willingly attend a clinic, but many will be upset and find it a humiliating experience. After treatment it is important to have several follow-up visits to the clinic to exclude persistent infection, because mere absence of symptoms does not mean that it does not exist.

Drugs and drink

There has been an increasing use of drugs and alcohol among young people in recent years, probably reflecting the increasing use of mood-altering drugs and alcohol in the population in general. In the past there was a marked excess of male over female drinking in adolescence but this has largely disappeared. As the alcohol consumption in teenagers increases so more teenagers are presenting with alcohol-related problems. In addition there has been increasing concern among adults about solvent abuse. The prevalence is not known, since in most instances professional help is not sought.

The peak age for solvent abuse is 13–15 years, with a higher incidence in boys. Parents may be unaware that their child is glue-sniffing, but it should be thought of if the child appears drunk or develops a rash around his mouth or nose. Most adolescents who abuse solvents do so intermittently in groups, possibly to express their rebellious feelings or to identify with their peers. They seldom become physically damaged or become psychologically dependent. However, a few abuse solvents when they are alone on a regular basis for the euphoric effects or as relief from stress. These often have disturbed family backgrounds and are more prone to physical or psychological complications. The latter group are more likely to need psychiatric referral.

Most drug-taking in young people is experimental: it is not uncommon for students, for instance, to develop acute alcohol poisoning merely because they are ignorant of the likely effects of the large amounts of alcohol they consume, but they are unlikely to wish to repeat the experience. The opportunities for students to use drugs, particularly cannabis, are widespread, but most surveys of the extent of the use are based on questionnaires and so can only be speculative. It is a common belief that the use of drugs facilitates self-examination, and students may experiment with them for this reason; or they may merely be used as a weapon to provoke parental anger, or as an expression of their frustration at what they see as the inadequacies of the society around them.

An adolescent who is having difficulty in coping with his work, or in relating to his peers because of depression or personality problems may resort to more serious misuse of drugs than his colleagues. He will find it comforting to be accepted by a group outside 'straight' society which provides a means of escape from the pressures which he finds himself unable to respond to adequately. If the effects of drug-taking are experienced as pleasurable, then drug-taking is reinforced, likely to be repeated, and likely to become a habit.

There is an association between drug-taking and delinquency, but no indication that the relationship is causative.[17] Rather it seems likely that both drug abuse and juvenile delinquency are accounted for as facets of the same sociopathic personality.

Treatment in the short term is concerned with acute intoxication with drugs or alcohol, and with secondary complications; for

instance infection after injections, overdoses, and withdrawal symptoms (including fits).
Success in withdrawing from drugs and alcohol in those who are dependent will depend largely on their motivation. It is usuaily best carried out in hospital where social, personality, and psychiatric factors involved can be teased out; and an appropriate programme with attention to these factors can be instituted.

Pregnancy and abortion

Schofield found little evidence to suggest that promiscuity among adolescent girls had increased in recent years. However, as shown in Table I, there has been increasing use of abortion, under the 1967 Act, as a solution to the problem of unwanted pregnancy.

Year	All births, stillbirths and abortions (thousands)	Abortions (thousands)
1972	100.3	20.3
1973	97.5	23.4
1974	94.1	24.6
1975	89.2	25.0
1976	83.5	25.0
1977	80.1	24.9
1978	82.1	25.5
1979	87.8	28.1
1980	92.5	31.2

(Office of Population Censuses and Surveys, Birth Statistics 1980 England and Wales, Government Statistical Service)

Table I. — Births and abortions (under the 1967 Act) to residents of England and Wales aged under 20 years, 1972–80

Schofield found that only a low percentage of sexually experienced adolescents used contraceptives, and that girls became pregnant for one of several reasons. Some girls who have been deprived of affection actively want to get pregnant, so that they will have someone to love and someone who loves them and depends upon them. Others may be afraid to refuse sexual intercourse because they believe that their boy-friend's affection depends upon it. For others sexual intercourse is unpremeditated and they are unprepared, whilst others have the minimum of information about sexual matters and believe that infrequent sexual intercourse cannot result in pregnancy.
Some girls resist the idea of taking oral contraceptives because they are diffident about going to a clinic or a doctor, or because they believe that to take 'the pill' is an admission that they will expect and will permit sexual intercourse to occur: this they or their peers

may regard as immoral or 'tarty'. Wolfish,[18] in the Teen Clinic of the Hospital for Sick Children in Toronto, found that in five years only two of the girls who received contraceptive advice became pregnant. The adolescents in his clinic who became pregnant had little knowledge of how to prevent it.

The realization by an adolescent girl that she is pregnant is usually a devastating one: she will feel that she has let her parents down, and may be afraid to tell them. She may feel trapped, or that her friends despise her or are laughing at her. What previously was an unlikely event which happened to other people becomes an unmistakable fact from which she cannot escape and which requires her to make an important and irrevocable decision. The doctor must decide whether or not to recommend termination of the pregnancy, and he must help the girl to decide for herself whether or not she wants to have her baby. Because she fears that her parents may reject her, she is vulnerable, and may be more easily pressurized by her parents or her boy-friend into seeking an abortion which she does not want. It is the doctor's task to ensure that the decision she reaches is her own. She will require counselling and support whether she has an abortion or continues the pregnancy.

If the decision to have an abortion is made in an unhurried and careful way, with the girl taking responsibility for it, and if it is done for the best reasons rather than because her parents are manipulating her into it, then the subsequent feelings of guilt and remorse will be less. The question 'why did she become pregnant when she didn't want a baby?' should be asked, and this may involve discussion and insight into her relationship with her boy-friend. Disturbed girls may require psychiatric treatment; these can be identified during abortion counselling. It is important to discuss future contraception at this time.

If the adolescent decides to have her baby, she will need support and practical help. What is involved in having a child fostered or adopted should be discussed, and if she decides to look after the child herself she will need financial and other support. It is helpful to involve a social worker to assess each girl's position, and provide the maximum of support.

Russell[19] reports that those pregnant girls who are under the age of 16 years are twice as likely as older teenagers to delay seeking advice until after the twelfth week of pregnancy. This may reflect a denial of the pregnancy or an attempt to conceal it, and may increase the risks of termination and lead to poor antenatal care in a continuing pregnancy. Pregnancy carried to term or termination of pregnancy in teenagers are rarely associated with maternal deaths, but neither is without risks. If the pregnancy continues to term most young girls have their babies without trouble, but there is an increased incidence of pre-eclamptic toxaemia in this age group, while anaemia and low birth weight babies are common (Russell[20]). These findings may be related to poor social conditions or inadequate antenatal care. The adolescent girl's education usually ceases as the pregnancy progresses, and it is not often resumed. Her marriage prospects are also greatly altered.

In his personal series of 50 teenage patients who had had therapeutic abortions, Russell stressed the risk to future pregnancies because of the danger of cervical tears in this age-group. They seem to be more common than in older patients, and may prejudice the chances of future pregnancies continuing to term. Similarly infection after abortion progressing to endo-salpingitis or salpingo-oophoritis will reduce the chances of future conception. These are particularly important considerations in girls who have yet to begin their families.

The Lane Committee (1974)[21] reported that major emotional disturbance is rare following termination and there is usually a sense of relief. It recommended against termination contrary to the girl's wishes but concluded that it was justified in the majority of girls under 16 years whether there was mental instability or not, on grounds of immaturity and attendant risks to health.

Studies of longer-term psychological effects are mainly based on older women. In Kaye and Shapira's review of the literature (1967)[22] it was found that 85 per cent of cases after abortion had a good outcome, 10–15 per cent experienced severe self-reproach and regrets, while 1–2 per cent developed definite psychiatric illness although not necessarily connected with the termination.

It has been reported that those teenagers carrying their babies to term are different from those requesting abortion. They have more school difficulties, a greater degree of emotional pathology, and more support from family and boy-friend.[23]

It is important to take time and care in assessing the adolescent's feelings and relationships, her resources and support network, in deciding how best to help her to reach her decision.

Contraception

Obviously it is far better than either of the above alternatives if unwanted pregnancies can be avoided, and advice about contraception should be given after abortion or delivery. Some doctors seem to think that by refusing to give contraceptive advice to teenagers, they will change their sexual habits, but this is unlikely. It is important, however, when giving advice, to discuss with the adolescent her relationship with her boy-friend, and to allow her to ventilate her feelings about sexual intercourse. Is she asking for 'the pill' merely to conform to the behaviour of her friends, or because she is afraid to refuse to have sexual intercourse? Does she feel that premarital sexual intercourse is morally wrong? If she chooses 'the pill' in preference to a mechanical method of contraception, is it because she is afraid to touch her vagina? In this way psychosexual difficulties can be discovered and often helped.

If contraception is thought to be appropriate, the advantages and disadvantages of the different methods should be discussed. The oral contraceptive is the safest from the point of view of preventing pregnancy, and most adolescents find it the most acceptable method. The diaphragm has fewer side-effects, but requires too much planning and forethought for most teenagers.

Among women using intrauterine contraceptive devices, there is an increased risk of young nulliparous girls developing pelvic inflammatory disease.[24] These devices should therefore be avoided if at all possible.

References

[1] Tanner, J.M. (1962): *Growth at Adolescence*. Oxford: Blackwell Scientific Publications

[2] Dalton, K. (1960): Effect of menstruation on schoolgirls' weekly work. *British Medical Journal*, *1*, 326

[3] Dalton, K. (1960): Schoolgirls' behaviour and menstruation. *British Medical Journal*, *2*, 1647

[4] Dalton, K. (1961): Menstruation and crime. *British Medical Journal*, *2*, 1752

[5] Snaith, R.P. (1981): *Clinical neurosis*. Oxford: University Press

[6] Bruch, H. (1978): *The Golden Cage: the enigma of anorexia nervosa*. London: Open Books

[7] Crisp, A.H. (1965): Clinical and therapeutic aspects of anorexia nervosa. *Journal of Psychosomatic Research*, *9*, 67–78

[8] Stokoe, I.H. (1969): Atypical mononucleosis and glandular fever. *Journal of the Royal College of General Practitioners*, *17*, 340

[9] Dunnet, W.N. (1963): Infectious mononucleosis. *British Medical Journal*, *1*, 1187

[10] Laufer, M. (1975): *Adolescent Disturbance and Breakdown*. Harmondsworth: Penguin Books

[11] Henry, W.D. (1973): Some aspects of adolescent psychiatry. *The Practitioner*, *210*, 21

[12] Blos, P. (1962): *On Adolescence*. New York: Free Press of Glencoe

[13] Hadfield, J.A. (1962): *Childhood and Adolescence*. Harmondsworth: Penguin Books

[14] Meyerson, S. (1975): Adolescence and Sexuality. In *Adolescence, the Crises of Adjustment*. London: Allen and Unwin

[15] Rutter, M. (1976): Adolescent turmoil: fact or fiction? *Journal of Child Psychology and Psychiatry*, *17*, 35–56

[16] Schofield, M.G. (1965): *Sexual Behaviour of Young People*. London: Longmans Green

[17] Kraus, J. (1981): Juvenile drug abuse and delinquency: some differential associations. *British Journal of Psychiatry*, *139*, 422–430

[18] Wolfish, M.G. (1973): Adolescent sexuality. *The Practitioner*, *210*, 326

[19] Russell, J.K. (1983): School pregnancies — medical, social, and educational considerations. *British Journal of Hospital Medicine*, *29*, 159–166

[20] Russell, J.K. (1974): Sexual activity and its consequences in the teenager. *Clinics in Obstetrics and Gynaecology*, *1*, 683
[21] *Report of the Committee on the Working of the Abortion Act* (1974) (Cmnd. 5579). London: HMSO
[22] Kaye, D.W.K. and Shapira, K. (1967): Psychiatric sequelae of termination of pregnancy. *British Medical Journal*, *1.299*, 82–3
[23] Freeman, E.W. and Rickels, K. (1978): Adolescent contraceptive use: current state of practice and research. *Obstetrics and Gynaecology*, *53*, 388
[24] Booth, M., *et al.* (1980): Effect of age on pelvic inflammatory disease in nulliparous women using Copper 7 intrauterine contraceptive device. *British Medical Journal*, *281*, 114

4.4
The young adult

John C. Hasler

The young adult in society

It is important that general practitioners should be aware of the implications of the social environment for medical care, if they are to comprehend the problems and opportunities which face them. In spite of developments in the undergraduate curriculum of medical schools, teaching about sociology and the environment still plays a relatively small part. Yet, without an understanding of the broader aspects of the circumstances in which our patients live, we cannot hope to achieve further major advances in primary medical care. This chapter deals with the physical, psychological and social aspects of the developing young adult, and begins with marriage and the foundation of the new family.

Marriage. – Marriage is a major milestone in the social development of the individual. The nature of marriage, like most other social institutions, is constantly changing. Throughout this century the age for marriage of both men and women has been falling. Although the divorce rate has quadrupled in the United Kingdom during the past quarter of a century, this has been matched by an increase in remarriages. In 1974 there were some 113.5 thousand divorces in England and Wales, and some 121 thousand remarriages (of one or both parties).

The roles and relationships of married partners are affected by legal, religious and social factors.[1] In the last century the roles of the man and the woman were more clearly different and these differences have gradually merged although the extent to which they have done so in an individual union varies considerably. The role of the man has not altered to a significant degree, but the change for the woman has been marked. The development of her legal rights has finally culminated in legal equality. Better educational facilities and, most important of all, efficient contraception have contributed to the married woman's opportunities. Conjugal roles have been described as being scattered between two extremes.[2] At one end of the scale there are segregated conjugal roles, in which the wife is responsible for running the home and family in the traditional way while the husband is the breadwinner, and often follows his own interests with other members of his own sex. At the other end of the scale there are joint conjugal roles where all family activities are shared. The wife often pursues her own occupation and the husband will be involved in day-to-day domestic matters. These couples often entertain friends at home but may be distant to neighbours. By and large 'working-class' couples adopt segregated, and middle-class couples shared, roles.

These roles describe something of the expectations which the partners have of marriage. Sexual satisfaction appears to be less important for couples with segregated roles, compared with those with joint roles. The expectations of couples in the latter category may be so high that they cannot be achieved, creating frustrations and unhappiness. As well as expecting a fulfilling sex life, joint-role partners are often anxious about whether their children are being brought up correctly. All of these behaviours and expectations are in part a reflection of the culture of the middle-class family. Pregnancy, childbirth and motherhood often present problems for the professional woman who may resent being forced into a segregated role, albeit temporarily. Hence the frequent desire to return to work as quickly as possible.

Joint roles are more common where the partners have occupations of equal status. That the wife is more likely to have economic independence, means that she can leave home more easily if the marriage breaks down, than a woman in a segregated-role family who may have no choice but to remain with her husband. These two types of partnership roles are obviously extremes. Most couples will be somewhere between the two.

A new marriage affects not only the two partners but the families of origin of the partners as well. This may produce discord, but the availability of parents may be an important support for young mothers.

The choice of a mate is affected by a number of factors, including religion, social class and geographical limitations. A study in England and Wales[3] examined education and occupation in fathers of brides and bridegrooms and showed that similarities were greatest at the extreme ends of the social scale. Educational equality appears to reduce the problem of social inequality. Susser and Watson[1] describe the concept of marriage isolates, wherein marriages are more likely to take place between individuals from certain defined groups, although increased mobility has now tended to reduce this.

It is important to remember that, despite the unprecedented popularity of marriage in our society today, many individuals live their lives as single people. For the most part those who do not get married in our society remain single by choice. Whatever the psychological grounds for their decision, or sometimes the ethical grounds for them, these individuals are able to live full lives which are rewarding both for themselves and others. But because marriage is the norm in our society, the single person is still seen as a deviant, and may suffer from the stigma of his or her single status. This is a hidden source of stress, of which the doctor should be aware. It is a different sort of stress from those who are single, but not from choice: the widowed, or those whose marriages have been dissolved. Such individuals may experience a prolonged bereavement, the divorced no less than the bereaved (see chapter 3.3). Homosexuals have yet another set of problems with which to deal. Sometimes the homosexual may remain single, forming a series of short-lived relationships. Often the homosexual couple will show a life-long stability not dissimilar from that of the heterosexual married couple. But homosexuals, despite the protection of their own subculture, and the sense of security which they may derive from their group of friends, will suffer from all the stress of a more or less undeclared stigma. The general practitioner must be aware of these stresses, and must be prepared to discuss them openly with the patient. It is important to remember that homosexuality is not universally regarded as a form of illness, but as simply another way of expressing human sexuality, and love.

The young family. – For many couples their new marriage will coincide within a year or two with new occupations and will usually be followed relatively soon by the arrival of children. These steps of creation and expansion are steps of increased status in society. Pregnancy, childbirth and parenthood, although natural steps in themselves, are often responsible for health problems. New occupational responsibilities or the responsibilities of parenthood may create stress problems. The comparative isolation of the basic family unit is an aspect of modern society. This also has implications for health. Certain families may differ from the standard pattern: one-parent families may have serious problems, as may those with exceptionally large numbers of children or those with none.

The environment. – Some kind of stimulation and interaction with others is an important need for human beings. Isolation is likely to produce problems, for example in the case of mothers with young children who may be cut off from their families of origin, or from the neighbourhood in which they grew up.
Fanning[4] examined the consultation patterns of 558 Service families living in flats and houses in Germany. They were standardized by social class and income and were included in the study only if their occupation of a house or flat was by chance (i.e. by their turn on the waiting list). The differences in rates of first attendance by the general practitioners showed an increase

in morbidity of 57 per cent in the flat families compared to the house families. In the young women genito-urinary disorders were twice as common in flat dwellers compared with house dwellers and appeared to be associated with the incidence of psychoneurotic disorders. These latter disorders also showed a marked discrepancy, between flat and house dwellers, mainly in women between 20 and 29 in whom the rate was between 2 and 3 times higher. This was found to be more marked the higher the woman lived in the block of flats. Monotony and boredom were felt to be factors and lack of communication between flat dwellers was contrasted with the much closer relationship between the house dwellers.

Women immobilized by young children are very dependent on their surroundings, and opportunities to meet neighbours are important. On the other hand, too much proximity can also be a disadvantage: the lack of privacy including poor soundproofing, and screaming young children may create more stress for the young mother.

An important aspect of the newly married's life will be the likely move and establishment of a new home which may be many miles from their parental homes, with the new couple needing to establish their own way of life. Bain and Philip[5] investigated a cohort of one hundred consecutive families containing 347 individuals for a period of one year after registration with a practice at Craigshill Health Centre. The cohort had a significantly higher number of 16-30 year-olds than the total practice population but both cohort and practice consisted largely of young adults and children. Nearly half the patients consulted within three months of registration, Only 21 per cent of these young adults did not consult at all during their first year. All families had a higher consulting-rate than the mean rate for the practice as a whole and the rates from social classes 4 and 5 were higher than social classes 1, 2 and 3. The most common presenting symptom of the adults was mental disorder and these disorders also produced the greatest number of consultations during the one year study period.

A study of the patients who stayed with the practice showed that the consultation-rates of the adults for psychiatric and respiratory illness and ill-defined conditions fell to a rate similar to the rest of the practice during the following two years. Bain and Philip came to the conclusion that where families have recently moved and where there is a background of stress there will be an increased demand on doctors. They observed that much of a general practitioner's time is spent dealing with problems of living rather than with ill health as such.

Morbidity

The broad (morbidity) classification groups shown in Table I reveal certain interesting features. Confirming previous impressions the episode-rate for mental disorder was over twice as high for females as for males in the 15 to 44 age-group. This difference persisted into the older age-groups. In both sexes the main diagnoses in this category were anxiety and depressive neuroses and physical disorders of presumably psychogenic origin. The biggest problem in the respiratory diseases was disease of the upper respiratory tract. There was a large discrepancy between the sexes for genito-urinary disease: the main problems in the women were acute cystitis, amenorrhoea, hypomenorrhoea, dysmenorrhoea and vaginal discharge.

The section on prophylactic procedures and other medical examinations showed a large difference between the sexes which only occurred in the 15 to 44 age-group. This was largely accounted for by antenatal and postnatal care and advice on contraception. So far as the men were concerned most episodes were for medical

Int Class No.	Disease or condition	Episodes by sex and age			
		M 15-24	M 25-44	F 15-25	F 25-44
290 - 315	V Mental disorders	69.6	115.9	176.7	281.8
320 - 389	VI Diseases of the nervous system and sense organs	88.0	100.7	110.2	117.1
460 - 519	VIII Diseases of respiratory system	317.0	283.1	402.8	354.5
580 - 629	X Diseases of the genito-urinary system	15.9	21.6	282.6	273.4
680 - 709	XII Diseases of the skin and subcutaneous tissue	154.1	112.0	186.9	144.9
710 - 738	XIII Diseases of the musculo-skeletal system & connective tissue	58.7	117.4	65.0	126.2
780 - 796	XVI Symptoms and ill-defined conditions	110.2	117.2	176.4	180.1
N800 - N999	XVII Accidents, poisoning and violence	198.3	130.1	95.4	82.3
	XVIII Prophylactic procedures and medical examination	96.1	89.7	560.6	411.9

Table I. – Episode rates per 1,000 population for 15 to 44 age-group

examination of some kind and for immunization or vaccination. There was a small number of health education and instruction episodes for both sexes, the women again being involved approximately twice as often as the men.

Morrell and Wale,[6] studying the way patients responded to symptoms of illness, examined health diaries kept by 198 randomly chosen women between the ages of 20 and 44. This group was investigated because of the high demands on the general practitioner and/or the belief that a better understanding of their behaviour would aid a more rational response to their demands for care for themselves and their children. Symptoms were recorded in the diaries on one day in three but only one symptom episode in 37 led to a consultation. The women were also asked to complete an anxiety questionnaire and the study demonstrated that high users of general-practitioner care were high recorders of symptoms and that both the recording and reporting of symptoms was related to objective measures of anxiety. Symptoms presenting to the general practitioners were also analysed and it was confirmed that the patients were selective in determining which symptoms to present. Even a minor shift from self-care to doctor care could make intolerable demands on the general practitioner service.

Dunnell and Cartwright[7] carried out a survey in which they examined some aspects of consumption of medicines both in relation to conditions and symptoms, and in relation to professional treatment and self-medication. Adults were chosen at random from twelve constituencies in England and Wales and two in Scotland. In the 21 to 34 age-group 35 per cent of those interviewed described their health as excellent and 34 to 38 per cent as good. (21 to 24: 34 per cent; 25 to 34: 38 per cent.) More than half of all the adults said they had taken or used some medicine during the twenty-four hours before being interviewed. For every prescribed item in the previous two weeks, there had been two non-prescribed items. People were questioned about the absence or presence of specific symptoms during the two weeks and by and large women reported more symptoms than men. In the 21 to 24 age-group there was no difference with a mean of 4.1 reported symptoms for men and 4.2 for women. But between 25 and 34, the mean number for men was 2.8 and for women 4.4. Women also consumed more medicines than men at all ages.

When drugs acting on the central nervous system were examined, it was found that a tenth of the adults had taken a sedative drug during the two-week period. In the young adult group (21 to 35), approximately 10 per cent reported sleeplessness (which increased in the older age-groups) and 26 per cent reported 'nerves', depression, or irritability (which decreased in the older age-group). Four per cent of those aged between 25 and 34 had taken sedatives, sleeping tablets or tranquillizers (this also increased in the older age-groups). The potential danger of consumption of these drugs by drivers was emphasized.

In general it seemed that the threshold level at which patients with symptoms decided to consult a doctor, compared with a previous study five years before,[8] had fallen, certainly in relation to feelings of depression and difficulty in sleeping. Yet as the authors pointed out, there was no indication that general practitioner's consultation rates were increasing: indeed they seemed to be falling.

Mortality

Some information about the health of young adults in the United Kingdom is contained in a recent publication on *Prevention and Health* from the Department of Health and Social Security.[9] In 1973, life expectancy for males at age 15 was 56 years and for females was 61 years. Compared with 100 years ago the mortality in every age-group up to 35 was one-tenth or less. Maternal mortality has fallen dramatically from 40 to 45 deaths per 10,000 pregnancies in 1928-1935 to 1 death per 10,000 pregnancies in 1974. This is an early example of medical audit with collection of data on maternal deaths since 1952 and subsequent improvement in several aspects of maternity care, notably nutrition, prevention of pre-eclamptic toxaemia, blood transfusion, anaesthesia and antibiotics.

In 1972, 3.6 per cent of all deaths were in the 15 to 44 age-group, with cancer, accidents and heart disease accounting for over half of these. As people move from young adulthood to middle age, the most important single cause of death for men is ischaemic heart disease and for women is cancer, with breast cancer the single most important cancer. Death-rates for carcinoma of the lung in women and ischaemic heart disease rose during 1963-1973 in the middle age groups.

There has been a fall in the birth-rate by approximately 172,000 from 1964 to 1974 although there are suggestions it may shortly start rising again. In 1974 the birth-rate was 13 births per thousand. Self-poisoning has been increasing – mainly in young women, and is now the commonest cause of admission of such women to acute medical wards. There has been a reduction in the numbers of men smoking, although more women have been taking it up. One estimate suggested that over 1,000 foetal and infant deaths in Britain in 1970 were associated with smoking in pregnancy.

The position in relation to road traffic accidents gives cause for concern. The age-group 15 to 24 is at greatest risk and one in every 50 school-leavers will be killed or seriously injured on the road before he or she is ten years older. Although the stricter arrangements for dealing with drunken drivers produced an initial improvement this seems to be reversing. The compulsory wearing of seat belts, which has been shown to be beneficial, is currently under review.

The general picture

In summary the vast majority of young adults become established in an occupation, get married and start a family. This usually involves a move away from the locality of the parents. After childbirth the woman spends most of her time at home, at least for several years while the children are growing up. It is suggested that this restriction to the home, and isolation in it, and the demands of a young family are partially responsible for the incidence of psychoneurotic complaints. It is an age when the man is seen comparatively infrequently by his general practitioner, while the attendances of women are to a large extent related to the prevention of, desire for, or management of, pregnancy and childbirth, and to anxiety and psychoneurotic problems.

Despite low levels of mortality in the young adult, ischaemic heart disease and cancer begin to become significant problems in middle age and many deaths in these fields are due to habits and health factors established early in adult life. Although numerically small, the young adult is the most common victim (and perhaps also the most common cause) of road traffic accidents. The early rehabilitation of such individuals, giving due attention to their reintegration into social and family life, is a crucial factor in the quality of the rest of their lives.

Implications for the primary health care team

In this age-group there is not only a marked discrepancy between the sexes in the amount of care provided but in the nature of that care. One of the most striking features of the primary care of women is its preventive aspect whether it be prevention of conception or the prevention of complications of childbirth. Why is a similar provision of preventive care not available for men, many of whom are destined to die before they reach retirement? Much of the morbidity of middle and old age is predicated by the habits established in youth. Why are self-injurious habits and patterns of living not tackled early? There is an important role here for the general practitioner in health education. But if he is to pursue these policies of prevention, he must take stock of the social and environmental aspects of his patients' way of life in a new and challenging way.

Contraception. – During the past few years there has been an increasing awareness of the hazards of overpopulation. In 1700, the population of Great Britain was 7 million, in 1850 it was 20 million and in 1971 it was 54 million. The density of population in England and Wales has been calculated at 323 people per square kilometre, the third highest in the world, exceeded only by Taiwan and Bangladesh. If the birth-rate continues at the past rate, approximately ten more cities the size of Liverpool will be needed by the year 2000. The greater the population, the greater the likelihood of overcrowding and pollution and the greater the strain on resources.

In July 1975, contraception was made available free of charge to all patients under the British National Health Service. Yet the provision of free contraception is of little use unless doctors, health visitors and nurses are prepared to adopt a positive attitude towards family planning. The effect of a combined positive and planned population policy has been demonstrated in Aberdeen where there has been a liberal contraception, abortion and sterilization policy for the last ten years with excellent maternal and infant mortality figures and a falling birth rate.

A survey by Cartwright and Waite[10] in 1967-1968 showed that only 51 per cent of general practitioners would raise the subject of contraception with an unmarried girl who had a baby although by 1970/1 the figure had risen to 73 per cent, but the figures were lower for patients who did not show obvious need for family planning advice. General practitioners and all members of primary health care teams have a duty to make known their interest and concern in this field to all their patients. They can make use of posters and individual literature to new patients registering with them. The health visitor and doctor during their routine post-natal services should raise the subject automatically without being asked. They must be sensitive to the possible contraceptive need of any fertile girl whom they see.

Undoubtedly in the past some of the popularity of Family Planning Association clinics was due to the inadequate service provided by primary health care teams. General practitioners are now paid for providing contraceptive services (an interesting example of a number of item-of-service payments to doctors to encourage preventive medicine). It should be possible for at least one member of every group practice to fit intra-uterine devices and diaphragms. Moreover, as has been demonstrated in a recent article by Newton and his colleagues[11] specially trained nurses are perfectly capable of supervising oral contraception and inserting intrauterine devices.

Abortion. – The introduction of the 1967 Abortion Act meant that with an increasing demand for abortion, family doctors had to clarify their own attitudes towards the problem. Howard[12] describes the emotional pressure on the doctor because of the ease with which the doctor can identify with a pleading patient and because of a sense of guilt or failure when a woman for whom one is providing contraception becomes pregnant. There is often a demand for help but not for understanding. Cartwright and Waite[13] carried out a postal survey of 900 general practitioners in England and Wales, of whom 601 replied. It appeared that, compared with an earlier survey in 1967-68, there was a more liberal attitude. They estimated that the mean number of patients referred to the National Health Service for abortion by each doctor was 5.0 in the twelve months preceding the study. It is not known how many of these were subsequently carried out. The study illustrated the arbitrary way in which the barriers operate both in general practice and in hospital. Variations of attitude between the age, sex and marital status of general practitioners were small but geographical differences were much more significant both among general practitioners and gynaecologists. A majority of general practitioners wanted more facilities for abortion.

General practitioners should be in a good position to help their women patients come to the right decision over whether or not to seek abortion. Cartwright and Waite pointed out that the general practitioner's role was that of arbiter as to whether or not a patient reached a gynaecologist. The two roles may interfere with each other. Yet it seems that even in their role of arbitration and referral agency doctors often do less than justice to the problem. How often do referral letters arrive in gynaecology clinics with full details of all the relevant social, psychological and environmental factors? Referral letters merely asking for a termination to be considered, without an attempt to examine the patient's problem in the light of her own needs and the general practitioner's attitude, do not help specialists.

Childbirth. – General practitioners are only too aware of the changes that have taken place in obstetric practice in the last decades in the United Kingdom. Whereas many general practitioners in the past had a large obstetric practice, a number of factors have altered the general practitioners' role in the care of the pregnant woman.

The number of deliveries has fallen in the last few years in many practices while the categories of women recommended for specialist booking has risen. The increase in the number of obstetric beds has meant that these recommendations can be put into effect. The criteria for specialist booking are largely based on features of pregnancy and the pregnant woman that have been shown to produce a higher than average risk to the mother. The general practitioner has been reduced to a provider of antenatal care in many instances, while looking after fewer and fewer women for the actual delivery. Once the woman has had her baby the policy is often to send her back to her home or general practitioner maternity unit. The future of the general practitioner practising care during delivery seems assured only in those situations where a general practitioner and specialist maternity unit are combined or where the patients are so far from the specialist maternity unit that some kind of local unit is essential. General practitioners and district midwives seem uneasy about the future. Obstetrics is a field which requires both personal care and technical expertise. There is no doubt that specialist units provide the latter and no-one disputes the value of modern advances in technical obstetrics. Yet anxieties are voiced by mothers that maternity care has become too impersonal, and that their bodies seem to belong to the hospital rather than themselves, for what is, after all, a natural process. Various writers, both doctors and mothers, have emphasized the vulnerability of mothers, and the inability of those mothers to talk to doctors and midwives looking after them.

Integrated general practitioner and specialist units would seem to provide the best of both worlds. It is conceivable that the pendulum may swing back in the future and more deliveries will be under the care of general practitioners again without an increase of perinatal mortality but with a more personal element. In the meantime general practitioners must be aware of potential problems affecting maternal emotions and perhaps play a more active role in initiating discussions of these matters with consultant obstetricians.

This chapter is not the place for a detailed examination of antenatal care and booking policies with which all family doctor obstetricians should be familiar. One important aspect of prevention deserves comment. A small but important minority of women of childbearing age are not immune to rubella although it is possible that this number will fall following the policy of immunization against rubella in the early teens. It should be standard practice for rubella serological tests to be carried out as part of routine antenatal blood tests and for immunization to be offered to all susceptible women following delivery: a similar policy may well be linked with the provision of contraceptive services.

Some mothers are affected emotionally more than others, and of direct concern to all general practitioners is the difficult problem of puerperal depression. A general-practice study carried out in Plymouth[14] analysed 112 patients during pregnancy and the puerperium. The aim was to determine the extent to which puerperal depression could be predicted. Four factors were found to be significant: the absence of the husband from home at the time of birth, low tolerance to suffering as indicated by attitude to dysmenorrhoea, low tolerance to suffering at a previous birth, and an ambivalent attitude towards or an inability to accept the pregnancy, during the second trimester. Another study in Wales[15] examined the incidence and severity of depression in 99 mothers and 77 fathers before and after the birth of their child. The incidence of depression remained uniformly constant throughout the antenatal and postnatal period and did not increase in the puerperium: 10 per cent of the mothers were moderately depressed and 3 per cent severely depressed. A Beck Depression Inventory was used to detect the depression. A significant difference was found in mothers, compared with fathers and nulliparous women. The mothers showed an increase in irritability, fatigability, work inhibition and loss of libido both during the pregnancy and for twelve months afterwards. Doctors and health visitors must be alert to any evidence that problems may arise after childbirth, giving extra attention to mothers at risk (see Chapter 3.3).

Psychoneurosis and stress

The second national morbidity study (Table I) showed that there were 281.8 episodes per 1,000 population classified as mental disorders in women aged 25-44, over twice the rate for men of the same age. Many general practitioners are concerned at the amounts of psychotropic drugs they prescribe, and in the young adult age-group, the mother with small children under school age seems particularly at risk. Hemmed in by toddlers, often isolated from other adult company in the day time, and sometimes with difficulty in adjusting from her previous occupation to a life of constant demand, it is small wonder that many women seek help. Medication is one way that doctors attempt to provide that help. A symposium[16] in 1972 sponsored by the Department of Health and Social Security examined the medical use of psychotropic drugs. The point was made that modification of the patient's environment is often impossible whereas it appears relatively simple to modify the patient's reaction to her environment. Parish[17] carried out a comprehensive survey of the prescribing of minor tranquillizers from 1965 to 1970. In a survey of general practitioners in a midland industrial city he found some 14 per cent of the 20 to 35-year-old women were on psychotropic drugs, and this proportion increased in the older age-groups. The numbers of patients receiving psychotropic drug therapy increased rapidly from the age of 18 to 25 years. In an examination of family neurosis Ryle[18] has argued that for the person with more complicated problems, individual psychotherapy can offer a possibility of help, and with limited resources, a strong case can be made for concentrating on the young (see Chapter 3.2).

It seems that general practitioners have three options. First they may prescribe a considerable number of minor tranquillizers, attempting to listen to some of their patients' problems and enlisting the help of their psychiatric colleagues for the more difficult problems. Secondly they can examine other ways of coping with tension and stress, with less emphasis on psychotropic drugs and more on helping people to understand and help themselves. For many doctors this commitment in time and ability would be difficult and the provision of counselling services in practices is an extension of primary care that might be examined with benefit. Thirdly, doctors may look a little harder to see whether some social and environmental problems, such as the physical and intellectual isolation of young mothers, could be influenced with more joint action by doctors, health visitors, social workers, architects, planners and voluntary workers.

This community role for general practitioners has been little explored in the past. Perhaps with the advent of Health Care Planning Teams more may be achieved. The possibilities of joint action by general practitioners and community physicians are many and challenging.

Sexual problems

During the last few years general practitioners have found that an important part of their work with young adults has been trying to help with sexual difficulties. Education for doctors in this field has hitherto been inadequate and attempts are now being made to remedy this in postgraduate and continuing training for general practice. Some of these problems will be relatively straight forward and an understanding family doctor with a reasonable knowledge of sexual techniques will be able to deal with them. Some problems will be more complex and require more time and expertise than the family doctor will have to give and will often be an introduction to more fundamental difficulties in the marriage relationship.

The general practitioner should be able to discuss sexual

problems without inhibitions. To do this he will need to understand his own feelings and the way in which his approach and attitude influences his relationship with the patient. He needs to understand the physical, psychological and social aspects of sexual relationships and functions, the common difficulties of men and women, and the way in which counselling can help couples. The reader is referred to a selected bibliography,[19,20,21] and Chapter 3.61. For those doctors unable to provide the time and expertise, and for more complex problems the marriage guidance services and to an increasing extent psychiatric services provide expert help in most areas. Marriage Guidance Counsellors are now working in a few health centres and group practices.

Screening and detection of problems

After an initial enthusiastic vogue in the sixties, screening is now being examined more critically and realistically. McKeown[22] contributing to a collection of essays on screening in 1968, pointed out that biological and economic criteria should be established before screening is introduced. The natural history of the disease must be known, the effectiveness of early treatment must be established and early identification must be possible. It is essential to ensure that screening will make better use of limited resources than competing medical measures.

Hypertension. – The undoubted risks facing people with raised blood-pressure levels are well known and the situation is summarized in the recent report on *Prevention of Coronary Heart Disease* from a joint working party of the Royal College of Physicians of London and the British Cardiac Society,[23] sent to all general practitioners by the chief medical officer of the Department of Health and Social Security. Raised blood pressure is common and the risk increases continuously over the whole observable range of levels. Severe hypertension produces a specially high risk of stroke and left ventricular failure, but the commoner moderately raised levels contribute more to the occurrence of coronary heart disease. The reader is referred to Chapter 3.80 for a more detailed consideration of this subject.

The conclusions of the joint working party were that definite evidence of a particular dietary regime in reducing the incidence of coronary heart disease would not be available in the foreseeable future, but that there was sufficient evidence to suggest that saturated fat intake should be reduced and that there should be some replacement by foods high in polyunsaturated fats, although the Department of Health's advisory panel did not agree with the latter proposal. There was general agreement that population screening for plasma lipids was not justified but that there were certain high-risk groups who merited it. These were those people with strong family histories of premature coronary heart disease or hypercholesterolaemia, and those with several other risk factors.

The general practitioner, if he follows these recommendations which seem eminently sensible, will have to look again at his records system. He can and should arrange for laboratory investigation of cholesterol and triglyceride levels for children (and siblings if appropriate) of all his patients with premature coronary heart disease. But he will not be aware of many of his young adult patients whose parents or siblings have died young or who have evidence of coronary heart disease because they will be registered with other practices. It should become a matter of routine for patients registering with a practice to complete a short questionnaire on their medical and family history (and their smoking habits) and for family doctors to be much more conscientious about recording family histories in the records.

Having identified those at risk all general practitioners should be able to have plasma cholesterols carried out on them and many people would now regard 250 mg/dl as the upper limit of normal. Many laboratories will now carry out lipid profiles which includes plasma triglyceride levels; for the latter, it is important to take fasting blood. A triglyceride level about 150 to 170 mg/dl is considered raised.

The joint working party emphasized that the prevention of coronary heart disease in the community is predominantly the role of the general practitioner, and that selective health examinations for the high risk patient is reasonable medical practice.

Diabetes mellitus. – The sequelae of diabetes mellitus are well known both in relation to coronary heart disease as an additional risk factor and in relation to other organs, notably the peripheral blood vessels, kidneys, eyes and nerves. For the purposes of screening, glycosuria is not in itself an adequate measure because of the variations in renal threshold. The incidence is relatively low in early adult life and there seems to be general agreement that routine screening of this age-group would not be justified. (The reader is referred to Chapter 3.80.).

Cervical cancer. – It is still not entirely clear whether carcinoma-in-situ or the abnormal cells identified by the cytologist are the same disease as invasive cervical cancer but it seems likely. The number of smear-positive women proceeding to invasive cancer is not known. The number of women dying from cervical cancer in England and Wales is between 2,000 and 2,500 annually, and the great majority of women dying are aged over 45. Allowing for several years to pass from the appearance of abnormal cells, it has been suggested in the past that the priority of screening should be in women aged 35 and over. (In the NHS payment for such screening is made only in respect of women aged 35 years and over unless the woman has had three or more pregnancies). The response rates in general, however, have shown much higher figures in younger woman than in the middle-aged. Those quoted by Knox[24] from data provided by Cochrane showed 74 per cent response in women aged 25 to 34, compared with 64.9 per cent response for women aged 35 to 44. These fell gradually until for women aged 65 to 69 the figure was 21.2 per cent.

Wachtel[25] pointed out that the immediate results in all mass-screening centres are a yield of large numbers of unsuspected cases of carcinoma-in-situ and dysplasia, and again describes the greater participation of younger women. The worst defaulters come from the highest risk group, although smaller and more close-knit communities may achieve better results.

The latest information on cervical screening has come from the Walton report,[26] which describes the fall in incidence of cancer of the cervix in several Canadian provinces but is unable to conclude whether or not some of this is due to screening. Unpublished data apparently show an association between percentage change in mortality from carcinoma of all parts of the uterus and the screening rate. The incidence in Canada of abnormalities drops from 5.5 to 0.5–0.7 per 1,000 for women who have been screened at least once. The suggestion is that if two satisfactory smears are negative then repeat smears need only be done 3-yearly in women under 35 and less often subsequently.

The lessons for family doctors seem increasingly clear. Opportunity should be taken of offering cervical smears to all women attending for contraceptive advice and postnatal examinations. After one or two negative smears, further ones need not be done more often than every three years. This practice should be adopted from early in the young woman's life in spite of the DHSS policy on payment. The peak incidence of carcinoma-in-situ is in the third decade. Particular attention must be paid to women in the high-risk category because they are least likely to attend for screening: those in lower social groups, sexually active early and with multiple partners and pregnancies. Once again primary care records are inadequate and must be structured to ensure that all appropriate women are examined and re-examined at appropriate intervals.

Breast cancer. – Unfortunately there seems no immediate likelihood that effective screening for breast cancer will become available in the near future.[27] It is, however, reasonable to use such opportunities as postnatal examinations (in women who are bottle feeding), oral contraceptive 'check ups' and occasions when cervical smears are being taken, to palpate breasts and to teach women the art of self examination.

Health awareness and the young adult

We are left with the inescapable fact that much morbidity and mortality are related to the way we live, and that it is unlikely that some dramatic cure for cancer, heart disease, bronchitis, or strokes will appear on the horizon. In these circumstances as doctors we are left with the choice of either continuing in our traditional way, largely waiting for our patients to consult us, or adopting a more positive role in identifying and helping people to understand their own health and hazards. If doctors are to move in this direction, then it is logical that doctors in primary care should be principally involved. Preventive medicine and advice cannot be entirely disentangled from care of the patient when he is ill and it is likely to be more successful if done on a local or personal basis. Moreover, general practitioners have a great asset in the United Kingdom: the registration of patients produces an identifiable population at risk. If primary care teams are to be involved in some kind of educational role for these populations then the young adult would seem to be the priority age-group. School children should be involved increasingly with health awareness in schools and once middle age has come it may be too late.

A few practices have tried some kind of health education programmes. Hasler[28] described a short course of evening sessions provided by a group of doctors with a health visitor and district nursing sister. Pike[29] has examined the consumer demand for health education by a survey of practices in various parts of the country: 534 questionnaires were analysed. Half the population did not think that doctors had a duty to keep them well but the majority were eager to have education for health – a number of popular topics were listed. About 90 per cent gave doctors and clinics as their first choice to find helpful advice about health.

Richards[30] emphasizes that health education is a wide embracing term and that the aims are more than mere imparting of information, but involve bringing about favourable changes in behaviour and response to health services. It must involve a wide understanding of education, and social, psychological, cultural, economic, political and organizational facets of life. It is a two-way process involving working with and through people and, as in the field of medical education, too many programmes have been devised without clear objectives. During the earlier part of the century there was comparatively little need for incorporation of social and behavioural science into health education programmes, but now that most of the improvements in health from better sanitation and immunization procedures have been achieved, an increasing proportion of morbidity is man made and requires a new approach that needs an understanding of local cultural traditions and behaviour.

It seems there are both parallels with, and implications for, general practice training. It is increasingly understood that educational objectives must be set and that assessment is part of the educational process. Attitudes will not be altered by an authoritarian dogmatic approach but by alternative approaches, often involving small groups. Health education is in some ways an unfortunate term conjuring up images of films of the dangers of venereal diseases and posters emphasizing the dangers of flies in kitchens. Perhaps what young adults need is greater awareness of health with an emphasis on positive aspects and not a long list of forbidden vices. If we agree that some kind of action is necessary, then it is relatively easy to look at the important facets to be covered.

There is a general view that saturated fats should be reduced in the community and a rather more controversial view that they should be replaced to some extent by polyunsaturated fats. Maintenance of desirable weight is equally important and reduction of sugar and alcohol may be important measures in themselves. The importance of high-roughage diets should also be stressed. Smoking has been incriminated as an important factor in a number of major diseases and every effort must be made to eliminate this in the young person. Physical activity and regular exercise should be promoted and people encouraged to look at their particular stress factors. People should be made aware of important symptoms needing medical attention in relation to heart disease and cancer, and in particular what the local practice policy is for measurement of blood pressures, cholesterol levels, cervical smears and the like in asymptomatic people.

The general practitioner does not have to shoulder the burden on his own. One of the health visitor's major tasks is preventive medicine and health education and it will often be appropriate to involve nurses and midwives as well. Dietitians are now providing a community service in some health centres. Health education officers are available at area health authorities as an important resource. It is important to provide a working framework in which the young adults can meet, possibly in the form of regular small groups, rather than merely attending lectures. Assessment although difficult, must be tackled.

Conclusion

There is considerable potential for the continuing care of young adults by general practitioners, who should:

1. Continue to provide an effective antenatal and postnatal system of care while pressing for more integrated specialist and GP obstetric units and initiating more research into emotional and psychological hazards of childbirth.
2. Continue to develop a comprehensive family planning service based on each group practice.
3. Examine their policies for the management of minor psychoneurotic illness, particularly in relation to the mothers of young children.
4. Develop an ability to deal with the more common psychosexual problems and requests for termination of pregnancy.
5. Consider how they may act to remedy local environmental factors which produce ill health.
6. Encourage self-reliance among patients in the management of minor, self-limiting and non-serious conditions.
7. Take the opportunity to record the blood pressure of every patient who attends.
8. Establish which patients are at risk of developing ischaemic heart disease: these are patients who have positive family histories, are diabetic, smoke, are overweight and take little exercise.
9. Offer these patients a selective medical examination including estimations of plasma cholesterol or lipids.
10. Endeavour to carry out a mimimum of two cervical smears on every woman patient, using family planning and postnatal attendances as opportunities.
11. Discuss with other members of the primary care team the setting up of health awareness groups and initiating studies into the effectiveness of these groups.
12. Create efficient records systems to enable these policies to be carried out.

Many doctors will argue that these suggestions are impracticable, unnecessary and unrealistic. Yet those doctors who see themselves as most overworked are in a sense the ones who most need to reappraise their method of primary care. There is little doubt that unless general practitioners increasingly adopt a more positive attitude to health, as opposed to disease, little impact will be made on morbidity and mortality. Doll,[31] writing on the effect of the environment on health, comments that we need to learn to control our social environment and that the social factors are hard to modify. He concludes: 'Doctors can no more avoid tackling them now than we could avoid the problem of polluted water in the nineteenth century'.

References

[1] Susser, M.W. and Watson, W. (1971): *Sociology in Medicine.* 2nd ed. London: Oxford University Press

[2] Bott, E. (1975): *Family and Social Network.* London: Tavistock Publications

[3] Berent, J. (1954): Social Mobility and Marriage: A Study of Trends in England and Wales. In *Social Mobility in Britain.* ed. Glass, D.V. London: Routledge and Kegan Paul

[4] Fanning, D.M. (1967): Families in Flats. *British Medical Journal, 4,* 382

[5] Bain, D.J.G. and Philip, A.E. (1975): Going to the Doctor – attendances by members of 100 families in their first year in a new town. *Journal of the Royal College of General Practitioners, 25,* 821

[6] Morrell, D.C. and Wale, C.J. (1976): Symptoms perceived and recorded by patients. *Journal of the Royal College of General Practitioners, 26,* 398

[7] Dunnell, K. and Cartwright, A. (1973): *Medicine Takers, Prescribers and Hoarders.* London: Routledge and Kegan Paul

[8] Cartwright, A. (1967): *Patients and their doctors.* London: Routledge and Kegan Paul

[9] Department of Health and Social Security (1976): *Prevention and Health: Everybody's business.* HMSO

[10] Cartwright, A. and Waite, M., (1972): General Practitioners and Contraception in 1970–71. *Journal of the Royal College of General Practitioners,* Supplement 2, Vol. 22

[11] Newton, J. *et al* (1976): Nurse Specialists in family planning. *British Medical Journal, 1,* 950

[12] Howard, Geraldine (1969): In *Problems over Abortion in Birth Control Clinics. The Abortion Act 1967.* London: Pitman Medical

[13] Cartwright, A. and Waite, M. (1972): General Practitioners and abortion. *Journal of the Royal College of General Practitioners,* Supplement 1, Vol. 22

[14] Blair, R.A. *et al* (1970): Puerperal Depression. *Journal of the Royal College of General Practitioners, 19,* 22

[15] Dewi Rees, W. and Lutkins, Sylvia G. (1971): Parental depression before and after childbirth. *Journal of the Royal College of General Practitioners, 21,* 26

[16] The Medical Use of Psychotropic drugs (1973). *Journal of the Royal College of General Practitioners,* Supplement 2, Vol. 23

[17] Parish, P.A. (1971): The Prescribing of Psychotropic drugs in general practice. *Journal of the Royal College of General Practitioners,* Supplement 4, Vol. 21

[18] Ryle, Anthony (1967): *Neurosis in the ordinary family.* London: Tavistock Publications

[19] Friedman, L.J. (1962): *Virgin Wives.* London: Tavistock Publications

[20] Courtnay, M. (1969): *Sexual Discord in Marriage.* London: Tavistock Publications

[21] Tunnadine, L.P. (1970): *Contraception and Sexual Life.* London: Tavistock Publications

[22] McKeown, T. (1968): *In Screening in Medical Care.* London: Nuffield Provincial Hospitals Trust

[23] Report of a Joint Working Party of the Royal College of Physicians of London and the British Cardiac Society (1976): Prevention of Coronary Heart Disease. *Journal of Royal College of Physicians,* Vol. 10, No. 3, April 1976

[24] Knox, E.G. (1968): Cervical Cancer. In *Screening in Medical Care.* London: Oxford University Press for Nuffield Provincial Hospitals Trust

[25] Wachtel, E. (1973): Screening for Cervical Cancer. *The Practitioner, 211,* 137

[26] Cervical Cancer Screening Programs (1976). *Journal of the Canadian Medical Association, 114,* 1003

[27] Greening, W.P. (1973): Mammography. *The Practitioner, 211,* 143

[28] Hasler, J.C. (1968): Health Education by Community Health Team. *British Medical Journal, 3,* 366

[29] Pike, L.A. (1971): The Consumer demand for health education. *Journal of the Royal College of General Practitioners, 21,* 156

[30] Richards, N.D. (1975): Health Education: Methods and Effectiveness. *Social Science and Medicine*, *9*, 141

[31] Doll, Sir Richard (1975): The effect of changes in the environment on the health of the community – and epidemiologist's view. *Journal of the Royal College of General Practitioners*, *25*, 326

4.5
Antenatal and postnatal care

David Morrell

The consultation

The provision of good antenatal and postnatal care involves patient and doctor in between twelve and twenty consultations over a period of six to eight months. If this care is provided by the patient's general practitioner it gives him a unique opportunity to get to know his patient in the context of her family and community. Of equal importance, it improves the patient's knowledge and expectations of her doctor.

Antenatal consultations differ from most others in a variety of ways: they can be planned to allow more time and structured to encourage discussion over a wide area of social as well as medical problems and the patient will often discuss her anxieties, hopes and ambitions. The antenatal consultation lacks the challenge of the normal surgery consultation when the patient presents with symptoms and the doctor is expected to identify the problem and provide a cure. In pregnancy, the diagnosis is not in doubt and the care provided is more in the nature of a partnership. It is concerned not with an episode of illness but in planning an important human event. In the second or subsequent pregnancy, the antenatal consultation introduces another opportunity. It is a time when an older sibling can visit the surgery unmolested, watch the doctor examine the mother, be at ease with the doctor, and become involved in the preparations for the new baby.

Who cares?

Childbirth is probably the most important event in a woman's life. It is a physical, emotional and social experience. If the words 'continuing personal care' or 'family doctoring' have any meaning or value at all it is surely at this stage in a family's development, and yet in the last two decades, particularly in urban areas, not only has hospital confinement become the rule but antenatal care has been increasingly taken over by the hospital specialist. The general practitioner in many places having diagnosed pregnancy refers his patient to the specialist. He is, usually, handed back a live mother and baby about six months later having taken no part in preparing himself or the patient for the care he is then expected to provide for the emergent family. In some group practices one of the doctors 'does' all the obstetrics. This effectively prevents the patient from receiving continuing care from her own personal doctor.

A variety of forms of shared antenatal care have been tried over the last two decades in which the general practitioner sees his patient in his surgery between consultations at the hospital and a variety of obstetric liaison records have been developed. These work fairly well in rural areas where specialist and general practitioner are well acquainted and staff changes are minimal. In urban areas where large antenatal clinics are staffed by many doctors in training posts who never get to know the patients or the general practitioners, there are frequent misunderstandings and, sometimes, friction.

For a number of years some obstetricians, some general practitioners and some patients have become increasingly dissatisfied with this service. Pressure groups have appeared among patients clamouring for a return to home confinements, only to find that general practitioners with the requisite skills and recent experience are now becoming uncommon. There can be little doubt that with recent technological advances hospital confinement is safer for mother and baby and, in some cases, less painful and that the home is no place to deal with such unpredictable events as fetal distress or post-partum haemorrhage. At the same time, there is also little doubt that the well-trained general practitioner is the right person to prepare his patients for motherhood and to provide the continuity of care which extends from the antenatal period through confinement to the postnatal period, family planning, and care of the infant in the early years of life. The problem facing those concerned with providing for the needs of expectant mothers is that of marrying the advances of modern obstetrics with the concepts of continuing care in modern general practice.

In attempting to solve this problem it is helpful to list the needs of the expectant mother and family and try to relate these to the skills of those available to provide care:

PATIENT'S NEEDS	PROVIDER
At the onset of pregnancy	
Assessment of physical and psychological fitness for pregnancy, childbirth and motherhood	General practitioner
Assessment of personal and social implications of pregnancy and motherhood	Health visitor

PATIENT'S NEEDS	PROVIDER
Identification of factors making patient vulnerable to medical complaints of pregnancy	General practitioner Obstetrician
Antenatal period	
Regular supervision of physical and mental health	General practitioner Midwife
Recognition and management of complications of pregnancy	General practitioner Obstetrician
Identification of social problems likely to occur in the first year of the infant's life	Health visitor
Opportunities to learn about pregnancy, childbirth and motherhood, and to discuss anxieties	General practitioner Health visitor
Intranatal period	
Access to modern knowledge and aids in delivery	Obstetrician Midwife
Postnatal period	
Close supervision with opportunities to discuss anxieties and learn skills of motherhood	Midwife Health visitor General practitioner
Advice concerning future pregnancies	General practitioner

As a result of such an exercise it is possible to identify the roles of those concerned in providing care in pregnancy.

The obstetrician has a role in identifying individuals who are vulnerable to complications of pregnancy. With the support of the hospital midwives using modern techniques he is responsible for the conduct of labour. He has also an important educational role in updating the primary health care team in their knowledge and skills of antenatal care. The health visitor is important in the antenatal period in identifying those who are vulnerable to social problems and in preparing the patient for motherhood. The general practitioner provides continuity of medical care and must clearly work closely with the health visitor. The role of the community midwife is difficult to define. She has many of the skills of both the general practitioner and health visitor but does not provide the continuity of care which goes forward into the early years of life. She is of crucial importance in the management of labour in hospital and in providing the compassionate care which some mothers feel is lacking in large obstetric units. In general practice, she provides for the needs of those who are delivered at home and the increasing number who are discharged early from hospital. For both these groups she needs close contact with the mothers in the antenatal period.

The organization of obstetric care varies in different practices depending on local conditions. But bearing in mind the needs of the expectant mother, it would seem essential for the general practitioner and health visitor to play a major role. Recently, a number of experiments have been reported from large cities where obstetric care has been carried out in general practitioners' surgeries with the specialist available for consultation. In these studies, the patients have the benefit of care from their own general practitioner, health visitor and midwife and in almost all these experiments the patient has been custodian of her own obstetric records. In most cases the patient has been delivered in hospital but has frequently returned home early and received continuing care in the early postnatal period by her own primary care team.

Antenatal care

The diagnosis of pregnancy

Most pregnancies are diagnosed when the patient reports that she has missed a menstrual period. Unmarried mothers, however, are prone to present some other symptom such as nausea or headache and may even on direct questioning not admit to amenorrhoea. In patients who normally have regular periods, six weeks' amenorrhoea in the absence of other possible causes, such as a sudden change in environment or an acute emotional upset, is almost diagnostic of pregnancy. If there is nausea or breast tenderness and if the patient has been enjoying unprotected intercourse then this tends to confirm the diagnosis. In a primigravida, pelvic examination at this stage will usually be sufficient to confirm the diagnosis by eliciting softening of the cervix and uterine enlargement. Pelvic examination at this stage of pregnancy is almost certainly without danger and it has the advantage of confirming the duration of gestation and excluding any pelvic pathology. In patients who have been taking oral contraceptives shortly before pregnancy, it is particularly important to establish the duration of gestation as the normal cycle pattern may have been disturbed by the hormones.

If the doctor is in doubt about the pregnancy, he may arrange to see the patient two weeks later or carry out a pregnancy test on the urine. This is available in most district hospitals and some general practitioners do these tests in their side room. A variety of tests are available but usually consist of adding a drop of urine on a slide to a suspension of erythrocytes or latex particles coated with human chorionic gonadotrophins. Precipitation of the erythrocytes or particles is a negative result. In view of the different tests available, however, it is always important to follow closely the manufacturer's instructions.

Once the diagnosis of pregnancy is established, an opportunity is made to take a full history and carry out a full physical examination designed to establish the patient's fitness for pregnancy and childbirth. Nowadays, the past medical history frequently reveals no serious illnesses but it is important to ask specifically about any history of rheumatic fever, tuberculosis and urinary-tract infections. A record is also made at this time of any drug allergies or previous blood transfusions. In taking the family history, there should be enquiry about diabetes, epilepsy, any congenital diseases and any family history of deafness or blindness. The social history is designed to evaluate the effect of the pregnancy on the family and includes the mother's and father's attitude to the pregnancy, the housing and financial situation and personal family resources which are locally available. In some practices, the social history may be taken separately by the health visitor.

Physical examination usually starts with a general assessment of the patient's build — is she tall or short, fat or thin? This may be followed by detailed examination working from the head down. Inspection of the teeth provides an opportunity to give positive advice concerning the need for dental surveillance during pregnancy. In a similar way, examination of the breasts for any abnormal lumps gives an opportunity to introduce the subject of breast feeding. This is followed by examination of the chest which is routine but rarely productive and careful examination of the cardiovascular system to exclude any cardiac murmurs and hypertension. If a murmur is heard, it is important to identify its nature. All diastolic murmurs require referral to a cardiologist. Not infrequently systolic murmurs are detected. In these cases it is important to ascertain that the patient has no symptoms of cardiac disability, such as shortness of breath on exertion. Many of these murmurs are of little significance and in the absence of symptoms may be noted and reviewed later in pregnancy.

The abdomen should be examined for signs of enlargement of the liver, spleen and kidneys, and, where the pregnancy is sufficiently advanced, to confirm the duration of gestation. If a pelvic examination has been carried out to diagnose pregnancy, this need not be repeated, but if the patient complains of excessive vaginal discharge a swab may be taken. Examination is completed by observing the presence or absence of varicose veins in the legs.

After the physical examination, 20 ml of blood is taken for examination of haemoglobin, blood group and rhesus factor, the presence or absence of rhesus and rubella antibodies and examination for any past evidence of syphilis such as WR or VDRL. A mid-stream specimen of urine is usually also obtained at this time and examined for significant bacteriuria. Following the examination, the patient should when dressed have a further opportunity to sit down with the doctor and ask any questions or express any anxiety. Where it is justified the doctor should reassure the patient that she is physically fit to undertake a pregnancy. He may give advice on diet, emphasizing the dangers of obesity and the importance of an adequate intake of protein and vitamins. He may advise the patient to take adequate exercise and should particularly reassure her that she can continue to have normal sexual relationships. This is also an opportunity to advise against smoking, taking unprescribed medicines and alcohol in excess.

The detailed organization of antenatal care will vary from one practice to another. It is important, however, for all general practitioners involved in providing antenatal care to be able to identify at an early stage in pregnancy those who are likely to need the resources of the obstetric specialist. The following groups may be recognized:

Primigravida. — Patients in their first pregnancy have not yet proved their ability to undergo a normal labour and were at one time regarded as needing specialist care. Much of the anxiety about these patients was concerned in the past with the adequacy of the pelvis which is rarely in doubt today in the presence of a normal foetal presentation. Their propensity to toxaemia of pregnancy is an additional hazard, but this again is much less common than in the past. Many primigravida can be safely confined in general-practitioner obstetric units. Consultation with the specialist is desirable at about the thirty-sixth week of pregnancy.

Elderly primigravida. — It is well established that in a first pregnancy increasing age increases the risks of both pregnancy and delivery, in particular with respect to pre-eclamptic toxaemia, and uterine inertia in the mother and prematurity and congenital abnormality in the foetus. For this reason primigravidae over the age of 35 merit special attention throughout both pregnancy and delivery.

Intercurrent illness. — In some patients intercurrent illness may determine the place of confinement. Patients suffering from diabetes, hypertension, epilepsy, schizophrenia, valvular heart disease, to give but a few examples, should be confined in specialist units and should receive antenatal care by obstetrician and general practitioner working very closely together. In some cases, such as diabetes, other specialists will also be involved. Patients of abnormally small stature should also receive special attention and deliver in specialist units.

Past obstetric history. — This may be an indication for extra care in the antenatal period and delivery in a special unit. A history of miscarriage in the first trimester is an indication for care during this time, while second trimester miscarriage or recurrent miscarriage may indicate the possibility of an incompetent cervix which can be dealt with surgically. A past history of toxaemia, hypertension, ante- or post-partum haemorrhage deserve particularly careful antenatal observation in the third trimester and delivery in a specialist unit. A past history of stillbirth or delivery of a small-for-dates baby demand meticulous attention to fetal growth in the third trimester of pregnancy.

Family history. — A family history of diabetes may suggest the possibility of a large but immature baby. A family history of congenital defects, twinning, etc., should lead to special care in the antenatal period, and in some cases, amniocentesis or advice from a geneticist may be necessary.

Social history. — There is good evidence that babies born to mothers whose own childhood has been unhappy or resulted in separation of them from their parents at an early age and babies born to mothers under the age of 20 are more likely to suffer from battering, cot deaths and behaviour disorders. Identification of these mothers in the antenatal period makes it possible for the general practitioner and health visitor to anticipate trouble and provide extra help at this time and in the postnatal period. Low socio-economic status is also associated with complications in labour and problems in the first year of life.

Problems of gestation. — Uncertainty concerning the date of the last menstrual period not uncommonly occurs when patients have irregular cycles or after oral contraception. These patients need close observation, and ultrasound examination early in pregnancy will clarify the duration of gestation.

Continuity of care in pregnancy

The provision of continuing care in pregnancy is usually described in terms of the action to be taken at the various antenatal visits which take place at monthly intervals up to the twenty-eighth week, two-weekly intervals from then until the thirty-sixth week and then weekly until term. These details can be obtained from standard textbooks in obstetrics. This chapter is concerned more with the continuity of care which the general practitioner can provide at this time and which facilitates the early identification of deviations from normality. In broad terms, it is concerned with monitoring the health of the mother through pregnancy and into the postnatal period and monitoring the growth of the fetus in the uterus and subsequent extra-uterine development into infancy. It is also concerned with monitoring the physical relationship of the mother to the fetus in pregnancy and the physical and emotional relationships which develop subsequently in the context of the family.

Monitoring maternal health. — In the first three months of pregnancy many women feel nauseated in the morning and unusually tired. Occasionally vomiting in the morning or, rarely, all day long becomes a problem. Patients should be reassured that this does not mean that there is anything wrong with the pregnancy and that indeed it is associated with the hormones that the body is producing to accommodate the pregnancy. They can also be told that it will almost certainly disappear by the sixteenth week. Taking a cup of tea and a biscuit before rising can be helpful in alleviating the symptoms. There is disinclination to use drugs at this stage in pregnancy, but if symptoms persist meclozine hydrochloride (Ancoloxin) 25 mg can be helpful and has been used for over three decades without any evidence of teratogenicity.

Later in pregnancy, the mother usually feels well and monitoring her physical health will depend on recording a number of serial observations.

Weight gain. Maternal weight gain is an important indicator in pregnancy. In the first three months there may be little change in weight. Subsequently, the mother may be expected to gain about 5 lb (2.5 kg) per month. Failure to gain weight in the absence of dieting may indicate retarded fetal growth, particularly in the last trimester of pregnancy. Excessive weight gain in the third trimester may indicate fluid retention and impending toxaemia. Obese patients in pregnancy need dietetic advice on carbohydrate restriction and some may be able to maintain their weight at a reasonably stable level despite fetal growth and development. The assessment of changes in weight in pregnancy must be made in relationship to diet and other observations such as the presence of oedema or a rise in blood pressure.

Following delivery sudden weight gain may be associated with puerperal depression and obsessional eating. The postnatal period is a time for special vigilance concerning maternal weight and eating habits which may be changed radically by the arrival of a new baby.

Haematology. Anaemia in pregnancy is relatively uncommon today. An initial measurement of haemoglobin is followed by further measurements at twenty-eight and thirty-six weeks. Most general practitioners routinely prescribe iron and folic acid to be taken daily during pregnancy. In African immigrants sickle-cell traits are looked for in early pregnancy. If present, specialist's advice should be sought. In rhesus-negative mothers, antibodies are always looked for and can be prevented in subsequent pregnancies by the injection of anti-D gammaglobulin in the immediate postnatal period. If post-partum haemorrhage occurs, the haemoglobin is measured postnatally and monitored until it returns to normal. Severe iron-deficiency anaemia in pregnancy not responding to iron by mouth will require parenteral administration and, if discovered late in pregnancy, the transfusion of packed red cells.

Urinalysis. A mid-stream specimen of urine is examined at the beginning of pregnancy for asymptomatic bacteriuria, which, if present, needs treatment. Subsequently, any symptoms of urinary-tract infection lead to further bacteriological examination. In treating bacteriuria, it is important to avoid using drugs which may affect the fetus. Amoxycillin or metronidazole are the drugs of choice. Regular examination of the urine for protein will help to detect toxaemia of pregnancy and may alert one to the possible presence of asymptomatic urinary-tract infections.
Glycosuria is not uncommon in pregnancy due to the kidneys developing a low renal threshold for glucose. This finding should lead to examination of further specimens and if this persists a glucose-tolerance test will exclude the possibility of diabetes. Postnatally, urinalysis is required if there has been any evidence of toxaemia of pregnancy and microbiological examination if there has been a urinary-tract infection in the antenatal period.

Measurement of blood pressure. This is carried out routinely in pregnancy. Frequently, the blood pressure is low in early pregnancy and to obtain an accurate diastolic reading it is important to flex the patient's arm slightly while taking the recording. In very fat patients a relatively high value for systolic pressure may be obtained, and here serial measurements are particularly important. A rise in blood pressure in the third trimester should always attract attention and in cases where toxaemia of pregnancy is suspected daily recordings by the practice nursing sister may form part of the continuing care. In some cases where complete rest is recommended these recordings may be taken in the patient's home. At the postnatal visit, the blood pressure is recorded and in patients who have had toxaemia long-term follow-up may be desirable. When the blood pressure remains high postnatally, contraceptive hormones should be avoided as a method of family planning.

Dental care. Even today, many patients are frightened of the dentist. The need for dental care in pregnancy may be stressed and the fact that advice has been taken verified at subsequent antenatal visits.

Care of the breasts. — The benefits for the infant of breast feeding may be discussed at the first antenatal visit and subsequently reinforced during pregnancy. In mothers who reject breast feeding at the outset it is often worth exploring the reasons for this. Some of them may arise from ignorance or false attitudes to motherhood or sexuality and if carefully explored can be helpful in understanding the mother's approach to pregnancy and possibly helping her to adjust to the situation. While encouraging breast feeding, one should warn mothers that establishing feeding may not be easy in some cases and that the crucial period is usually the time when they are discharged from hospital. As they begin to resume their normal activities at home, there may be a temporary mismatch between the infant's demands and the mother's ability to respond. The health visitor has an important part to play at this time. Cracked nipples may cause special problems in breast feeding and can be avoided in some cases by antenatal preparation designed to harden the nipples. Vigorous drying of the nipples at bath time with a rough towel may be helpful. In the immediate postnatal period, the use of a silicone barrier cream or Tinct Benz Co may sometimes be helpful if the nipples become sore. Should an abscess develop, the use of an antibiotic with particular activity against the staphylococcus such as flucloxacillin is indicated.

Patients who decide not to breast feed may ask for tablets to prevent lactation. The use of hormones at this time is generally contra-indicated because of the added risk of thrombo-embolism when they are employed. The patient may be advised to support the breasts firmly and reduce her salt and fluid intake to a minimum. In rare cases where drugs are required a diuretic may be helpful or failing this bromocriptine (Parlodel) 2.5 mg twice daily for 14 days.

Care of the perineum. — Most women in pregnancy experience a vaginal discharge in excess of their normal in the non-pregnant state. This is due to the hyperaemia of the vagina which occurs during pregnancy. Excessive discharge, particularly if it is itching or offensive, should lead to investigation by culture from a charcoal swab which can be transmitted to the laboratory in Stuart's medium. The infection should then be treated appropriately and both nystatin and metronidazole are safe to use during pregnancy.

Following delivery, perineal lacerations are treated by regular salt baths, and at the postnatal examination the perineum should be carefully inspected for any signs of persistent infection and palpated for tenderness. Six weeks postnatally the perineum has usually returned to normal but persistent tenderness may indicate the need for a further examination one month later. In these cases, it is wise to advise the mother to abstain from sexual intercourse until the perineum has returned to normal as dyspareunia may lead to fear of intercourse, vaginismus and a situation which may be very difficult to cure.

At the postnatal examination, enquiry is made about stress

incontinence and if vaginal examination reveals a lack of power in the levator muscles, the patient may be advised to carry out perineal exercises to strengthen these muscles. Patients should usually be given positive advice about when it is appropriate to resume sexual intercourse as many are in doubt.

Gastro-intestinal problems. — Many patients experience constipation in pregnancy. When possible, this is best relieved by the use of bulk purgatives. Heartburn may be troublesome in later pregnancy and may be relieved by raising the head of the bed, taking the main meals without fluid and drinking between meals and the use of simple antacids such as magnesium trisilicate mixture.

Haemorrhoids may be troublesome in pregnancy and need symptomatic treatment in ensuring a regular soft bowel motion and possibly the use of suppositories or ointment, such as Anusol HC. They usually resolve rapidly following delivery.

A fissure in ano may present in the postnatal period due, presumably, to distention of the anus at the time of delivery. This will usually heal if the bowels are kept regular and well lubricated by, for instance, liquid paraffin emulsion and local lubricants applied prior to defaecation. Surgical treatment is rarely necessary.

Musculo-skeletal problems. — Many patients suffer from backache in late pregnancy. This is due to the abnormal lordosis which is necessary for them in order to maintain their centre of gravity. In obese patients, it may be anticipated and sometimes prevented by the use of a well-designed obstetric corset. In some patients, acute pain may be experienced due to separation of the symphysis pubis in late pregnancy. There is usually localized tenderness on pressure over the symphysis in these cases. This can only be treated by rest.

Varicose veins commonly develop in pregnancy. They should be treated by support stockings or tights.

Social and psychological problems

Almost all mothers experience some anxiety as to whether their child will be physically and mentally normal. At each antenatal visit, the doctor should reassure the mother that everything is normal and should be prepared to discuss any anxieties. In some cases, such as patients over 35 years of age or patients with a family history or past obstetric history of congenital abnormality, such anxiety may be fully justified. In consultation with the obstetrician amniocentesis may be indicated in some of these cases.

Mothers' knowledge about pregnancy and childbirth varies widely and they are exposed daily to the propaganda, not all of which is well-informed, of women's magazines, their neighbours and their family. Recent studies have shown that many women fear that sexual intercourse during pregnancy may be harmful to the fetus and others become concerned about changes in their sexual feelings in pregnancy. Some are concerned about drugs which they have inadvertently taken early in pregnancy or about their cigarette or alcohol consumption. A well-organized antenatal clinic will provide mothers with opportunities to discuss these problems. Where it is possible, it is advantageous to involve the father in antenatal care, even if he attends on only one occasion. This provides an excellent opportunity to explore the hopes and fears of the family. In some cases, the arrival of another baby presents serious social or financial problems and this is particularly so in the case of unmarried mothers. In such situations the practice health visitor has an invaluable contribution to make.

Postnatally, the doctor is privileged to observe the development of a new family or the addition to an established family. At the postnatal examination and subsequently at visits to the well-baby clinic he should enquire about the way the family is responding to the new arrival. A period of depression or emotional lability in the mother is almost normal in the immediate postnatal period but may need some explanation to the confused husband. Equally, the husband may feel deprived when his wife focuses all her attention on the newborn baby and a few words of advice to the mother may avert marital disharmony.

Monitoring the Growth of the Foetus and Infant

At the same time as the doctor monitors the health of the pregnant mother, he is also involved in monitoring the development of the foetus and subsequently the newborn infant.

Vaginal bleeding in pregnancy. — In the first trimester of pregnancy the major risk to the fetus is of abortion. Spontaneous abortion probably occurs in about one pregnancy in six and in the majority the cause is not known. Bleeding in early pregnancy can only be treated by rest. If the bleeding is accompanied by pain and dilatation of the cervix, an abortion becomes inevitable. In suitable social circumstances this may be treated at home but in some cases hospital care is needed particularly if the bleeding is heavy or continuous. Bleeding in late pregnancy indicates abruptio placentae or placenta praevia and in all cases needs specialist advice. Occasionally, bleeding in early pregnancy may come from a cervical erosion which can be demonstrated by speculum examination.

Fetal growth. — It is always useful to assess uterine size by pelvic examination at the outset of pregnancy. The difference in size between an eight- and twelve-week pregnancy is obvious on pelvic examination at this time whereas the difference in gestation later in pregnancy on abdominal examination may be much less easy to judge.

Maternal weight gain in later pregnancy is an important indicator of fetal development and failure to gain weight in the absence of any cogent reason is usually an indication of failure in fetal growth. Measurement of fetal growth by successive measurements of the uterine height above the symphysis pubis is, after a period of disdain, attracting increasing attention. The full benefits of serial measurements can only be obtained if they are made each time by the same observer. After about twenty weeks, the uterine height in centimetres above the symphysis is about 4 cm below the expected period of gestation in weeks. Serial measurements can detect a failure in uterine growth and if this is associated with a failure of maternal weight gain it has serious implications for the fetus.

Ultrasound offers a new method of measuring fetal growth. It is most accurate between the twelfth and twentieth weeks of pregnancy. It should be carried out in patients in whom there is some doubt about the date of the last menstrual period and in patients in whom there is a discrepancy between the expected and observed state of gestation. Similar measurements in late pregnancy can help to identify fetuses which are failing to develop and help to clarify when active intervention in initiating labour is desirable.

Failure of fetal growth in late pregnancy is usually associated with placental insufficiency. There is as yet no perfect test of placental insufficiency but serial tests of urinary oestriol excretion may be helpful. This requires a 24-hour urine specimen and there is often delay in obtaining the results. New methods of investigation using radioimmunoassay techniques have been developed for measuring plasma oestriol and human placental lactogen. Both investigations if carried out at intervals are useful in indicating placental insufficiency. Clinical evidence of failing fetal growth will lead to advice from the obstetrician who may recommend one or other of these tests depending very often on the resources available or admission to hospital for 24 hours for fetal monitoring.

Following delivery, the general practitioner is equally concerned with the development of the newborn baby. This may be expected to regain its birth weight by about ten days and subsequently to gain about 300 g per week during the first six weeks. At this time, it is usual for the general practitioner to carry out a developmental assessment.

Monitoring the relationship between mother and baby

In the antenatal period this is concerned mainly with the physical relationship between the fetus and its mother. It is important, however, particularly in early pregnancy not to ignore the emotional aspects. Is the baby wanted and planned, or is it causing an unpremeditated marriage or simply a reminder of a disastrous sexual relationship? If the general practitioner knows the answers to these sorts of questions, he is better placed in planning his care for the mother both during pregnancy and in the postnatal period.

During pregnancy, the need to observe and record the physical relationship between mother and fetus becomes particularly important after the thirty-fourth week. Up to this time, the presentation of the fetus is often unstable. By the thirty-fourth week most fetuses will have adopted a cephalic presentation and in primigravidae the head will become engaged in the pelvis by about the thirty-sixth week. An unstable or breech presentation after the thirty-fourth week calls for specialist assessment, as also does an unengaged vertex presentation in a primigravida at the thirty-eighth week. Abdominal examination at this stage will usually suffice to ascertain the presenting part and whether or not the head is engaged, but if in doubt a vaginal examination will usually resolve any doubtful cases.

In the case of a persistent breech presentation, the obstetrician may attempt an external cephalic version or may accept the patient for breech delivery. In the latter case, it is wise to obtain an X-ray of the pelvis to ensure that it is of adequate size. Rarely, it may be necessary to carry out elective caesarian section.

The mother is naturally interested to know about the presentation of her baby. In the case of a persistent breech presentation it is important to discuss this in detail because many mothers have great anxiety at the prospect of a breech delivery.

Time may be set aside during the last few weeks of pregnancy to discuss delivery. Most mothers may attend antenatal classes but are often left with uncertainties. Should they have an epidural anaesthetic? Should their husband attend? Will they be allowed to hold their baby after delivery? Will they feel an episiotomy, etc.? It may be helpful to liken labour to an activity such as climbing Everest. It is hard work and at times painful but the reward far exceeds the effort and pain expended.

Following delivery, all mothers should have an opportunity to cuddle their baby and put it to breast as soon as possible. The general practitioner although he may visit his mothers in hospital will, in some cases, not be involved in her care until she is discharged from hospital. He then has an opportunity to visit at home and see how the new baby is fitting into the family. At this stage, the practice health visitor has a major part to play and it is here that the attached health visitor will benefit from her prior contact with the patient in the antenatal period. On returning home, the breast-feeding mother may encounter some difficulties as she becomes more active physically. She needs reassurance at this stage and encouragement to increase her fluid intake and, if possible, spend an hour or two on the bed each afternoon.

During the early weeks after delivery, the mother is likely to be very preoccupied with her new infant. She may also be moody or depressed. This is a time when the father may feel confused and out of it and should be encouraged to take an active part in tending to the new infant, such as bathing, changing nappies, etc. The first few weeks after delivery can cement or shatter a marriage and the general practitioner and health visitor have a special responsibility to see that the former occurs.

Conclusions

Pregnancy, delivery and the immediate post-partum period have been described in this chapter as an integral part of the continuing care provided by the general practitioner. Improved technology in the delivery suite indicates that hospital is the ideal place for confinement although it may make care rather more impersonal. This makes it more important for the patient's personal doctor to be involved in the antenatal and postnatal period as in many cases only he can offer true continuity of care. The precise roles of general practitioner, health visitor and community midwife at this time have not been clearly defined. It is doubtful if a firm definition of roles in this situation is helpful. Each of these members of the primary health care team is capable of providing most of the services described. What is important is to provide continuity of care and use the skills available in the most productive way.

4.6
The middle years

Julian Tudor Hart

Death and disability in middle age

The child who succeeds in being born without any obvious gross defect can now expect to live about 70 years for a man, 75 for a woman. As he reaches adolescence, marginal risks of malignant disease recede, and the risks of violent death merge with problems of behaviour and social adjustment. The content of primary care comes to centre on these, on transient, usually self-limiting and self-contained, episodes of illness. Death is hardly thought of, and fear of it is a sign of emotional immaturity. The engineering aspects of medical care can be almost ignored, and the doctor as priest can flourish.

In men, 5 per cent of deaths occur from birth to 39 years; from 40 to 64 they leap to over 30 per cent. Equivalent figures for women are 4 per cent and 14 per cent. By age 65, 12 per cent of men and 33 per cent of women have been widowed. Chronic disability accelerates in the same way. At ages 15 to 44, about 10 per cent of men and 8 per cent of women have some limiting longstanding illness; at 45 to 64, these proportions rise to 25 per cent in both sexes.

Risks of death and chronic ill health are strongly related to social class, and the social character of a practice largely determines the burden of organic disease seen by the doctor. Death rates below age 65 are 75 per cent higher for unskilled labourers than for higher managerial and professional men. Limiting longstanding illness is 2½ times as common in men of the same groups, and three times as common in their wives.

The ideas outlined in this chapter are derived from and apply to general practice in the National Health Service; in which there is functional and professional separation of primary from hospital care; in which access to hospital specialists is normally by referral through a general practitioner; in which everyone, well or ill, has access to their own doctor with minimal financial barriers; in which each general practitioner has a more or less stable list of patients for whose care he is continuously and fully responsible; in which the general practitioner is paid for that personal responsibility rather than for individual items of service; and in which an entire generation of doctors and patients has been adapted to this experience for nearly thirty years. It is important to bear this in mind, since these assumptions cannot be made in most other countries of the European Common Market, the USA, or the 'white Commonwealth'. Ideas in the context of the National Health Service may have wholly different meanings and implications, or may not be feasible at all, in other contexts.

Death, chronic disability, and the reasonable fear of these are therefore the inescapable background to medical care in middle age, the more so because at this time the over-riding aim of all diagnosis and treatment is still to preserve life, whereas in old age this is supplanted by the aim of improving its quality.

In a specially threatening way, continuing care in middle age is fraught with uncertainty, ambiguity and error. The immature patient and the immature doctor are alike unable to tolerate such uncertainty, and in middle age the vain attempt to prove negatives takes off for its costly and futile journey through the hospital departments.

'Multiple pathology'

The patient's problem must be evaluated in physical, psychological and social terms; not one, but all three always. In this sense, even in younger patients, the pathological background is always multiple, and the search for alternative psychological or somatic morbid states misconceived. Hospitals dealing only in episodes of sickness may be able to evade the consequences of their simple and one-sided diagnoses, but in primary care problems must either be solved (or at least recognized) in their true complexity, or endured until they are buried. Either as cause or effect, neurotic symptoms tend to be associated with somatic symptoms. In random samples from the general population, those with psychiatric illness have 55 per cent more major physical illness, and are seven times more likely to have two or more major physical illnesses.[1]

Certain emotional states lead to awareness of bodily function normally unnoticed, which together with the patient's ideas of pathology may lead to permanent fearfulness; in terms of the information available to the patient, these fears are rational. To an even greater extent, there is association both of cause and effect between psychological and somatic disease, and social problems. The association between social class and mortality has been referred to. Of clients newly presenting to a social service department in London, not referred from doctors, 47 per cent had major physical illness or disability, and 16 per cent major mental illness. Presented symptoms do not, of course, fully reflect symptomatic illness in the population.[2]

A generally increased level of symptoms in all dimensions is clearly related to subsequent mortality, particularly in early middle age, but less so later on. In men in active work aged 35 to 54 at entry, mortality was more than twice as high in those with high scores on the Cornell Medical Index (a rating of symptoms across a wide range of variables); little association was found in those aged 55 to 69 at entry. Known biological risk factors (cholesterol, blood pressure and weight for height), on the other hand, had high predictive value for mortality in both age-groups.[3]

In middle age, not only are all symptoms more common, and more often associated either causally or coincidentally with serious disease, but so are the irreversible complications of prolonged asymptomatic deviations from normal physiological values of arterial pressure, cholesterol, glucose, and cervical cytology.

The dimension of time

Hospital care is episodic. Whilst hospital doctors are more aware than they were that each episode is only one stage in the life of the patient and the natural history of his illness, the high intensity of hospital care tends to compress investigation to a short time without reliable data from the past or opportunity for easy revision during an observed future. Although hospital doctors gain advantage from their relative abundance of peer criticism, they see neither the origins of illness nor the remote consequences of their actions, and are under pressure to reach a clinically respectable diagnosis before discharge. In general practice the term 'back pain ?cause' is a good diagnosis in the absence of confirmatory signs of disc protrusion; it has the great merit of not obstructing the later diagnosis of spinal cord tumour or whatever. Such naive truthfulness is difficult in hospital, where each episode must be neatly packaged and dispatched back to primary care, and waiting and seeing is not officially admissible.

Primary care diagnosis can be experimental. The most likely, or sometimes the most important, of the several hypotheses generated by the first consultation, can be reviewed after hours, weeks, or months of further history, with or without various planned interventions, and a sequence of simple but critical investigations. The process is thrifty in everything but time; a repeated return to the history from a sequence of separate angles.

The initial hypotheses can also be more economic than those required for good specialist care in hospital; they can be tried for reasonable fit into an already familiar story, then relegated to the most remote periphery of possibility, or pursued with determination in the light of that story.

Of course, if the story has not already been recorded accurately, if it lacks quantified baseline values, if good records are simply not read when the time comes for later decision, or if, in the absence of any records worthy of the name, the story has been simplified to a mnemonic caricature, then the whole of this advantage is thrown away. It is replaced by its opposite, cocksure assumption that the present must be a simple projection from the past, without any search for evidence. Since most disorders are either self-limiting, or progress rapidly to self-evident diagnosis and a shift to hospital care, slipshod investigation, data-recording, and data-recall have an astonishing capacity to survive, equalled only by the patients to whom they are applied.

If records truly represent those fragments of the patient's life observed in 10 or 20 years of continuous care, and are fully used in conjunction with current and retained impressions of the patient's language, personality, and motivation, they give the practitioner an immense diagnostic advantage. They narrow the field of possible hypotheses to the few that make sense in that private context, and suggest particular ways of testing them over appropriate periods of time. They give the confidence necessary to battle on for evidence when that is needed, and to resist pressure from patients and relatives for futile shopping-around when it is not; and the means to change one's mind, as one must often do, on evidence rather than impulse.

The engineer model

Forced to analogy, most of us would probably still choose engineer rather than priest. For all its failings, engineering is the power of all men to change the world, priesthood a means of enduring it unchanged.

Real advances in medicine have come from regarding man as a particular kind of machine; they will continue to do so at higher levels of complexity. What particular kind of machine? Beautiful, precious, a dynamic equilibrium of contradictory processes, wonderfully equipped with sequentially protective mechanisms of self-regulation. Our necessarily crude interventions must be applied with the greatest caution and respect. They can be justified only by real evidence that they do more good than harm, not only in terms of immediate effects, but also of remote consequences. We are ruled as much by custom as by reason, and custom is historically evolved. The history of medicine is not only the history of cure and care, but also of the appearance of cure and the appearance of care. The separation even now of illusion from reality is difficult and complex, the more so because we are hedged about by the customary expectations of our colleagues and our patients. The subject of our engineering is enormously complex, our knowledge of it is still vastly exceeded by our ignorance, yet what is known is already far greater than any of us can know. It is no use taking fright at this and deciding that life would be simpler if we were priests. We have to learn to be engineers in human biology, medical scientists capable of adapting the theoretical advances of science to the specific people and populations for whom we are responsible, in such a way that the course of events is actually changed.

It is true that the engineering model suggests a passive role for the patient, a present feature of care most urgently requiring change. The human machine has a brain and a voice, which of all protective and self-regulating mechanisms are the most valuable to life and health. 'Listen to the patient', said Charcot, 'he is telling you the diagnosis'. Not only can he tell us the diagnosis, he can and must work jointly with us on the plan of treatment. Our fault lies not in the engineering model, but in that style of education that teaches fascination with disease verging on love, and detachment from patients bordering on contempt.

Continuing care of the middle aged requires hatred of disease and attachment to patients, powerful enough to sustain painstaking work over decades, going far beyond response to presented symptoms, actively pursuing health conservation. We may call this a style of anticipatory care.[3]

Patterns of consultation, morbidity and mortality

In the age group 45 to 64, cancers and acute myocardial infarction each account for about one-third of all deaths, but for fewer than 1 per cent of people consulting an average general practitioner in one year. Cerebrovascular accidents cause over 8 per cent of deaths, but less than 0.5 per cent of people consulting. Even if we lump together all the presenting (not casually detected) risk factors for myocardial infarction – obesity, hypertension, diabetes mellitus, peripheral arterial disease and angina pectoris – they account for only 8 per cent of people consulting.

The distribution of sickness is different from the distribution of causes of death. The main causes of prolonged disability also differ from the main immediate causes of consultation. Transient minor disorder tends to displace severe but stable chronic disability. Consultations tend to be concentrated at the inception of major disability, and at points of instability during its subsequent course.

Serious disorders may be endured over long periods with little medical supervision. Moreover, the doctor is not only a direct source of care and cure, but also the sole gateway to the rest of the NHS, to sick status and the social insurance connected with it. He is consulted for all of these things, so that the relevance of consultation in general to the conservation of health may become very indistinct when viewed in standard teaching-hospital terms.

Nearly every process in the NHS starts from a transaction, in which a patient with a problem enters the system through a primary-care consultation where he seeks its solution. If each immediate problem is dispatched as quickly and simply as possible, to the apparent satisfaction of the customer in the most superficial terms, isolated from preceding and subsequent consultations by failure either to record the current episode accurately or to review the story so far, the episode can be no more than itself; and in itself it will most often be trivial. A style of consultation that is all tactics and no strategy, that aims only at the immediate satisfaction of presenting complaints, moving as quickly as possible to next business, has a trivializing effect on the whole of our work. It ensures not only that about 80 per cent of our task is beneath the notice of the kind of medicine we still learn in teaching hospitals, but also that no other kind of medicine can be developed to replace it. The solution does not lie in teaching us how to deal with episodes in clinically trivialized isolation while remaining contented with our lot. It lies in bringing the episodes together into a connected story relevant to the conservation of the patient's health, the most exciting aim that is possible in medicine. It lies in harnessing the immense inertial force of transactional care (people generate large and small problems all the time and will continue to do so) to life-long conservation of health.

Constraints on the shift from episodic to anticipatory care

Major outcomes – death or serious irreversible disability – are for the most part preceded by a more or less prolonged period of accumulating but reversible risk. Some of these prodromes – for instance, those of chronic middle and lower respiratory disease – lead to symptoms which prompt consultation. The doctor may then already choose to go beyond episodic transaction to anticipatory care; he may be more concerned with remote consequences than is the patient, and less satisfied with apparently quick symptomatic solutions based largely on the natural tendency of most acute episodes to remit without treatment, or in spite of it. The same is true of a wide range of common and important disorders: early alcoholism and drug dependence, sickness-seeking neuroses, recurrent urinary tract infection in women, occupational dermatitis, chronic low back pain, obesity, piles, and some forms of psychotic illness. Other prodromes are either not associated with symptoms, or only fortuitously associated. They are found only by looking for them in the course of some standardized investigation: high arterial pressure, cholesterol, impaired glucose tolerance, early renal failure, in-situ carcinoma of the cervix, and bladder cancer in those exposed to occupational carcinogens. Finally there is that most potent and curious risk factor of all for lethal disease, smoking; never complained of, always significant, without doubt reversible – but how?

Just over two-thirds of people aged 45 to 64 consult their general practitioner at some time in each year, a remarkably constant figure in many different countries and cultures. There is less evidence about the number who do not consult over 5-year spans, but this is probably seldom more than 15 per cent or less than 5 per cent. Few non-consulters will suffer from the symptomatic prodromes, except for psychotic illness. Probably more than 90 per cent of the population will therefore be covered by a system of health supervision based on normal consultations, over 5-year spans.

Anticipatory care of symptomatic prodromes requires the planned, rational approach already outlined in Part 3 of this book. Diagnosis will depend on a branching decision-tree, each fork of which is based on some kind of verbal, clinical, laboratory or radiological measurement. Treatment will require titration of a drug or procedure against a measured outcome; even 'better, worse, or the same' is in this sense a measurement. There is no evidence that rational anticipatory care is less laborious and time-consuming than episodic symptomatic care; it nearly always requires more history and other data collection, more follow-up, and much more communication both ways with the patient. It may reduce subsequent consultation for problems that persist because they have been evaded, rather than solved or acknowledged as insoluble; but even this is uncertain, since many patients will reward an ineffective doctor by attempting to cope unaided with their own complaints. It almost certainly reduces medication, but the savings from this will not go to assist the primary care team. Good anticipatory care increases work load, with consequences for each practice and for the NHS as a whole.

The constraints of time in present general practice are severe. Buchan and Richardson[4] showed an average face-to-face time of 5 minutes in over 2,000 consultations by 22 general practitioners, with half of them lying in the range 2.8 to 6.3 minutes. The average time in the 45 to 64 age-group was 5.4 minutes, with 28 per cent more time spent on history, 10 per cent less on examination, and 20 per cent less on advice, than the average for all ages. There was no difference in time taken for men and women, but patients of professional and managerial class got 50 per cent more time on history than all other social classes, and 3½ times as much time on indirect consultation (about other members of the family) and social chat. These authors concluded that 'if more clinical responsibility is to be placed on the family doctor and his team, if that team is to accept the challenge of preventive medicine, if comprehensive health records are to become a reality, the objective of at least 10 minutes per consultation should be a top priority'.

It is only necessary to consider the data required for rational management of such common conditions as obstructive airways disease[5] or hypertension to see that such work cannot be contained within these time limits. Apart from antibiotics, safe and effective use of nearly all drugs depends on the repeated titration of dosage against measured response, desired or otherwise; such measurements take time. The clinical quality of consultation within present constraints is always precarious; there is good evidence of this even in the best teaching practices.[6]

To some extent these constraints can be overcome by reduction of minor and casual work load, by improved organization, and by delegation of work to ancillary staff. There is sound evidence for a nation-wide decline in home visiting which still continues, and this certainly makes more 'office' consultation time available. There is also some evidence of declining 'office' consultation rates in some practices; this cannot yet be assumed to be a national trend, and may in part reflect decasualization by the spread of appointment systems. There is some evidence that the large differences in work load between practices and between areas are linked with high morbidity and mortality, and certainly with the social composition of practice populations. Those populations most in need of good anticipatory care are also those of high work load, constrained resources, and low patient expectation.[7] Improvements in organization tend to attract more work load, from within the population and perhaps by extending it. Work becomes more efficient, but it also increases, since slipshod practice repels serious custom while encouraging casual, superficial complaint. High-speed, low-quality general practice is ineffective in changing outcomes of illness, but high-quality care cannot compete with it in economy of time and resources, a fact not lost on the many governments since the Insurance Act of 1912 that have ignored the squalor of urban industrial general practice, with a canny appreciation of the high yield of primary care for social morale, despite low clinical effectiveness.

Generally speaking, improvements in organization lead to doing things well that previously were not done at all; in a capitation system, that represents no saving either in time or treasure. Typewritten referral letters lead to keeping copies and filing correspondence in date order, so that hospital letters are not only kept but read, using up more doctor's time. Efficient filing and record-keeping means that the doctor makes and reads notes instead of 'keeping it all in his head': more doctor's time. Flow-charts in A4 size records, for sequential weight, peak expiratory flow rate, arterial pressure, or centile progress charts in infancy greatly extend the quality and speed of decision-making, but they involve huge amounts of staff time to set them up, and a continuous state of alertness by doctors to maintain them: more doctor's time. Use of age–sex registers, preferably with a rapid data-recall system such as feature-cards, is almost indispensable for rational planning of care in whole populations, if we are to stop depending entirely on patient initiative, but they are costly in time and labour to establish, and add yet more to the daily chores of the office staff. All of these are ways of doing new things better, rather than old things more efficiently.

Delegation of work

Anticipatory care is not feasible without extensive delegation of work to ancillary staff, particularly of clinical measurements. It seems doubtful whether the initial assessment of newly presenting illness can be called delegation. No new episode in any age-group is wholly predictable, and if medical training confers any diagnostic advantage the patient should have it. If it does not, we had better change that training to make it more effective. Once that assessment has been made, however, a competently and fully performed checklist approach delegated to a nurse, can for the first time release the doctor to work out an individual plan of treatment for each patient, with audit of outcome. This can only work for conditions that are common, that feature quantified variables, and for which standardized diagnostic and treatment packages have been validated by evidence of controlled trials and studies of natural history in whole populations. For practice populations under 5,000, these include (in middle age) the control of treated or observed hypertension in the diastolic range 100+ mm Hg, all forms of obstructive airways disease, and urinary-tract infection. In populations larger than this, the number of insulin-dependent diabetics is sufficient to justify elaboration of a 'follow-up package' of the same kind. Between them, these cover quite a lot of middle-age chronic morbidity. Similar packages can be devised for control and observation of rheumatoid arthritis treated by penicillamine, but again the numbers are small.

Delegated elements of these packages can relieve doctor time in any situation where they arise. Delegated tasks may include the taking of venous blood, measurement of height and weight, calculation of weight-for-height formulas, measurement of arterial pressure, quadriceps circumference, haemoglobin, erythrocyte sedimentation rate (ESR), audiometry, visual fields, visual acuity, peak expiratory flow rate with calculation of expected rate for age, sex and height, cervical smears, skin scrapings, blood smears, bacteriological swabs, incubation and reading of urine dipslide cultures and other routine urine analyses, suture of small wounds, removal of stitches, ear-syringing: so much, in fact, that six doctors working to a good but routine diagnostic standard should keep four nurses busy most of the time. In smaller units the flow of delegated work is much more uneven and difficult to plan economically. All this greatly enlarges the scope, effectiveness, and satisfaction of clinical work in primary care, but there is no net gain in time. The doctor can concentrate on effective history-taking and decision-making, but he will still be seeing the same 15 or 20 patients each session, will still begin to wilt after the 21st patient, and will still feel the constraints of time. He is using his improved resources to do more and do it better, not to take on a larger caseload.

Flagging systems for patients with certain chronic conditions that have a single valid tracking variable (weight, arterial pressure, peak flow rate) may, with constant vigilance, ensure that they seldom see the doctor without previous measurement of that variable by a nurse. This permits the doctor, perhaps for the first time, to stick to the rules of good but simple clinical medicine. Many of us, including myself, could not do clinical work of high quality when we worked on our own; we took calculated risks, stole time from the many to give to a few patients of special concern, and even then sporadically, as circumstance permitted. Delegation of clinical work to ancillary staff has made simple but good clinical care available to all patients, all the time, in a way that was not previously possible. In my experience, however, it has not permitted either a saving of medical time over-all, or an enlargement of the population cared for.

There are many good doctors who do not agree with this view. These differences of opinion are in part differences of experience, depending on differing social composition of practice populations, and on local customs that largely dictate what the public expects of its doctors. On present evidence it seems wise to conclude that the doctor who wishes to steer the style of care beyond immediate response to presented symptoms, to a planned strategy of anticipatory care, will be very lucky indeed if he can cope with more than 2,000 to 2,500 patients at risk, even with maximum ancillary staff backup.

Relation of hospital to primary care in middle age

An important regional variable is the quantity and quality of available hospital care, and the extent to which this may usurp the primary care function or, on the other hand, fail to provide all the services appropriate to primary care. This is certainly an important factor determining apparent optimal practice size.

Only 6 per cent of hospital admissions are to general-practitioner beds in cottage hospitals. Elsewhere, admission procedures include information from the practitioner, which may or may not be acted upon. For emergency and some planned admissions, there is some continuity from primary care to the inception of the hospital phase. Although about 7 per cent of hospital inpatients are visited at some time while they are in hospital by their general practitioner, few of these visits involve any co-operation in planning current or future care. Care after discharge is often not planned at all, but just happens. Routine outpatient follow-up is usual, apparently to ensure against failure of the practitioner to continue observation or treatment. This is an invitation to abdicate responsibility, and hypertensives, diabetics, and other patients with common chronic disorders may slide into more or less permanent hospital care, usually by a succession of junior staff. Where the patient returns to general-practitioner supervision, there may be a more or less prolonged, wasteful and confusing duplication of effort and advice. This may be reduced by stating clearly in referral and admission letters that return of the patient to primary care as soon as possible will be welcomed, and that full responsibility will be accepted for continued observation and treatment. Better still is participation by the practitioner in formulating a treatment plan for the patient while still in hospital. It is still as exceptional for consultants to accept this, as it is for general practitioners to propose it. The situation varies from one area to another; where such a style of work does not exist, it may be encouraged by greater telephone contact or general-practitioner visiting during admission, but time constraints will make this difficult.

Patients should be contacted one way or another within a week of discharge, to confirm that treatment established before admission has been maintained, and that changes have been incorporated into a new treatment plan agreed and understood by the patient.

Diagnosis and plans for action

In the young, disease still tends to be a transient intrusion in an otherwise healthy life. Prospects for total recovery are usually good, and the patient is emotionally, socially, and occupationally more or less mobile, so that all options for treatment are open. In the aged, a mode of thought that in any way considers disease separate from its individual human substrate is impossible: clinical decisions are increasingly subordinate to other personal considerations, and options for treatment are narrowed by the shrinking adaptability of the patient, the diminishing scope of cure, and expanding need for the management of failure and death.

As middle age advances, moving from the cure-orientation of youth to the care-orientation of old age, it encounters first narrow, then broadening, salients of tissue senescence. It brings to these encounters the accumulated damage of inhaled tobacco and industrial pollutants, unbalanced energy intake and expenditure, maladaptations of arterial behaviour and clotting mechanisms, and varying burdens of unhappiness too late for correction. Both the asymptomatic precursors, and the symptomatic effects of most disorders of middle age are graded characteristics, continuously distributed, and much less easily defined than hospital experience tends to suggest. This is clearly true of the cluster of disorders around premature vascular senescence: obesity, diabetes mellitus, angina pectoris, claudication, myocardial and cerebral infarction, sudden cardiac death, hypertension, and deep venous thrombosis and embolism. It is true of the menopause. It is true of rheumatic disease. It is true of nearly all psychiatric disorder. It is not as yet true of the cancers, partly because we know too little of their precursors and untreated natural history, partly because we have so far been unable to use what we do know, to develop an effective anticipatory style.

In these circumstances, diagnosis is not an exercise in description, but the first stage in the elaboration of a plan for action. Unless this plan includes personal and social components, it is unlikely to be sufficiently comprehensible or relevant to sustain the motivations of either doctor or patient over the many years of effort required for the conservation of health in middle age. Whether treatment plans are elaborated in or out of hospital, the practitioner should be the guarantor that they include these personal and social components in a realistic way, and that patients have the opportunity to share in decisions that must ultimately become their own.

Active participation of the patient in diagnosis and management depends on five factors:

1. Assurance of continuity of personal advice
2. Understanding that diagnosis, prognosis, and management decisions are all based on probability rather than certainty, and that all biological measurements show within-subject variability and some degree of technical error
3. Understanding of the natural history of the untreated condition
4. Understanding that there are no effective treatments without risk, and that all management of illness depends on benefit balanced against potential loss
5. Understanding of the limits of and criteria for self-management.

This joint approach by doctor and patient is unfamiliar to some doctors and to many patients. A successful shift away from dogma and *ex officio* authority depends on the creation of a new implied contract between care-giver and care-receiver, and an altogether higher level of understanding on both sides than that to which we have been accustomed. In some patients this cannot be achieved; in many more it may be obstructed by initial fears that, in encouraging a less one-sided and dogmatic style, the doctor is withdrawing guarantees of interest and support. Some patients who most vocally demand the right to run their own illnesses are in the event unable to cope with this responsibility, and reveal this by resorting to multiple sources of advice in a search for certainties that cannot exist. Others, with poorer command of information and less confidence in communication, are more familiar with the uncertainty of everything in life except death, are more tolerant of error, and understand more easily that they share the National Health Service with other people. These limitations of attitude and information can be overcome, but not by ignoring them.

Continuity of personal advice

This cannot simply be a matter of making the same personal doctor available at every consultation. One traditional form of continuity depended on restricting advice to the idiosyncrasies and prejudices of one doctor, backed up by an 'ethical' system wherein all other staff and colleagues supported that advice without regard to circumstances or their own opinions. This eventually became a form of religious observance, in which the personal doctor made himself indispensable, the patient became totally dependent, and other health workers were denied the right to think for themselves. The price of such unrestricted 'clinical freedom' was the bondage of patients and staff within interlocking blocks of personal dogma, fortified by self-fulfilling prophecies, immune to criticism, and relieved only by presenile eccentricity. The British primary care system, with stable lists and powerful pressures against competition, has been particularly subject to this style of mutually agreed suppression of criticism and isolation from new evidence. New entrants to general practice with most to gain and least to lose from a more open approach, have a responsibility to overcome this tradition.

Within a primary care group, there needs to be broad agreement on diagnostic and treatment policies for the main categories of more common disorders. The apparently infinite diversity of diagnostic and treatment options is spurious, reflecting a largely illusory diversity of drugs, and excessive respect for personal opinions that are not backed by evidence. Evidence derived from whole, free-living populations in our own culture (rather than hospital series with an unknown bias of selection) is the only possible basis for the definition of rational diagnostic categories, with agreed criteria and terminology. Such evidence is available only from a small number of classical studies, which should become known to all general practitioners. There are more controlled trials of different treatments, at least of drugs; for surgery they remain very incomplete, nor are we in a position to apply them directly. Few controlled trials, however, take account of the effects of different methods of care sustained over years rather than days or weeks, or relate to ultimate outcomes rather than immediate side-effects and relief of symptoms. Adequate controlled studies in this sense are again few and classical; they permit the rational discussion of a fairly small body of commonly agreed evidence.

Such rational discussion is seriously impaired by the absurd multiplication of brand names, inconsequential molecular variants, and one-sided or inflated claims resulting from the promotion of drugs as commodities for a mass market, rather than precision tools to be used selectively and with caution. Faced with organized pressure favouring spendthrift prescription, alongside snap diagnosis and superficial evaluation, general practitioners should organize counter-pressure of their own by group discussion aiming at agreed group policies. Books such as this are a possible point of departure, not to be followed slavishly, but as an agreed basis for discussion; the exact point of departure is less important than agreement to travel and to arrive. Of course, agreement may prove to be a decision to differ, but at least after discussion such differences should no longer be idiosyncratic, defensible only in the magical terms of personalities of individual doctors. Differences could then be based on interpretation of evidence (including personal experience) that can be rationally defended in discussion.

Clinical continuity

Continuity of care is not a sentimental or genteel adornment of a hard but independently effective clinical machine. It is not a *de luxe* option, to be indulged when the going is easy, and stripped off when it is hard. Without continuity clinical medicine becomes a wasteful and dangerous mess. This truth must be re-asserted again and again, because real continuity is nowhere securely rooted as a norm of clinical behaviour. Our customs derive from the handling of discrete, self-contained hospital episodes, artificially severed from their origins, their consequences, and often even internally divided by specialty. The customs of general practice are in this respect better, but depend on personal attitudes rather than methods of organization and recording. They therefore fail to survive transposition to group practice and rotation of duties, that are bound to replace single-handed practice. Continuity held in the head is tied to intuitive clinical methods; as these are supplanted by more structured styles of treatment and diagnosis, the old continuity is lost also. We have to devise new ways of ensuring continuity linked at each step with clinical methods, so that one cannot proceed without the other.

This clinical continuity has three dimensions: continuity with the past, with the future, and a harmony of management of concurrent problems.

Continuity with the past: data recording and retrieval.– Traditionally, this is established by the history. Because of the habit of managing discrete episodes, it is re-established over and over again. Though this is a wasteful, and to some patients exasperating, method, it has the apparent merit of training the patient to discard what appears to be irrelevant in the story, so that a readily classifiable clinical problem emerges more and more clearly and conveniently for the doctor. Even in the short run, this can be grossly deceptive; the apparent clarity of diagnosis is an artefact, the result of excessive haste in getting away from the jumble of reality. In the long run, it eliminates from the available record the earliest indications of future problems, as they were expressed when they occurred; it throws away the immense advantages the practitioner can have in supplementing a verbal history by careful retrospective study of records. Failure to record histories fully, failure to communicate such records effectively to colleagues sharing the care of the patient, failure to read recorded histories that are available, and failure to believe them if they conflict with a preferred current assessment – all these appear to justify themselves both by their immediate convenience, and by their simplifying effect on the data. In fact, they lead to incomplete, irrelevant or wrong diagnosis, and suppress recognition of the true complexity of continuous anticipatory care.

Clearly this is mainly a problem of data recording and data recall. What data, and how should it be recorded and recalled? For men and women in the age-group 45 to 64, one can devise a checklist of baseline data required for anticipatory care, justified either by their value for preventive action, or for more rapid, accurate and appropriate diagnosis in the event of later symptoms. These are shown in Table I.

	Interrogation	Examination	Investigation
Initial data	Forenames Original surname Date of birth Smoking: age started and peak rate Any important thing you have not told me, you think I should know	Height Squints, pupils, fundi, ptosis Peripheral pulses Heart sounds and murmurs Finger clubbing	
Cumulative data	Acquired names Addresses Occupations Hospital operations, admissions, and major illnesses Immunizations Allergies and drug intolerance Current smoking Current medication	Weight Blood pressure Pulse rate Peak Expiratory Flow Rate or FEV1 Electrocardiogram Urine: dipculture dipstick (Breast lumps) (Haemoglobin)	Chest x-ray Cholesterol Creatinine

	(Menstrual history and current menstrual pattern)	(Pelvic examination and cervical smear)
	(Obstetric history)	
(women only)		

Table I.– Baseline data for anticipatory care in age-group 45 to 64

Nothing is easier than listing such minimum data requirements, and nothing more difficult than actually acquiring and recording them in a form readily accessible for subsequent care. This list could be extended indefinitely by including everything that might conceivably improve the apparent quality of care. Even stripped to necessities, it presents serious problems of gratuitous workload, which in our system must be added to the existing and inescapable obligation to respond to presented illness from the whole registered population.

The items included are those that have been found useful in industrial practice over twenty-five years. The physical signs are mainly useful as baselines. Did this man always have clubbed fingers, persistent crackles at the left base of the lung, or unequal pupils? He will not know the answers himself, at least not reliably. Are the minor changes in the ST segment of this electrocardiogram taken after an episode of chest pain, a new and significant feature, or were they already present 10 years ago? A few are important for all future management: a high plasma creatinine in late middle age, without other symptoms of renal failure, demands a permanent warning flag on the notes to prevent intoxication by drugs cleared in the kidney, or use of tetracycline which may precipitate frank uraemia. Signs of aortic valve incompetence without symptoms will affect subsequent dental care, and increase alertness for septicaemia. One or two are vital: diastolic blood pressures as high as 180 mm Hg can be sustained without any symptoms whatever, and routine measurement in this age-group is the only way to ensure complete ascertainment of all those seriously (not marginally) in need of treatment.

In most cases none of these enquiries or measurements will prove very useful, let alone vital, to future care. Compared with crude symptom-response, the improvements in outcome will no doubt be marginal, but the margin will include real people, people we know. It is a scheme for detecting needles in haystacks. The contribution of doctors to health generally is marginal, less important than housing, education, social happiness or misery; but we are doctors, and it is our job to make the fullest possible contribution within those rather narrow limits. We are by profession needle-seekers, we get satisfaction not only by finding but by searching well, and should be able to accept realistic expectations on the diagnostic yield of screening procedures, without losing motivation.

It is beyond question an advantage, in interpreting an electrocardiogram recorded for diagnosis of recent chest pain, to have access to a pre-ictal recording; yet this advantage will be obtained only by routinely recording electrocardiograms on all those at risk, and keeping them available in the record. This and other measurements can be made without excessive strain by having a standard work-up of each practice in-migrant in this age-group, and of all patients as they reach their 45th birthdays. The work of accumulating complete data on the entire age-group within (say) 1 to 5 years, is in my opinion beyond the resources of any normal practice, and should not be attempted. Recording of blood pressure alone is feasible, and gives a good diagnostic yield. Case-finding of this sort will roughly double the number of known hypertensives, regardless of diagnostic criteria. If conservative criteria are used (in this age-group, a phase V diastolic pressure of 105+ mm Hg sustained over three readings, in both sexes) treatment of asymptomatic hypertension has a dramatic effect on the incidence of stroke, and probably a marginal effect on mortality from coronary thrombosis. Similar screening for glycosuria, with or without modified glucose tolerance tests, has also doubled the known cases of diabetes mellitus, but the consequences are not the same. Although knowledge of the presence of asymptomatic glycosuria is certainly useful in future management, its reversal by treatment has not been shown to have any effect on outcome by reducing the main complications of diabetes.[8] A search for glycosuria should therefore not be a part of a minimum case-finding programme, though it certainly should be included in any full screening programme.

Collection even of the simplest standardized data from an entire age-group in a practice is difficult enough; to record them in a way that encourages subsequent up-dating and permits easy retrieval, is even worse, not least because we have no well-established model to imitate. It is difficult if not impossible to modify the standard octavo sized record envelope so that personal data unrelated to symptoms can be conveniently grouped, easily updated and clearly presented, without duplication in the clinical record. A number of more or less successful attempts to do this have been made, mostly using over-printed immunization summary cards or treatment summary cards which are available through family practitioner committees. Another alternative is a patient-held record, along the same lines as the maternity co-operation card.

Those who have converted practice records to the A4 size have a much smaller problem: the standard sheets for these include one fairly well designed for precisely this purpose. Although introduction of these has now been postponed indefinitely by the DHSS on grounds of cost, it is difficult to believe that the octavo envelope can last more than another ten years. Even with drastic pruning of hospital reports, well-kept clinical records over 15 or 20 years, together with electrocardiogram envelopes, summary cards, and 10 to 25 double-sided octavo continuation cards, are more than a gusseted cardboard envelope will stand. However this may be, for the time being each group has to reach its own decision on a uniform recording system that can be efficiently used by the whole medical team, so that information elicited becomes permanently available.

Continuity with the future: planned continuing management and compliance.– Diagnosis in all significant dimensions must be followed by a plan for treatment. It may be possible in some frequently recurring and fairly uniform situations (for example, frequency and dysuria in women, or exacerbations of chronic productive cough in men) for this plan to be a more or less automatic and standardized consequence of the diagnosis. If responsibility is shared within a group, agreement on some such standard sequences is essential. Each new consultation may result either in continuation of the plan unchanged, or initiation of a new phase. Decisions can be made more often than consultations if patients are drawn into management of their own illness, and the criteria for various contingent decisions are explained and understood. Whoever takes the decisions, they cannot be made rationally if more than one variable is altered at a time, or if observations are too few to allow for the variability inherent in the case. A rational plan for management is experimental, and the rules are not different, only the scale. This is true not only of hypertension or airways obstruction, where we have a quantified physical variable; it is true of all biological variables, and psychosocial variables.

Figure 1 shows a pattern of variability for 48 consecutive measurements of arterial pressure, made over a period of nine years in a woman aged 41 at the outset. The horizontal line represents the treatment aim of 100 mm Hg diastolic pressure; clearly, this was a difficult case. Based on these measurements, the arrows show 11 points at which decisions were taken to initiate new drugs or resume old ones; many more decisions were taken to change dosage. How meaningful could these decisions be, based on such infrequent glimpses of such an unstable variable?

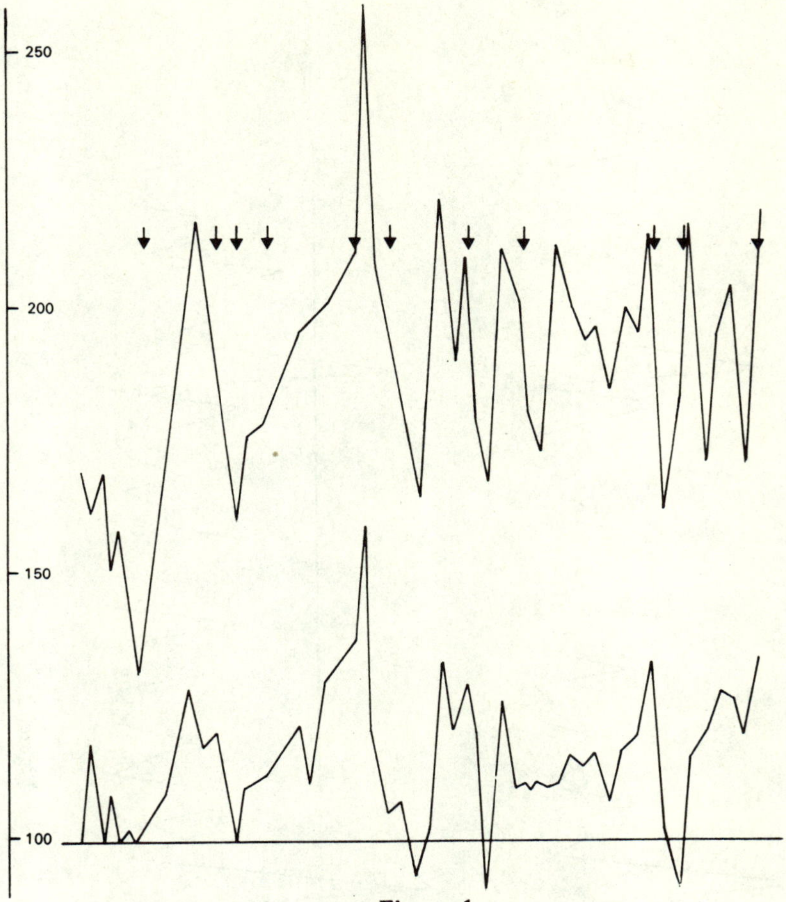

Figure 1

Figure 2 shows the pattern of variability found in repeated measurements in a single resting subject, on 48 consecutive days. He is not hypertensive and the measurements are not affected by treatment. Since raised pressures show a variability from day to day and from hour to hour no greater and no less than normal pressures, this variability must be borne in mind in planning the management of hypertension. The full implications of this are rarely considered. Patients who show little variability can be managed reasonably well with standard techniques (one consultation = one measurement = one decision), but in the many who are less stable, new methods must be devised. Once nurses are well trained, it becomes possible to prescribe more diagnosis, not just drugs. We write (on a prescription pad) 'BP x 10 before next consultation please' and leave it to the patient to arrange with the nurse a convenient time to come up during the next three weeks for the measurements to be done; we can then build the next decision on rock instead of sand.

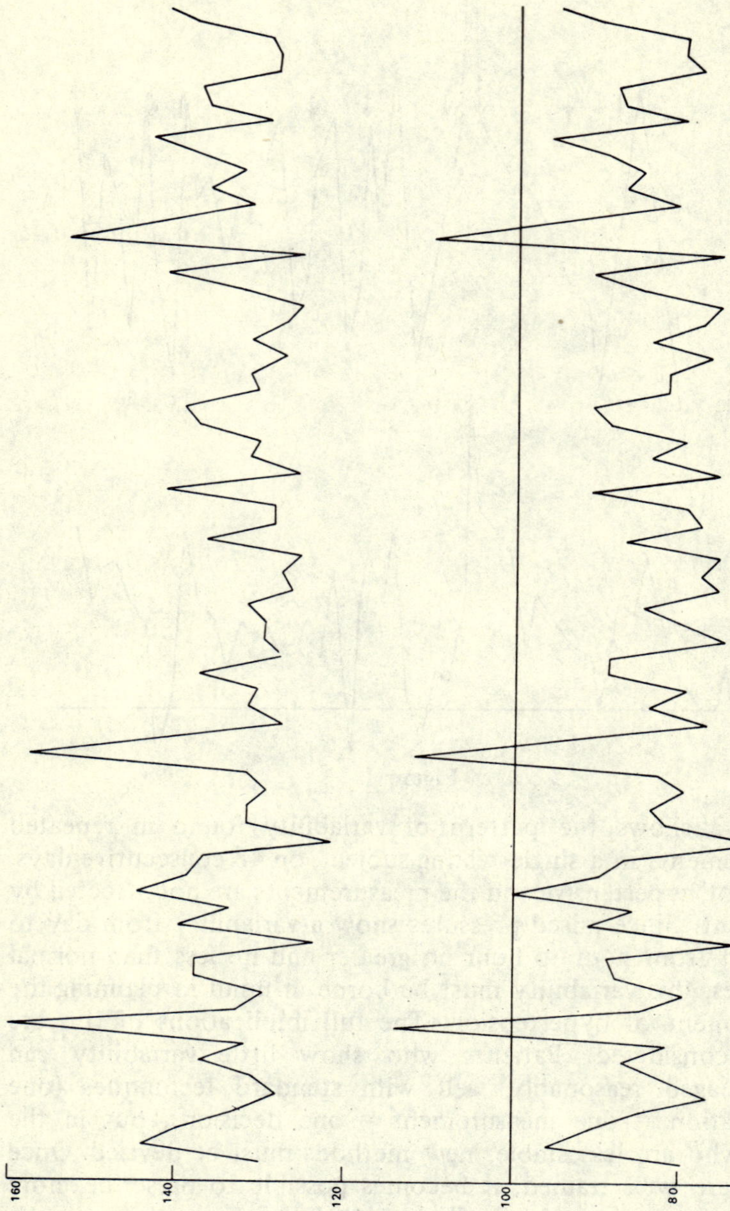

Figure 2

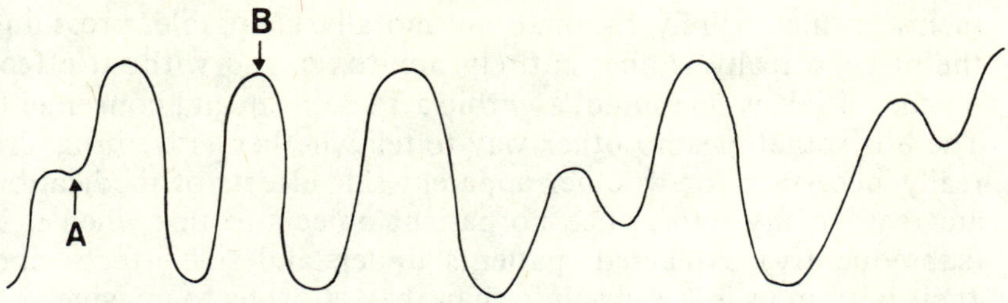

Figure 3

Figure 3 shows a theoretical pattern for any variable in which deviations beyond a certain point, or combined with certain symptoms, are perceived as signs of illness requiring action: say, arterial pressure, pulse rate, plasma glucose or uric acid, peak expiratory flow rate, or haemoglobin. If a first observation is made at point A, the deviation is small, the physical sign is negative, no intervention is made and the measurement will not be repeated. If it is made at point B, the deviation may be assumed to be significant, acted upon, and repeated. When it is repeated, its value is likely to be closer to the mean, so the action, whatever it was, will appear effective. Even if the value happens again to be high, the self-fulfilling nature of the prophecy will not be disturbed; increase the dose my dear, and come and see me again next week. Sooner or later it will be down! Diagnosis and treatment neatly packaged at one consultation commonly create just such a situation. It is subject to no effective audit because the management plan is a passive, transactional response to symptoms and the expectations of patients, not a mutually planned experiment with defined aims and a frequency of measurements related to their known accuracy and variability.

This criticism is equally true of softer measurements, as in observations of mood. Tricyclic antidepressants may appear remarkably effective, even when habitually used in doses repeatedly shown by controlled trials to be useless. The illusion may be created either by short follow-up or, more commonly, by extending the diagnosis of depression, and thereby the indications for treatment, to include large numbers of self-limiting mood changes, or normal responses to painful events, often not disclosed.

Planned management of any continuing illness generally requires more observation and less intervention than custom demands. Whenever possible, changes in management should be made singly, and the experimental use of placebos over short periods seems to me entirely rational and morally justifiable, providing the placebo really is one: entirely non-toxic, and without effect on the variables measured; ascorbic acid is cheap and convenient. There is sometimes no other way to tell whether active drugs are really necessary, or whether apparent side-effects of medication are real. In my experience no patient objects to this when it is (subsequently) explained; patients understand side-effects, and their faith in us is less absolute than they allow us to imagine.

Poorly planned and performed measurements are one obstacle to effective care, and are usually accepted as our own error. The other is failure of patient compliance, and is seldom accepted as a medical responsibility at all. One study showed that one-fifth of a group of diabetics were having either double or a half of their prescribed dose of insulin.[9] Another showed that more than one-third of patients have stopped antibiotic treatment within four days, and do not complete a prescribed course.[10]

Compliance is worst, though often most necessary, where treatment is aimed at precursors of illness in a patient without symptoms, as in all hypertension short of the malignant phase; here, symptoms are not only not relieved by medication, they are often worsened by it. Where a fairly long latent period precedes the useful effect of a drug, as in antidepressants, D-penicillamine for rheumatoid disease, or cromoglycate in extrinsic asthma, similar problems may arise. As more of the precursors of symptomatic illness become known and reversible by treatment, the problem of securing compliance without the sticks and carrots of symptom relief will increase.

A strategy of general practice that responds only to symptoms can depend entirely on patient-initiative. It is the patient's job to complain, and ours to respond thereafter. If he does not complain, or having complained, fails to follow advice, the fault is his entirely. We have our work cut out merely to meet presented demand, without looking for more. In a capitation system such as ours, with few fees for service, this approach can provide a good living, but only limited care to a population. That large majority of people who have learned their small value in the world market, who accept dangerous adventures in nicotine and alcohol as life itself, and whose response to fear is denial, cannot reach us as customers, except for salvage. Few people lack intelligence (and they have the right to care as good as anyone), but nearly all lack information. We know more than they do about their health, and to the extent that this is so, initiative and responsibility must lie with care-givers at least as much as with care-receivers. It is not possible to base a preventive or anticipatory style of care on unplanned symptom-response; there has to be a large element of organized, doctor-initiated care.

Where the progress of illness is unrelated, or very indirectly related to symptoms, organized follow-up is essential. The models for this, of which we already have experience, are antenatal care and the follow-up of tuberculosis in chest clinics. Both of these include forward planning, a checklist approach to basic data collection, fail-safe devices so that default is noticed and acted upon, and an active search for illness and its precursors.

Applied to the management of continued actual or precursor illness in middle age, this principle may require two organizational forms. First (and mainly) we need methods for noting default in relation to individuals with important disease; secondly, we may need methods for management of groups: those with hypertension, diabetes mellitus, chronic lung disease, or any other condition likely to occur in sufficient numbers in the population at risk to justify grouping.

The organization of special clinics is a great advantage in permitting greater delegation of diagnostic work to nursing staff, giving a firm base of checklist data, together with the extra time needed to give flexible and truly personalized care by the doctor. Defaulters are perceived easily and the reasons for non-compliance can be sought effectively. Hypertension, on a definition of diastolic pressure sustained at 105 mm Hg for 40 to 64 year olds, or 100 mm Hg under 40 years (in both men and women), presents sufficient numbers to make such clinics feasible in every general practice, even single-handed. With a minimum of four consultations a year, and allowing for more frequent consultations in those not yet stabilized or out of control, in our practice we have found a monthly case-load of about 20 consultations per 2,500 patients at risk (all ages) just about right for a full evening's work.

There are, however, serious limits to this clinic approach. Only chronic obstructive airways disease or, in practices of 5,000 or more, diabetes mellitus provides numbers of this order. Chronic bronchitis, emphysema and asthma can be so disabling that consultations are difficult to plan ahead on a regular basis. Even hypertensives, normally without symptoms, will consult for other things at other times, or wish to raise different problems when consulting at a special clinic. A clinic system of data collection and recording must be flexible enough to accept other complaints when they are offered (thus greatly improving compliance), and also be adaptable to isolated, unplanned consultations.

Control of individual, less common conditions is more difficult. There are three main techniques for doing this: review of defaulted appointments, control of repeat prescriptions, and flagging of records. Defaulted appointments can be reviewed quickly by the receptionist at the end of each office session. She should have a good nose for what is going on, and knowledge of the significance of different diagnoses sufficient to alert the doctor on her own initiative after important default. Since the records will already have been extracted for the appointed consultation, a check on decisions made at the last consultation is easy.

In repeat prescribing where the patient approaches nurse or receptionist directly, records should be extracted and an entry made, unless some other control system (patient-held treatment card, ledger or computer) is in operation. The date of the last consultation should be checked, and staff must be encouraged to refer these patients to see the doctor if they are in any doubt at all, not only for psychoactive drugs and hypnotics, but for steroids, bronchodilators, diuretics and antihypertensives, where patients have not been seen for three months or more. Staff will do this only if they are confident that doctors will accept the extra workload willingly.

Flagging of records means the attachment of markers, colour-coded for diagnosis, to patients belonging to groups requiring special action or alertness at every consultation. This can be done by sticking coloured tape on the top margin of octavo envelopes, or on the spine of A4 folders. Such labels are fairly durable, and there has been a standard Royal College of General Practitioners colour code in use for the past twenty-five years, though still not widely recognized. Their disadvantage is that they cannot easily be removed, and diagnostic groups often prove less static than practice planners anticipate. It is important not to enlarge the number of categories without good reason; the more there are, the less attention will be paid to them by anyone other than their practice-parent.

Sustained motivation

This more structured, yet flexible, style required for continuous health care is not too difficult to describe, or even to initiate, at least piecemeal; but to maintain it, give it roots so deep and so tough that it becomes irreversibly established custom for care-givers and expectation for care-receivers, demands a lifetime of sustained work. This motivation must somehow be communicated to the whole primary care team, and to the population it serves. It is easy to devise programmes of prevention and anticipatory care but, if they are to be consistently performed, health workers must be convinced of their usefulness, and a decisive majority of the people must turn away from episodic relief of symptoms to the conservation of their health with skilled advice.

Several studies have shown that a majority of patients would welcome such a shift in the style of care. Patients will not and should not accept simple abdication from responsibility for apparently minor illness, with exhortations to increased self-care, unless this is accompanied by a positive extension of care in new directions. Provided such an extension does in fact occur, our experience has been that the shift away from simple symptom-response is welcomed.

For example, it is now clear that the treatment of menopausal symptoms by prolonged oestrogen replacement (natural or synthetic) increases the risk of endometrial carcinoma from 4- to 14-fold[11] and significantly raises levels of clotting factor VIII,[12] which is a major risk factor for coronary heart disease, and is probably responsible for the increased risk associated with oral contraception. There is also evidence of increases in ovarian and breast cancer rates in women on hormone replacement therapy.[13] Though oestrogens certainly relieve the symptom of menopausal flushing, the effect of placebos is also dramatic.[12] These risks have got to be discussed openly and in a balanced way with patients before starting treatment; the patient, and only the patient, has a right to decide just how intolerable her symptoms are, and to make her decision. The risks must be presented in a meaningful way. Our experience has been that patients welcome this information and make sensible use of it.

The main difficulty is not one of communication with patients, but of ourselves possessing accurate information that we can give them. It is not enough to use one simple analogy to cover all cases (e.g.: 'Well, it's safer than driving to London'), regardless of its accuracy. Some order of magnitude must either be given, or at least considered by the doctor. When we do not have such information, or when it simply does not exist, there seems no ethical alternative to saying so. We have found that the fairly small number of women whose lives are really intolerable because of these symptoms, readily accept short courses with minimal dosage and incomplete remission, rather than importuning for prolonged and fully suppressive treatment, as they formerly did. Often we have found that what was most needed was reassurance that flushes are in no way connected with high blood pressure, and are not the precursors of stroke. Given five or more years of sustained educational work, patients do accept a shift from episodic care, and cease either to expect or demand a label and a drug for each and every complaint.

In the same way, we have to remember, and in some form acquaint our patients, with the known risks of psychotropic drugs. Benzodiazepine tranquillizers, even if subjectively satisfying, can cause personality changes quite opposite to those intended, causing aggressive behaviour at worst, and passive capitulation at best. The risks of monoamine oxidase inhibitors are well known, and they are now used with caution, but tricyclic antidepressants are used on a vast and still increasing scale, with an ever-increasing diversity of molecular variants creating even greater confusion, with benefit to no-one but their promoters. In patients with known cardiovascular disease, amitriptyline increases the incidence of sudden unexpected death fourfold, compared with similar but untreated controls.[14] The makers recommend that these drugs be avoided in the presence of ischaemic heart disease; yet in whom (in this age-group) can we be sure this is absent?

The responsibility for deciding the balance between risks and benefits of treatment is a heavy one, and cannot be taken by doctors alone. Where there is real doubt that even small risks can be justified, patients will on the whole accept waiting and seeing, providing they are given knowledge of the likely natural history of their condition, and the known hazards of treatment on the one hand, or inactivity on the other. For nearly thirty years medical care in Britain has ceased to be a commodity. It is now rare for patients to offer money for more energetic or effective treatment, and private practice is used not to obtain exceptional skills, but in the main to secure rapid access to normal skills. We no longer derive any economic advantage from the mystification of medicine, or from pretending that we can do things that are as yet not possible. We underestimate the difference this has already made to our own attitudes to care, and to the expectations of our patients. Steady educational work within a population has in many practices already created a situation where doctors can discuss freely with their patients the limitations of symptom-response transactions. It is not difficult to understand that checking the oil from time to time may be both cheaper and easier than buying a new engine every 25,000 miles, and human engines are often not available at any price.

Of course, there are difficulties in this approach. Some of these derive from the expectations of patients, and from their lack of knowledge. Low intelligence is often assumed or perceived as an obstacle; yet it is a curious fact that doctors explain more to patients they consider more articulate, and give least advice and information to those considered inarticulate.[15] Our communication with our patients might benefit from the golden rule of television educators: never underestimate the intelligence of the public, but never overestimate its knowledge.

A further difficulty is our own slender knowledge of the confidence limits of both diagnosis and treatment. This field, if not actually concealed, is usually badly taught, and is very incompletely researched. The only recent and fairly comprehensive review of the reliability of clinical methods, data, and judgments, by Koran[16] deserves to be better known. Take the fairly common example of gall-stones, which are directly or indirectly responsible for about 1 per cent of all deaths. They are found in about one-quarter of all post-mortem examinations, six times more often than evidence of cholecystectomy. Probably at least one in five of all middle-aged people have stones that are either silent or only occasionally troublesome. If they develop virtually any persistent or recurrent abdominal symptom, cholecystography is likely to lead to a diagnosis of clinically significant gall-stones, quite possibly leading to cholecystectomy.[17] This operation carries a minimum average mortality of 0.5 per cent, even as a planned procedure, and mortality from gall-stones and/or cholecystectomy is highest where cholecystectomy is most often performed.[18] If we are to help our patients to use the health service safely, effectively, and with reasonable economy, we must ourselves know facts of this kind and be able to discuss them in a balanced way with our patients.

This shift in the perception of medical science from mystified certainty to quantified probability and doubt is bound to take time, and while it may be quickly or even eagerly accepted by some, it will be bitterly resisted by others. This is as true of our colleagues, both doctors and other health workers, as of our patients. The transition will be quicker and less painful if both staff and patients can be drawn into the discussion and planning of new health strategies applied in local terms, and are given the information needed to understand its rational basis. It has to be remembered that the teaching of nurses has been even more hierarchical and dogmatic than the teaching of doctors, and older nurses particularly need a good deal of help to tolerate a more critical attitude.

Conclusion

I have not sought in this chapter to mention more than a few of the infinite variety of disorders and management problems found in middle age. The treatment is lopsided, with a heavy emphasis on health maintenance and the prevention or anticipation of disease, rather than methods of recognizing and handling episodes of illness quickly and efficiently. This is not because I discount the value of accurate responses to acute symptoms, but because this has already been taught to the readers of this book, and can to some extent be taken for granted (though this is a dangerous assumption in all of us).

Primary care presents a heavy new burden every day, of only partly predictable content; this must be dealt with before anything else can be thought of. The elaboration of new strategies must come afterwards, and too often it does not come at all. Practice planning that is geared only to survival ultimately kills the doctor (intellectually, if not always physically) as well as the patients. The large and growing number of doctors who have in various ways begun this process of reorientation toward anticipatory care, will end on a common pathway whatever their point of departure. The starting point will depend on the nature of local problems and the clinical skills and interests available, and it matters little what it is. The critical matters are to know roughly where we are going, and be determined to arrive.

References

[1] Eastwood, M.R. and Trevelyan, M.H. (1972): Relationship between Physical and Psychiatric Disorder. *Psychological Medicine*, *2*, 363

[2] Daly, M.B. and Tyroler, H.A. (1972): Cornell Medical Index Response as a Predictor of Mortality. *British Journal of Preventive and Social Medicine*, *26*, 159

[3] Van den Dool, C.W. (1973): From Multiple Screening to Anticipatory Medicine. *Allgemeinmedizin international*, *3*, 100

[4] Buchan, I.C. and Richardson, I.M. (1973): *Time study of Consultations in General Practice*. Scottish Health Service Studies no. 27. Edinburgh: Scottish Home and Health Department

[5] Gregg, I. (1975): The Treatment of Asthma. *The Practitioner*, *215*, 520

[6] Marsh, G.N., Wallace, R.B. and Whewell, J. (1976): Anglo-American Contrasts in General Practice. *British Medical Journal*, *1*, 1321

[7] Hart, J.T. (1976): General Practice Workload, Needs and Resources in the National Health Service, *Journal of the Royal College of General Practitioners*, *26*, 885

[8] Jarrett, R.J. and Keen, H. (1976): Hyperglycaemia and Diabetes Mellitus, *Lancet*, *ii*, 1009

[9] Stewart, R.B. and Cluff, L.E. (1972): quoted in Lancet, ii, 695

[10] Mattar, M.E., Markello, J. and Yaffe, S.J. (1975): quoted in Lancet, ii, 539

[11] Ziel, H.K. and Finkle, L.D. (1975): Increased Risk of Endometrial Carcinoma among Users of Conjugated Oestrogens. *New England Journal of Medicine*, 293, 1167

[12] Coope, J., Thomson, J.M. and Poller, L. (1975): Effects of 'Natural Oestrogen' Replacement Therapy on Menopausal Symptoms and Blood Clotting. *British Medical Journal*, *4*, 139

[13] Anthony, H.M. (1976): Age-specific Incidence of Cancer of the Endometrium, Ovary, and Breast in the United Kingdom and the United States. *International Journal of Epidemiology*, *5*, 231

[14] Moir, D.C. *et al.* (1972): Cardiotoxicity of Amitriptyline. *Lancet*, *ii*, 561.

[15] Joyce, C.R.B., Caple, G., Mason, M., Reynolds, E. and Mathews, J.A. (1969): Quantitative Study of Doctor-Patient Communication. *Quarterly Journal of Medicine*, 38, 183

[16] Koran, L.M. (1975): The Reliability of Clinical Methods, data, and judgments. *New England Journal of Medicine*, *293*, 642 and 695 (2 parts)

[17] Annotation (1976): When do gall-stones matter? *Lancet*, *i*, 1061

[18] Vayda, E. (1973): A Comparison of Surgical Rates in Canada and in England and Wales. *New England Journal of Medicine*, *289*, 1224

4.7 Old age

J.S.K. Stevenson

When Kemp[1] took a new look at geriatrics in 1965, he expressed the opinion that most doctors thought of old people as medical nuisances. This he felt explained so much of the medical neglect seen and the indifference shown, and gave rise to many of the comments that were heard. He suggested that the problems presented by advanced old age were so new that it was understandable that doctors had not adjusted to them emotionally. In addition he wrote that most of us have a secret or declared fear of this phase in our lives.

Yet despite the impossibility of having a personal view of age and ageing, in good time to do something about it, the first essential, particularly for doctors, is to face up to the reality of large numbers of old people, rather than to pretend or argue that they do not exist. The profession must give the lead to the community to think carefully about standards of care and concern for the elderly patient.

Since the establishment of the National Health Service in 1948, our society has changed markedly, and in particular the role of the individual and the structure of the family. Despite the upward trend in marriage rates, the declining birth rate has led to a situation in which fewer children have been born to take responsibility for the greater number of people who now live into old age and require support.

Although mortality rates have remained almost stationary since the middle of this century, it must be assumed that the present investment of resources, devoted to the study of diseases of middle age, will eventually exert its effect on over-all mortality and thus increase average life expectancy. This poses many problems in providing services of all kinds, but it is of the utmost importance in relation to the likely pattern of continuing care for older people.

Some demographic facts and projections

The present high proportion of older people in the population is due to several factors.[2] The decline in mortality rates, especially of infants, children and young people at the end of last century, the continuing high birth rates during the late Victorian era, and further improvements in life expectancy during the first half of this century have all meant that a higher proportion of our present population has survived to age 70 and beyond. Furthermore, as the generation depleted of males by the 1914-18 War progressively passes from the population structure, the proportion of males to females in the elderly population will become slightly higher.

Another factor is the reduction in the birth rate that occurred during the years of economic depression, between the two world wars. The survivors of these smaller birth groups are now in middle age, and although this has the effect of increasing the proportion of old people in the population at present, as they, themselves, pass into the retirement group, the total number of elderly in the population during the latter part of the century will be reduced. Although this will eventually produce an over-all reduction in the proportion of elderly, the actual number of those over 75 will increase. This group contains the very old and frail and a high proportion of widows and widowers living alone. It is well recognized that extreme old age, bereavement and loneliness, not only carry particularly high risks, but the greatest need for medical and social services.

The effect of these projections, for the Scottish elderly population, has been strikingly illustrated by Williamson.[3] He has kindly authorized the use of the histograms – figures 1-3. The projections for the elderly populations of other parts of the United Kingdom are similar.

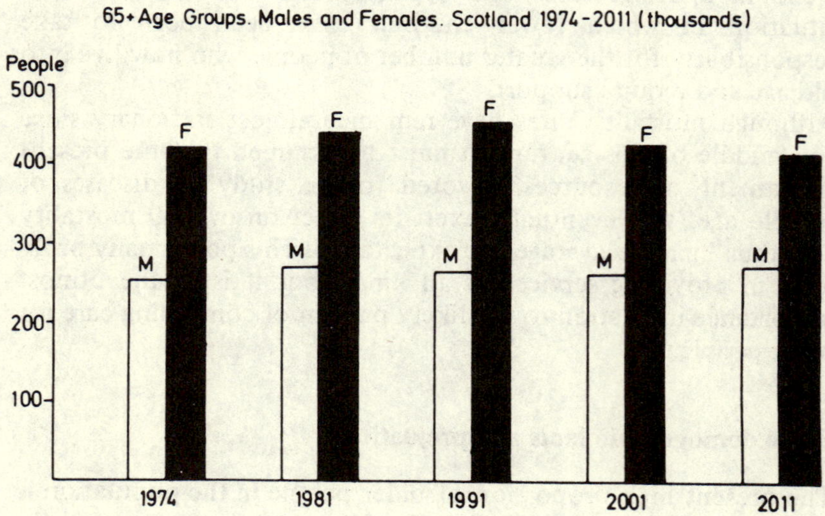

Figure 1

75+Age Groups. Males and Females. Scotland 1974 - 2011 (thousands)

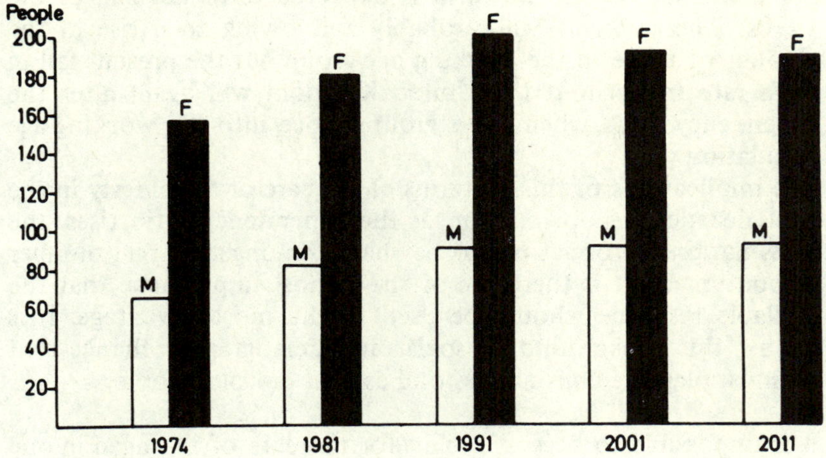

Figure 2

85+Age Groups. Males and Females. Scotland 1974 - 2011 (thousands)

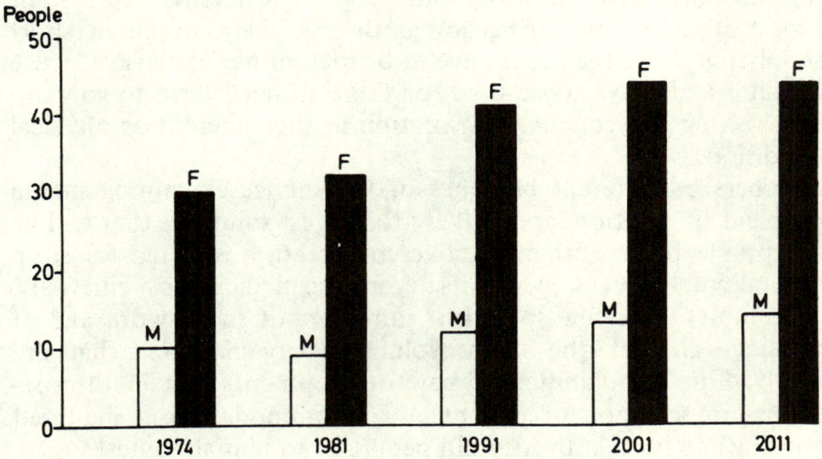

Figure 3

Another important factor is the ratio of the dependent population, (infants, children of school age and those in the retirement age-group) to the rest. This is called the dependency ratio and is expressed as follows:

$$\text{Dependency ratio} = \frac{\text{Number of children under working age + persons of retirement age}}{\text{1,000 persons of working age}}$$

In 1941 the ratio was 488/1,000; in 1969 it was 655/1,000. Some further rise in the ratio is expected until the end of the 1970s. Thereafter it will probably fall owing to a rise in the number of those in the working age-group but the present fall in birth rate throughout the United Kingdom will again alter the dependency ratio when these groups move into the working-age population.

The implications of this, in terms of the care of the elderly in the next decade, are obvious for, as the dependency ratio rises, the gross national product has to be shared amongst a larger number of consumers. It is therefore of the utmost importance that the available resources should be used to the most advantage. It is against this background of social and demographic change that we must plan the continuous total care of our old people.

It is impossible to suggest a plan for the care of the aged in one particular service section while ignoring the effect that this may have on another. In no other field of care is an understanding of the interdependence of services more important than in the care of the elderly. A good example is the provision of sheltered housing and local authority old people's residential homes. In times of economic stringency both are likely to be in short supply but, since the needs have to be met, either expensive, acute hospital beds have to be used, or those in need have to go without, risking subsequent deterioration in their mental or physical condition.

Members of different branches of the service examining such a problem in isolation, are unlikely to suggest solutions that will be acceptable to the others. Active co-operation is called for from general practitioners, specialists in geriatric medicine, psychiatrists, community medicine specialists, directors of social work and of housing, and of the many voluntary organizations that are involved in the planning of new developments and in the pre-admission selection of patients for accommodation in sheltered housing and local authority old people's residential homes.

For the purposes of this chapter, however, it is intended to examine only the role of the general practitioner and the primary care team in the continuous care of elderly patients. It is therefore appropriate to examine some of the present criticisms levelled specifically at this branch of geriatric care.

The present organization of general practice

The organization of general practice in the United Kingdom has been geared to a system of care that is dependent upon patient-initiated demand. It is well known that this is inappropriate in meeting the medical and social needs of the elderly.

The trend towards group practice from centralized consulting premises, the growth of appointment systems, the use of repeat prescriptions in place of consultations, and the general practitioner's changing attitude to personal doctoring and to home visiting in favour of surgery consultations, may all be potential barriers between older patients and their general practitioners. The remoteness of some of the newer housing estates, coupled with transport difficulties, makes access to the general practitioner and the pharmacist more difficult, especially for the very old. When elderly patients are discharged from hospital or from convalescence, faulty communication among hospital doctors, general practitioners, health visitors and social workers can disrupt the continuous care that is necessary – sometimes with most unfortunate results. Insufficient attention is paid to the need to show older patients how to deal with emergency situations and in making sure that they can summon help easily when it is required.

As a result of these deficiencies there are substantial amounts of unmet need and of unknown morbidity among the elderly population. This can be worse in highly populated areas, where both the private citizen and the caring professional may more easily escape from their responsibilities. The controlling effect of public and professional opinion in maintaining higher standards of care in smaller closeknit communities is likely to be very real.

It is to the ultimate benefit of patients that there should continue to be a variety of choice between different forms of practice organization. Most practices, however, need to take care and thought to ensure that the advantages they have are not counteracted by possible disadvantages: large groups though efficiently organized may tend to become impersonal; small partnerships though well integrated may lose personal contact in delegated out-of-hours emergency work; single-handed practitioners though knowing their patients well may have difficulty in ensuring adequate supporting nursing and health visitor services.

The role of the primary care team in the continuing care of the elderly

In 1959, Ashworth[4] concluded that it is the general practitioner's responsibility to see that all forces are mobilized to keep the elderly patient healthy and happy at home. Forsyth and Logan[5] found that the range of services and extent of patient care varied directly with the personal interest of the general practitioner. The report of the Royal College of Physicians of Edinburgh,[6] saw the aim of geriatric care as the maintenance of independent comfort and contentment in patients' own homes, and, when independence begins to wane, the support of such patients by all means necessary for as long as possible.

The planning necessary to meet these aims was summarized by Warren[7] in 1964:

> In order to assess the adequacies of plans now being made, we need to know much more about the medical, social and economic indications for and against the alternative types of care which can be provided in hospitals, in institutions and in the home. Well designed, controlled trials are needed to see how we can best meet the diverse and complex medical, psychological and social needs of elderly people.

Since Warren's plea for more planned research in the care of the elderly, some progress has been made.

In their review of geriatric care in general practice in 1973, Elliot and Stevenson[8] suggested that the time had now come to take stock of this in looking to the future. The fact that emerged most strikingly was that there were many old people in the community who either had difficulty in getting about, or suffered from defective vision or hearing, or were depressed, or had other mental instability. Many of these disabilities had been found to be treatable, some with relative ease. Groups had been identified as being at special risk: those recently bereaved, those living alone, and the very old. It was clear that self reporting, by the geriatric patient, of illness or disability could not be relied upon. This was thought to be due to the high prevalence of locomotor difficulties or depressive illness, although many old people saw their medical and social problems as being part of the business of growing old, and therefore put up with them.

It was concluded that a system of geriatric care was needed that would (i) identify the elderly in a community, (ii) sort out those in need from those at risk, and (iii) meet the requirements within the resources available. The importance of continuing surveillance of the group, and of those who would be recruited to it, was stressed, but there must be greater co-operation and flexibility among general practitioners themselves in setting up an organization for general practice that would consider, amongst its priorities, such things as the zoning of practices and transport for patients.

Although general practitioners are paid more for looking after patients over the age of 65, this additional payment does not necessarily guarantee improved service to these patients, because the present system relies primarily on the self-reporting of illness. Rather the reverse holds true, in that practitioners who provide a comprehensive caring service for their older patients, seeking out their medical and social problems rather than waiting for these to be reported at times of crisis, are at a financial disadvantage, compared with their colleagues who rely on giving attention solely at these times. One of the defects of the pay structure for general practitioners in the National Health Service is that preventive care often goes unregarded in purely financial terms.

A suggested scheme for the continuous medical and social care of the elderly in general practice

The flow chart (Figure 4) represents a possible scheme for the continuous medical and social care of the elderly in the community.

The team policy – a word of caution

Although it is accepted throughout this chapter that the primary care team provides the basis for acceptable medical and social care for elderly patients, it would be naive to assume that all that is required is to establish teams in the community and let them get on with it. The importance of understanding the difficulties that can all too easily arise in such teams, has been rightly stressed by Taylor and his colleagues.[9]

To obtain optimum output from any group of people working together, certain standards must be observed. There should be unity of direction. One person or one committee should be responsible for formulating the aims of the group as a whole and for co-ordinating them. Each member of the team must also understand, and contribute towards, these aims in whatever role is assigned to him.

If it is accepted that larger multi-disciplinary groups provide care most economically, then an understanding of at least the basic principles of modern management theory and techniques should be understood by the whole group, and at least one of the constituent members should be identified as having special knowledge and skills in this field.

Management begins with division of labour and delegation of work. Therefore each member of the team must clearly understand that his or her efforts are contributing to the aims of the group. There are also certain members of any team whose duties may be subject to continuing change. The fact that a job has been done in a certain way for many years makes any suggestion of change difficult, since it may appear to hint at previous inefficiency. There must therefore be close consultation before the introduction of any new method of work, and care should always be taken to avoid giving the impression that change implies criticism of those who have previously been doing their jobs to the best of their abilities – often with insufficient information as to what the object of the exercise was.

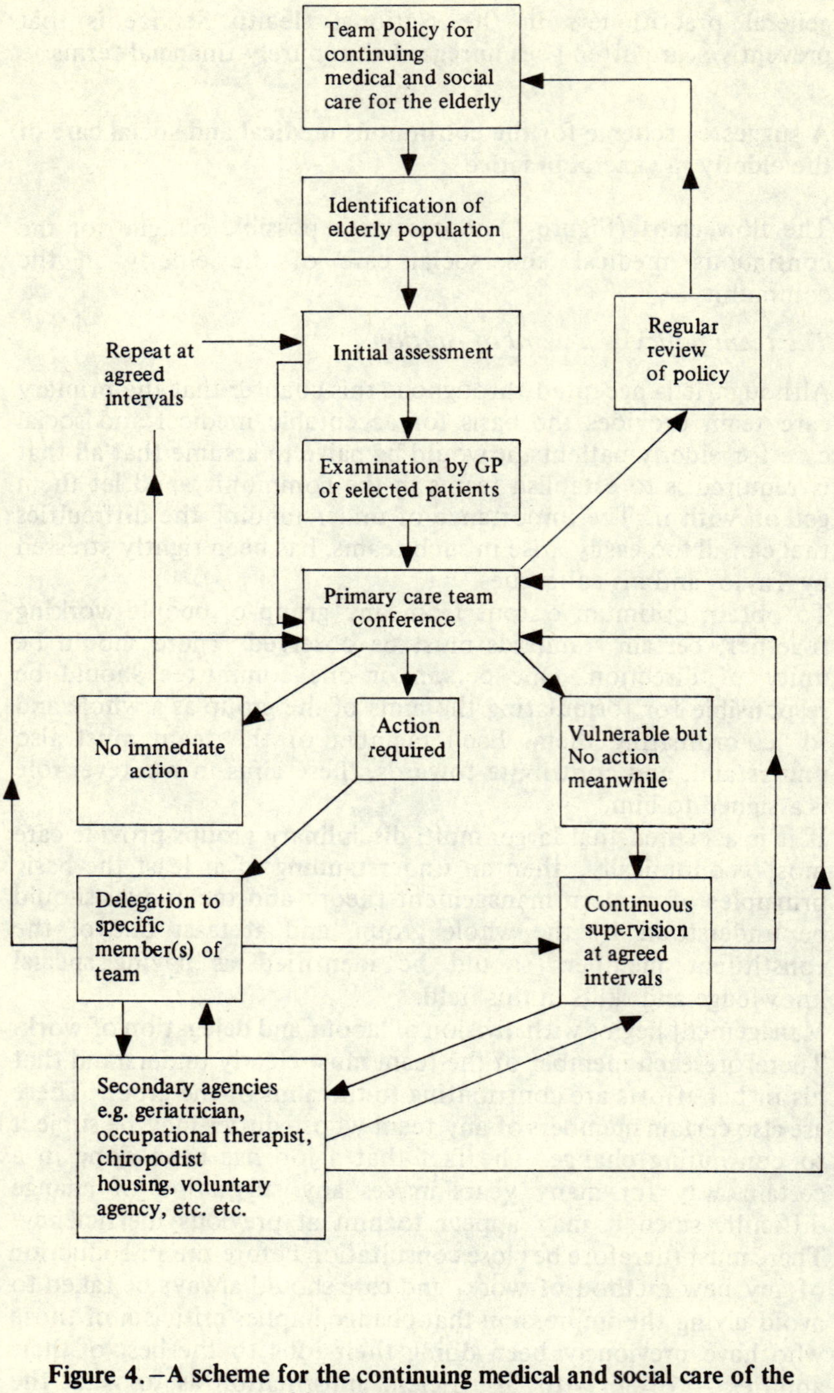

Figure 4. –A scheme for the continuing medical and social care of the elderly in general practice.

All groups who work together for any length of time establish working habits that should be regularly reviewed and assessed if the work of the group as a whole is to expand and develop. If, as a result of this probing, the role of anyone within the group is altered, then the new role must be clearly defined so that the team member not only knows what to do, but can exert more control over the way that he or she does it. The individual must also attach importance to this new role and sense that others respect the work that he or she does.

Members of a primary care team who are aware of these difficulties and face up to them are most likely to provide optimum care for the elderly and achieve the greatest satisfaction from their work.

Identification of elderly persons

Before discussing a suggested programme for continuing care in old age, it is important to consider how the elderly in any practice can be identified. Increasing numbers of general practitioners keep age/sex registers and thus the identification of those over retirement age is easy. For those without an age/sex register, serious thought should be given to creating such a record, although the initial work involved is painstaking and time-consuming and may require extra secretarial help. Once the register is completed, it is easily kept up to date. There are many different types of age/sex register, but perhaps the easiest to manage has a card index system in two sections: one for males and the other for females. Many general practitioners have been greatly helped in setting up age/sex registers by the staff of primary care divisions of health boards or Family Practitioner Committees. Others, tackling specific research projects, have had a sum of money included in their research grants, specifically earmarked to establish an age/sex register for the population under study.

Initial assessment

Once the number of elderly persons in the practice has been defined, the next stage is to ascertain the needs of the group as a whole. This is the stage of assessment and it can be competently undertaken by a health visitor or a district nursing sister. Some have questioned the professional expertise required to identify obvious medical and social needs amongst older patients. They have suggested that untrained case-workers could be used to alert the professionals regarding priority cases, at least in the initial stages of any geriatric care programme. For the purposes of this chapter, however, it is assumed that the initial assessment will be made by a health visitor or a district nursing sister, who may either make an initial visit to the patient's home – probably the best method – or the patient may be invited by letter to attend a specific health visitor/district nursing sister clinic at the group practice or health centre.

Questionnaires, such as the one suggested in the appendix (modified from that used in Stokoe's practice[10] and incorporating the mental health questionnaire validated by Milne and his colleagues[11]), have been found useful in this initial assessment. They can be completed by the trained health visitor or district nursing sister, any difficulties being reported to the responsible general practitioner. Completed initial assessment questionnaires form a useful subject for discussion among team members at subsequent case conferences. They can be printed in such a way as to fold in two, to fit the patient's medical record envelope.

If patients of 70 and over are chosen, Anderson[12] found that the person undertaking the initial assessment obtained great satisfaction. It is also likely that considerable ill health will be uncovered and that between 25 to 50 per cent of all patients visited will require help, to meet some newly discovered need. Anderson also suggested that the person performing the initial assessment should probably not be the general practitioner. He is associated in the minds of the elderly with disease, and thus his uninvited appearance in the house may not only cause apprehension but the suspicion that illness has occurred and that someone has complained. On the other hand the district nursing sister or health visitor is not viewed in this light.

Once the initial assessment has been completed, the elderly in the practice can be classified into three broad groups: (i) the able, i.e. those who are healthy and contented and not yet in need of any special assistance; (ii) the vulnerable, i.e. those who are coping with some medical, psychiatric or social disability but who will require periodic supervision to ensure that they are able to remain independent; (iii) the disabled, i.e. those who are found to have some medical, psychiatric or social disability that calls for immediate action.

It is debatable whether the whole elderly population should be offered a medical examination by the general practitioner. Where this has been done, a high compliance rate has been found. The desire of elderly patients to be medically examined increases with age, but it may be felt that the additional work involved in offering a screening programme to the entire elderly population would be too great. Instead, it may be decided that scarce manpower resources should be directed at the vulnerable and disabled groups. Whatever is decided, it is important that time should be set aside to enable the elderly patient to be seen unhurriedly. For this reason it is advisable that only four to six elderly persons be asked to attend at each special clinic. This can be done, either by sending a personal letter inviting the patient to attend at specified times, or by the health visitor calling with the appointment card and explaining what will be involved. It is best to avoid the times of the year when the practice is likely to be busy. These, in fact, are usually times when colder weather keeps the elderly indoors. It thus suits everyone to organize any screening programme in the period between late spring and early autumn.

Screening programme for selected elderly patients

At the clinic the patient can be enrolled by the practice secretary who can start by checking that the patient's name, address and other personal particulars agree with those on the practice records. The patient should then be seen by the practice or district nursing sister. She should record the patient's weight and compare it with any previously recorded measurement. The patient's vision should then be tested with Snellen type – with glasses if worn. The ears should be examined with an auriscope for the presence or absence of wax, and the mouth inspected for dental caries, ill-fitting dentures or any other abnormality. The nurse should then measure the blood pressure, examine the urine for the presence or absence of sugar and albumin and take a sample of blood for simple haematological examination.

The patient should next be seen by the general practitioner whose examination should be concerned particularly with:

1. Any disorders of locomotion – inspecting the hands and feet, including simple tests of function such as hand movements, observing the gait, asking the patient to do knees bend and to lift the hands above the head.
2. Any evidence of heart failure, chronic bronchitis, weight loss, anaemia or malnutrition.
3. Simple tests of memory and orientation.
4. Evidence of depression, elicited by questioning about mood, sleep patterns, feelings of inability to cope and observing any agitation.
5. A review of medication.

At screening clinics for elderly patients, Thompson [13] found that the new diseases diagnosed fell into three main categories:

1. Conditions that were remediable: e.g. depression, anaemia, heart failure, hernia, uterine prolapse, urinary infection, prostatic hypertrophy, diabetes mellitus, faecal impaction, gout, thyroid disorders and osteomalacia.
2. Conditions that may be alleviated: e.g. deafness, chronic respiratory impairment, foot defects, arthritis, anxiety, visual defects, dyspepsia, Parkinson's disease, varicose veins,

prostatic carcinoma, cervical spondylosis, diverticulitis, postural hypotension, trigeminal neuralgia and Paget's disease.

3. Conditions that required symptomatic relief and social support: e.g. carcinomatosis, dementia, hemiplegia, vertebro-basilar ischaemia and gangrene.

After the screening examination has taken place, the general practitioner should be in a position to compile a problem list showing any action that is required. These recommendations should be made available for discussion at the next practice meeting, following the screening clinic, and the most appropriate member of the practice team can be charged with the responsibility for initiating appropriate action, and reporting back to the group. It is important that any decision taken is noted in the patient's records, and the matter put on the agenda for a subsequent meeting, when progress can be reported.

Individual roles of members of the primary care team

Although deficiency in geriatric care cannot be attributed simply to an abdication of responsibility by the younger generation, it is undoubtedly true that the increasing mobility of labour, especially in cities, has led to a greater isolation of old people from close family contact. The effect of this has been to create a demand for services based in the home, to replace some of the functions formerly provided by members of the extended family. As Kemp[1] has written: 'When it is possible to provide for the ageing person a complete supporting background or one which is adequate, then old age progresses normally and problems are unlikely to arise'. He concludes: 'It is an interesting thought that the volumes that have been written and spoken on this matter can all be rendered unnecessary by the existence of an effective daughter.'

In looking at the individual roles of the non-medical members of the primary care team, it is a useful exercise to ponder what the effective daughter can provide for her elderly parent in a very real and continuing way. No team of people can replace her, however hard they may try, but if the community is attempting to provide a substitute for her, then these are some of the attributes that an effective daughter may have.

She provides a nursing or caretaking service which the elderly parent accepts as of right in return for the care given to the effective daughter in childhood and adolescence. Her presence in the home guarantees that there is someone there who is uncritical of the domestic circumstances. She is familiar with the places in which domestic articles are kept and is a medium for getting shopping done in accordance with what the elderly person would have bought for her or himself. She is able to carry out the requests and recommendations of the general practitioner, district nursing sister or health visitor without the elderly person having to be appealed to for decisions. She copes with the elderly person's laundry and can remove soiled linen and clothing without embarrassment. She is likely to have insight into what pastimes are most enjoyed by her parent, whereas professional persons may often make unrealistic suggestions that the patient is too polite to refuse.

She provides a good listening service, which is especially important to the elderly person who may well be reminiscing about things in the distant past. She is also a link with events taking place outside the home, in which the elderly patient may no longer be able to participate, and she provides a news service about relatives, neighbours, local changes and other day-to-day items of interest. She decides when professional help is needed and is able to summon it. She also fetches any drugs that are prescribed, and takes responsibility for ensuring that they are taken in the right doses and at the right times. In short, she provides an environment for her parent that cannot be given by unrelated professional persons. Society must take this into account when assessing her value, even in monetary terms. The sacrifice that she is making, however willingly, must restrict the opportunities that are available for her to pursue a career in her own right. It may well be that part of this sacrifice is to accept a life of less interest and quality for as long as her parent may live.

If the concept of substituting professional persons for the effective daughter is taken as one of the main objectives of the primary care team, so as to provide continuing care for the elderly person living at home, then the individual role of each member of the team becomes much clearer.

The home help

The home help is placed at the top of the list because her role is undoubtedly the most important in the continuous care of the elderly, and especially the very old and frail. Her importance stems from the fact that she spends more time in the company of the patient than any other member of the team, and also that the ideal home help comes nearest to compensating for the absent effective daughter – often giving out-of-hours support beyond the call of duty. In addition to housework, cooking and shopping, she can collect drugs from the pharmacist and pensions from the post office. She can summon help when this is required and, perhaps most important of all, she provides company and often keeps the housebound patient in touch with local happenings.

Close bonds often develop between elderly patients and their home helps and many old people express feelings of insecurity when their home help is away for even short holiday periods. The importance of good home helps maintaining contented older patients in the secure environment of their homes cannot be over-emphasized. Indeed, it is doubtful if the full potential of the service has yet been reached. With further training, and at little extra expense, the duties of the home help could surely be extended and even expanded. Such an acquisition of new skills would undoubtedly lead to an upgrading of responsibilities that would enhance the status and importance of this under-rated member of the primary care team.

The district nursing sister

The role of the district nursing sister is perhaps the easiest to define since she is involved in traditional nursing duties that are well recognized by both the professional and the lay person. She provides the nursing component of the absent, effective daughter, and is often assisted by ancillary workers such as bath attendants. She liaises, principally with the health visitor, in meeting the material needs of the elderly patient at home. She may, for example, arrange for the patient to be provided with a bedpan or commode, or suggest that the patient's home, especially the bathroom and lavatory, be fitted with suitable wall attachments and handrails to allow handicapped old patients a much fuller use of the available accommodation. She may also arrange for the supply of aids, such as Zimmer walking aids, specially adapted kitchen tools and equipment, bookrests, special chairs or wheelchairs. With the health visitor, the district nursing sister can also play an important part in the initial assessment of physical needs in the elderly, but she will be mainly involved in the continuing supervision of the group at greatest risk: the very old and handicapped, especially those living alone.

The health visitor

The health visitor can exert her influence in three main ways. She can play an important part in the initial and ongoing assessment of the needs of the elderly in the practice and in their subsequent management and supervision. As she is by training a health educator, she is the most appropriate member of the team to instruct the patient in matters of prevention and the maintenance of good health. Since most old people live on relatively low fixed incomes she can advise on the best buys in food, clothing, heating and furnishings. She can also ensure that the temperatures in the living room, and especially the bedroom, are adequate, and she can advise on safety, by inspecting the home for potential hazards, such as long flexes to electrical equipment, inappropriate bathroom heaters, oil heaters, electric blankets, gas cookers operated from slot meters, highly polished floors and ill-fitting carpets, especially those on stairs and in poorly lit rooms. The health visitor is the most appropriate person to act as the link between the primary care team and the social services.

The social worker

The contribution that the social worker could make to the care of the elderly is obvious. It is therefore unfortunate that there are so few who are permanent members of primary care teams. The wide-ranging responsibilities that have been thrust on them by reorganization, the inevitable changes in personnel due to promotion – often sadly into administration – and the abandonment of professional specialization have all been factors diminishing this contribution. If, however, the social work profession is able to recruit trained staff of high calibre to its ranks, the structure of social work could become more stable and social workers, themselves, might be made to feel more secure in their dealings with the medical profession.

The present gulf that exists between the two professions is both unnecessary and wasteful of precious resources. There are two ways by which this gap might be bridged and thereby improve the service provided. One would be the return to some form of social work specialization; the other would be to create a structure of promotion that would allow at least some social workers to achieve high status and adequate remuneration while remaining in active, professional contact with the people whom they seek to serve.

Such an experienced medical social worker would be a boon to the primary care team. If she specialized in the social care of the elderly, her expertise could be shared among several primary care teams, to whom she would act as consultant. She would work in close collaboration with her health visitor colleagues, in the identification of the patient's social needs but her principal role would be the assessment of their social functioning. She would give guidance on budgeting, pensions, special benefits and other supporting facilities. She would also liaise with the various voluntary organizations interested in the welfare of the elderly, arranging such things as meals on wheels, holiday placements, attendances at lunch and social clubs and visits to the housebound by voluntary workers.

The general practitioner

The general practitioner need not necessarily lead the team, but in many cases he will be expected to do so. His role will therefore involve him as a clinician, an organizer and a supervisor. As clinician, he will be expected to compose his diagnoses in physical, psychological, personal, family, and social terms, and when he intervenes therapeutically he must be familiar with the pharmacological hazards of prescribing for elderly patients, as discussed later in this chapter. As an organizer he must realize the difficulties that older patients can have when trying to cope with modern general-practice organization. For example, with a little foresight and imagination, a rigid appointment system, that may act as a barrier for older patients, can be altered with little difficulty to one that meets their particular needs. The practice policy for home visiting must take into account transport difficulties for the elderly population, and the fact that, as a group, older patients under-use the services of their doctors, often requiring more attention than they seek.

To simplify his role as supervisor he should give thought to the introduction of a special geriatric record card that would undoubtedly enhance the prospects of optimum continuous care. The same card would be used by all the members of the primary care team. This should ensure that omission in recording is minimized; furthermore, it could act as a check that appropriate action had been taken.

The general practitioner must also accept responsibility for regular review of the services offered. This need not be unduly formalized, but the team should develop enough confidence in itself to allow its members to criticize constructively the quality of care provided and examine methods of work, in the light of reasoned argument for change. No-one likes change, but since improvement can only come about by change, this must be faced. A healthy inward-looking group is the one most likely to succeed in getting the best results for the patient. The general practitioner could therefore act as the catalyst for such group reaction, by actively encouraging comments about his particular contribution to the care of the elderly in the practice.

Practice secretaries and receptionists

Much of the initial contact that elderly patients have with their practice is through the practice secretaries and receptionists. To many older patients a long-serving practice secretary or receptionist may well be the best known member of the team. It is therefore important that junior secretarial and reception staff be trained how to talk to and deal with elderly patients. Steps should be taken to explain the difficulties that older patients may have in contacting the practice, either in person or by telephone. They may, for example, have difficulty with their hearing, or their vision and be slow in movement and in thought. These factors must be taken into account when dealing with the elderly, and if any secretarial buffer exists to protect the doctor, this should be played down when older patients telephone or call at the practice centre.

It is also important that the secretary or receptionist is made to feel an important member of the team, by being given recognition for the skilled work that she does. She should be given the opportunity to attend practice meetings and discuss her contribution to the care of the elderly. This is especially important if changes in her role are being contemplated by other members of the team.

Voluntary Workers including the good neighbour

No-one in any community should be absolved from the responsibility of looking after the aged. Although there are professionals who have a clear duty in this field, their effectiveness in densely populated areas, where the problems of ageing are seen at their worst, is less than in small towns and rural communities. Since the urban primary care team is seldom identified with any particular community, the individual members can much more easily assume a degree of anonymity which dilutes their influence. This also applies to the private citizen, who can in cities more easily escape from any caring obligation to the elderly. It is also less likely that any local group will come together to exert pressure directly or indirectly when services are found to be inadequate.

To combat these deficiencies in our urban areas, many voluntary agencies have sprung up in the field of geriatric care to champion the cause of the elderly in the country as a whole. These agencies encompass such diverse interests as housing, sheltered warden-supervised accommodation, transportation of patients to day hospitals, lunch clubs, holiday homes, travel concessions, pre-retirement courses, leisure and employment opportunities for the elderly, and the funding of research into their special problems.

The services that they provide are clearly important, and it is therefore essential that at least one member of the primary care team should know precisely the range of services available in the area served by the team. That person would normally be the social worker, but in her absence the health visitor should undertake this duty. She should also become known personally to the members of the voluntary agencies, who may wish to contact her from time to time, when the support of the primary care team is required.

Apart from the organized voluntary agencies, essential material and psychological support is often given to the elderly in the community by neighbours, ministers of religion, and groups of young people. Such involvement, by individuals and groups, should be fostered locally by primary care teams and, where appropriate, their opinion should be canvassed when any changes in the service are being discussed.

The specialist in geriatric medicine

One of the most important roles of the geriatrician is to act as a support to the primary care team. In some areas he attends the group practice or health centre in his clinical capacity, seeing selected patients, advising about assessment, continous supervision programmes and in some cases prosecuting research in collaboration with members of the team. The team looks to him or her for advice about the selection of patients for day centres, pre-retirement programmes, sheltered housing, inpatient and outpatient medical assessment and establishing priorities for those requiring less urgent admission to long-stay hospitals or homes. The geriatrician should also play a leading role in in-service training programmes, suggesting the content of these from his knowledge of recent advances in the specialty.

Other professionals involved in the continuous care of the elderly

These include physiotherapists, occupational therapists, speech therapists, dietitians, chiropodists and visitors to the blind and partially sighted. Of necessity, these workers will require to share their expertise among the elderly patients served by several primary care teams, but their very necessary contribution should never be forgotten when considering the continuous care of the elderly in the community. It is therefore important that they be invited from time to time to practice meetings when matters relevant to them, and their work, are being discussed.

The team concept

The preceding sections describe the roles of many people, any of whom may work together in a variety of combinations to form a team to help the elderly. There are, however, few instances when all need to be involved, and many when in any event all will not be available. In larger group practices with health visitor and district nurse attachments, teams may be more easily formed and readily identifiable than in situations where the general practitioner works single-handed with little or nothing in the way of employed or attached staff. The concept of the team can nevertheless be applicable to any form of practice organization. It is for the general practitioner with his responsibility for providing all necessary medical care for his patients to decide how he can best communicate with and encourage the co-operation of other relevant workers in providing total care for his patients, and especially his elderly ones.

Prescribing for the elderly

Any programme of continuing medical care of the elderly must contain a general policy for the diagnosis and drug treatment of the common conditions met with in this age-group. It is not intended to list these systematically in this chapter, but rather to concentrate on the principles of management and particularly on the pitfalls of long-term drug therapy. The basis for sound therapy in the elderly is the same as in any other age-group. It is dependent on taking a full and careful history and making an accurate diagnosis. Since, in the aged, multiple pathology is the rule rather than the exception, it is advisable to list the diagnoses in order of importance. This is not always easy, but the necessity to make accurate diagnoses is obvious if a reasoned plan of therapeutic action and management is to be made.

Once the diagnostic list has been completed, the practitioner must decide on his course of management. It is important for him to realize that he need not necessarily aim at total symptomatic relief with drugs: indeed he might well discover some conditions that could best be helped by stopping drugs altogether. Only some elderly patients will require drug therapy, whereas others can be relieved by the mobilization of resources that are at the command of other members of the primary care team. When the doctor does decide that drugs are necessary, it is important for him to make the regime as simple as possible. The fewer drugs he prescribes the better, as it is well known that the incidence of adverse reactions rises with the number of drugs used. Trouble is most likely to arise with drugs like digitalis, thyroxine, hypnotics and psychotropics which require careful adjustment of the dose to achieve correct therapeutic response. Barbiturates are particularly prone to cause confusion in the elderly and tricyclic antidepressants have cardiotoxic effects which tend to be more pronounced in the older age-group.

Somewhere between 7 and 15 per cent of hospital admissions are attributable to drug reactions and it is known that drug-induced morbidity and mortality are much more common in the elderly than in any other age-group. If there is any doubt about the safety of any drug or combination of drugs. it is prudent to seek advice about this; it may also be lifesaving.

If drugs are necessary, those chosen should be suitable for the elderly patient. Certain drugs have a cumulative toxicity, when their excretion or breakdown is impaired by diseased organs or in very advanced old age. Drugs that are prescribed for old people should be acceptable to them. There is no point in prescribing large pills for someone who cannot swallow them. Drugs should be dispensed in suitable containers that can be easily opened and should be labelled with clear instructions that can be easily read. Most doctors prescribe safely for their elderly patients from a range of drugs with which they have become thoroughly familiar. The danger comes when new medicaments are added to the range. It is at such times that caution should be the watchword. It is also important that the regime of drug therapy be reviewed at regular intervals, to ensure that all prescribed preparations are still necessary. This is especially so when tranquillizers and hypnotics have been prescribed.

One of the commonest drugs used in geriatric practice is digoxin and this provides an illustrative example of the dangers of drug therapy in the elderly. Digitalis intoxication is common. Its symptoms include nausea, loss of appetite, weakness and apathy, vomiting and, commonly, the onset or worsening of heart failure. Elderly patients, even when not in heart failure, have a higher blood concentration of digoxin than younger patients. This is due to their smaller body size, to diminished urinary excretion and to the fact that the half-life of digoxin is increased by 50 per cent in patients between the ages of 25 and 75. The manifestations of incipient digitalis toxicity in the elderly may be very misleading. Nausea may be the sole feature, or the patient may present with vague ill health or even confusion. Digitalis preparations are unnecessarily, and often dangerously, prescribed for old people presenting with tachycardia, which may be due to anaemia or thyrotoxicosis, or with dependent oedema, due to lymphoedema or varicose veins. Toxicity to digoxin develops in 8 to 20 per cent of hospital patients and mortality ranges from 7 to 50 per cent in different reported series.

A common clinical sign of digitalis intoxication is atrial fibrillation, with a ventricular response of under 50 beats per minute, accompanied by ectopic ventricular beats. Other arrhythmias, suggestive of digitalis intoxication, need electrocardiography for their recognition. During long-term digitalis therapy, the maintenance of normal plasma potassium is all-important. Low potassium levels may be produced by the use of powerful diuretics, or may already exist as a result of dietary deficiency, or of chronic diarrhoea resulting from abuse of purgatives; conditions not uncommon in the elderly.

When given by mouth, atropine-like substances increase digoxin absorption, and may enhance the likelihood of toxicity. On the other hand, metoclopramide (Maxolon) decreases absorption, so that the effect of the digoxin is reduced or even abolished. Synergistic reactions occur when propranolol (Inderal), ephedrine, or aminophylline are taken with digoxin. The combination of propranolol and digoxin causes increased bradycardia, whilst the combination of ephedrine or aminophylline with digoxin produces increased ventricular excitability.

Postscript

The scope of work undertaken by doctors is continually evolving to meet the changing needs of society. On the one hand, the range reflects the profession's responses to scientific discovery; on the other, it indicates the extent to which national policies on the provision of medical care have materialized in practice. In most instances the pattern and speed of this evolution are controlled by the monetary demands of an authoritarian medical profession, but there are areas of care in which society itself becomes the main instigator for change. Such an area is the care of the aged. With a few notable exceptions, medical men of power and influence have not recognized the claim of geriatric medicine for its fair share of academic, research and service resources. It is sad to realize that the acceptance of geriatric medicine as a distinct discipline continues to be a matter for professional debate and that there are still some medical schools without independent departments of geriatric medicine. Unless the care of the aged is accorded the same status as the care of the young, how can students of medicine and other allied professions be expected to acquire during their formative years appropriate attitudes to the care of the elderly? It is the responsibility of the middle-aged and young in any society to provide a comprehensive and humane system of continuing medical and social care for its elderly. If they fail in this task they, themselves, may live long enough to regret it.

References

[1] Kemp, R. (1965): *A New Look at Geriatrics.* London: Pitman Medical

[2] Thomson, Jean (1970): The Growth of Population to the End of the Century. *Social Trends*, No. 1. Central Statistical Office, HMSO pp. 21–32

[3] Williamson, J. (1976): Problems in care of the elderly. *Health Bulletin*, *34*, 312

[4] Ashworth, H.W. (1959): The Care of Old People in General Practice. *Medical World*, *91*, 314

[5] Forsyth, G. and Logan, R.F.L. (1964): Medical technology and the needs of chronic disease. *Journal of Chronic Diseases*, *17*, 789

[6] Royal College of Physicians of Edinburgh (1963): *The Care of the Elderly in Scotland.* Edinburgh: Royal College of Physicians

[7] Warren, M.D. (1964): Demands and needs for inpatient care for elderly people. *Medical Care*, *2*, 113
[8] Elliot, A.E. and Stevenson, J.S.K. (1973): Geriatric Care in General Practice, *Journal of the Royal College of General Practitioners*, *23*, 615
[9] Taylor, C., Busby, J.C., Huntley, J. D. *et al.* (1955): The Health Centres of Harlow – an essay in co-operation. *Lancet*, *ii*, 863
[10] Stokoe, I.H. (1971): Care of the Elderly, *Update Plus*, *1*, 677
[11] Milne, J.S., Maule, M.M., Cormack, S. and Williamson, J. (1972): The design and testing of a questionnaire and examination to assess physical and mental health in older people using a staff nurse as the observer. *Journal of Chronic Diseases*, *25*, 385
[12] Anderson, Sir Ferguson (1976): *Practical Management of the Elderly.* 3rd ed. Oxford: Blackwell Scientific Publications
[13] Thomspon, M.K. (1975): *In Screening in General Practice.* Ed. C.R. Hart, p.141 Edinburgh: Churchill Livingstone

Appendix

Initial assessment questionnaire

Date

Names Surname
Forenames

Address

Married/Single/Widowed/Divorced

Date of birth

Previous occupation
Spouse's previous occupation

Religion

Numbers in household Males
Females

Medical assessment

General physical condition	Good/neglected
Body build	Thin/average/obese
General health	Good/moderate/bad
State of nutrition	Good/poor
State of skin	Normal/abnormal/clean/dirty
Evidence of anaemia	Yes/doubtful/no

Vision (using newspaper)	Good/impaired/nil With glasses/without glasses
Hearing	Good/impaired/nil
If impaired or nil is there any ear wax?	Yes/no
Teeth – own – dentures	Satisfactory/unsatisfactory Satisfactory/unsatisfactory
Bowel habit	Continent/incontinent
Bladder habit	Continent/incontinent If incontinent - day/night/both Frequency/dysûria
Mobility indoors	Unlimited/limited/chairbound/bedfast
Mobility outdoors	Unlimited/limited
Foot defects	Present/absent
Joint pains/stiffness	Present/absent If present, specify
Hemiplegia	Present/absent
Contractures	Present/absent
Oedema	Present/absent
Cough	Present/absent
Spit	Present/absent
Dyspnoea on moderate exertion	Present/absent
Smokes cigarettes	Yes/no
Pressure sores	Present/absent
Current medication	Yes/no If yes, understands dosage of each drug Yes/no
Appliances	None/stick/tripod stick/walking aid

Comment

Mental health

'Some of the questions I am going to ask are about things like memory and concentration and may seem a little different from the things a doctor usually asks.'

Questions to assess dementia:

1. What is your full postal address?
2. How long have you been living at this address?
3. What day of the week is it today?
4. What month are we in?
5. What year is it?
6. How old are you?
7. When is your birthday?
8. What year were you born?
9. Just making a guess – about what time is it just now?

(Each wrong answer scores 1. Sum error score. 0-1 = no mental impairment: 2 = possible chronic brain syndrome: 3 = definite chronic brain syndrome.)

Questions to assess depression or anxiety:

'These questions are about how you are feeling in yourself.'

1. Have you any anxieties or problems that worry you at present? If yes
   - (i) Are you feeling very upset by this?
   - (ii) Is there any other particular worry bothering you at present?
2. (i) Are there times when you feel anxious without really knowing why?
   - (ii) Are you distressed by silly pointless thoughts that keep coming into your mind against your will?
3. Have you any fears that tend to haunt or worry you?
4. What interests have you? (sewing, knitting, TV etc.)
   (If none) Have you lost interest in almost everything?
5. Do you look forward to things?
   (If not, or doubtful) Does the future seem pointless?
6. Do you find it a bother to do the things you are able for? If yes
   - (i) Does even the thought of having to do anything feel an effort to you?
   - (ii) Do you sometimes have to push yourself to start even the simplest task?

7. (Ask women)
Do you tend to cry any more often than you used to?
(Ask men)
Have you ever felt like crying?
(If yes) Have you felt more like crying recently than you used to in the past?

8. (i) How are you in your spirits today? Are you quite happy or do you feel down in your spirits?
(ii) Have your spirits been good or poor lately?
(iii) Have your spirits ever been so low that you have just sat for hours on end?

9. (i) How are you sleeping just now?
(ii) Do you feel rested when you rise in the morning?
(iii) Has your sleep been good or poor during the past 12 months?

10. Do you sleep with or without sleeping tablets?

11. Have you felt nervous or depressed at any time during the past 12 months?
(If yes) (i) Do you feel better or worse now compared to then?
(ii) Were you able to cope adequately with your everyday life when you were like this?

12. Are you being given any medicines, tablets or capsules to soothe your nerves or make you less depressed?
If yes. Do you know what you have been given?

13. (i) Do you enjoy your food?
(ii) Has your appetite been good or poor lately?

14. Would you say that you are content with your present way of life?
Do you have doubts about this?
Are you dissatisfied?

Comment

Social assessment

Housing	Flat/tenement/house/other
Stairs	Yes/no – If yes, approximate number

Number of rooms	
Toilet	In house/outside/shared
– easily accessible	Yes/no
State of house	Clean/Neglected
Lighting	Good/bad
Cooking facilities	Good/bad
House heating	Good/bad
Power	Gas/electricity/coal/other
Any accident hazards	Yes/no – if yes, specify
Clothing	Good/adequate/poor
Bath	Yes/no
Able to use bath unaided	Yes/no
Laundry arrangements	Satisfactory/unsatisfactory
Social contacts	Adequate/inadequate
Social support	Relation(s)/home help/health visitor/district nurse/social worker/volunteer/meals on wheels/social club
Capacity for self care	Dress – yes/no/partial Undress – yes/no/partial
Cooks for self	Yes/no/partial
Feeds self	Yes/no/partial
Shops for self	Yes/no/partial
Can summon help in emergency	Yes/no
Finance	Adequate/inadequate
Comments	

4.8
Terminal care and bereavement

Derek Doyle

Death is not a medical defeat but failure to relieve the suffering of the dying could be regarded as professional failure. Terminal care affords the doctor, and probably the general practitioner more than any other, a challenge only equalled by its immeasurable personal rewards. It tests his skill as clinician and communicator, the warmth of his personality and the depth of his faith or philosophy.

There is no standard practice but there are well established principles which enable individualized care to be tailored to the ever changing needs of each patient.

General principles

Terminal care must be total care, not only physical, emotional and spiritual, but seen in the context of a family or community itself grieving, sometimes growing in stature and never likely to be the same again. Failure at all times to recognize and care for each facet of a patient's life may easily lead to total failure for all concerned. Hence, tempting as it may be to rely on drugs for pain and symptom control, terminal care is most certainly not an exercise in clinical pharmacology.

Terminal care is team care, capitalizing on the skills and experience, the strengths and even the frailties of doctors, nurses, para-medicals and invited clergy who make up the primary care team. As the strain of a mortal illness is a burden carried by the family, as well as the patient, so is their care the responsibility of all who have skills and compassion to share.

Terminal care is palliative care, unashamedly not aiming for cure but a continuing development in evolution of the professional care offered from the outset of the illness — sometimes energetic, always positive, preferably planned.

Terminal care myths

'Most patients prefer to die in hospital or hospice.'
Only in this century has the position changed from 70 per cent dying at home to 70 per cent dying in hospital but the reasons are complex social ones and in no way reflect the expressed wishes of patients but rather the characteristic unselfishness the dying display in seeking to save families additional work and strain. That more than half would elect to remain at home might be seen as evidence, if ever it were needed, that more understand fully what is happening than we realize. The patient who, until recently, has always been happy to go to hospital for sophisticated diagnostic or therapeutic procedures and now needs persuasion to do so is saying something to his doctor and his family if only they can hear it.

'Most patients don't know how serious it is.'
The doctor who genuinely believes this is suffering from delusions of grandeur or unable to come to terms with his own discomfiture in the presence of death. Every study carried out has shown that though just under 50 per cent of patients have, at some time, been given an explicit explanation of the diagnosis and prognosis, close on 90 per cent of the intellectually intact are fully aware of their condition but deliberately and often quite skilfully keep it from families and doctors alike. They speak of their sinister suspicions during the initial diagnostic stage, the period of optimism or denial as matters improve, and the reawakening of suspicions or fears as doctors become more secretive, families more tense, therapeutic activity less energetic and their physical wellbeing diminishes.
No misunderstanding could be more dangerous for the doctor, himself being considered by the patient, but often reluctant to give any hint of the fatal outcome for fear of removing 'hope'. All he may be achieving is enhanced fear based on ignorance, further loneliness and isolation of someone who, more than at any other time in life, needs loving, understanding companionship. How right Hippocrates was in saying: 'Young men fear death, old men fear dying'. Few dread the end of life, much as they may resent its premature timing, but fewer still can face dying with pain, secret fears and unexpressed feelings.

'Most patients tell you their problems in their own time.'
The man with a myocardial infarction will not be slow to describe his pain, often in graphically accurate and helpful detail. The one with metastatic carcinoma may never mention pain (particularly when his doctor has been unskilled in relieving it), his fears (especially when the doctor acts as though he should not have any), or his faltering faith. The nearer he gets to death, the less will he mention and the more he will bear in silence. At any one time he will usually

have five symptoms he may report with modest encouragement, but five others which trouble him deeply but cannot be mentioned lest they be considered trivial or waste the precious time of a doctor who signifies he would rather not know.

'*Good terminal care demands so much time.*'
It demands that time be spent but often much less than would willingly be put aside by the doctor for marriage counselling, or the health education of his patients. The dying have a deeper understanding of the value of time, and its scarcity, than many others and ask only that the doctor give a few minutes of undivided attention to what troubles *them* rather than what interests or rewards *him*. 'Tell me exactly how you are feeling and what you would like me to do for you if I am able', is more helpful and encouraging than the 'Hello, how is the pain today?' for a patient now thankfully free of pain but terrified by the less professionally interesting nausea, constipation, anorexia, weight loss, panics and distancing from God.

'*The terminally ill prefer to be sedated.*'
Five per cent certainly do but the others prefer alertness provided the long day is not punctuated by pain and vomiting or saddened by the embarrassed despair of relatives who often need the support of the doctor more than they do. There is no question that some doctors sedate with phenothiazines and benzodiazepines because of their own professional bankruptcy, and a third of relatives will ask for sedation to spare them embarrassing conversations made all the more painful because they, long ago, put an embargo on the patient being told the truth and now they, and the patient, must live a lie.

'*The dying prefer to be on their own.*'
Perhaps doctors have come to associate dying with single rooms from their early hospital days but it is rarely the wish of a well-cared-for patient to be set apart in this way. Most would rather remain with or near to others so long as their suffering does not upset these companions, for death, as they so well know, will soon separate them from the comradeship in tribulation which makes life so precious.

'*Children are upset by being with the dying.*'
Perhaps some are but not so much as being kept in the dark about what is happening, allowed to ponder and suffer alone whilst the adults go about their work in sadness and silence. Beyond question most children do more for the happiness of the dying patient than the doctor can do, and themselves mature as they learn so early in life that even in death can a person grow in stature and loveliness.

Co-operation with professional colleagues

With hospital colleagues. — Though 90 per cent of the final year of life is usually spent at home, there are obviously many contacts with hospital colleagues who understandably are sometimes more concerned with pathology-orientated therapy than the general practitioners and equally hesitant about discontinuing out-patient follow-up.

Each must know what the other is doing and *saying*, what each is planning and anticipating, and what each hopes to achieve. The hospital specialist will often have more expert knowledge of the condition and its modern management (particularly in the radio-therapeutic or cytotoxic management of cancer) but his judgement must take into account the total picture of patient and family often available only through the general practitioner. A death-bed should not become the battlefield where opposing views are fuelled by professional recriminations. As the hospital doctor has a responsibility to report what the patient was told, how he reacted and what therapy may achieve as well as the most recent biochemical results, so the general practitioner must update the hospital on his patient's fears, the family reactions and interactions and his own, independent recommendations. In the same way that no hospital should send a letter saying merely . . . 'A further course of chemo-therapy was given', neither should the general practitioner send a note . . . 'Worth tapping this effusion?'. Whether so much should be committed to paper when it could more easily be said on the telephone is debatable. Perhaps general practitioners should give ex-directory numbers to selected colleagues, and consultants set aside one hour per week for general practitioners to telephone them.

With nursing colleagues. — Without doubt community nurses, particularly when members of primary care teams, should be informed of patients entering the terminal phase even if their visits and ministrations are not yet needed. Extensive experience of a hospice-based advisory home care service has convinced the writer that nurses are usually called in too late when even by advice alone they would have made a useful contribution earlier on. As they would be the first to point out, they are not 'hand-maidens to the medical profession' but fellow professionals and better able to advise on oral hygiene, dietary alterations, prevention and treatment of pressure sores, and often better able to explain details to relatives in a language more easily understood.

They can support doctors but only as much as they are respected and supported in this testing work.

With hospice colleagues. — There are now many hospices and home care services in Britain, each with a body of experience and expertise which can enable practitioners to give better care at home, some able to admit for skilled palliation and rehabilitation even of the terminally ill, and a few with the complete armamentarium for pain relief. Each doctor should familiarize himself with their facilities, their operational policy and their staff. Like any specialist service their value rests in the skilled use of their expertise and the quality of relaxed co-operation which can be developed.

With clerical colleagues. — In recent years dying has become 'medicalized' and death 'institutionalized' and many ministers and priests feel left out, their role difficult to define, their contribution either not recognized or not appreciated. This is sad because, no matter what their previous depth or detail of faith, 75 per cent of the dying spontaneously turn to questions of faith or philosophy — the meaning of life, the presence of God, the mystery of suffering, the possibility of forgiveness or reconciliation. The good minister, like the complete doctor, often has a rich understanding of a family and its resources — knowledge which can only enhance the care everyone is trying to give. Where possible it seems both right and natural, with the patient's consent, to share this care with the clergy explaining what medical support hopes to achieve, and what help the minister or priest can give the primary care team. Just as doctors are now being better trained in giving terminal care, so are our clerical colleagues. For both it should be generous and unashamed, as natural to speak of spiritual problems as physical ones.

With para-medical colleagues. — Much more use could be made of community physiotherapists than is usually done and equally of the wide ranging skills of occupational therapists in the provision of aids and adaptations, the 'total' assessment of physical and social problems, and the benefits of activities which will lessen the greatest problem of the dying — boredom! The better is the pain and symptom control, the longer most patients will survive, but the greater may be the sense of personal uselessness and worthlessness, and the more they will relish something to restore this sense of worth.

Planning good terminal care

Terminal care can, to a large extent, be planned. It need not be an exercise in crisis intervention. Several studies have shown that in fact the fatal outcome was recognized on average twelve to thirteen months before, allowing plenty of time for all concerned to plan carefully. Because a patient is, rightly, still attending for chemotherapy it can at the same time be recognized and the knowledge shared between colleagues that the final stage is approaching. Some guidelines are helpful here:

1. One person, preferably his own doctor, should assume by mutual consent the responsibility for co-ordinating the care. On no account should home visits be done by any or all of the partners at random with all the possibilities of different explanations, advice and regimes.
2. Each member of the primary care team must accept responsibility for the passing on to colleagues of all information considered relevant, as soon as possible.
3. The patient should, as a routine, be discussed at regular team meetings and a check list used to ensure that every aspect of care, of patient and family, is dealt with and each knows his role and responsibility.
4. Problems can be anticipated. Commodes can be ordered before the patient falls 'en route' to the toilet, sheepskins before he is permanently in bed, Zimmers before walking is well nigh impossible etc. Arrangements can be made for soiled linen, community or hospice volunteers brought in as 'sitters' before the relatives become exhausted, respite admissions arranged, families gently but authoritatively forewarned about developing symptoms, the sick-room furnished downstairs and so forth.
5. Discussion with specialist or hospice colleagues before anticipated problems arise can prepare for different pain problems, domiciliary visits, serious bereavement reactions. For example, it may be predicted that a patient with a pancreatic carcinoma infiltrating the first lumbar vertebra will suffer pain which a coeliac plexus block will help. The local pain relief clinic can be contacted to ascertain their referral and admission procedure. Paraplegia from spinal cord compression would in some areas be dealt with by the radiation oncologists, in others by the neurosurgeons. Foreknowledge will make for speedier relief should this complication occur.
6. Bereavement, as will be discussed later, cannot be abbreviated but undoubtedly can be mitigated by skilled anticipation. It begins when the relative first realizes that he or she is to lose a loved one. Its care and management start at the same time.

Symptom control

By popular usage terminal care has come, perhaps unfortunately, to mean care of the cancer patient and occasionally those with end-stage cardiac, respiratory or neurological disease. These are, of course, those with the most protracted terminal phase and cancer patients have been shown to have many more symptoms than any other group, though often easier to control than the crippling dyspnoea in someone with chronic obstructive airways disease, or the terrifying helplessness of the motor neurone disease patient. In the sections which follow each of the commonest problems — expressed symptoms and unventilated distresses — are discussed in outline with suggestions and guidelines on management.

ANAEMIA

Most patients will have adapted to a low Hb and often repeated blood tests, the prescribing of iron and the giving of blood transfusions are done more for the doctor's morale than the patient's wellbeing. Red cell concentrates given to the dying are not tonics but useful only when dyspnoea is thought to be due more to the anaemia than anything else. Sending a frail and frightened patient back to hospital for a transfusion which will not improve his quality of life is unfair to the patient and the junior hospital doctor who must also learn that there comes a time when good intentions may amount to meddling.

ANOREXIA

Causes:

1. Oral candidiasis (present in 75 per cent of patients often without white plaques).
2. Chronic constipation.
3. Uninteresting, unimaginative food, in too large helpings, offered only at standard meal times.
4. Unpleasant odours in the environment.
5. Nausea and vomiting.
6. Excessive medication and/or dry mouth (itself usually drug-induced).
7. Depressive state.
8. Hypercalcaemia or uraemia.

Management:

1. The only proven 'tonic' is a steroid, preferably prednisolone 5 mg tid or dexamethasone 2 mg each morning.
2. Encourage fluids but allow the patient to eat what he fancies, when he fancies, on the smallest plate, remembering that the nearer he is to death the colder must be the drink and the only meal may be his breakfast. Most will manage porridge, even at night, and many live for weeks on four-hourly ice-cream, chilled custard, or ice-cubes of their favourite 'tipple'.

ANXIETY

Anxiety in the dying is normal and not usually pathological, usually related to unrelieved or unexplained problems and more helped by realistic understanding and reassurance and company, than sedative anxiolytics or incomprehensible platitudes.
Each symptom usually has a significance to the patient different from its meaning to their doctor. To the patient dyspnoea is 'suffocating to death', dysphagia 'starving' or 'choking', haemoptysis 'bleeding to death', and a bad dream, panic or loss of memory 'mental change'. He may see sweating (as in liver secondaries or in oat cell bronchogenic carcinoma) as 'consumption' and his steatorrhoea as infectious to the family sharing the toilet.

Management:
1. At each consultation elicit what troubles the patient and what he attributes it to, then explain, reassure or at least show that every anxiety is worth reporting and taken seriously.
2. The best 'anxiolytics' are those which relieve the distresses whether analgesics for pain, steroids for anorexia, laxatives for constipation or anti-emetics for vomiting.
3. When a true anxiolytic is needed, decide between a once daily long half-life one (e.g. diazepam [Valium] 10 mg each night) or short half-life benzodiazepines (e.g. lorazepam [Ativan] 0.5–1 mg sub-lingually) prn. the continually frightened, restless patient in the final stages of life is best helped with diazepam (Valium) suppositories 10 mg daily. (See Figure 1.)
4. When pain is sufficient to merit an opiate, or dyspnoea the cause of anxiety, low dose opiates are better than any other anxiolytics (e.g. morphine solution 5 mg every four hours or morphine sulphate [MST] 10 mg twelve-hourly).

BOREDOM

This has been referred to above. It is best relieved by giving the patient useful, rather than merely time-filling activities. Much encouragement is needed in education of the relatives before the patient will return to knitting, cataloguing recipes, polishing the silver, updating the address book, preparing the vegetables, choosing paint colours, completing the magazine rack, or whatever, interspersed with TV, radio, colour magazines (rather than heavy books) and the carefully rationed visits of friends who know how to bring news rather than be entertained and, so important, know when to go.

Figure 1. — Benzodiazepines and metabolites: half lives

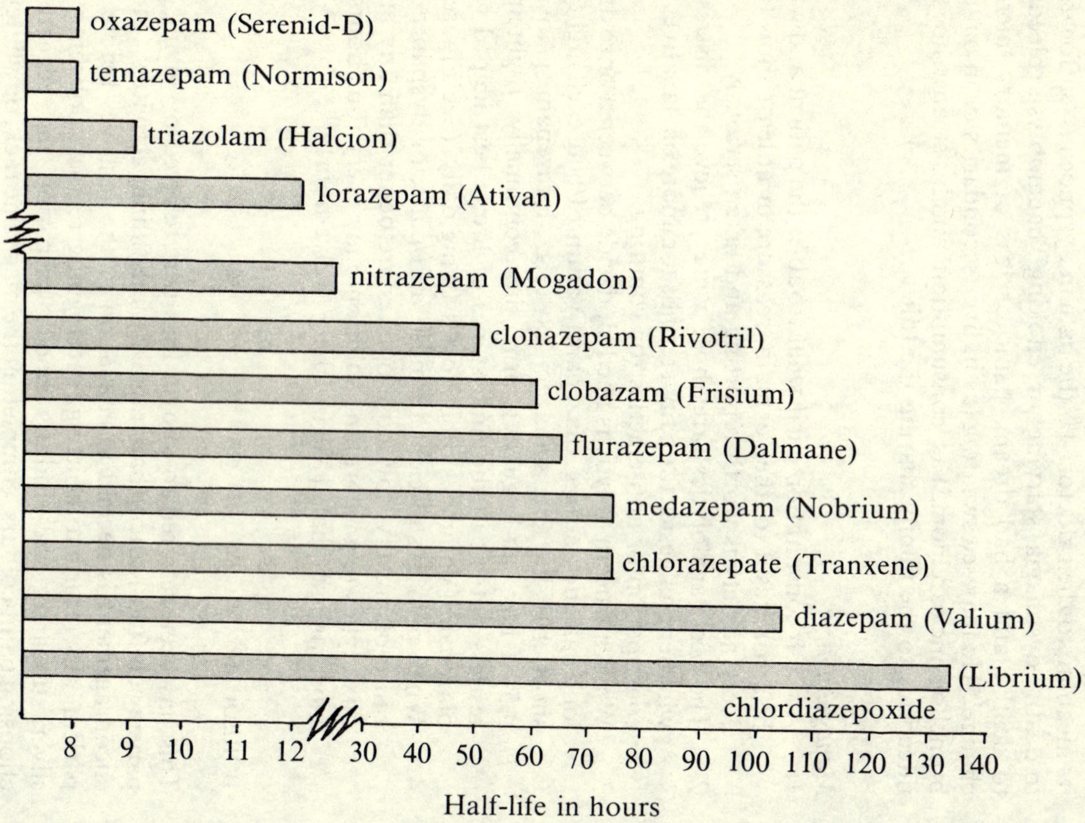

CONFUSION

This occurs in not less than 25 per cent of patients, can be caused by almost any of the commonly prescribed drugs, is usually worse at night or when the lay-out of a room is changed, and often alarms the relatives sufficiently for them to ask for the patient's admission. It is important to diagnose or exclude:

— hypercalcaemia
— hyponatraemia
— reversible anaemia
— drug effects (including excessive sedation)
— hepatic damage
— cerebral metastases.

Management:

1. Treat any remediable cause, for example:
   — dexamethasone for raised intra-cranial pressure
   — high-dose steroids for toxicity from hepatic secondaries
   — modification of drug regime
   — correction of hypercalcaemia.
2. Try thioridazine (Melleril) 10–25 mg tid, chlorpromazine (Largactil) 10–25 mg tid.
3. Reassure and support the relatives who may see it as impending psychiatric breakdown.

CONSTIPATION

Sadly often regarded as unimportant by doctors, this is a problem in not less than 75 per cent of patients and is the commonest cause of nausea and vomiting in the terminally ill. Its causes are usually obvious.

Management:
By this stage it is usually impossible for the patient to take a high roughage diet and resort must be made to appropriate laxatives. *They are always necessary in patients on opiates.*
Do a rectal examination and define:

(a) whether the rectum is loaded with faeces;
(b) whether it is empty or ballooned suggesting faecal impaction above the examining finger;
(c) whether it is empty and collapsed.

For (a) one must prescribe arachis oil retention enemata nightly for two nights with a bisacodyl (Dulcolax) and a glycerine suppository on the following two mornings until the rectum is empty. Faecal expanders by mouth are contra-indicated because they will merely expand the rectal lump into an even more impossible mass to express or remove manually.

For (b) give a combined faecal expander/peristaltic stimulant (Dioctyl) each night and a daily rectal examination to gauge progress.

For (c) do no rectal treatment but rely on appropriate regular oral laxatives, for example sodium picosulphate, lactulose (Duphalac), Dioctyl, senna extract.

CONVULSIONS

In patients not previously known to be epileptic, these occur in 10 per cent of terminally ill cancer patients, usually as a result of cerebral metastases. Understandably they often lead to a plea for admission but this is not always necessary.

Management:

1. Supply diazepam rectal tubes (Stesolid) (10–20 mg) and instruct willing relatives in their use, explaining that they work within ten to fifteen minutes and remain effective for close on three hours — a useful effect when a doctor cannot hope to be there within minutes to give IV diazepam (Diazemuls).
2. If the convulsions are seen to be due to rapidly rising intracranial pressure, give IM or IV dexamethasone (Oradexon) 16 mg followed by oral dexamethasone 8 mg daily in divided doses.
3. Put the patient onto regular anti-convulsants, for example phenytoin (Epanutin) 300 mg daily p.o. or IM phenobarbitone daily if unable to swallow.

COUGH

Even in patients with bronchogenic carcinoma or chronic obstructive airways disease, though dyspnoea is common, cough is most unusual but easily controlled.

Management:

1. Exclude a super-added infection which, except in the last days of life, is worthwhile treating with an appropriate antibiotic, simple physiotherapy and good nursing.
2. Dry, irritating, non-productive cough may occasionally be stopped with codeine or pholcodine linctus, methadone (Physeptone) or an opiate but is better managed with 0.25 per cent bupivacaine (Marcaine) via a nebulizer every four hours. The equipment is often obtainable on loan from a chest unit, physiotherapy department or hospice.
3. Tenacious sputum responds to humidification (using sterile water rather than bupivacaine in the nebulizer), or simple glycerine-based expectorants.

DEPRESSION

The features of both endogenous and reactive types are no different from at any other time in life but the increased incidence of the reactive type is usually evidence of poor pain and symptom control *or* long-term opiate use. Their fewer adverse effects probably make the tetracyclics, e.g. mianserin (Norval, Bolvidon) 60–100 mg nightly, preferable to tricyclics but the sedative effects of the latter, particularly amitriptyline (Tryptizol, Lentizol) and clomipramine (Anafranil) are useful for agitated, insomniac, depressed patients.

DIARRHOEA

True diarrhoea occurs in only 4 per cent of patients. It should be considered as spurious until proved otherwise.
There appears to be nothing to choose between kaoline, codeine phosphate and diphenoxylate (Lomotil) but loperamide (Imodium) has a speedier action and may usefully be given on a 'prn' basis. It also appears to act upon the anal sphincters and may therefore have a useful role in controlling faecal incontinence.

DYSPHAGIA AND DYSPEPSIA

The principal causes at this stage are:

1. *A blocked Celestin or Atkinson tube*
   If a Celestin tube has been inserted to relieve dyspagia problems may arise with the tube blocking perhaps because the patient has eaten white bread, failed to take an effervescent drink before and after each meal, or failed to liquidize some bulky food.
2. *Candidiasis* — descending from the oral pharynx. This is common, can become symptomatic within twenty-four hours, and can be present when oral candidiasis appears to be under control. It responds to continuing nystatin mouth drops swallowed after oral hygiene, combined with ketoconazole (Nizaran) 200–400 mg daily.
3. *Post-irradiation oesophagitis* will usually clear spontaneously, helped by simple antacids or in severe cases with the use of carbenoxolone (Pyrogastrone) sucked qid.
4. *Invasion of the lower third of oesophagus by oesophageal/gastric carcinoma* — sometimes helped by cimetidine (Tagamet) tablet/syrup (200 mg qid) or ranitidine (Zantac) (150 mg bd) if gross hepatic involvement is proven.

5. Extra-oesophageal pressure from mediastinal adenopathy, sometimes responds to mediastinal irradiation or dexamethasone (4–6 mg per day).

DYSPNOEA

Potentially treatable conditions should be excluded:
— cardiac failure
— pleural effusion
— chest infection
— reversible anaemia
— elevation of the diaphragm by ascites
— mediastinal adenopathy

Management:
The management of each is standard, with either radiotherapy for the adenopathy or dexamethasone (Oradexon) (6–8 mg per day), but drainage of an effusion (provided it is not caused by mesothelioma) only when it is thought to be the principal or only cause of dyspnoea. After drainage the instillation of thiotepa, C-parvum, tetracycline, or talc powder may prevent re-accumulation. Each tapping of a mesothelioma effusion is liable to lay down tumour seedings in the needle tract.

Non-specific management:
1. Prednisolone 20–30 mg/day in divided doses.
2. Low-dose morphine relieves tachypnoea and is strongly recommended (morphine solution 2.5–5 mg 4-hourly).
3. Lorazepam (Ativan) sub-lingually (0.5–1 mg) prn for panic dyspnoea or daily diazepam (Valium) (5–10 mg).
4. A table fan at the bedside.

The doctor has an obligation to give details of the site of an effusion and any other cause of dyspnoea to the nurse. She will know to nurse the patient with an effusion on the same side and expect distress when he is moved onto the contra-lateral side. The patient with a bronchogenic carcinoma may be easier when recumbent or sitting in a reclining chair whilst the one with chronic obstructive airways disease will be propped up and need supervised oxygen therapy.

FUNGATING TUMOURS

The principal physical problems are odour and haemorrhage. The former may be reduced by bismuth-iodoform paste (BIPP) applied directly to the tumour and left undisturbed for three to four days; by the use of metronidazole (Flagyl) tablets daily allowed to dissolve in the tumour; by natural yoghurt supplied daily and by the provision

of an activated charcoal dressing (Denidor, Actasorb) applied on top of other dressings in use.
Capillary ooze from a fungating tumour can be controlled, or at least kept out of sight, by non-adherent dressings or controlled with daily soaks of 1:5000 silver nitrate solution applied to the tumour. Relatives should be discouraged from using household aerosol air-fresheners which, from then on, will come to be associated with this sad time.

HAEMORRHAGE

1. *Haemoptysis* occurring in spite of palliative radiotherapy (the first line of treatment) will require heavy sedation using diazepam rectal tubes (Stesolid) instilled by the relatives, IV diazepam (Diazemuls) by the doctor or high-dose diamorphine injection.
2. *Haematuria* is sometimes reduced by daily noxytiolin (Noxyflex) bladder instillations or daily bladder lavage with 1:10,000 silver nitrate solution.
3. *Haematemesis*, like haemoptysis, calls for sedation as an emergency, but careful consideration rather than automatic hospital referral if death is likely to occur within hours.

HALITOSIS

By its unpleasantness and embarrassment for all concerned, this often isolates the patient from his relatives and friends.

Causes:
1. *Bad oral hygiene* (often made worse by the dry mouth produced by drugs).
2. *Poor dental hygiene* (which many dentists would deal with in a patient's home).
3. *Chest pathology*, whether a bronchogenic carcinoma or bronchiectasis.
4. *Cesspool halitosis*, particularly with carcinoma of stomach and linitis plastica.

Management:
In addition to the obvious recommendation of mouth freshening sweets and lozenges, the doctor may wish to try:
1. Metronidazole (Flagyl) 100 mg tid for odours from the lungs.
2. Metoclopramide (Maxolon) 10 mg tid or domperidone (Motilium) 10–20 mg tid to accelerate gastric emptying.

HICCUPS

It is worthwhile trying:
1. to encourage better fluid intake in the uraemic patient;
2. chlorpromazine (Largactil) 10–25 mg prn;
3. haloperidol (Serenace) 1–2.5 mg prn;
4. metoclopramide (Maxolon) 10 mg or domperidone (Motilium) 10–20 mg prn;
5. re-breathing into a polythene bag;
6. phenol infiltration around a phrenic nerve as a last resort.

INCONTINENCE (URINARY AND FAECAL)

Urinary incontinence is encountered at some time or other in between one-third and one half of all patients with terminal carcinoma, and double incontinence in about 15–20 per cent. Many families will tolerate the former but, even with special laundry facilities available, few will accept the latter. Sadly, though the causes may be obvious, there is little one can do except:
1. Exclude urinary tract infection, faecal impaction, and excessive sedation.
2. Catheterize using a 5 ml bulb silicone-coated catheter and arrange for weekly lavage with water if there is no infection or debris, daily lavage with 0.2 per cent chlorhexidine or 0.5 per cent citric or 0.5 per cent acetic acid if there is infection, and lavage with noxythiolin (Noxyflex) if haemorrhage is occurring.
3. Exclude faecal impaction as a cause of faecal leak, try intermittent loperamide (Imodium) or create constipation with codeine phosphate and have the community nurse evacuate the rectum twice weekly.

INSOMNIA

The principal causes in someone previously a good sleeper are:
1. *Inadequately relieved distresses* (particularly pain) or anxiety.
2. *Unrecognized depression* where insomnia is often the first, and for some time, the only feature.
3. *Nocturnal frequency* which may respond to emepronium (Cetiprin) 200–400 mg at night.
4. *Night sweats* particularly in those with oat cell bronchogenic carcinoma, hepatic metastases and any of the reticuloses. Cimetidine (Tagamet) 400 mg nightly or ranitidine (Zantac) 150 mg nightly are very effective. Failing them the doctor would try indomethacin (Indocid) 50–100 mg nightly, or propanalol (Inderal) 40 mg.

When all else fails, one resorts to a short half-life benzodiazepine (temazepam, triazolam) or a sedative anti-depressant (amitriptyline, clomipramine). The agitated, aggressive patient with personality change more evident at night is usually helped by pericyazine (Neulactil) 10–20 mg or by chlormethiazole (Heminevrin) 50–100 mg, and the patient in his final days and suffering pain benefits from methotrimeprazine (Veractil, Nozinan) 50 mg. Fortunately terminal illness is not a contra-indication for a tipple of their favourite whisky, still the best sedative we have.

NAUSEA AND VOMITING

Patients may tolerate vomiting if they have no persistent nausea but sadly we are more often defeated by nausea than by any other symptom in the dying. The causes are legion (and paradoxically investigations may never reveal a cause) but particularly important in the dying are:

— constipation
— hypercalcaemia
— anxiety state
— raised intra-cranial pressure
— sub-acute obstruction
— hepatic metastases

the opiates (see later) contrary to what is often believed are seldom the cause when the right dose has been attained.

After attempts to correct any of the above causes it will be necessary to use a single anti-emetic in 80 per cent, two drugs (one centrally-acting, one gut-acting) in a further 15 per cent and no anti-emetics at all but rather high-dose dexamethasone in the others in whom no cause could be found. The steroid routine is 24 mg by injection on the first day, 20 mg by injection on the second day, 16 mg by injection on the third day, then oral (Oradexon) 8 mg per day thereafter.

Having decided, often empirically, which group of anti-emetics to use, central-acting or gut-acting, the choice of drug is usually more dependent on side-effects than anti-emetic efficacy.

Central-acting:

1. Haloperidol (Serenace) 0.5–1 mg tid is useful, only minimally sedative, and rarely produces extra-pyramidal effects at that dose.
2. Prochlorperazine (Stemetil) 5–25 mg tid and chlorpromazine (Largactil) 10–25 mg tid are equally anti-emetic but sedative and produce extra-pyramidal effects.
3. Methotrimeprazine (Veractil, Nozinan) 25–50 mg tid or more frequently is an excellent anti-emetic (and analgesic) but exceedingly sedative.

4. Droperidol (Droleptan) 5 mg qid is better than haloperidol (Serenace) but very sedative.
5. Cyclizine (Valoid) 50 mg and thiethylperazine (Torecan) 6.5 or 10 mg are useful when nausea and vomiting are related to movement, the former more sedative than the latter, a much under-valued drug.

Gut-acting:

1. Domperidone (Motilium) 10–20 mg available as tablet, injection and syrup and as a 30 mg suppository would appear to have the edge on metoclopramide (Maxolon) because of freedom from Parkinsonian features and its effect on the oesophageal gastric sphincter.
2. In a patient with a proven gastric carcinoma both cimetidine (Tagamet) and ranitidine (Zantac), initially by injection, will often stop both vomiting and nausea.

OEDEMA

1. *Unilateral arm oedema* (lymph oedema) often benefits from the use of an intermittent compression pump (Flowtron) obtainable from physiotherapy departments.
2. *Bi-lateral arm oedema* is always part of the syndrome of Superior Vena Cava obstruction calling for radiotherapy if available, a trial of dexamethasone (8 mg per day in divided doses) or the advice of an oncologist on possible chemotherapy.
3. *Unilateral leg oedema* — if not due to DVT there must be a venous and/or lymphatic obstruction near the iliac vessels requiring urgent radiotherapy or chemotherapy. Steroids and diuretics have no place.
4. *Bi-lateral leg oedema* — whilst cardiac failure will be managed routinely, hypoproteinaemia is not amenable to treatment at this stage and resort will have to be made to pelvic or para-aortic irradiation and spironolactone (Aldactone) (100–400 mg daily) occasionally augmented with frusemide (Lasix) 250 mg daily.

PAIN

In spite of this being associated in most people's minds with cancer, and probably the feature most feared, it continues to be inadequately diagnosed and treated. Some of the reasons for this are:

1. It is chronic pain, and not acute, and therefore the onset is indeterminate, the pattern variable, the description often vague, and the mood of the patient depressed and unco-

operative. It is too easy to assume that 'no pain reported' means 'no pain present' when in fact he has given up speaking of it because of previous professional failure or indifference and he has programmed himself to believe it must be suffered as an inevitable feature of his cancer.

2. Analgesics are used at the dose and frequency employed in acute pain whereas high doses may be required, usually at shorter intervals, because of changed metabolism.
3. Co-analgesics are not employed appropriately.
4. Agonists and partial antagonists are employed concurrently.
5. The place of neurolytic procedures ('nerve blocks') is not considered often enough nor the benefits of palliative radiotherapy.
6. It is not recognized that *every* patient is suffering more than pain — he has other physical, emotional, social and even spiritual problems — and preoccupation with the role of analgesics to the exclusion of other 'pains' is doomed to failure.

Diagnosis of pain:
It is a good rule to assume until proved otherwise that a patient with metastatic carcinoma has pain though in fact it effects only about 70 per cent and is very severe in only 10–15 per cent.

1. Remembering that many have multiple pain from multiple causes, attempt to define the site, cause and intensity of each:
   — bone pain
   — visceral pain
   — nerve entrapment pain
   — colic
   — skin (hyperaesthetic) pain
   — muscle pain
   — joint pain
   — raised intra-cranial pressure pain
2. Trust clinical judgements more than investigations which should only confirm. Pain may arise in bone metastases before a bone scan is positive and long before a straight film reveals anything (though the alkaline phosphatase and/or isoenzymes may assist). Headache from raised intra-cranial pressure cannot wait for a positive CT scan, nor can treatment be withheld for pain in expanding hepatic metastases until an ultrasound has been done. If in doubt about the pattern of pain and its response to treatment, get the patient to complete a pain chart for *each* type of pain.

Specific treatment of pain

Where possible treatment should be specific rather than non-specific though frequently this is impossible.

Bone pain:

(a) Palliative radiotherapy, effective within three to four weeks, is the first line of treatment.

(b) Prostaglandin bio-synthetase inhibitors (NSAIs) should be given in maximum dose unless specifically contra-indicated and continued indefinitely.

(c) Medium-strength or strong analgesics will usually be required at least until the irradiation has taken effect — obvious by the onset of adverse effects of the analgesic because pain, the physiological antagonist of the opiates, has been removed.

Visceral pain:

This refers to the pain caused by stretching of liver and renal capsules by metastatic deposits. It may be of two types — the constant ache over the affected organ or the sudden intense pain, sometimes associated with shock and collapse, caused by haemorrhage into a deposit. The latter constitutes an emergency in terminal care.

(a) Strong analgesics will almost always be needed.

(b) Steroids, initially by daily IM injections then orally, will help to relieve the acute inflammatory reaction. Probably the best preparation is IM methyl prednisolone sodium succinate (Solu-Medrone) 125 mg per day for six days.

(c) Continuing pain in an otherwise relatively well patient merits the advice of a pain relief clinic on a para-vertebral block.

Nerve root compression:

This is suggested by any unilateral pain down one or two adjacent dermatomes, the radiation clearly defined by the patient, usually worse on coughing or sneezing. Similar but more persistent pain occurs in post-thoracotomy wounds, after irradiation or surgery producing scarring.

(a) This is an indication, 'par excellence', for a nerve block which can be expected to relieve pain for eight to twelve weeks and often longer.

(b) Steroids, e.g. prednisolone 20–30 mg daily in divided doses, assist by reducing perineural oedema.

(c) The dysaesthetic element in the pain requires a tricyclic anti-depressant such as amitriptyline 50–75 mg nightly (Tryptizol, Lentizol).

(d) A medium or strong analgesic until at least a nerve block has been carried out.

Raised intra-cranial pressure:

It should be noted that cerebral tumours, whether primary or secondary, are not in themselves indications for dexamethasone which should be reserved for patients with clinical evidence of raised intra-cranial pressure, focal neurological signs and secondary epilepsy. Like all 'life-support systems' they are easy to start and difficult to discontinue.

(a) Dexamethasone (Oradexon), initially 16 mg per day, in divided doses and then reduced over two to three days and maintained at 8–10 mg per day.
(b) Simple analgesics may be more effective than narcotics and are worth trying first. Narcotics, if needed, are more likely to produce respiratory depression in such patients if there is co-existing chronic obstructive airways disease or other serious respiratory embarrassment. When pain is not relieved it is worth checking it is not caused by bone secondaries in the skull requiring palliative radiotherapy and prostaglandin bio-synthetase inhibitors.

Skin (hyperaesthetic) pain:
This appears to be more of a problem with patients with melanomatosis, the reticuloses, and oat cell bronchogenic carcinoma. All the skin is extra-sensitive to light touch, making nursing difficult and heavy bed clothes uncomfortable.

(a) The concomitant use of a low potency centrally-acting analgesic (e.g. paracetamol) and a peripherally-acting one (e.g. aspirin) is often more effective than a single agent.
(b) Occasionally propranolol (Inderal) 10 mg tid or cimetidine (Tagamet) 200 mg tid help.

Colic, muscular and joint pain:
Colic is unusual in the terminally ill even in those with sub-acute intestinal obstruction. The clinical picture and management of all three types differ in no way from standard practice.
When specific treatment is not possible, the doctor prescribes the mild-strength analgesics up to their maximum recommended dose. When pain recurs he moves to the medium-strength analgesics and again builds up to their maximum dose. When pain breaks through yet once more he moves to the strong, narcotic analgesics but continually reviews where the indications exist for other co-analgesics, nerve blocks, radiotherapy or anti-depressants. (See Figure 2.)

Analgesic equivalents (See Table I)

Much unnecessary confusion arises in moving from the medium-strength to the strong analgesics. One simply converts to the stronger drug using the equivalent table and gives a modest increase in dose. For example, a patient experiencing pain on dipipanone (Diconal) 20 mg qid is on the equivalent of 10 mg × 4 of oral morphine. Because that 40 mg is inadequate he requires 60 mg per

Analgesic			*Oral morphine equivalent*	*Ratio to oral morphine*
dipipanone	(Diconal)	10 mg	5 mg	2 : 1
papaveretum	(Omnopon)	10 mg	5 mg	2 : 1
pethidine		100 mg	12 mg	8 : 1
dihydrocodeine	(DF 118)	30 mg	3 mg	10 : 1
dextromoramide	(Palfium)	5 mg	15 mg	1 : 3
methadone	(Physeptone)	5 mg	7.5 mg	1 :1.5
phenazocine	(Narphen)	5 mg	25 mg	1 : 5
buprenorphine	(Temgesic)	200 μg	12 mg (approx.)	1 : 60
diamorphine	(Heroin)	5 mg	7.5 mg	1 :1.5
diamorphine injection		5 mg	15 mg	1 : 3

Table I. — Analgesic equivalents (to be used only at appropriate prescribing intervals)

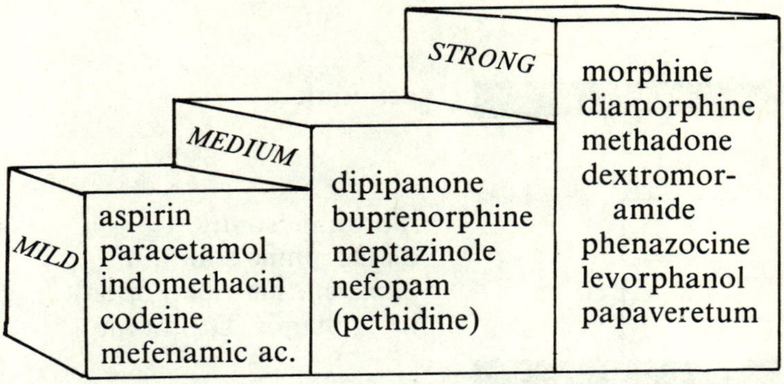

Figure 2. — Terminal care: analgesic ladder (non-specific therapy)

day, given as morphine solution 10 mg every 4 hours if the pain is developing rapidly, or MST 30 mg 12-hourly if more slowly.

Period of analgesic efficacy

The frequency of administration is dictated by the period of efficacy and not by domestic and nursing routine, and is often briefer than in acute pain. (See Figure 3.) For example, morphine and diamorphine solutions require to be given 4-hourly round the clock, dipipanone 6-hourly, methadone 8-hourly initially then often increased to 6-hourly. Even MST may occasionally have to be given 8-hourly though *never* more frequently.

Morphine and diamorphine:
Much experience convinces the writer that many myths still surround the use and dangers of the opiates which might better be started much earlier than is often the case. Terminal care is, par excellence, the indication for their use.
Without doubt there is nothing to choose between these drugs in analgesic efficacy but only their potency and solubility, diamorphine being much more soluble. In current practice, morphine is the drug of choice by mouth, made up as a simple solution, or with the preservative chloroform water, or syrup, whilst diamorphine is best reserved for injections, up to 1000 mg being capable of dissolving in only 1.6 ml of water.
Morphine solution should be used:

(a) 4-hourly (including 2a.m.) until analgesia has been achieved and only then can a double dose be tried at 10p.m. omitting the 2a.m. dose.
(b) For patients whose analgesic requirements are changing rapidly.

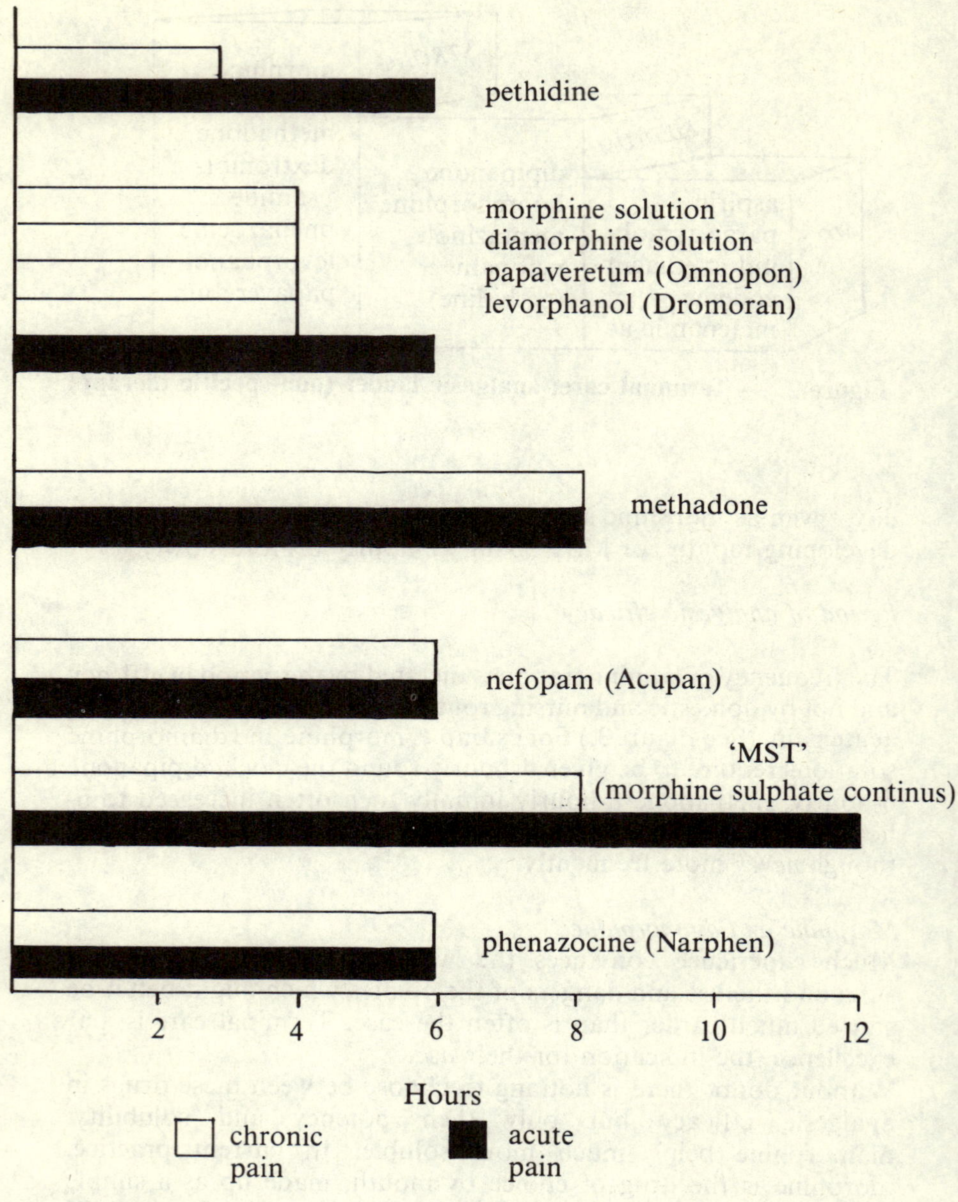

Figure 3. — Terminal care: analgesic efficacy (orals)

Controlled-release morphine (MST Continus) should be used:

(a) When analgesic requirements have been defined (see above).
(b) When recent dose increases have been infrequent and widely spaced.
(c) 12-hourly in most cases, simply dividing the daily intake of morphine solution (or its equivalent) by two.

Adjuvant laxatives are always necessary with both forms.

Diamorphine sub-cutaneous:
The battery-powered 'syringe-driver' capable of injecting a day's supply of sub-cutaneous diamorphine has changed the face of modern terminal care, enabling many to stay at home when previously they would have required 4-hourly visits by community nurses. They have also contributed to reduce use of morphine suppositories useful as they still are in general practice.
A syringe is loaded with a 24-hour supply of diamorphine calculated on the basis of oral morphine 3: sub-cutaneous diamorphine 1, a butterfly needle inserted sub-cutaneously and left in situ for three or four days, and the syringe-driver carried in a holster, pocket or bag.
It is indicated in preference to 4-hourly injections in:

(a) Patients unable to swallow oral morphine solution or tablets.
(b) Patients unreliable in their compliance.
(c) Patients whose pain is, for some reason, poorly controlled on oral medication.

Agonists/partial antagonists:
Though the agonists (morphine, diamorphine, dextropropoxyphene, codeine) are not completely antagonized by the partial antagonists — pentazocine (Fortral), buprenorphine (Temgesic) and meptazinol (Meptid) — it is advisable *never* to use agonists and partial antagonists concurrently.

Co-analgesics:
Many have already been mentioned. Their use is one of the 'secrets' of good analgesia in the dying — antibiotics for secondary infection, anti-depressants for dysaesthesia, diazepam for muscle spasm, chlorpromazine for tenesmus, strangury and pelvic pain, steroids for nerve entrapment and lymphoedema, etc.

Neurolytic procedures:
Patients who might profitably be referred to a pain relief centre or hospice colleagues for advice include those with:

(a) Pancreatic carcinoma (coeliac plexus block).
(b) Unilateral chest/abdominal wall pain (intrathecal/epidural block).
(c) Perineal pain (caudal block).

(d) Pancoast tumour (epidural steroid injections).
(e) Recto-anal pain (coeliac plexus block).

PRURITUS

Useful measures to relieve itch include:

1. Sodium bicarbonate washes every hour or so.
2. Cholestyramine (Questran) 1 sachet bd provided the patient can tolerate the taste and there is no steatorrhea.
3. Prednisolone 30 mg per day (or dexamethasone 4 mg per day, in divided doses).
4. Eurax HC cream bd.

However, like many symptoms, it is more usually helped by good nursing and understanding.

SORE MOUTH

It cannot be stated strongly enough that oral candidiasis, characterized in these patients by a red, sore, spongy mouth *without* white plaques, occurs in 75 per cent of the dying and needs energetic treatment with nystatin (with dentures out) and the dentures cleaned nightly in half-strength domestic bleach.
Non-specific therapy includes:

(a) Aschurt's Medium used as a mouthwash 4-hourly.
(b) Hydrocortisone (Corlan) pellets 2.5 mg sucked qid.
(c) Carbenoxolone pellets (5 mg) sucked qid.

SWEATING

Those with active hepatic metastases, fulminating oat cell bronchogenic carcinoma, and some of the reticuloses, may sweat so much that bedding requires to be changed frequently and both patient and family are embarrassed.
Worth trying are:

1. Cimetidine (Tagamet) 200 mg tid or 400 mg nightly or ranitidine (Zantac) 150 mg bd.
2. Indomethacin (Indocid) 25 mg tid or 100 mg nightly.
3. A table fan playing by the bedside.

WEAKNESS

It is tempting but wrong to assume that nothing can be done for this symptom. There is still a place for excluding hypokalaemia, hypercalcaemia, and treatable infection, for seeking the guidance of a physiotherapist or occupational therapist, or for the assistance of a local hospice in encouraging mobilization and the restoration of the sense of usefulness in spite of the advanced state of disease.

Miscellaneous matters

Much has been said about the terminal care of patients with malignant disease. The same principles apply to those with any other pathology.

Important principles in all care are:

1. Do only such investigations as *may* enable the treatment to be changed for the better and never to disguise the doctor's sense of helplessness.
2. Involve the patient in all decision-making as a member of the team.
3. Pay more respect to the *quality* of life than its *prolongation* without quality.

The doctor's bag

Drugs of value for 'emergencies' encountered in terminal care which might usefully be carried in a doctor's bag include:

1. Hyoscine hydrobromide 0.4 mg for the 'death rattle'.
2. Injection dexamethasone (Oradexon) 16 mg.
3. Injection methyl prednisolone (Solu-Medrone) 125 mg.
4. Injection diamorphine HC1 30 mg.
5. Injection haloperidol (Serenace) 10 mg.
6. Injection methotrimeprazine (Nozinan) 50 mg.
7. Injection domperidone (Motilium) 20 mg.
8. Diazepam rectal tubes (Stesolid) 2 × 10 mg.

Bereavement

Grieving starts when the diagnosis was first suspected or confirmed, not after death. It carries a definite morbidity and even mortality and merits professional attention though sadly many doctors fail in this respect, preferring to regard it as 'something we all have to go through'.

The care of the bereaved can, to a certain extent, be planned, performed and monitored scientifically as well as compassionately.

Factors affecting grief reaction

1. *Time to prepare for the death.* Sudden, unexpected death produces the profoundest reaction whereas time well spent with, for example, the cancer patient will reduce the reaction. Every relative of someone dying unexpectedly should be considered as 'at risk'.

2. *Griever's sense of usefulness.* The more a relative has been able to care for the deceased, the less the reaction. This has important implications when so often doctors succumb to pressures to hospitalize the dying or fail to educate relatives in simple home nursing.
3. *Griever's perception of personal support received.* Well-conducted studies have confirmed that relatives' *perception* of support received is more important than the amount of support given and this obviously will relate to personality.
4. *Previous personality and help.* Those with extrovert personalities usually suffer the most reactive depression but, predictably, those with a dependent personality will intuitively seek someone else on whom to lean. Those with inflexible, obsessional traits will find adapting and coping difficult.
5. *Quality of relationship with the deceased.* The poorer the relationship (though often vehemently denied afterwards) the worse the prognosis much as the doctor may be aware that secretly the griever had longed to be freed from an unsatisfactory marriage. It cannot strongly enough be stated that in all grief there is, often unjustifiably, an element of guilt.

Prediction of grief outcome

The doctor, armed with these factors, can obviously prepare and predict. No one is better qualified by his knowledge of personality, relationship and coping ability.

Sadly most people feel they must conform to social norms. They must return to work as if nothing had happened, appear relaxed when racked with remorse, be brave when they would rather cry with despair, feign activity when they cannot concentrate on anything, profess faith when God seems far from loving and approachable.

At all costs we must enable and encourage grievers to be themselves, at least with their doctors, and not stifle or deny their inner turmoil.

Features of grief

More than 50 per cent of the bereaved experience many of the same symptoms suffered by the deceased in their first months of loss. They must be taken seriously when they report palpitations, breathlessness, chest tightness, weight loss, anorexia, dyspnoea and dysphagia.

If they have persuaded the doctor to join with them in a well-intentioned fabric of lies with the deceased, they will find it difficult for years to come to know whether they themselves can now trust his explanations and his honest integrity.

Ninety per cent will suffer disturbed sleep patterns in the first six months with frequent wakening, vivid dreams involving their loved ones and bouts of misery (not to be confused with true depressive state). More than 50 per cent will have auditory and/or visual hallucinations of the dead one, but fewer than 10 per cent will mention this for fear of being labelled psychotic. Simple explanation of these phenomena, *in advance*, saves much sadness and silent fear.

Stages of grief

1. Period of relief.
2. Period of relaxing.
3. Period of resenting.
4. Period of remembering.
5. Period of repairing.

1. *Period of relief.* This follows immediately on the death and usually lasts no more than days, characterized by happiness for the deceased coupled with personal relief. There is much gratitude for the care-givers and a pervading sense of unreality and numbness. Visits by the doctor will be appreciated but soon forgotten. Hypnotics demanded by the relatives rather than the bereaved will seldom work but be taken as a token of the doctor's continuing role.
2. *Period of relaxing.* This follows the funeral and usually only lasts as long as near relatives can remain with the widow or widower. There is a sense of support and shared pain, preoccupation with practical problems and the danger of precipitate decisions about house-selling, emigrating etc. Inappropriate advice is often given to get rid of visible reminders of the deceased and the doctor should exert his full influence to ensure that photographs, letters, trophies etc., are kept and treasured for the time when the world, but not the widow(er) has forgotten he ever existed.
3. *Period of resenting.* This dates from the departure of family and lasts anything from three to four months coinciding with the end of 'acceptable grief' in our modern society. There is a profound sense not only of loneliness but aloneness, of insecurity and self-pity, with much criticism both of self and the professional helpers.

   The suffering is heightened by others describing how well the griever looks, failing to ask how she is, coupled by embarrassing invitations to resume social and church activities, when she is fearful of returning to the empty house.

4. *Period of remembering.* This starts at approximately three months and continues for a further twelve to fifteen months with constant reminiscing and reliving of events before the death, coupled with a conscious effort to recapture the happier emotions of the past. A time of great despair is six to seven months, marked by the peak in suicide attempts.
5. *Period of repairing.* No longer does the past seem more attractive than the future and slowly the griever begins to make a deliberate effort to think positively about his/her resources and skills. New interests, hobbies and friendships are cultivated and at each consultation with the doctor some new evidence can usually be elicited. Nevertheless anniversaries, particularly birthdays, Christmas and the date of the death, remain extremely painful yet often ignored completely by other family members and even the doctor.

Bereavement support by the doctor

The following guidelines may assist:

1. Visit as soon after the death as possible to remind the patient of continuing support and concern. The visit can usually be a very short one.
2. Visit again, allowing sufficient time, when the relatives plan to leave and be positive in advice, emphatic in advising against precipitate action and reassuring about professional concern for his/her own health.
3. Arrange a visit/consultation for three months and at that time conduct a careful physical examination giving opportunity for the patient to express fear and suppressed emotions. Take pains to explain the features of 'normal' grief, because probably no one else will!
4. Find an opportunity for a further consultation three months later when the world accepts her 'everything is fine' but experience shows that she is most at risk.
5. Keep a diary of dates of deaths of patients in the practice for planned follow-up for the first year. On an average list this will amount to fewer than ten immediate relatives annually.
6. Make use of CRUSE or any other bereavement service in the area no matter how enthusiastic are the members of the primary care team about bereavement support.

It is useful to remember that grief is like a surgical wound — painful and ugly at first, gradually fading but still easily damaged and hurt, never disappearing and always a permanent reminder of a time of pain, shock, change and fear. Time does not heal — it only makes the scar less visible to onlookers!

The two principal tasks of a doctor caring for the bereaved are firstly, to reassure and educate them about the 'normality' of much that they are suffering, and, secondly, to be on the alert for abnormal reactions. Just as terminal care can usually be planned, so can much bereavement support.

Further reading

Bond, M. (1979): *Pain: Its Nature, Analgesics and Treatment.* Edinburgh: Churchill Livingstone.

Doyle, D. (1984): *Palliative Care: The Management of Far Advanced Illness.* London: Croom Helm.

Doyle, D. (1984): *Coping with a Dying Relative.* London: McDonald Publishers.

Hinton, J. (1979): *Dying.* London: Penguin Books.

Parkes, C.M. (1975): *Bereavement.* London: Penguin Books.

Saunders, C. and Baines, M. (1983): *Living with Dying.* Oxford: OUP.

Saunders, C. (1978): *The Management of Terminal Disease.* London: Edward Arnold.

Stedeford, A. (1984): *Facing Death.* London: William Heinemann Medical Books.

Twycross, R. and Lack, S. (1984): *Symptom Control in Far Advanced Cancer: Pain Relief.* London: Pitman.

Wilkes, E. (Ed). (1982): *The Dying Patient.* Lancaster: MTP Press.

4.9 Welfare and charitable organizations

This list comprises some of the major national organizations which exist to provide information and help for specific groups of patients and their relatives and professionals caring for them. The addresses of regional and local organizations and branches of national organizations can often be found by reference to area social work offices.

Alcoholism	National Council on Alcoholism 3 Grosvenor Crescent London SW1X 7EE Tel: (01) 235 4182
Blindness	Royal National Institute for the Blind 224 Great Portland Street London W1N 6AA Tel: (01) 387 5571
Cancer	The Marie Curie Foundation 199 Sloane Street London SW1X 9RF Tel: (01) 235 3336
Chest and heart diseases	Chest and Heart Association Tavistock House North Tavistock Square London WC1H 9JE Tel: (01) 387 3012
Coeliac disease	The Coeliac Society P.O. Box 181 London NW2 2QY Tel: (01) 459 2440
Cystic fibrosis	Cystic Fibrosis Research Trust 5 Blyth Road Bromley Kent BR1 3RS Tel: (01) 464 7211

Deafness	Royal National Institute for the Deaf 105 Gower Street London WC1E 6AH Tel: (01) 387 8033
Diabetes	The British Diabetic Association 10 Queen Anne's Gate London W1M 0BD Tel: (01) 323 1531
Disablement	Disabled Living Foundation 346 Kensington High Street London W14 8NS Tel: (01) 602 2491
Epilepsy	The British Epilepsy Association Crowthorne House New Wokingham Road Crowthorne, Berks RG11 3AY Tel: (034 46) 3122
Haemophilia	Haemophilia Society P.O. Box 9 16 Trinity Street London SE1 Tel: (01) 407 1010
Ileostomy	Ileostomy Association of Great Britain and Ireland 149 Harley Street London W1 (No telephone) *Also at* Leslie S. Kingston Esq. The Central Office The Drove Kempshott Basingstoke, Hants RG22 5LU Tel: (0256) 21288
Leukaemia	Leukaemia Research Fund 49 Great Ormond Street London WC1N 3JJ Tel: (01) 405 0101
Migraine	British Migraine Association 'Evergreen' Ottermead Lane Chertsey, Surrey KT16 0HJ Tel: (093) 287 3242
Multiple sclerosis	Multiple Sclerosis Society of Great Britain and Northern Ireland 4 Tachbrook Street London SW1 Tel: (01) 834 8231

Muscular dystrophy	Muscular Dystrophy Group of Great Britain Natrass House 35 Macaulay Road London SW4 0QP Tel: (01) 720 8055
Parkinson's disease	Parkinson's Disease Society 81 Queens Road London SW19 8NR Tel: (01) 946 2500
Rheumatism and arthritis	British Rheumatism and Arthritis Association 1 Devonshire Place London W1 Tel: (01) 935 9905
Spastics	The Spastics Society 12 Park Crescent London W1N 4EQ Tel: (01) 636 5020
Spina bifida	The Association for Spina Bifida and Hydrocephalus Tavistock House North Tavistock Square London WC1H 9HJ Tel: (01) 388 1382
Tinnitus	British Tinnitus Association 105 Gower Street London WC1E 6AH
Widows	Cruse: The National Organization for Widows and Their Children Cruse House 126 Sheen Road Richmond, Surrey Tel: (01) 940 4818

4.10
The continuing care of patients with chronic disorders

J.J.C. Cormack and C.J. Watkins

A large part of this book is concerned with responding to the common symptoms of illness presented in general practice (Part 3). With the increasing number of individuals living to old age the general practitioner is becoming increasingly involved in the continuing management of patients suffering from chronic disorders. In managing this type of illness he must have a clear understanding of the natural history of the diseases he is treating so that he can make a prognosis of the complications and likely outcome of the disease. His treatment will then be directed to reducing the number of complications and if possible achieving a more favourable outcome. By virtue of the fact that he is easily accessible to his patients, provides continuing care often over a period of many years and is well placed to identify the social and psychological constraints within which his patients live, he is uniquely placed to undertake this task.

The area of continuity of care (which, along with ready accessibility for the purpose of diagnosis, provides the hallmark of effective general practice) is dealt with in Part 4, largely on an age-group basis. Because this is not a conventional disease-orientated textbook we have deliberately refrained from attempting to lay down prescriptive approaches for the follow-up of classical 'diseases' once diagnosed. Many of the conditions with which we deal are self-limiting (e.g. tonsillitis, depression or backache), while there are others (such as migraine or osteoarthrosis) where a pattern of remissions and exacerbations may make an 'on demand' pattern of consultation the most effective form of care.

This chapter is concerned with the way in which the general practitioner can use the continuity of care he offers to improve the prognosis of chronic illness within his practice population. His effectiveness depends on his understanding of chronic illness, the resources that he has at his disposal for effective management and his knowledge of how these resources can be most usefully deployed.

There are a number of conditions in which regular planned follow-up, once a diagnosis is established, provides the best way of preventing secondary damage and caring for existing disability where natural remission is not to be expected and cure is not practically possible – for instance hypertension and diabetes.

There is, as yet, little consensus about the best long term management of many chronic conditions. The fact that little agreement exists should act as a stimulus to further research and the development of fresh ideas on the organization of care. The authors of this chapter are aware of the dangers of blind conformity to untested criteria for high quality care, or some kind of 'check list' medicine. Nevertheless, there are examples of medical care where there is an agreed good standard of practice and where a check list or aide-mémoire type of record are of proven value – most notably in obstetric care, but also on the assessment of paediatric development (see Chapter 4.2) and in the care of the elderly (Chapter 4.7). We are encouraged by these examples to attempt to set out in this chapter in schematic form for a number of selected conditions what are necessarily only broad guidelines, but guidelines nonetheless which may provoke thought and controversy and, we hope, the sort of dialogue between readers and editors which contributes to the dynamic development of the work.

Organization

In organizing continuing care, as opposed to simply responding to patient need or patient demand, it is necessary to identify those conditions which will be helped by this approach, to define such conditions clearly and to decide the objectives of this type of care. Once the conditions are selected the patients 'at risk' must be identified. This will involve setting up some form of a register – whether a disease index, computer file, tagged records or by modifying an existing age-sex register will depend on the inclinations and resources of the practice concerned.

The initial listing of patients suffering from selected diseases will almost certainly be incomplete, but over a period of one to two years, it should be possible to identify the majority of patients in the practice in any given category, provided doctors, nurses and secretarial staff can all be involved in and understand the importance of the exercise. The medical records can be marked with a coloured tag, or contain a list of chronic diseases, prominently displayed, to remind the general practitioner at the time of consultation of the conditions from which the patient suffers, which may need review at regular intervals.

Long term follow up can usefully be recorded on specially designed flow sheets within the record, both to provide a check list aide-mémoire and to make easily available in sequential form measurements such as blood pressure, blood glucose levels, peak flow meter readings, etc. Examples of these, for diabetes mellitus and cardiac failure are shown in Figures 1 and 2.

The decision whether to see patients in defined categories of follow-up in special clinics (e.g. antenatal clinics) or 'ad hoc' in the midst of ordinary surgeries is one which must be made individually. There are good arguments for and against both types of approach and either can be made to work equally well. Optimum intervals between review appointments must be determined individually and policies have to be made about 'chasing up' defaulters — policies which can strike a balance between the practitioner's proper concern for providing continuity of care and the patient's right not to attend (even if regular attendance is considered to be medically in his own best interest).

Repeat prescriptions

In many chronic conditions the patient's most frequent contact with the doctor is at second hand, when he gets a repeat prescription without seeing the practitioner. The whole phenomenon of repeat prescriptions has been researched and described in detail[1] but it still gives rise to feelings of guilt, which may reflect the doctor's need to be needed rather than rational concern for optimal care. An adult asthmatic patient, for instance, may be dependent on bronchodilators, but provided his requests for such therapy reflect regular use and the system of recording such prescriptions ensures that increasing use can be detected, there is no reason why that patient should not continue to receive such prescriptions without adding to his proper dependence on an effective drug a more questionable emotional dependence on his doctor.

Self care and independence may involve taking prescribed medication and some conditions may remain stable for years without face-to-face consultation being either necessary or desirable. Repeat prescribing is not by itself bad medicine — repeat prescribing without proper recording and monitoring is.

Follow-up and the hospital

Where long term hospital care is involved it is important to examine the reasons and come to an agreement with consultant colleagues about the most effective way of providing for the patient's needs.

For the patient the authority of the 'white-coated' doctor may be therapeutically important and in some instances the technical facilities of the hospital may be necessary. The consultant may need to see the patient for the purposes of teaching or research, and such needs are legitimate, but should be admitted overtly. All too often, however, hospital follow-up is delegated to rapidly changing junior staff and continuity is sacrificed for a spurious appearance of technical efficiency.

The general practitioner should be alert to this form of dis-

Ideal Wt. ______________________ Name ______________________

Diet Cals. ______________________

Gms. CBH

Diabetes review flow sheet

Date							
Symptoms							
		Right	Left	Right	Left	Right	Left
Visual acuity							
Cataract							
Fundal Changes	Dots						
	Blots						
	New vessels						
	Exudates						
Pulses	Post.tib						
	D. pedis						
Ankle jerks							
Vibration sense							
Fine touch							
Urine	Glucose						
	Protein						
	Blood						
Blood	Glucose						
	Urea						
Blood pressure							
Weight (Kgs)							
Home urine testing							
Drug therapy							
Assessment							
Plan							

Figure 1

Name:	Periodic assessment	Cardiovascular disease flow sheet
Date		
Symptoms		
Smoking		
Weight (Kgs)		
Pulse (Radial)		
Optic fundi		
Blood pressure		
JVP (raised or normal)		
Chest/heart		
Liver palpation		
Oedema (ankle or sacral)		
Urine Protein Blood		
Blood Urea Sodium Potassium Creatinine		
Chest X-ray		
E.C.G.		
Other investigations		
Assessment		
Plan		

Figure 2

continuity and take steps where possible to arrange for a more satisfactory system — either by offering to continue follow-up himself, re-referring the patient if necessary, or by offering some form of shared care — as obtains notably in the field of obstetrics. Shared care may also be of value for such chronic conditions such as diabetes mellitus and epilepsy, where it has been shown that the close contact between the specialist and generalist may be useful in reviewing the management of these groups of patients.

Objectives

The objectives of providing continued care for such disorders fall into two categories:

1. general
2. individual

The *general objectives* should ideally be agreed as matters of practice policy, and while these vary with different conditions, they include in broad terms:

(a) the early detection of complications,
(b) adjustments in treatment to prevent complications,
(c) co-ordination of general practitioner and hospital specialist care,
(d) the application, as and when appropriate, of proven recent advances.

The *individual objectives* will be governed by the family, psychological and social circumstances of the patient, including his age and the availability of support. Few doctors would wish to modify the treatment regime of a woman of 80 with high blood pressure because of the appearances of arterio-venous nipping in the fundi, but the same changes occurring in a woman of 40 would give rise to much greater concern. The widower of 70 with chronic bronchitis who has been unable to give up his cigarettes will be unlikely to be denied this source of comfort even though it may shorten his remaining span — or at least the admonition to cut down or stop will hardly be delivered with the vehemence directed to his similarly affected son of 35.

The following suggestions for long term management are therefore not to be taken as hard and fast prescriptions, but rather guidelines round which individual practitioners and practices can build their own policies, always interpreting them in the light of individual objectives.

Diabetes

The objectives are:

1. to check on diabetic control,
2. to detect complications as early as possible and to attempt to slow down their rate of progress.

Unless the general practitioner is confident in his ability to identify diabetic retinopathy, the most serious correctable complication in insulin dependent diabetics, these patients are best followed up by the specialist.

Patients controlled on diet alone or on diet plus an oral hypoglycaemic agent, once stabilized, should be seen in the early stages after initial diagnosis at intervals of approximately three months in the first year, and thereafter annually.

The *history* should include:

1. General wellbeing,
2. Changes in weight,
3. Reports of skin or urinary infections, or pruritis,
4. Reports of angina pectoris or intermittent claudication.

The *examination* should include:

1. Inspection of the patient's urine and weight record,
2. Visual acuity,
3. The optic fundi,
4. Legs and feet for any signs of muscle wasting, or ulcers, and loss of sensation with particular attention to light touch, joint position and vibration,
5. Blood pressure, standing and lying.

The *investigations* indicated are:

1. Fresh specimen of urine for sugar, ketones and albumin,
2. Blood for random blood sugar,
3. Blood urea and creatinine every two years,
4. Chest X-ray every five years.

In presence of complications

1. Retinopathy

Background

This is benign but may become proliferative.

- Check visual acuity and blood pressure four times a a year.
- Treat hypertension vigorously.
- Check cholesterol and triglyceride levels.

Proliferative

Very likely to lead to visual impairment.

- Check visual acuity and blood pressure *monthly*.
- Refer to eye or diabetic specialist if visual acuity declines
- Treat hypertension vigorously.

2. Nephropathy

- Control glycosuria.

—Frequent dip slides – treat if infected.
—Blood urea and creatinine and full blood count once or twice per year.
—Treat hypertension vigorously.
—Assess 24 hour urine protein loss.

3. Neuropathy: Peripheral, Mononeuritis, Ocular, Autonomic
—Consider insulin treatment if on oral hypoglycaemics.
—Check full blood count and B_{12} and folate annually.
—Check feet and footwear frequently.

4. Arterial disease

—Treat hypertension.
—Check nutrition of feet.
—Advice on hygiene and feet.
—Advice on smoking.
—Chest X-ray and E.C.G. annually.
—Fasting cholesterol and triglycerides (repeat every two years if raised).
—Possibly low animal fat diet.
—Consider surgical opinion.

Hypertension

The objectives are:

1. to assess and attempt to control the level of the blood pressure,
2. to assess and attempt to postpone the development of complications.

The intervals between visits will be determined largely by the success or otherwise in achieving the desired level of blood pressure for the individual patient. Once this is reached and provided there are no troublesome side-effects of treatment, follow-up should generally be at three or four monthly intervals, though with older patients (over the age of 65) a six monthly or even annual visit may well suffice.

At each visit the *history* should include:

1. General wellbeing,
2. Any history of breathlessness,
3. Any history of chest pain.

At each visit the following should be *examined*.

1. Weight,
2. Pulse rate (if on beta-blockers),
3. The level of the blood pressure.

In addition, at *yearly* intervals:

1. urine should be tested for albumin and sugar,
2. the fundi should be examined for signs of retinopathy,
3. the lung bases should be examined for crepitations,
4. serum potassium should be estimated if the patient is on diuretics.

Every *two to three years* a chest X-ray should be taken to check on heart size, and blood urea and creatinine measured.

Asthma

While in the long-term management of diabetes or hypertension the intervals between reviews are largely indicated by the doctor, in the management of asthma the indications for review will be determined by the occurrence of acute episodes or deterioration in routine control of the condition experienced by the patient (or his parents) or by an increasing rate of request for repeat prescriptions, monitored by the doctor.
The objectives of review will include:

1. assessment of airways obstruction,
2. reinforcement of education on the correct use of inhalers:
   (a) technique
   (b) frequency
   (c) prophylactic application
3. assessment of the indications for introducing (or withdrawing) sodium cromoglycate, steroids by inhalation, or oral steroids,
4. checking the patient's knowledge of emergency management.

1. *Airways obstruction*. This should be measured by peak expiratory flow assessment with a Wright Peak Flow Meter or Gauge. It is usual to take the best of three readings, explaining that it is the force of expiration and not its duration that is being measured.

2. *Education on inhaler usage*
(a) The patient should be asked to demonstrate his technique. With aerosols the points to watch are correct timing of pressure on the aerosol can at the time of inhalation, and complete sealing of the mouthpiece with the patient's mouth. The latter point is also of importance when using a spinhaler or rotahaler.
(b) If bronchodilators are being administered by aerosol it should be checked that the dosage is two puffs, the second administered five minutes after the first. The maximum safe does is 10 puffs per 24 hours.

(c) It should be checked that the patient knows to use his aerosol as soon as he suspects that he is getting wheezy – not to wait until the attack builds up. If attacks are precipitated by exercise, two puffs administered 10 minutes before the exercise is due to begin can prevent an attack.

3. *Progressive treatment.* If bronchodilators appear to be ineffective on their own, sodium cromoglycate should be introduced for a four week spell initially. The usual starting dose is four spincaps a day (which can be increased in serious cases up to 6-8 per day). If this is effective a gradual stepwise reduction may be tried till the lowest effective dose is found.
If response to sodium cromoglycate is poor it should be discontinued and a trial of steroids by inhalation is then indicated (two inhalations 3-4 times a day).
With both sodium cromoglycate and steroid inhalations it is important to stress that these are for regular use as prophylaxis and not for intermittent use as treatment. A helpful hint is to advise the use of the bronchodilator inhaler 10 minutes before the steroid inhaler, to ensure the maximum effect of the steroid inhalation.

4. *Emergency treatment.* Asthma can still be fatal: it is important that patients should know how to summon medical aid rapidly in an emergency. This involves checking that the patient knows the arrangements for emergency cover in the practice and what number to phone. Some hospital units have a policy of permitting direct admission without referral of patients with an acute exacerbation of asthma.
It is helpful to give patients their own supply of oral prednisolone (along with a steroid card to carry), with written instructions, such as:

> 'It is safe to use your inhaler up to 10 puffs every 24 hours.
> If: 1. your inhaler is giving no relief, or
> 2. the safe dose is being exceeded, then
> START Prednisolone tablets (four tablets per day) and consult the doctor.'

Chronic bronchitis

The objectives of the long term management of chronic bronchitis are:

1. the prompt treatment of exacerbations,
2. influenza prophylaxis.

The first objective may be obtained by giving the patient a supply of broad spectrum antibiotic (e.g. oxytetracycline or ampicillin) with written instructions:

'If your sputum becomes yellow or green, take two of your tablets every four hours until you have taken eight tablets; then take one tablet four times a day for the next four days. If your sputum does not clear in this time, or if you don't feel well, you should make an appointment to see the doctor.'

The second objective may be attained by notifying chronic bronchitic patients annually in the autumn, or by taking the opportunity of reminding such patients whenever they are seen that they should seek influenza immunization annually. This, of course, depends on the confidence with which the strain of influenza likely to be responsible for the current year's infection can be predicted, and the availability of suitable vaccines.

Treated thyrotoxicosis

Patients who have had ablative surgery or radioactive iodine for the definitive treatment of thyrotoxicosis should be reviewed annually to monitor the possible development of hypothyroidism. In Scotland there is a national computer-operated system whereby patients are alerted annually to consult their doctors, who are in turn provided with a standard check-list sheet and materials to take and send blood to the central laboratory – the results then being sent on to the G.P. who informs the patient (SAFUR – Scottish Automated Follow-Up Register).

A *history* should be taken with regard to:
—Diminished sweating
—Dry skin
—Cold intolerance
—Weight increase
—Constipation
—Hoarseness
—Paraesthesiae
—Deafness

The patient should be *examined* to detect:
—Slow movement
—Coarse skin
—Cold skin
—Periorbital oedema
—Slow pulse
—Slowing of ankle jerks

The *investigations* are:
—Thyroid function tests
—Cholesterol levels

Post gastrectomy follow-up

A patient who has had a gastrectomy may in the course of time develop anaemia, B_{12} deficiency or metabolic bone disease. With such patients an annual or two-yearly screening may be useful

1. to check general wellbeing,
2. to check: Haemoglobin, serum iron and serum B_{12}, alkaline phosphatase, serum calcium and serum phosphate.

If the alkaline phosphatase is raised or the serum calcium lowered, the hands, femurs and spine should be X-rayed to look for signs of osteomalacia and calcium and vitamin D therapy should be started.

Conclusion

In the management of patients with chronic disorders in general practice the management of the disease must never obscure the assessment and treatment of the patient. The formulas given in this chapter are simply outline suggestions to provide a framework; with each patient and on each occasion the individual objectives of the consultation must be remembered and tailored to suit the patient and his needs. System is helpful, but only as the servant of good sense.

Reference

[1] Balint, M., Hunt, J., Joyce, D., Marinker, M. and Woodcock, J. (1970): Treatment or *Diagnosis.* London: Tavistock Publications

Index

Because this book is primarily designed as a diagnostic tool for the general practitioner it is concerned with the interpretation of presenting symptoms. It has been suggested, however, that it would be useful to be able to refer to particular diseases and subjects and identify the chapters in which they are described. This index is designed to satisfy that need. Page numbers refer to the first page of the relevant chapter.